UNIGASTRO

DIGESTIVE DISEASES

2022-2025 Edition

UNIGASTRO

Coordinamento Nazionale
Docenti Universitari
di Gastroenterologia

EDITRICE GASTROENTEROLOGICA ITALIANA

Publishing manager: Rosa Incarnato

C.so di Francia 197, 00191 Roma
Tel. 06 36388336 – Fax 06 36387434
E-mail: info.egi@fastwebnet.it

Production and distribution
EDRA S.p.A.
Via Spadolini, 7
20141 Milano (MI)
Tel. 02.881841
Fax: 02 88.184.304
www.edizioniedra.it

Project manager: Arianna Ribichesu
Cover: Emanuela Contieri
Layout: Daniela Manunza

Printed in Italy in September 2022 by "Rotomail Italia"

ISBN 978-88-214-5635-0

CONTRIBUTORS*

Ludovico Abenavoli Montebianco - Professore associato
Università "Magna Graecia", Catanzaro

Alessio Michele Aghemo - Professore associato
Humanitas University, Milano

Domenico Alvaro - Professore ordinario
"Sapienza" Università di Roma

Bruno Annibale - Professore ordinario
"Sapienza" Università di Roma

Paolo Giorgio Arcidiacono - Professore associato
Università San Raffaele, Milano

Sandro Ardizzone - Professore straordinario
Università degli Studi di Milano

Alessandro Armuzzi - Professore ordinario
Humanitas University, Milano

Francesco Azzaroli - Professore associato
Università degli Studi di Bologna

Danilo Badiali - Ricercatore
"Sapienza" Università di Roma

Leonardo Baiocchi - Professore associato
Università Tor Vergata, Roma

Monia Baldoni - Ricercatore
Università degli Studi di Perugia

Michele Barone - Professore associato
Università degli Studi di Bari

Gabrio Bassotti - Professore associato
Università degli Studi di Perugia

Massimo Bellini - Professore associato
Università degli Studi di Pisa

Antonio Benedetti - Professore ordinario
Politecnica delle Marche, Ancona

Gaetano Bertino - Professore associato
Università degli Studi di Catania

Federico Biagi - Professore ordinario
Università degli Studi di Pavia

Livia Biancone - Professore ordinario
Università Tor Vergata, Roma

Stefano Brillanti - Professore associato
Università degli Studi di Siena

Elisabetta Bugianesi - Professore associato
Università degli Studi di Torino

Patrizia Burra - Professore ordinario
Università degli Studi di Padova

Emma Calabrese - Professore associato
Università Tor Vergata, Roma

Vincenza Calvaruso - Professore associato
Università degli Studi di Palermo

Giovanni Cammarota - Professore associato
Università Cattolica del Sacro Cuore, Roma

Flavio Andrea Caprioli - Professore associato
Università degli Studi di Milano

Marco Carbone - Ricercatore
Università degli Studi di Milano Bicocca

Vincenzo Cardinale - Professore associato
"Sapienza" Università di Roma

Fabiana Castiglione - Professore associato
Università "Federico II", Napoli

Roberto Catanzaro - Professore associato
Università degli Studi di Catania

Giulia Martina Cavestro - Professore associato
Università S. Raffaele, Milano

Nora Cazzagon - Ricercatore
Università degli Studi di Padova

Alessia Ciancio - Professore associato
Università degli Studi di Torino

Pierluigi Consolo - Professore associato
Università degli Studi di Messina

Vito Domenico Corleto - Professore associato
"Sapienza" Università di Roma

* MED/12 - Gastrointestinal diseases

CONTRIBUTORS

Saveria Lory Crocè - Professore associato
Università degli Studi di Trieste

Rosario Cuomo - Professore associato
Università "Federico II", Napoli

Nicola de Bortoli - Professore associato
Università degli Studi di Pisa

Giovanna Del Vecchio Blanco - Ricercatore
Università Tor Vergata, Roma

Alessandra Dell'Era - Professore associato
Università degli Studi di Milano

Alfredo Di Leo - Professore ordinario
Università degli Studi di Bari

Vito Di Marco - Professore ordinario
Università degli Studi di Palermo

Maria Pina Dore - Professore associato
Università degli Studi di Sassari

Leonardo Henry Umberto Eusebi - Professore associato
Università degli Studi di Bologna

Luca Fabris - Professore associato
Università degli Studi di Padova

Antonio Facciorusso - Ricercatore
Università degli Studi di Foggia

Massimo Claudio Fantini - Professore associato
Università degli Studi di Cagliari

Alessandro Federico - Professore ordinario
Università della Campania "L. Vanvitelli"

Walter Fries - Professore ordinario
Università degli Studi di Messina

Lorenzo Fuccio - Professore associato
Università degli Studi di Bologna

Pietro Fusaroli - Professore associato
Università degli Studi di Bologna

Armando Gabbrielli - Professore associato
Università degli Studi di Verona

Andrea Galli - Professore ordinario
Università degli Studi di Firenze

Edoardo Giovanni Giannini - Professore ordinario
Università degli Studi di Genova

Stefano Ginanni Corradini - Professore associato
"Sapienza" Università di Roma

Antonietta Gerarda Gravina - Ricercatore
Università della Campania "L. Vanvitelli"

Laurino Grossi - Professore associato
Università degli Studi di Chieti

Michele Pierluca Guarino - Professore associato
Università Campus Biomedico, Roma

Pietro Invernizzi - Professore ordinario
Università degli Studi di Milano Bicocca

Paola Iovino - Professore associato –
Università degli Studi di Salerno

Edith Lahner - Professore associato
"Sapienza" Università di Roma

Pietro Lampertico - Professore ordinario
Università degli Studi di Milano

Tiziana Larussa - Ricercatore
Università "Magna Graecia", Catanzaro

Giovanni Latella - Professore ordinario
Università degli Studi dell'Aquila

Francesco Luzza - Professore ordinario
Università "Magna Graecia", Catanzaro

Giovanni Egidio Maconi - Professore associato
Università degli Studi di Milano

Elisa Marabotto - Ricercatore
Università degli Studi di Genova

Santino Marchi - Professore ordinario
Università degli Studi di Pisa

Marco Marzioni - Professore associato
Politecnica delle Marche, Ancona

Manuela Merli - Professore ordinario
"Sapienza" Università di Roma

Stefano Milani - Professore ordinario
Università degli Studi di Firenze

Marco Montagnani - Ricercatore
Università degli Studi di Bologna

Olivia Morelli - Ricercatore
Università degli Studi di Perugia

Filomena Morisco - Professore ordinario
Università "Federico II", Napoli

Gerardo Antonio Pio Nardone - Professore ordinario
Università "Federico II", Napoli

Nadia Pallotta - Ricercatore
"Sapienza" Università di Roma

Alfredo Papa - Professore associato
Università Cattolica del Sacro Cuore, Roma

Roberto Penagini - Professore associato
Università degli Studi di Milano

Salvatore Petta - Professore associato
Università degli Studi di Palermo

Antonio Picarelli - Professore associato
"Sapienza" Università di Roma

Mariabeatrice Principi - Professore associato
Università degli Studi di Bari

Gian Ludovico Rapaccini - Professore associato
Università Cattolica del Sacro Cuore, Roma

Alessandro Repici - Professore ordinario
Humanitas University, Milano

Chiara Ricci - Professore associato
Università degli Studi di Brescia

Luigi Ricciardiello - Professore associato
Università degli Studi di Bologna

Lorenzo Ridola - Professore associato
"Sapienza" Università di Roma

Antonio Rispo - Ricercatore
Università "Federico II", Napoli

Marco Romano - Professore ordinario
Università della Campania "L. Vanvitelli"

Maria Grazia Rumi - Professore associato
Università degli Studi di Milano

Francesco Paolo Russo - Professore associato
Università degli Studi di Padova

Giorgio Maria Saracco - Professore ordinario
Università degli Studi di Torino

Giovanni Sarnelli - Professore associato
Università "Federico II", Napoli

Edoardo Vincenzo Savarino - Professore associato
Università degli Studi di Padova

Carola Severi - Professore associato
"Sapienza" Università di Roma

Gianluca Svegliati Baroni - Professore associato
Università Politecnica delle Marche, Ancona

Mirko Tarocchi - Professore associato
Università degli Studi di Firenze

Maurizio Vecchi - Professore ordinario
Università degli Studi di Milano

Angelo Viscido - Ricercatore
Università degli Studi dell'Aquila

Rocco Maurizio Zagari - Professore ordinario
Università degli Studi di Bologna

Fabiana Zingone - Ricercatore
Università degli Studi di Padova

TABLE OF CONTENTS

SECTION V
BILIARY TRACT AND PANCREAS

SECTION VI
GASTROINTESTINAL EMERGENCIES

PREFACE

We are glad to introduce the academics and the students attending the classes of Gastroenterology in the different integrated courses of the Medicine and Surgery degree to the tenth edition of the UNIGASTRO manual of Gastroenterology. Thanks to the success obtained by the previous edition, we publish both a coloured and an English version, which we hope to expand in the future.

The contents have been updated in order to keep offering a student-friendly manual that is permanently in line with the most recent research and pedagogical methodologies.

The structure of the book includes eleven Section Editors who had the responsibility to supervise their sections. Each chapter was assigned to two Authors of the UNIGASTRO Association. Inside the chapters, the learning objectives have been summarised on the first pages to provide the students with a study guide, while essential key concepts and up-to-date bibliographical references are shown at the end.

The book is made of both a paper volume and multimedia contents, that are accessible directly from the UNIGASTRO website through a password printed on the inner part of the volume cover. Converted from the flash technology to the more advanced HTML5 language, these contents offer an interactive experience to the students, who gain access to a multitude of clinical cases, diagnostic procedures, and supplementary in-depth analyses. The multiple-choice questions discuss all the topics contained in the manual and each of them presents five possible answers, with a sole correct answer. The questions have been renewed entirely and are available in the English version too.

Heartfelt thanks to all the Authors, to the Section Editors, to all the Editorial Board members for their work, and to EDRA S.p.a.

Patrizia Burra, Marco Romano, Carmela Loguercio

ABBREVIATIONS

A

AAA abdominal aortic aneurysm
AAG autoimmune atrophic gastritis
AAT α1-antitripsin
ABC airway, breathing, circulation
ABCD adiposity based chronic disease
ACLF acute on chronic liver failure
ADEX aberrantly differentiated endocrine exocrine
AHF acute hepatic failure
AIH autoimmune hepatitis
AJCC American Joint Committee on Cancer
ALD alcohol-related liver disease
ALF acute liver failure
ALFSG Acute Liver Failure Study Group
ALP alkaline phosphatase
ALT alanine aminotransferase
AMA anti mitochondrial antibodies
ANA anti nuclear antibodies
ANCA anti-neutrophil cytoplasmic antibodies
AP acute pancreatitis
APC adenomatous polyposis coli
ASBT apical bile salt transporter
ASH alcoholic steatohepatitis
ASLC acute self-limiting colitis
ASPEN american society for parenteral and enteral nutrition
AST aspartate aminotransferase
AUDIT alcohol use disorders identification test

B

BA bile acids
BCLC Barcelona Clinic Liver Cancer
BE Barrett's oesophagus
BED binge eating disorder
BMI body-mass index
BOBOCAT Benign Barrett's and Cancer Taskforce
BSEP bile salt export pump
BSFS Bristol Stool Form Scale

C

CA cholic acid
CASR calcium-sensitive receptor
CCA cholangiocarcinoma
CCA cholangiocarcinoma
CCK cholecystokinin
CD Crohn's disease
CDAI Crohn's disease activity index
CDCA chenodeoxycholic acid
CDP contractile deceleration point
CEA carcinoembryonic antigen
CFTR cystic fibrosis transmembrane regulator
cGMP cyclic guanosine monophosphate
CH cholesterol
CIC chronic idiopathic constipation
CMV cytomegalovirus
CNS central nervous system
COPD chronic obstructive pulmonary disease
CP chronic pancreatitis
CPMR cholangiopancreatography magnetic resonance
CRC colorectal adenocarcinoma
CRISPR clustered regularly interspected short palindromic repeats
CRP C-reactive protein
CSI cholesterol saturation index
CT computed tomography

D

DAA direct antiviral drugs
DAO diamineoxydase enzyme
DBE double-balloon enteroscopy
DCA deoxycholic acid
DCI distal contractile integral
DEXA dual-energy x-ray absorptiometry
DGGE denaturing gradient gel electrophoresis
DIC disseminated intravascular coagulation
DILI drug-induced liver injury
DL distal latency

DLBCL diffuse b large cell lymphoma
DMV dorsal motor nucleus of the vagus
DRESS drug reaction with eosinophilia and systemic symptoms syndrome

E

EAS external anal sphincter
EBV Epstein Barr virus
ECG electrocardiography
ECL enterochromaffin like
EEC enteroendocrine cells
EGDS oesophagogastroduodenoscopy
ELF enhanced liver fibrosis
ELISA enzyme-linked immunosorbent assay
ELTR european liver transplant registry
EMA anti-endomysium antibodies
EMR endoscopic mucosal resection
ENS enteric nervous system
EoE eosinophilic oesophagitis
EPT oesophageal pressure topography
ERCP endoscopic retrograde cholangiopancreatography
ESD endoscopic submucosal dissection
ESR erythrocyte sedimentation rate
ESWL extra-corporeal shock wave lithotripsy
EUA exploration under anesthesia
EUS endoscopic ultrasound scanning

F

FAP familial adenomatous polyposis
FD functional dyspepsia
FGF fibroblast growth factor
FHVP free hepatic venous pressure
FIAF fasting-induced adipocyte factor
FIT fecal immunochemical test
FNH focal nodular hyperplasia
FOBT fecal occult blood test
FODMAPs fermentable oligo-, di-, mono-saccharides and polyols

G

GALT gut-associated lymphoid tissue
GEJ gastro-oesophageal junction
GEP gastroenteropancreatic
GERD gastro-oesophageal reflux disease
GI gastrointestinal
GIB gastrointestinal bleeding
GIP glucose dependent insulinotropic polypeptide
GIST gastrointestinal stromal tumour
GLP glucagon-like peptide
GM gastric metaplasia

H

HAV hepatitis A virus
HBV hepatitis B virus
HCC hepatocellular carcinoma
HCl hydrochloric acid
HCV hepatitis C virus
HDL high-density lipoprotein
HDV hepatitis D virus
HE hepatic encephalopathy
HEV hepatitis E virus
HLA human leukocyte antigen
HNPCC hereditary non-polyposis colorectal cancer
HPV human papillomavirus
HRM high-resolution oesophageal manometry
HRS hepatorenal syndrome
HSV herpes simplex virus
HVPG hepatic venous pressure gradient

I

IAS internal anal sphincter
IBD inflammatory bowel diseases
IBS irritable bowel syndrome
IC ischaemic colitis
ICCA intrahepatic cholangiocarcinoma
IEM ineffective oesophageal motility
IFI indirect immunofluorescence
IFN interferons
IM intestinal metaplasia
IMMC interdigestive migrating motor complex
INR international normalized ratio
IPAA ileal pouch-anal anastomosis
IPMN intraductal papillary mucinous neoplasm
IRP integrated relaxation pressure

L

LES lower oesophageal sphincter
LKM anti liver/kidney microsome

LMWH	low-molecular-weight heparins
LPAC	low phospholipid-associated cholelithiasis
LPL	lipoproteinlipase
LS	lynch syndrome

M

MALT	mucosa-associated lymphoid tissue
MANEC	mixed adeno-neuroendocrine carcinoma
MCN	mucinous cystic neoplasm
MELD	model for end-stage liver disease
MEOS	microsomal ethanol oxidizing system
MICOL	Multicentric Italian Cholelithiasis
MMC	migrant motor complexes
MNA	mini nutritional assessment
MOFS	multiple organ failure syndrome
MRCP	magnetic resonance cholangiopancreatography
MRI	magnetic resonance imaging
MUST	malnutrition universal screening tool

N

NAC	n-acetyl-cysteine
NAFLD	non-alcoholic fatty liver disease
NASH	nonalcoholic steatohepatitis
NCTP	sodium taurocholate cotransporting polypeptide
NEN	neuroendocrine neoplasms
NERD	non-erosive reflux disease
NES	night eating syndrom
NETs	neuroendocrine tumours
NRH	nodular regenerative hyperplasia
NRS	nutrition risk screening
NSAIDs	non-steroidal anti-inflammatory drugs
NSE	neuron-specific enolase
NUCs	oral antiviral agents

O

OCT	optical coherence tomography
OLT	orthotopic liver transplantation

P

PanIN	pancreatic intraepithelial neoplasia
PBC	primary biliary cholangitis
PCR	polymerase chain reaction
PDFF	proton density fat fraction
PEG	polyethylene glycol
PET	positron emission tomography
PG	prostaglandins
PL	phospholipids
POEM	peroral endoscopic myotomy
PPIs	proton pump inhibitors
PSC	primary sclerosing cholangitis
PSS	porto-systemic shunts
PT	prothrombin time
PVT	portal vein thrombosis
PYY	peptide yy
PanIN	RAST radioallergosorbent test

R

RCD	refractory celiac disease
RSCS	ectosigmoidocolonscopy
Rx	radiography

S

SAAG	serum-ascites albumin gradient
SBFT	small bowel follow through
SBP	spontaneous bacterial peritonitis
SCAD	segmental colitis associated with diverticulosis
SCFA	short chain fatty acids
SGA	subjective global assessment
SIBO	small intestinal bacterial overgrowth
SIRS	systemic inflammatory response syndrome
SMA	anti smooth muscle antibodies
SOD	sphincter Oddi dysfunction
SPC	stellate pancreatic cells
SPEM	polypeptide-expressing metaplasia
SPTs	solid pseudopapillary tumours
SRUS	solitary rectal ulcer syndrome
SSA	somatostatin analogues
SSRIs	selective serotonin reuptake inhibitors
STC	slow transit constipation
SUV	standardized uptake value
SVR	sustained virologic response

T

TFF	trefoil peptide
TGF	tumour growth factor
TGGE	temperature gradient cell electrophoresis

TIA	transient ischaemic attack
TIBC	total iron binding capacity
TLESR	transient lower oesophageal sphincter relaxation
TLRs	toll-like receptors
TMA	transcription-mediated-amplification
TNF	tumour necrosis factor
TNM	tumour, lymph nodes, metastasis

U

UC	ulcerative colitis
UDCA	ursodeoxycholic acid
UDCA	ursodeoxycholic acid
UES	upper oesophageal sphincter
US	ultrasonography

V

VC	virtual colonoscopy
VCE	videocapsule endoscopy
VIP	vasoactive intestinal peptide
VLC	video-laparoscopic cholecystectomy

W

WD	Wilson's desease
WHO	world health organization
WHVP	wedged hepatic venous pressure

Z

ZES	Zollinger-Ellison syndrome

CHAPTER 1

MALNUTRITION AND OBESITY

Massimo Bellini

LEARNING OBJECTIVES

- To know the main clinical pictures related to eating disorders.
- To know how to recognize and interpret a condition of malnutrition and identify its causes.
- To know the pathogenetic mechanisms of being overweight or obese, the clinical implications and the main therapeutic strategies.

This chapter deals with nutritional disorders, namely, clinical conditions, in which there is a lack of or an excess of energy and nutrients. According to a recent classification by the European Society for Parenteral and Enteral Nutrition (ESPEN) guidelines, malnutrition/undernutrition can be defined as a nutritional disorder characterised by the lack of nutrients and energy, and an overweight or obese condition as an excess of intake of nutrients and energy.

MALNUTRITION/UNDERNUTRITION

Malnutrition, which can be caused by fasting, pathological conditions, and ageing, results from a reduced intake of nutrients, which determines primarily an alteration in body composition (reduction of lean body mass) and in metabolically active mass. This leads to a reduction in the physical and mental activity of the patient, with a consequent worsening of the clinical picture.

The definition of malnutrition has been the object of great debate within the major international nutrition societies (American Society for Parenteral and Enteral Nutrition [ASPEN]/European Society for Parenteral and Enteral Nutrition [ESPEN]/Italian Society of Artificial nutrition and Metabolism [SINPE]).

The Global Leadership Initiative on Malnutrition (GLIM) has proposed a definition that combines at least one of the parameters of phenotype a) with one of the aetiological criteria in point b):

a) unintentional loss of weight, reduction in the BMI, or reduced muscular mass;
b) reduced consumption or absorption of food and pathologies related to acute or chronic inflammation.

This definition attributes an important role to the presence of an inflammatory condition. In fact, three different subtypes of malnutrition are distinguished:

- malnutrition caused by a concomitant pathology with inflammation;
- malnutrition caused by a concomitant pathology without inflammation;
- malnutrition without a concomitant disease.

The first subtype can, in turn, be present in an acute form, characterised by an intense inflammatory response, or in a chronic form in which the inflammatory response is mild. Clinical examples of the acute form are patients admitted to the intensive care unit for acute pathologies or trauma, or patients undergoing major surgery. Conversely, the chronic form is associated with cachexia, defined as a complex metabolic syndrome associated with a disease and characterised by muscle loss with or without loss of fat mass, and weight loss. It is most frequently present in patients with terminal diseases complicated by a catabolic inflammatory response, such as neoplasia, chronic obstructive pulmonary disease (COPD), chronic intestinal inflammatory diseases, cardiac insufficiency, and renal insufficiency.

Malnutrition without inflammation is induced by a disease in which inflammation does not constitute an important pathogenetic element. Examples of pathological elements underlying this condition are dysphagia, short bowel syndrome, neurological syndromes such as stroke, Parkinson's disease, amyotrophic lateral sclerosis, dementia, and psychiatric disorders.

The third form (malnutrition without concomitant disease) refers to conditions characterised by lack of food (malnutrition from starvation), typical in developing countries, or socio-economic or psychological conditions in which not only the calorie

*The Author would like to thank Prof. Monica Nannipieri for her precious assistance.

intake but also the quality of the food plays an important role.

However, as far as the diagnostic criteria for malnutrition are concerned, there has been great debate within the international scientific societies (ASPEN/ESPEN/SINPE).

The ASPEN guidelines consider the presence of at least two of the following factors to be diagnostic:

a) low energy intake;
b) accumulation of liquids;
c) decrease in hand strength;
d) decrease in muscular mass or subcutaneous fat;
e) weight loss.

On the basis of this definition, the ESPEN guidelines propose two diagnostic alternatives:

a) a BMI <18.5kg/m2;
b) spontaneous weight loss (>10% of the initial weight independent of time or >5% in the previous 3 months) associated with a BMI evaluated in relation to age (<20kg/m2 if <70 years of age or <22kg/m2 if over 70 years of age) or to a lean mass index (fat-free mass index [FFMI] obtained by dividing the lean mass by the square of the height) <15 and 17 kg/m2 in women and men, respectively.

According to the EWGSOP2 and GLIM guidelines, Dual X-ray Absorptiometry (DXA) is one of the most preferred diagnostic methods for measuring muscle mass, even if the circumference of the calf can be used as an alternative way of measuring the peripheral muscular mass.

Malnutrition identified on the basis of the FFMI measured by means of DXA is defined as Malnutrition-DXA.

Together with the morphological and instrumental assessment, in making the diagnosis it is important to use validated questionnaires. These are aimed at quantifying the nutritional risk, and therefore helping the clinician to make a clear diagnosis.

The most widely used questionnaires are:

- SGA (Subjective Global Assessment), which includes history taking (weight loss, food intake, gastrointestinal (GI) symptoms, changes in functional capacities). It is an objective examination of muscle mass and fat mass, and identifies the presence of edema;
- MNA (Mini Nutritional Assessment), which is especially useful in the elderly, includes history taking (appetite, weight loss, basic diagnosis, motor activity, neuropsychiatric problems) and calculating the BMI;
- MUST (Malnutrition Universal Screening Tool) is a questionnaire developed by the British Association for Parenteral and Enteral Nutrition that takes into account the BMI, percentage of weight loss, and reduction in calorie intake correlated with the disease;
- NRS-2000 (Nutrition Risk Screening) is an instrument for evaluating the risk of malnutrition in hospitalized patients. It includes weight loss, reduction in calorie intake, BMI and the severity of the underlying disease.

The evaluations provided by these questionnaires include both the causes (reduced nutritional intake, severity of the basic pathology) and the consequences (weight loss, reduction in BMI) of malnutrition. Therefore, in order to plan the best therapeutic strategy for the patient, especially if hospitalized, together with evaluating muscle mass, cognitive capacity and efficacy of the patient's immune system, it may be necessary to associate that evaluation which is relative to calorie intake/absorption and that related to the presence of an underlying inflammatory condition.

Using more complex diagnostic techniques, such as computed tomography (CT), magnetic resonance imaging (MRI), positron emission tomography (PET), and Dual-energy X-ray absorptiometry (DEXA) should be limited to selected cases due to their elevated cost. Bioelectrical impedance analysis, on the other hand, is a low cost method able to give quantitative, if less precise, indications as to the content in the body of lean and fat mass.

OBESITY/OVERWEIGHT

Obesity is a chronic clinical condition with a complex aetiopathogenesis consisting of an excessive accumulation of adipose tissue, which can negatively influence the state of health. The factors that contribute to obesity interact and adapt to the environment and the culture, and evolve over time. Obesity is the leading cause of modifiable death worldwide, common among children and adults of both sexes. Obesity and overweight, initially considered to be problems of only rich countries, are also increasing in low- and middle-income countries, and are now recognised as real public health problems. According to the data published by the World Health Organization (WHO), the number of obese people in the world has grown exponentially since 1980. In 2014 over 1.9 billion adults were overweight, among which 600 million were obese. The estimates of WHO, announced on World Obesity Day-2021, reveal that

50% of the world adult population and 30% of children and adolescents are overweight or obese. In Italy 18 million (35.5%) adults are overweight and 5 million obese, that is one out of ten. Furthermore, 3 children out of 10 (29.8%) are overweight and among these 1 is obese (9.4%). It is foreseen that child obesity will increase by 60% in the next decade, reaching 250 million children by 2030.

The seriousness of the problem is correlated with the comorbidities that are associated with this chronic pathology. Just think that in Europe being overweight and obesity are responsible for about 80% of the cases of type 2 diabetes, for 55% of arterial hypertension cases and 35% of cases of ischaemic heart disease. This all brings about 1 million deaths and 12 million sick people every year.

It was long thought that at the basis of obesity there were only inappropriate dietary choices and a lack of physical activity. In reality, even though these two factors have a notable pathogenetic importance, recent evidence in the literature reports obesity as being a multifactorial clinical condition caused by the interaction of environmental, socio-cultural, physiological, clinical, behavioural, and genetic, epigenetic and metabolic factors.

Moreover, the complexity, interaction and frequent chronic trend of all these factors explains the difficulty in treating obesity and makes the classic therapeutic model inadequate, as it is based exclusively on a diet being understood merely as calorie restriction.

Furthermore, there is unanimous agreement among the major scientific societies that obesity is a chronic disease and that it should be treated as such. In fact, a recent consensus conference proposed Adiposity Based Chronic Disease (ABCD) as a definition for obesity.

There are numerous environmental factors involved in the genesis of obesity, defined as a disease: a sedentary lifestyle, (prolonged television viewing, computer use etc.) and excessive food consumption (in particular food with a high energy content, hyper caloric, with elevated palatability and consumed in ever-increasing amounts). Since not all people exposed to these risk factors become obese, genetic factors play an important role. In fact, numerous genes related to obesity have been identified. Although singularly they have a negligible effect, when operating in association and in synergy they can play a very relevant pathogenetic role. It is highly probable that obesity genes act not only on the homeostatic regulator of energetic equilibrium but also on the neural circuits involved in the interactions with an obesogenic environment, including the circuits at the basis of the decisional process based on reward, that is "craving". Understanding the mechanisms underlying obesity appreciates the role of the neural system as a control centre of appetite. In the central nervous system, there is a circuit located principally in the hypothalamus. It regulates the relationship between the consumption of nutrients and energetic consumption, integrating the hormonal signals coming from the periphery that communicate with the rest of the central nervous system. A key function of the hypothalamus is to detect deficiencies in consumption of nutrients in both the short and the long term, and translate them into behaviors; interference with the normal functions of this hypothalamic circuit leads to impaired regulation of the energy balance. Therefore, the development of obesity has also been associated with altered responses at the level of the neural circuits. These modifications, similar to those induced by substances such as cocaine and heroin, are responsible for the compulsiveness of these subjects. The hedonic properties of food can stimulate food behaviour, even when the requisites of metabolic-energetic homeostasis have been met. Even before being tasted and absorbed, food can have potent effects on the brain's visual and olfactory stimuli. This is particularly important for people who live in an environment with high food availability and constant reminders of "appetising" food.

Neuroradiological studies have identified various nodes and key cerebral networks that are influenced differently by visual food stimuli under fasting conditions, weight loss, re-feeding, overeating and exercise. Instead, it remains to be demonstrated whether the complex neural system responsible for controlling the consumption of food also has a role in controlling the intake of specific nutrients (e.g. carbohydrates, fats, proteins).

Obesity as a Risk Factor for Developing Metabolic Pathologies

Increasing scientific evidence has reported the association between overweight/obesity and the development of metabolic and neoplastic pathologies. An association has been demonstrated between the development of insulin resistance, Type 2 diabetes mellitus, dyslipidaemia, metabolic associated fatty liver disease (MAFLD), cardiovascular disease and arterial hypertension. Additional pathological conditions for which obesity represents a risk factor are polycystic ovary syndrome, obstructive sleep apnoea syndrome

and gallstones. Furthermore, obesity is a risk factor for numerous types of cancer such as that of the colon or rectum, pancreas, liver, oesophagus, breast, kidneys, and endometrium. One out of five cases of cancer is related to obesity.
This explains the observation that obesity is associated with an increased risk of mortality. For each increase of 5 kg/m^2 in BMI over 25 kg/m^2, overall mortality increases by approximately 30%, vascular pathologies by 40%, and type 2 diabetes, and kidney and liver failure by 60%. Compared to having a normal weight or being overweight, average survival is reduced by 2-4 years for a BMI between 30 and 35, and by 8-10 years for a BMI from 40-45.

Anthropometric Parameters and Body Composition

The parameters used to identify the degree of being overweight and obesity are those of the BMI.
In clinical practice, the anthropometric parameters normally used are:

- weight measurement and height from which the BMI is calculated to define the degree of obesity without, however, distinguishing the distribution of fat;
- waist circumference as a parameter of the distribution of body fat;
- bioimpedance analysis for the evaluation of fat and lean body mass;
- measurement of skin folds (biceps, triceps, subscapularis, iliac crest), which is less often used than the other parameters and which enables evaluation of the thickness of subcutaneous adiposity.

The BMI (or Quetelet Index) is obtained by dividing the weight (kg) by the height (m) squared (kg/m^2) and classifies obesity into:

- Overweight: 25-29.9 kg/m^2;
- Grade 1 obesity: 30-<35 kg/m^2;
- Grade 2 obesity: 35-<40 kg/m^2;
- Grade 3 obesity: ≥40 kg/m^2.

However, the BMI has two important limitations. It is not a measurement of fat mass and it does not give information regarding the distribution of visceral and subcutaneous fat. Strong scientific evidence reports that it is the accumulation of fat at the abdomen that constitutes an important risk factor for developing metabolic and cardiovascular diseases, and that this risk is especially elevated in moderately obese subjects (BMI 30-35) and in those simply overweight (BMI: 25-29.9).
The distribution of adipose tissue evaluated by measuring waist circumference is an indicator of two forms of obesity: visceral or android obesity and subcutaneous or gynoid obesity
A more objective measurement can be obtained by calculating the ratio between the body circumference measured at the waist and hips. This ration, termed WHR (Waist to Hip ratio), refers to the following values in order to define the obesity phenotype:

- android obesity is when the WHR ratio is greater than 0.85;
- gynoid obesity is when the WHR ratio is less than 0.79.

It is well known that visceral obesity is associated with metabolic disorders such as type 2 diabetes, dyslipidemia, MAFLD, cardiovascular diseases. Gynoid obesity, in which the fat is prevalently distributed subcutaneously is not associated with risks of metabolic pathologies.
The abdominal circumference (measurement of the waist) is used to assess the amount of abdominal fat. According to WHO parameters, a large abdominal circumference is associated with the same risks as being overweight. This is therefore visceral obesity, when the waist size is greater than the following parameters:

- men >102 cm;
- women >88 cm.

It is however possible to have a body mass index within the limits suggested but an abdominal circumference greater than the values indicated above. For this reason, measuring the abdominal circumference is just as important as measuring body weight.

Sarcopenic Obesity

In recent years, on the basis of increased life expectancy and the prevalence of obesity in Western countries, interest has increased in sarcopenic obesity, a clinical condition characterised by the presence of excessive fat mass and a progressive reduction in skeletal muscle mass with a consequent reduction in strength and muscle function.
This condition can be observed in the elderly, people with Type 2 diabetes and COPD, and obese people with neoplastic diseases.
Figure 1.1 shows the main risk factors associated with sarcopenic obesity. A low-grade chronic inflammation the presence of insulin resistance, hormonal changes, and a reduction in physical activity are all at the basis of the relationship between sarcopenia and obesity. An increase in pro-inflammatory cytokines, oxidative stress, the presence of insulin resistance, hormonal changes, and a reduction in physical activity are at the basis of the

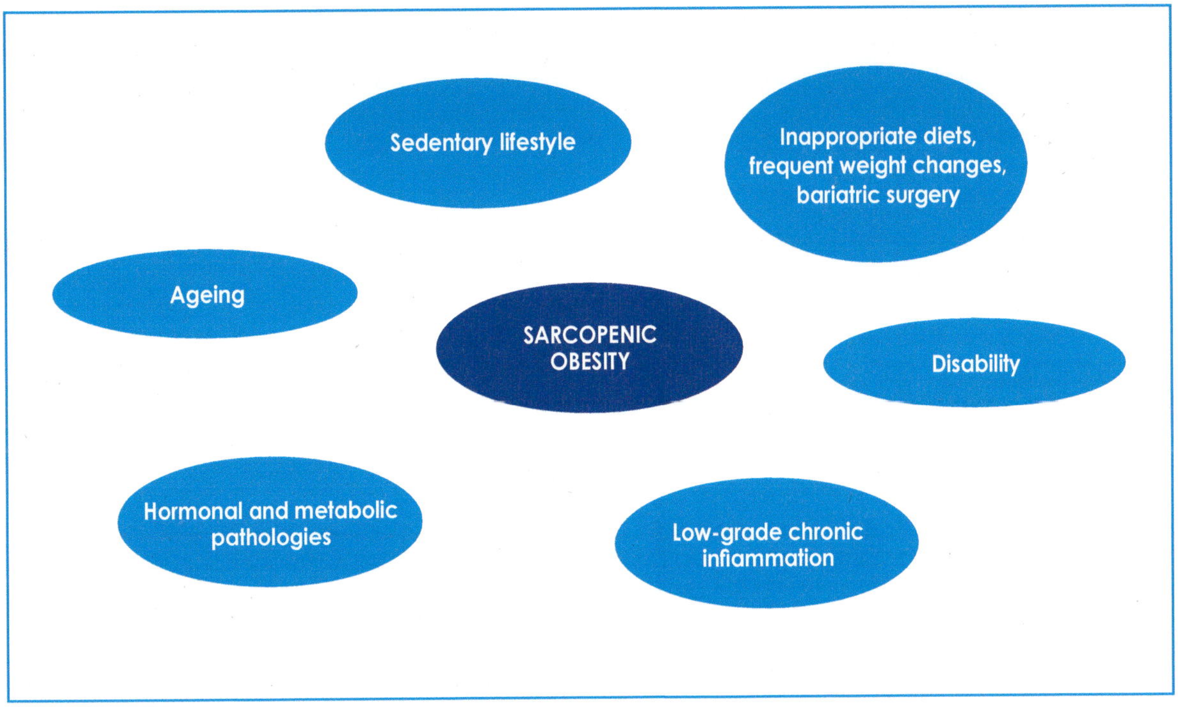

Figure 1.1 Risk factors for sarcopenic obesity. (Modified from Picca A. et al., 2018.)

relationship between sarcopenia and obesity. An increase in visceral fat, together with an increase in low grade inflammation, contributes to the development of sarcopenia. Therefore, while sarcopenia and obesity each represent a risk for the health of an older person, when combined, the risk for health and the onset of disabilities increase synergically. An in-depth evaluation of sarcopenic obesity should include measuring the anthropometric compartments and evaluating the physical performance of these patients. At present, the lack of a definitive definition of sarcopenic obesity does not permit establishing the objectives to be reached in the treatment of these patients, although, at present, weight loss obtained with an adequate diet and physical exercise seems to be the best treatment strategy also for sarcopenic overweight or obese subjects.

Obesity and Eating Disorders

Obesity is often linked to binge eating disorder and its numerous complications. Binge eating disorder (BED) and night eating syndrome (NES) are two forms of disordered food consumption associated with being overweight and obese. These disorders seem to be associated with an increase in weight over time, and a greater risk of diabetes and other metabolic dysfunctions. They also imply a greater risk of mental distress, including mood, anxiety, and sleep problems, as compared with obese people without BED. Treatment includes cognitive-behavioural therapy and interpersonal psychotherapy.

ORGANISATION OF THE PATHWAY OF CARE/TREATMENT

In order to define the severity of obesity, a classification system has been proposed. The Edmonton Obesity Staging System, irrespective of the amount of weight excess, takes into account metabolic, physical and psychological factors. This system has been shown to be more effective than the BMI in predicting mortality. Starting from this the Italian Obesity Society (SIO) has suggested an algorithm that identifies the preferred therapeutic option for the treatment of the obese patient (**Figure 1.2**).

In obesity, the aim of dietary treatment is to achieve and maintain weight loss to improve health and the altered metabolic parameters. Once these results have been reached, the objective is to maintain them in the long term.

The principal target of the therapeutic strategy regards the factors that influence and modify control of the regulation of the energy balance in the organism. An efficient approach to treating obesi ty should, above all, recognize that it is a progressive and chronic condition and, as such, needs therapeutic intervention that can last for the patient's entire life. Treatment cannot consist only in calorie restriction of a prescriptive type, but has to include interventions that bring about changes in behavior towards food and in lifestyle, and involve the activation of useful strategies for making the patient aware of the pathway they are taking, thus increasing their motivation to change. Long-term treatment is often complex and requires an integrated approach that uses the instruments available in a complementary manner, taking advantage of the various professional skills that share the same therapeutic objective. Efficient management of obesity implies setting up a personalized treatment plan tailored to the patient. The potential factors that contribute to weight increase, including food habits, physical inactivity, associated medical conditions and drugs, must be identified and addressed.

Lifestyle interventions including diet modification, physical activity for maintaining the results, behavioural therapy, food education, and counselling are among the strategies used today for the management of obesity. Another important point regards the expectations that the patients have regarding the healthcare pathway. These expectations are often greater than the results that can be realistically obtained and so it is necessary to define realistic objectives that produce health benefits. Aiming for 5% weight loss is clinically significant and can substantially reduce the risk of comorbidities.

As regards treatment of older obese patients, obesity influences not only morbidity and mortality but, above all, quality of life. In these cases interventions which induce weight loss can effectively lead to improved physical function. However, if based only on a dietary approach, they can negatively affect muscle and bone health, and produce other adverse effects.

Regular physical exercise associated with moderate calorie restriction has notable advantages

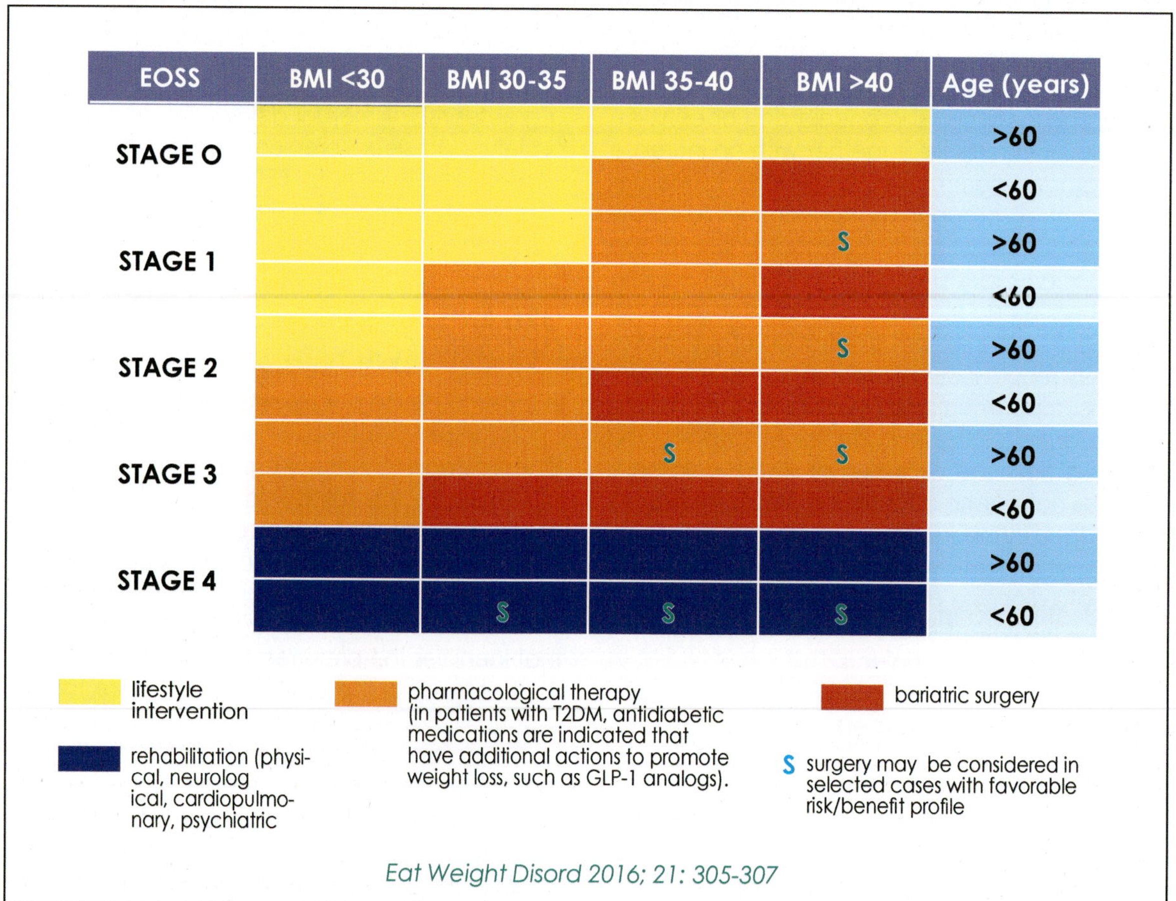

Figure 1.2 Algorithm for the treatment of overweight and obese patients. The therapeutic strategies are shown as a function of the EOSS disease stage (Edmonton Obesity Staging System).

for older people as it does for young adults. It has been demonstrated that the combined effect of dietary treatment and physical exercise improves pain and functional status in adults >60 years of age who have been radiologically diagnosed with osteoarthritis and physical disabilities.

PHARMACOTHERAPY

At present, diet, physical activity, and behavioural modifications constitute the cornerstones in the management of patients with disorders linked to nutrition. However, they are sometimes not sufficient. A greater knowledge of the control mechanisms regarding appetite control and energy consumption has brought about the development of new molecules, but the past history of anti-obesity drugs has taught us that the evaluation of their safety profile is a fundamental aspect to take into consideration. In fact, numerous medical solutions have been proposed over the years, with various having been promptly taken off the market due to their adverse side effects. For this reason, the regulatory authorities increasingly require a more in-depth assessment of the benefit-risk profile of new drugs.

Table 1.1 shows the main drugs available today that have been approved by EMA and/or the FDA. Other categories of medicines having potential anti-obesity effects are currently being studied, such as tesophensine, velneperit and beloranib.

At the moment in Italy, the drugs approved for the long-term treatment of obesity in adults are orlistat, liraglutide and an association of naltrexone/bupropion, indicated for patients with a BMI ≥30, or in overweight patients (BMI ≥27) with associated risk factors.

According to the guidelines of the Italian Obesity Society (SIO), the pharmacological therapy must be suspended if, after a period variable from 4 to 12 weeks, depending on the drug taken, a fall in body weight of at least 5% has not been achieved. On the other hand, they recommend continuing administration of the drug for more than 24 months (generally for weight maintenance) following discussion with the patient regarding potential collateral effects and the limitations of the pharmacological treatment.

The three active ingredients of the drugs available in Italy have different mechanisms:

- orlistat reduces the absorption of fats in the gastrointestinal tract. In particular, it blocks the lipase enzyme that breaks down the triglycerides taken with food in order to ensure their absorption. The adverse effects most frequently associated with this drug are gastrointestinal disorders (cramps, flatulence, fatty and oily stools, fecal incontinence) and reduced absorption of vitamins A, D and E.
- liraglutide is an analogue of the human glucagon-like peptide-1 (GLP-1), a hormone secreted by the L cells of the small bowel. It binds to the GLP-1 receptor, activating it. This induces an increase in insulin secretion by the pancreas, a reduction in gastric emptying and a central increase in satiety and a reduction in appetite and food intake. Possible side effects are nausea, diarrhoea, constipation, a slight increase in heart rate, all of which can be reversed by discontinuing the treatment.
- naltrexone and bupropion in combination increases the loss of calories and has effects on the sense of gratification associated with food intake. For these reasons it is able to reduce the appetite, making it easier to follow a low-calorie diet. Possible side effects are nausea, constipation, vomiting, dizziness and a dry mouth. In addition, it has also been associated with drowsiness and cases of loss of consciousness. This therapy is also not recommended for patients taking drugs that lower the epileptogenic threshold.

BARIATRIC SURGERY

Bariatric surgery is an additional therapeutic instrument in the management of severe obesity. It is considered a treatment option in eligible patients (BMI ≥40 in the absence of comorbidities or BMI ≥35 in the presence of comorbidities) to be used when other methods (restrictive diet, cognitive behaviour therapy) have not produced adequate results and when comorbidities associated with an increased risk of mortality are present.

The aim of bariatric surgery is to reduce comorbidities by means of restrictive or malabsorptive mechanisms, or both.

The types of bariatric surgery are:

- restrictive: based on the reduction of the gastric volume (lap-band, vertical gastroplasty and laparoscopic sleeve gastrectomy);
- malabsorptive: inducing a malabsorption provoking modifications of the intestinal anatomy, following which the absorptive capacity of the intestinal mucosa is confined only to the tract immediately before the ileocecal valve (50-100 cm) (e.g. biliopancreatic diversion and duodenal-switch, operations which are rarely carried

Table 1.1 Pharmacological treatments for obesity currently available and approved by EMA and/or FDA (modified from Garvey WT et al., 2016).

Active ingredient	Mechanism	Effect	Indications	Dose	Approval
Orlistat	Selective inhibition of pancreatic lipase	Reduced absorption and increased fecal excretion of food fats	In association with a hypocaloric diet for: - obese patients with BMI ≥30 or - overweight patients (BMI ≥28) with associated risk factors.	120 mg x 3/day	Approved by EMA and FDA. Available in Italy
Liraglutide	Agonism of GLP-1 receptor	Decrease in feeling of hunger and in desire for food	In association with a hypocaloric diet and increase in physical activity for - patients with BMI ≥30 - patients with BMI ≥27 and with comorbidities (prediabetes mellitus type 2, hypertension, dyslipidemia, obstructive sleep apnoea)	3 mg/day	Approved by EMA and FDA. Available in Italy
Naltrexone/ Buproprione	- Naltrexone: antagonism of opiate μ receptors - Bupropion: weak antagonism for dopamine receptors and inhibition of noradrenaline reuptake	- Reduction in appetite - Increase in energy consumption	In association with a hypocaloric diet and increase in physical activity for - patients with BMI ≥30 - patients with BMI ≥27 and with comorbidities (prediabetes mellitus type 2, hypertension, dyslipidemia, obstructive sleep apnoea)	32/360 mg/day (maximum dose)	Approved by EMA and FDA. Available in Italy
Lorcaserin	Selective agonism of 5-HT_{2C} receptor	Increase in sense of fullness	- patients with BMI ≥30 - patients with BMI ≥27 with at least one risk factor (diabetes mellitus type 2, hypertension, hypercholesterolemia)	10 mg x 2/ day	Approved by FDA (approval refused by EMA)
Phentermine/ Topiramate	- Phentermine: sympathetic-mimesis - Topiramate: inhibition of carbonic anhydrase and activation of GABA receptors	- Reduction in appetite - Increase in energy consumption	- patients with BMI ≥30 - patients with BMI ≥27 with at least one risk factor (diabetes mellitus type 2, hypertension, hypercholesterolemia)	3.75/23 mg/ day for 2 weeks (up to a maximum of 15/92 mg/ day)	Approved by FDA (approval refused by EMA)

out due to the serious side effects created by the malabsorption;

- mixed: the restrictive component (formation of a small gastric pocket) is combined with reduced absorption of food, diminishing the absorption of nutritive substances bypassing the duodenum and the first part of the jejunum (e.g. gastric bypass/Roux-en-Y and mini gastric bypass).

The gastric bypass is currently the most common operation carried out in subjects with severe

pathological obesity and/or a history of failure after restrictive surgery.
Bariatric surgical techniques are in continuous evolution to minimize the risks potentially associated with surgery and to obtain a better effect on the comorbidity associated with obesity.
In patients over 60 years of age with severe obesity, bariatric surgery can be considered in order to improve their quality of life.
The guidelines of the Italian Society of Obesity Surgery (SICOB) give the eligibility criteria for surgery. Surgery should be considered only after carefully evaluating the risks and benefits, including the risk of mortality. Furthermore, the guidelines have directed attention to the definition of the follow-up period after surgery. These are critical for good results, so as to consolidate the results from the surgery and avoid complications, above all those that are nutritional.

Teamwork
The healthcare workers involved in the therapeutic pathway should be fully aware of their responsibilities and those of other team members and exploit their individual skills in order to create effective interaction between the various professionals. It is essential to create a common language and culture within the entire team for efficient integration of the various responsibilities. The borders of the work of each team member should be clearly defined since confusion of roles can lead to failure of the treatment. An effective team is built by means of long and patient job training. Even if guidelines and protocols exist, the care pathway should be tailored to the individual patient, and continually updated on the basis of resistance, motivation, assertiveness, and difficulties encountered.

KEY CONCEPTS

- The goal of clinical nutrition is to prevent and treat malnutrition.
- Undernutrition and excessive nutrition can affect health status; malnutrition is associated with increased mortality and morbidity.
- A common nutritional terminology can be useful in clinical practice. A consensus on nutrition terminology can help to support and ensure appropriate shared care. The classification of malnutrition is very important to understand the complexity of the problem and to plan treatment.
- Malnutrition is associated with metabolic alterations, chronic inflammation, diseases and trauma.
- Obesity is a chronic disease resulting from the interplay of multiple factors. Obesity is associated with comorbidities that increase mortality and morbidity. Nutritional counseling is a part of obesity therapy.

REFERENCES

- Cederholm T, Jensen GL, Correia M et al. GLIM criteria for the diagnosis of malnutrition – a consensus report from the global clinical nutrition community. Clin Nutr 2019;38:1-9.
- Cederholm T, Barazzoni R, Austin P et al. ESPEN guidelines on definitions and terminology of clinical nutrition. Clin Nutr. 2017;36:49-64.
- Donini LM, Busetto L, Bauer JM et al. Critical appraisal of definitions and diagnostic criteria for sarcopenic obesity based on a systematic review. Clin Nutr 2019;39 (8):2368–2388.
- Linee guida SICOB (Società Italiana di Chirurgia dell'Obesità e malattie metaboliche) http://www.sicob. org/00_materiali/linee_guida_2016.pdf
- Santini F, Busetto L, Cresci B, Sbraccia P. SIO management algorithm for patients with overweight or obesity: consensus statement of the Italian Society for Obesity (SIO). Eat Weight Dis. 2016;21:305-7.

CHAPTER 2

GUT MICROBIOTA

Antonio Rispo

LEARNING OBJECTIVES

- To acquire knowledge on the composition and functions of human gut microbiota.
- To understand the importance of gut microbiota in health and disease.
- To know the principles of methods to analyze gut microbiota.

INTRODUCTION

The gastrointestinal (GI) system is a complex and constantly evolving ecosystem composed of components in a mutual relation with each other. It can be considered as a functional unit that works to absorb nutrients needed by the human body, and that prevents pathogenic microorganisms from entering the body.

One of the most important components of the GI system is the gut microbiota, which comprises the microbes living within the GI tract.

METHODS FOR CHARACTERISATION OF GUT MICROBIOTA

Standard microbiological culture techniques were the earliest methods for analysis of the gut microbiota. Their major limitation was that they were unable to detect the vast majority (70-90%) of the components of gut microbiota, because of their extremophile anaerobic nature. Because of this drawback, the contribution by such techniques to the characterization of intestinal microbiota composition has not been very relevant.

The subsequent use of methods not using culture techniques, but rather based on characterization of ribosomal RNA sequences – specifically, of its 16S part (16SrRNA) – by polymerase chain reaction (PCR) has advanced our knowledge of microbiota composition. Further methods gut microbiota analysis are denaturing gradient gel electrophoresis (DGGE) and temperature gradient cell electrophoresis (TGGE), which are based on the extraction, amplification, and subsequent electrophoretic analysis of cellular DNA, and fluorescence in situ hybridization (FISH), through which 16SrRNA is labeled with fluorescent material and subsequently identified.

The recent introduction of next generation gene sequencers (next generation sequencing - NGS), which differ from the classic sequencers both in the technology and the amount of data that they are able to collect for single analysis, has changed the scenario of gut microbiota analysis. Metagenomics indicates the use of these methodologies for the characterization of the composition of microbial species in biological samples.

In addition, the term metabolomics refers to the systematic study of the chemical fingerprints left by cellular processes of the host and intestinal microbiota, and the set of all metabolites produced by a biological organism.

In the near future, the metabolic profile will provide a snapshot of the body's physiology. One of the major challenges of systemic biology is to integrate data from metagenomics, proteomics, transcriptomics, and metabolomics to obtain an exhaustive overview of living organisms, and of gut microbiota in particular to better understand its functions.

GUT MICROBIOTA: OVERVIEW AND COMPOSITION

Gut microbiota consists of about 1014 microorganisms (progressively increasing in number from mouth to large bowel), 10-20 times greater than that of human cells, with a weight of nearly 1-1.5 kg and a total genetic heritage of more than 3.3 million genes (versus nearly 22,000 human genes). Gut microbiota is largely composed of bacteria; there are also viruses (especially bacteriophages), Archaea, and Eukaryota such as Fungi, Amoebozoa, Protozoa, and other microbes; very recent studies have highlighted the key role of these "minor" components (in particular fungi and viruses) in the pathogenesis of disease (e.g., inflammatory bowel disease).

Various factors, both in physiological (such as age, diet, genetic profile) and pathological conditions (infections, surgical interventions, use of antibiotics and proton pump inhibitors) can modify and/ or alter the gut microbiota composition.

Bacterial Gut Microbiota (Gut Bacteriome)
Gut bacteriome is composed of more than 1000 bacterial species. Thanks to the most recent methods of microbiota, characterization, four main bacterial phyla have been identified: Firmicutes, Bacteroides, Proteobacteria, and Actinobacteria, which account together for nearly 98% of intestinal microbiota, for a total of 11 divisions. Of these, Firmicutes and Bacteroidetes are the most numerous.
Firmicutes can be divided into two main groups: *Clostridium cluster XIVa* or *Clostridium coccoides*, and *Clostridium cluster IV* or *Clostridium leptum*.
The first group includes species of the genera *Butyrivibrio*, *Clostridium*, *Coprococcus*, *Dorea*, *Eubacterium*, *Lachnospira*, *Roseburia*, *Ruminococcus*. Beyond constituting a considerable part of the gut bacteria, this group includes several bacteria that produce short chain fatty acids (SCFA - *short-chain fatty acids*), in particular butyric acid, which provides a fundamental source of sustenance for colonocytes.
The second group includes species belonging to the genera *Anaerofilum*, *Clostridium*, *Eubacterium*, *Ruminococcus*. It is characterized by numerous extremophile anaerobic bacteria, and, like the first group, by SCFA producers, in particular the *Faecalibacterium prausnitzii*, a bacterium with important anti-inflammatory properties, whose drastic reduction has been exhaustively documented in inflammatory bowel diseases.
The second most numerous phylum is Bacteroidetes, including mainly gram-negative bacteria and obligate anaerobes.
Further minor bacterial phyla include: Actinobacteria, Cyanobacteria, Deferribacteres, Deinococcus/Thermus, Fusobacteria, Proteobacteria, Spirochaetes, VadinBE97, and Verrucomicrobia. Among Verrucomicrobia, Akkermansia muciniphila has important metabolic and immunological functions, and in particular its abundance is inversely proportional to various inflammatory conditions, such as obesity, type 2 diabetes mellitus and inflammatory bowel diseases.

Viral Gut Microbiota (Gut Virome)
Although human viruses have been considered as mere pathogenic organisms, recent methods of metagenomic analysis have shown that the human gut hosts predominantly bacteriophages, which have an active mutualistic role in the development and the homeostasis of gut microbiota.
Like bacteria, 1 g of faeces contains more than 109 virions, but, unlike bacteria, viral particles differ greatly between human subjects. Part of this variability is related to individual differences in bacterial colonization of the intestine.
Most intestinal viruses are bacteriophages, viruses that infect certain bacterial species. The first description of the gut virome was obtained through shotgun sequencing of virus-like particles (VLPs) from faecal samples.
Among the 1200 different virotypes analyzed, the Siphoviridae family is the most numerous, followed by Podoviridae.
Initial estimates of the abundance of the Microviridae family in the human gut microbiota were later resized and considered the result of a diagnostic artifact.
In any case, a new branch of the Microviridae family has recently been identified, which derives from the profages of genomes belonging to the Bacteroidetes.
The ratio of virotypes to bacteria is 10: 1 in oceanic marine environments, but nearly 1: 1 in the human intestine. This suggests that phages have a tamer attitude in the gut than in ocean ecosystems. In the gut this occurs in parallel with CRISPR (clustered regularly interspected short palindromic repeats) bacteria, which are involved in the development of our immune system to fight infections.
Recently, abnormalities have been found in the intestinal viroma of patients with ulcerative rectocolitis and Crohn's disease, diseases characterized by a diminished diversity of the bacterial microbiota (the diversity of the intestinal microbiota is an index of state of health).
Both diseases have been associated with a significant increase in Caudovirales bacteriophages. Furthermore, the data showed that this increase in virions is not secondary to alteration of the bacterial microbiota, but rather that alterations of the intestinal viroma can contribute to bacterial dysbiosis and intestinal inflammation.

Fungal Gut Microbiota (Gut Mycobiome)
Currently, it is not known precisely how many fungi make up the human gut microbiota. Fungi are detectable at different concentrations for each district, with a rising gradient from the mouth to the anus (from 102 in the stomach up to 106 in the colon. Although some may be pathogenic in other

organs (e.g., the lungs), they probably act as commensals, at low concentrations, in the gastrointestinal tract. In the healthy intestine, the dominant species are *Wallemia, Trichocomaceae, Rhodotorula, Saccharomycetaceae, Pleosporaceae, Agaricaceae, Metschnikowiaceae, Cystofilobasidiaceae, Ascomycota, Amphisphaeriacea.*

The presence of fungal species has been correlated with that of the bacteria. The presence of the genus *Fusarium* is positively correlated with that of *Syntrophococcus and Anaerostipes* (P=0.001), and that of *Pichia with Syntrophococcus* (P=0.001), while an interesting negative correlation between *Candida and Bacteroides* has been observed (P=0.001). The gut mycobiome can directly or indirectly interact with the host's immune system, potentially leading to exacerbation of numerous gastrointestinal diseases (e.g., inflammatory bowel disease).

FUNCTIONS OF GUT MICROBIOTA IN PHYSIOLOGICAL CONDITIONS

As recently discovered, the intestinal microbiota has fundamental functions in the maintenance of the homeostasis within our body, it is no longer considered a mere saprophyte, as in the past, but an essential inner component of our organism. Numerous processes the human organism is not able to do within our body are carried out by the gut microbiota. Therefore, the human body and the gut microbiota have been defined together as a "superorganism". The genes of gut microbiota ("gut microbiome") encode enzymes and other proteins involved in a variety of functions: the barrier, metabolic, and immune function.

Barrier Function

The gut microbiota is a component of the gastrointestinal barrier, together with the epithelial cells, the intercellular junctions, and the mucosal layer that covers the cells (physical barrier), and local immune system, blood flow, endocrine and neuroenteric systems, and digestive enzymes (functional barrier).

The gut microbiota contributes in several ways to protect the intestine against external pathogens. The SCFAs have a trophic function toward colonocytes coupled with a significant anti-inflammatory action. Furthermore, microbial derivates stimulate the expression of intercellular junctions (in particular, of tight junctions) and regulate the metabolism of the intestinal mucus.

Metabolic Function

The gut microbiota plays a fundamental role in the metabolism of nutrients within our body. The microbial colonization of the gut of germ-free mice was found to lead to an increase in weight and fat mass, regardless of the type of diet they were fed with. Gut microbiota can therefore considered a real "energy bioreactor" that produces energy from the nutrients ingested with food.

Most of the components of the gut microbiota reside in the colon, and metabolize the undigested foods in the small intestine, in particular fibers, polysaccharides, and plant-derived oligosaccharides. The gut microbiota metabolizes carbohydrates through an anaerobic process that produces gas derivatives and SCFAs, which are mainly composed of acetate (derivative of the fermentation of carbohydrates from the bacterial species of the colon, such as *Bacteroides, Clostridium, Bifidobacterium, Ruminococcus, Eubacterium*, etc.), butyrate (produced *Eubacterium, Coprococcus, E. rectale-Roseburia* and *Faecalibacterium*) and propionate (produced *Bacteroides, Propionibacterium* and *Veillonella*). The SCFAs are absorbed by the colonocytes, and sent to the liver, the muscular system, and the brain. Propionate and butyrate have a trophic action on colonocytes (synthesis of cell membranes), while propionate and acetate are used for gluconeogenesis and hepatic lipogenesis, respectively. The role of gut microbiota in protein metabolism is less relevant than in carbohydrate metabolism. Proteins arrive in the colon in reduced quantities, and the vast majority are of endogenous origin (e.g., digestive enzymes, biliary juice, products derived from enterocytes, etc.). Some bacteria, including *Bacteroides, Clostridium, Propionibacterium, Fusobacterium, Streptococcus* and *Lactobacillus*) can degrade them. This process leads to the production, of peptides assimilated by the microbiota itself, and of SCFA, but also of toxic metabolites such as phenols, indoles, ammonium, and derivatives.

Lipid metabolism is modulated by gut microbiota through several pathways.

The gut microbiota can deconiugate and hydroxylate bile salts, essential for lipid absorption. Also, gut microbiota influences the activity of lipoproteinlipase (LPL), which regulates the release of fatty acids from lipoproteins, through the downregulation of FIAF (fasting-induced adipocyte factor), which inhibits the production of lipoprotein lipase (LPL).

Furthermore, gut microbiota modulates lipogenesis by regulating insulin levels.

Finally, gut microbiota plays a role in vitamin metabolism, as the colonic microbiota is able to synthetize vitamin K and almost all the B group vitamins.

Immune Function

Although the fetus is almost sterile, our organism is colonized by gut microbiota after vaginal childbirth.

This contact stimulates maturation of the immune system. The molecular structures associated with microbes (MAMPs) are microbial particles that are identified by receptors (PRRs) found on enterocytes and dendritic cells of the intestine, i.e., the toll-like receptors (TLRs), with the maturation of cells and structures responsible for immune function (the lymphatic follicles and the B lymphocytes that mature in IgA-secreting plasma cells).

Lymphocyte subpopulations are stimulated by different bacterial species: for example, the segmented filamentous bacteria promote the differentiation of T helper 17 lymphocytes, while *Clostridia* assist in the differentiation of T cell lymphocytes.

KEY CONCEPTS

- Gut microbiota consists of the set of microbes residing within the gastrointestinal tract (bacteria, viruses, fungi, Archaea, parasites, and other microorganisms).
- Both physiological and pathological factors modify and / or alter the microbial composition of the gastrointestinal tract.
- The most reliable method to analyze the composition of intestinal microbiota is metagenomics via the use of genomic sequencing methods for characterization of the composition of microbial species in the biological samples.
- The intestinal microbiota has fundamental functions for the maintenance of homeostasis within our body. The genes that make up the gut microbiota ("gut microbiome") encode enzymes and other proteins involved in different functions: the barrier, metabolic and immune function.

REFERENCES

- Rothschild, D., Weissbrod, O., Barkan, E. et al. Environment dominates over host genetics in shaping human gut microbiota. Nature 555, 210-215 (2018). https://doi.org/10.1038/nature25973.
- Wibowo, M.C., Yang, Z., Borry, M. et al. Reconstruction of ancient microbial genomes from the human gut. Nature 594, 234–239 (2021). https://doi.org/10.1038/s41586-021-03532-0.
- Ianiro G, Tilg H, Gasbarrini A. Antibiotics as deep modulators of gut microbiota: between good and evil. Gut. 2016 Nov; 65 (11): 1906-1915. doi: 10.1136 / gutjnl-2016-312297. Epub 2016 Aug 16. PMID: 27531828.
- Rinninella E, Raoul P, Cintoni M, Franceschi F, Miggiano GAD, Gasbarrini A, Mele MC. What is the Healthy Gut Microbiota Composition? A Changing Ecosystem across Age, Environment, Diet, and Diseases. Microorganisms. 2019; 7 (1): 14. https://doi.org/10.3390/microorganisms7010014.
- Mukherjee PK, Sendid B, Hoarau G, et al. Mycrobiota in gastrointestinal diseases. Nat Rev Gastroenterol Hepatol. 2015 Feb;12(2):77-87.
- Norman JM, Handley SA, Baldridge MT, et al. Disease-specific alterations in the enteric virome in inflammatory bowel disease. Cell. 2015 Jan 29;160(3):447-60.
- Ni, J., Wu, G., Albenberg, L. et al. Gut microbiota and IBD: causation or correlation ?. Nat Rev Gastroenterol Hepatol 14, 573–584 (2017). https://doi.org/10.1038/nrgastro.2017.88.

CHAPTER 3

NUTRITION AND SUPPLEMENTS

Filomena Morisco

LEARNING OBJECTIVES
- To understand basic concepts on nutrition and food science in digestive disease.
- To connect notions of gastroenterology and human nutrition.

INTRODUCTION

Eating habits are essential for good health. The increasing prevalence of dysmetabolic diseases (diabetes, hypertension, obesity etc.) is driven by an unbalanced diet. Over the years, health care organizations around the world have striven to establish reference standards for a "healthy diet" with intake recommendations for micronutrients, macronutrients and calories distribution to optimize nutritional status. More recently, a new concept has emerged demonstrating that food and eating habits can modulate pathophysiologic mechanisms in body systems, properties that are particularly relevant for digestive function and the onset of gastroenterological diseases.

In fact, foods have bioactive molecular components that transform tissue and cellular molecular patterns that regulate gene and protein expression, oxidative state, inflammatory status and carcinogenic processes. Furthermore, the quantity and quality of food are fundamental for good functioning of digestive system and lowering the risk of the diseases. For example: 1) the quantity and quality of foods can determine the composition of the gut microbiota involved in the control of metabolic, inflammatory and immunological processes associated with gastrointestinal diseases; 2) the dietary habits of patients with non-alcoholic steatohepatitis (NASH) are characterized by a higher consumption of total calories, saturated fats and carbohydrates as compared to control subjects without the disease; 3) gluten free diet helps resolve the intestinal inflammation related to celiac disease; 4) a diet with adequate amounts of fibre and liquids can improve functional constipation.

These concepts must be part of the scope of the baggage of knowledge of a specialist in gastroenterology and applied in clinical practice, integrating a fundamental understanding of nutrition to manage (prevention and treatment) patients.

ALIMENTATION

Eating is a voluntary act by which an individual, through the ingestion of food and drink, brings energy and nutrients to the body. Eating is a complex process that presumes the integrity of functions such as introduction of food into the oral cavity, mastication, swallowing, digestion, intestinal transit, absorption and metabolism of nutrients. The desire to feed is induced by the need to maintain the energy balance and ensure the normal vital functions of an individual. The energy balance is maintained through the hunger-satiety circuit, a complex neuro-hormonal regulation, at the peripheral and the central level.

Several factors regulate the hunger-satiety circuit: environmental, gastro-intestinal and metabolic factors (**Table 3.1**). The environmental factors are controlled by the senses: smell, sight of a dish and talking about food. At gastrointestinal level it all starts with the release of ghrelin, a hormone which increases the sense of hunger. There are also other factors that act in the same way. In fact, when the level of cellular glucose declines the sensation of hunger increases. This also happens when the level of lipids inside the cells (lipoprivation) decreases. The brain evaluates the reduction of glucose at the blood-brain barrier, while the liver monitors both glucose and lipid reduction in the rest of the body. The hypothalamus produces two types of lipids that stimulate the hunger: the hormone containing melatonin (MCH) and oressin. In addition, the feeling of satiety is modulated by gastric distension, through the release of such hormones as cholecystokinin, GLP-1 (glucagon-like peptide-1), serotonin, insulin, glucagoneleged or through the blood levels of glucose, free fatty acids and amino acids, or through cognitive, psychological and social factors.

Eating disorders can modify the hunger-satiety circuit, both in excess, like increased frequency and

Table 3.1 Mechanisms of control of the hunger-satiety circuit.

	Orectic Effectors	Anorectic Effectors
Sensorial perceptions	Olfactory, gustatory, visual, tactile	
Mechanical signals		Gastric distension
Neurotransmitters	Adrenaline, noradrenaline, dopamine	Serotonin
Neuropeptides and hormones	Ghrelin, NPY, AgRP, MCH, orexin A and B, opioid system, endocannabinoids	POMC, CART, α-MSH, TRH, insulin, amylin, CCK, GLP-1, PYY, oxintomodulin
Cytokines		Leptin, adiponectin, TNF- α, IL-1, IL-6

Abbreviations: NPY: neuropeptide Y; AgRP: agouti related protein; MCH: melanin concentrating hormone; POMC: pro-opiomelanocortina; CART: cocaine and amphetamine-related trascript; α-MSH: α-melanocyte-stimulating hormone; TRH: thyrotropin releasing hormone; CCK: cholecystokinin; GLP-1: glucagone like peptide-1; PYY: peptide YY; TNF- α: tumours necrosis factor-α; IL-1: interleukin-1; IL-6: interleukin.

size of daily meals, or through default, such as decreased intake of food and / or other methods to reduce body weight by inducing vomiting or the use of anorectic, laxative or diuretic drugs.

Health presumes correct dietary habits, which dates back to the ancient Greek world. Unfortunately, in modern societies there is a high consumption of packaged foods, fast-food and soft drinks with a high content of saturated fats, cholesterol, sodium and simple sugars. Combined with sedentary habits, they are the cause of an increased risk of obesity, diabetes and cardiovascular disease, which are linked by a common pathophysiological mechanism that starts from insulin resistance and hyperinsulinemia.

Another important aspect of nutrition is the biomolecular properties food. Their bioactivity modulates the function of cells and organs and exerts genetic and epigenetic effects (nutrigenomics). There are several foods rich in bioactive components such as caffeine, polyphenols, carotenoids and glucosinolates. It has been demonstrated that these compounds are able to exert many activities, including antioxidant and anti-inflammatory activities, detoxification of enzymes, stimulation of the immune system, metabolic hormone modulation, antibacterial and antiviral activities and, finally, antiproliferative and pro-apoptotic activities.

NUTRITION

Nutrition is defined as the complex of biological processes that influences the growth, the development and the integrity of living organism in relation to energy, nutrients and other nutritional substances.

Nutrients are substances with a defined role in the physiological processes and human metabolism. They are grouped by their function, in macronutrients (carbohydrates, lipids, proteins) and micronutrients (vitamins and mineral salts).

The malnutrition, both for deficiency and excess, is associated with a reduced survival, worsening of the clinical outcome and quality of life. As consequence it's clear that nutritional status represents an important determinant of health status and the nutritional management of patients plays a primary role in the clinical practise.

Furthermore, the deficiency or the excess of specific nutrients influence specific physiological processes and the pathogenesis of many diseases. In particular, nutrition often has a crucial role in the pathogenesis and management of gastrointestinal disease. In celiac disease, for example, diet is the only helpful treatment.

Evaluation of the nutritional status includes clinical procedures that begin with the assessment of the adequate nutritional requirements, goals to reach and preserve health status and to define diet therapy for different diseases. Starting from the patient's medical and nutritional history and physical examination, the nutritional status evaluation relies on anthropometry, biochemical and functional tests and analysis of body composition.

Some biochemical tests are useful markers for nutritional status evaluation. However, their interpretation is often difficult and not always correlated to malnutrition. Biochemical tests allow to evaluate the lipid and glycaemic profile, nutritional proteic status, inflammatory state, immune function and principal micronutrients. Laboratory tests for the evaluation of nutritional status are:

- total cholesterol, HDL, triglycerides;
- glycaemia and insulinaemia;
- prealbumin, albumin, transferrin and immunoglobulin;
- erythrocytes, haemoglobin, leucocytes, platelets, prothrombin time;
- serum iron and ferritin;
- vitamin B12, folic acid and retinol binding protein (RBP);
- electrolytes (sodium, potassium, magnesium, calcium etc.) ;
- alkaline phosphatase and transaminases;
- pseudocholinesterase;
- thyrotropic hormone (TSH);
- urea nitrogen, azoturia, creatinine, creatinuria and uraemia.

Dynamometry or handgrip and indirect calorimetry are functional tests that evaluate malnutrition. Dynamometry is closely related to sarcopenia and it is recommended as a good measure of muscular strength. In indirect calorimetry, energy expenditure is calculated from the values of oxygen consumption and carbon dioxide production.

The energetic equivalent of oxygen consumption (VO2) and carbon dioxide production (VCO2) depends on quantity of carbohydrates, proteins and lipids oxidised. Protein oxidation is calculated from the nitrogen lost in the urine.

Body composition evaluation entails the study of the human body compartments that, in the bicompartmental model, can be divided in lean mass and fat mass, or the 5-compartment model that distinguishes total body water, protein mass, mineral mass, glycogen and fat mass (**Figure 3.1**).

NUTRITIONAL SUPPLEMENTS

Nutritional supplements are defined by the Italian Ministry of Health as "foodstuffs intended to complement the common diet and which constitute a concentrated form of nutrients, such as vitamins and minerals, or of other substances having a nutritional or physiological effect, in particular amminoacids, essential fatty acids, fibers and extracts of plant, both single or multi-composite, in premeasured forms". Importantly, supplements are not drugs but may be generically termed health enhancers.

Nutritional supplements usually come in tablets, sachets or vials. They can boost health by optimizing or promoting normal functioning of the body.

Supplements cannot replace a healthy and balanced diet but can be useful in specific conditions to compensate the lack of some nutrients.

Nutraceutical

The term nutraceutical was coined in 1989 by Stephen De Felice and was derived from the fusion of nutrition and pharmaceuticals. It refers to the study of the nutrients contained in foods that have beneficial effects on health. Nutraceuticals are, therefore, active substances of natural origin or synthesized and administered in pharmaceutical form. Examples are the □-3 fatty acids used in the prevention of cardiovascular diseases and the treatment of mild-grade dyslipidemia or, polyunsaturated fatty acids, monacolin, berberine, to reduce circulating cholesterol levels in association with hypolipidic and hypocaloric diets.

Probiotics and Prebiotics

In recent years the intestinal microbiota has assumed a central role in the pathogenesis of diseases

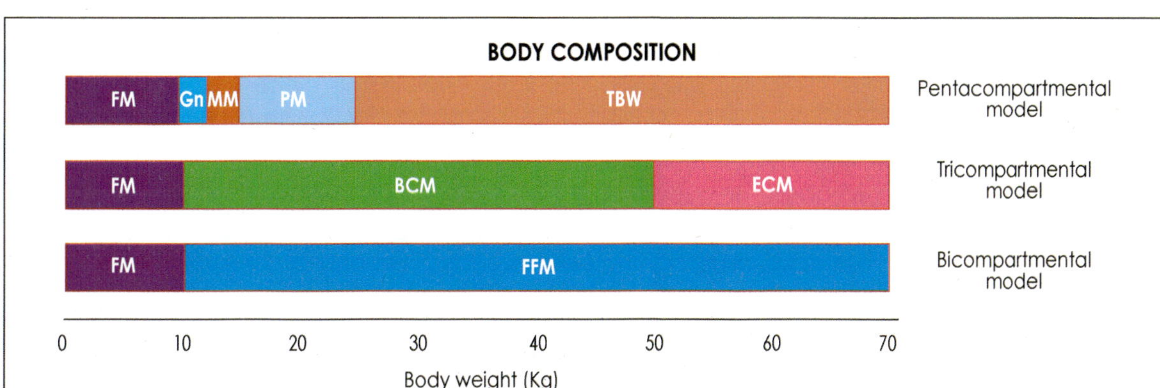

Figure 3.1 The body compartments. FFM, lean mass; FM, fat mass; ECM, extracellular mass; BCM, active metabolic mass; TBW, total body water; PM, protein mass; MM, mineral mass; Gn, glycogen.

and with it the use of supplements containing probiotics and prebiotics has spread.
The term "probiotics" refers to products containing a high number of live and active microorganisms that reach the intestine where they replicate and act on the equilibrium of the intestinal microflora through direct colonization. In clinical practice probiotics are often used for the treatment of acute diarrhoea to restore the physiological microbiota.
The term "prebiotic", instead, indicates indigestible components of foods that selectively promote the growth and activity of one or more bacteria present in the gut. In clinical practice, prebiotics are often used for treating irritable bowel syndrome or intestinal bacterial overgrowth syndrome (SIBO small intestinal bacterial overgrowth), which develops after surgery of the digestive tract.
In clinical practice, probiotics and prebiotics can be used together and so they are called symbiotics.

Supplements of Plant Origin

Supplements that are composed, exclusively or in part, of substances of vegetable origin are named botanicals. The use of plant extracts has gained widespread popularity because of commonly held, but not correct, idea that plant-derived products are free of harmful effects. Incorrect use of these products can trigger serious adverse events owing to the toxicity of some plants and potential interactions with drugs.
Nonetheless, many plant-based supplements are helpful in diseases of gastrointestinal tract. For example, silymarin, a derivative of milk thistle, a herbaceous plant commonly found in the Mediterranean basin, seems to have antioxidant and protective effects on the liver. Also, because of its digestive properties, ginger is often used for treating nausea or as prokinetic.
Summarizing: while nutritional supplements can be useful in many situations in clinical practice, they should not be considered as substitutes for drugs or a healthy and balanced diet.

KEY CONCEPTS

- Human nutrition is a complex act that, in addition to the primordial need to eat, is influenced by social, cultural and psychological factors. It ensures the individual's normal vital functions.
- Food, in addition to being the sources of nutrients, is a vehicle for bioactive molecules that interact with cells, organs and systems and positively or negatively influence cellular metabolic processes.
- Assessment of nutritional status is a clinical skill of the specialist in diseases of the digestive system and must be integrated in the diagnostic and therapeutic approach.
- Food supplements are food-based products that can be used to boost habitual diet, for a limited period of time, and to compensate for temporary deficiencies of specific nutrients. Food supplements are not intended as substitutes for a varied and balanced diet.

REFERENCES

- Federico A, Dallio M, Caprio GG, Gravina AG, Picascia D, Masarone M, Persico M, Loguercio C. Qualitative and Quantitative Evaluation of Dietary Intake in Patients with Non-Alcoholic Steatohepatitis. Nutrients. 2017;9(10).
- Livovsky DM, Pribic T, Azpiroz F. Food, Eating and the Gastrointestinal Tract. Nutrients. 2020;12(4):986.
- Tack J, Verbeure W, Mori H, et al. The gastrointestinal tract in hunger and satiety signalling. United European Gastroenterol J. 2021;9(6):727-34.
- Hamada Y. Objective Data Assessment (ODA) Methods as Nutritional Assessment Tools. J Med Invest. 2015;62(3-4):119-22.
- Rivellese AA, Annuzzi G, Capaldo B, Vaccaro O, Riccardi G. Nutrizione Umana. Idelson-Gnocchi 2017;17:275-306.
- Floch MH. The role of Prebiotics and Probiotics in Gastrointestinal Disease. Gastroenterol Clin North Am. 2018;47(1):179-91.

CHAPTER 4

NEW TECHNOLOGIES

Domenico Alvaro, Antonio Benedetti, Vincenzo Cardinale

LEARNING OBJECTIVES

- Know the terms and definitions used in the field of digital health, artificial intelligence (AI), big data, telemedicine, network medicine.
- Know the new tools for the acquisition and analysis of health and clinical data.
- Know the possible role of AI, telemedicine and radiomics in gastroenterology.

INTRODUCTON

Technological advancement is revolutionizing daily life globally. For a doctor, keeping up with the times today means knowing the potential of new technologies, knowing the meaning of terms commonly used in the domains of digitalization, big data, artificial intelligence (AI), telemedicine, and of data science.

In order to understand how medical practice and research in the various fields of reference are impacted by new technologies, we could consider a sort of stratification of complexity: the pyramid of new technologies. At the base operate digital systems for interfacing with the user and digital data storage (all data subject to digital transformation). In a layer of higher complexity, telematic infrastructures and services operate that can be connected to each other, for example radiology units, pathological anatomy, etc., which acquire and make complex data digitally usable, such as images. All this large amount of data (potentially big data) constitutes a resource that can be managed through the tools of AI, data science, to support the diagnosis and monitoring of patients. Finally, at the apex of this pyramid of complexity we can imagine an ecosystem for personalized medicine, in which the acquired and digitized clinical and instrumental data can be correlated with experimental data, such as multiomic characterization (genetics and genomics, transcriptomics, proteomics, metabolic), also using the precepts and methods of the network medicine, to return new information and knowledge useful for personalized medicine; for example the rapid and precise identification of patient candidates for 'target' therapies, the prediction of the histological and molecular characteristics of a pathology on the basis of radiological data (radiomics), the prediction of the risk of bleeding from oesophageal varices in hepatopathic patients etc. The new technological systems not only facilitate the acquisition and analysis of data, or the conduct of innovative research, but also represent an incredible tool for interfacing with users (general population, patients, specific categories etc.). Just think of telemedicine and the possibility of performing remote surgery using surgical robots and highly advanced connectivity systems.

Each important phase in the history of humanity and the technologies that guide it have pros and cons. With the advent of 'big data' today the risk is to spend more time managing information than planning future actions based on the 'insights' obtained. We have seen from the national and international news how the breach of the security of digital data, especially sensitive medical data, involves major problems in the functioning of health systems as well as representing violations of privacy with consequences for the individual. The need for data protection systems that are in step with technological advancement, which generates those data, is increasingly acute. Finally, there are philosophical and ethical problems in relation to the growing role of AI in daily life.

The medical student lives in a Copernican revolution of biomedical knowledge and the practice of the medical profession. Have an integrated vision of traditional medicine and digital health, consider the possibility that there may be a systemic approach to health and research, which has the same objectives as traditional medicine and public health, but which uses in a complementary way the traditional tools (visit, hospitalization, diagnosis etc.) and the tools of digital health, AI etc., are issues that the doctors of future generations will certainly have to implement. The goal of this chapter is to create a 'toolbox' glossary for the young doctor projected into a constantly evolving present and to bring some examples of the use of such tools in gastroenterology.

DIGITAL HEALTH

From a systematic review of the literature published in 2020, it emerged that there are 95 different definitions of 'digital health'. The results of this study show that in the field of digital health, the main focus is on health, rather than on technology. Under the concept of health, the emphasis is placed on the health and well-being of individuals and the population, rather than on diseases and patients. It is evident that in the concept of technology the emphasis is on (correct) use of technology, rather than its technical aspects. Based on the results of this study, it can be inferred that digital health is about the correct use of technology to improve the health and well-being of people at the individual and population level, as well as improve patient care through the intelligent processing of clinical and genetic data.
The rationale behind the adoption of digital health tools, and in particular of telehealth and telemedicine, became clear during the Covid-19 pandemic. 'Hospital-centered' health systems have failed to cope with the acute management of the Covid-19 pandemic and the simultaneous routine management of patients with other acute or chronic diseases. The consequences that the pandemic had on health were immediate, but they will also be present in the coming years, especially for millions of people suffering from chronic diseases. Therefore, the Covid-19 pandemic has speeded up the implementation of a model of health care, clinical management and scientific research based on the diagnosis, monitoring and control of the population outside the physical perimeter of hospitals and/or clinics: the digital health. Digital health is an emerging field of study at the intersection of healthcare, medicine, biomedical research and digital technologies, which has attracted a lot of attention in the last decade in many countries around the world. In 2019, the American Medical Association reported that companies invested billions of dollars in new digital health entrepreneurship. The FDA considers a wide range of technologies within 'digital health'; 'Mobile health', wearable devices, 'telehealth' and telemedicine, information technologies applied to the management of health data, and personalized medicine. WHO stresses that digital health can be beneficial to achieving sustainable development goals by making health and wellness services accessible with high standards for all people globally. A systematic review of the literature identified the following components of the digital health innovation ecosystem: 'e-health', 'm-health', 'health 2.0', telehealth and telemedicine, public health surveillance, personalized medicine, health promotion, self-tracking, wearable devices and sensors, genomics, medical imaging and information systems. Digital health uses not only electronic/digital data but also traditional data to serve healthcare and research. Today, AI and machine learning are used as essential tools in digital health, to be combined with information and communication technology (or technologies) (the infrastructure and components that enable computer science) and other technologies to solve problems of the general population and patients (**Figure 4.1**). 'eHealth' is another term related to digital health, used in particular in the UK and Europe, as an umbrella term encompassing telehealth, electronic health records and other components of health information technology.

TELEHEALTH AND TELEMEDICINE

Telemedicine seen as a remote mode of interaction aimed at maintaining health, to be implemented in society needs the complementary approach of health education aimed at patients and caregivers. This is why the broader term of telehealth has been coined, which includes telemedicine within it in a holistic approach to the person and well-being. Indeed, early and correct clinical management is only part of the effort needed to preserve individual and community health. In order to prevent disease risk factors, and to alleviate the harmful effects of sometimes subtle environmental causes, accurate information on health and environmental issues is also necessary. The US Health Resources and Services Administration distinguishes telehealth from telemedicine in its scope, defining telemedicine as pertaining to remote clinical services, such as diagnosis and monitoring, while telehealth includes preventive and health promotion, including education, training and training of patients and caregivers. WHO uses the term telehealth to describe all aspects of health care, including primary prevention care. By taking into consideration preventable non-communicable diseases, which represent the first challenge for global health for over twenty years, as these are due to the global spread unhealthy lifestyles, including diet, sedentary lifestyle, smoking and alcohol consumption, they can be fought by the dissemination of correct and precise infor-

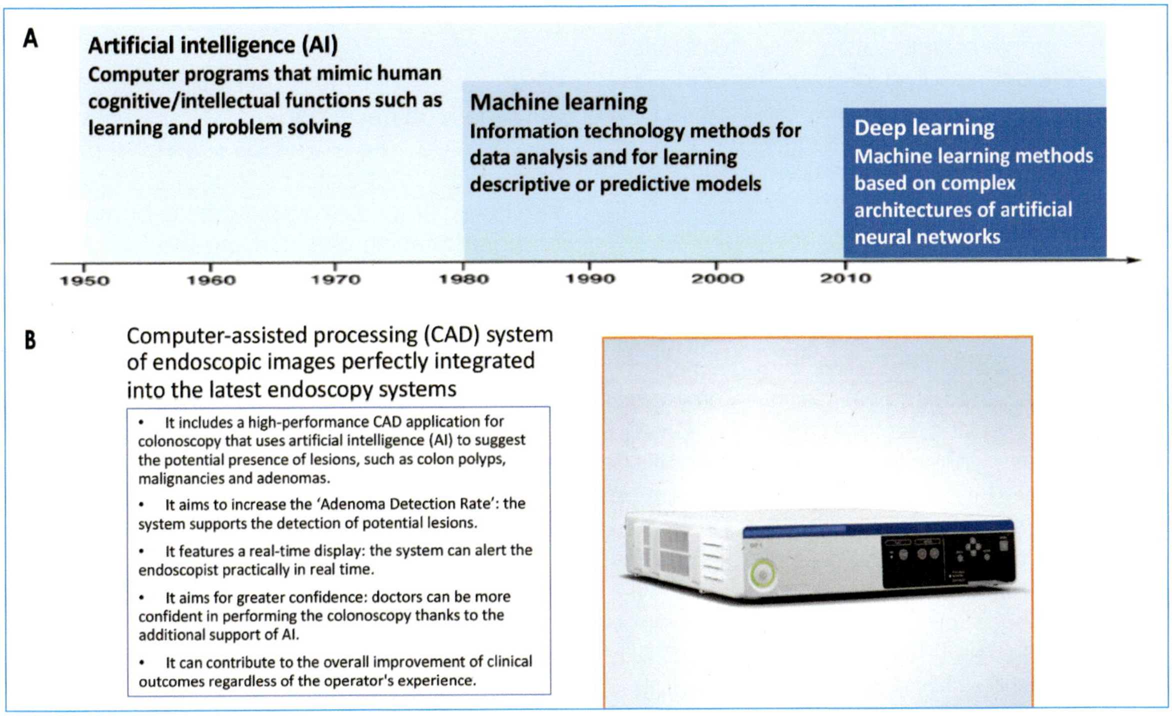

Figure 4.1 A) Evolution over time of artificial intelligence; B) instrumentation and functions of AI in lower digestive endoscopy.

mation and education on healthy lifestyles, as the WHO has been doing for years.
According to the Italian Ministry of Health 'The development of tools for Telemedicine allows both to find new answers to traditional problems of medicine, and to create new opportunities for improving the health service through greater collaboration between the various health professionals involved and patients'. Among the main reasons and expected benefits that drive the development and adoption of telemedicine techniques and tools, the Italian Ministry of Health includes: i) the equity of access to health care. For example, the equity of access and the availability of qualified health care in remote areas (sea, islands, high mountains, hinterland), in places of assisted health care residence, or in places of detention; ii) improving the quality of care by ensuring continuity of care, bringing the doctor's service directly to the patient's home, without leaving his or her office and without the patient being forced to move. Telemedicine could be the tool to meet the request for care of subjects suffering from chronic diseases, which can represent a priority area for the application of telemedicine models: telemonitoring can improve the quality of life of chronic patients through self-treatment solutions, remote management and monitoring, also for the purpose of early de-hospitalization. By way of example, it can also be used to support drug therapy to improve drug compliance; iii) the improvement of effectiveness, efficiency, and appropriateness: the optimal organization of health systems supported by information and communication technology (ITC), makes communication between the various actors usable and continuous and the continuous evaluation of process indicators. The consequences may be the targeted orientation of the providers towards an appropriate use of resources, the reduction of risks related to complications, the reduction of the use of hospitalization, waiting times, and the optimization of the use of available resources. Digital health and telemedicine are tools already used for management and research in the field of rare diseases. Within the European Reference Networks (ERNs) of the different types of rare diseases, every single doctor of any participating hospital/center can share diagnostic and therapeutic choices, which have no guideline support, with the best experts in the the most important European centers, through the interactive digital system of the Clinical Patient Management System (CPMS) (https://rare-liver.eu/healthcare-professionals/cpms). Furthermore, the creation of digitized European databases or registers is the only and real strategy, already in

place in the ERN RARE LIVER (ERN of rare liver diseases), capable of delineating the natural history of the different rare liver diseases through European multicentre prospective studies, and to help doctors and patients understand the prognosis of these diseases, and hopefully improve their therapeutic approach in the future.

The use of telemedicine has allowed in the first phase of the pandemic, the one characterized by the lockdown and limitations of movement on the one hand and the conversion of entire hospitals into Hub Covid on the other, to guarantee patients suffering from chronic gastroenterological diseases at least one remote assistance. E-mails, televisions, etc., while not replacing the 'traditional' visit, allowed the patient to have a discussion with the doctor, to check the analyzes and instrumental tests carried out and an indication of any changes to the therapy in progress.

STITCH (Sapienza information-based Technology InnovaTion Center for Health) in collaboration with industrial partners, it has designed an integrated 'telehealth' and telemedicine program for remote monitoring to tackle the Covid-19 epidemic. This far-reaching telehealth program will integrate telecommunications to provide accurate and precise medical information and education to a broad audience (potentially the general population), with a telemedicine platform for home point-of-care diagnosis and telemonitoring remote doctor, already developed and in use for cardiovascular diseases. In the future of telemedicine as in that of teleducation in medicine, innovation will be fundamental. To increase the confidence of telemedicine systems, the contribution of high definition and advanced internet systems will be important. Innovation in telemedicine goes hand in hand with digital innovation and the country's networking. As the evidence based medicine teaches, the tools in the hands of clinicians must be validated in broad contexts in which they will be used. Until a few years ago, the acquisition of big-data remotely was unthinkable, but above all the management of the enormous amount of data. With the advent of the analytical sciences of big data, machine learning and AI, telemedicine is ready to take a great leap into the future. As we have learned in the biomedical sciences, which often suffer from the failure to translate research into clinical application, it will be crucial to keep research and application linked in telemedicine as well. Without a contextual implementation of research strategies aimed at non-hospitalized patients, it is difficult to imagine a precision or personalized telemedicine.

AI

What do people mean by artificial intelligence (AI)? The term never had clear boundaries. When it was introduced in a 1956 seminal seminar at Dartmouth College, it was understood broadly as the strategies for making a machine behave in an intelligent fashion, like a human being. A major recent advance in artificial intelligence has been machine learning ('machine or deep learning'), which has been used in various technologies, such as spell checking, self-driving cars, and is often performed by computer systems called neural networks. Any discussion of AI is likely to include other terms as defined in the glossary below.

AI GLOSSARY

ALGORITHM A set of step-by-step instructions. Computer algorithms can be simple (if it's 3 p.m., send a reminder) or complex (identify pedestrians).

BACKPROPAGATION The way many neural networks learn. They find the difference between their output and the desired output, then adjust the calculations in the reverse order of execution.

BLACK BOX A description of some deep learning systems. They take an input and provide an output, but the calculations that occur in between are not easy for humans to interpret.

BIG DATA Term used to describe the exponential growth of data. Big data requirements are typically beyond the capabilities of commonly used software tools. In any case, it is necessary to reconsider the methods of circulation, collection, analysis and analysis of data.

DATA MINING It is the process of identifying patterns in huge amounts of data, that is, in big data. It is based on a combination of AI, machine learning and database.

DATA SCIENCE The field of study dedicated to the extraction of knowledge and 'insight' from data through scientific processes, algorithms, systems and methods. It unifies statistics, data analysis, computer science and related methods in order to understand and analyze real phenomena with data.

DEEP LEARNING As a multi-layered neural network becomes sensitive to progressively more abstract patterns. When analyzing a photo, the layers may respond first to the edges, then to the paws, then to the dogs.

EXPERT SYSTEM A form of artificial intelligence that attempts to replicate a human's experience in an area, such as medical diagnosis. Combine a knowledge base with a hand-coded set of rules for applying that knowledge. Machine learning techniques are increasingly replacing manual coding.

GENERATIVE ADVERSARIAL NETWORKS A pair of jointly trained neural networks that generates realistic new data and improves through competition. One net creates new examples (fake Picassos, say) as the other tries to detect the fakes.

MACHINE LEARNING Algorithms that find patterns in data without explicit instructions. A system can learn to associate input features such as images with outputs such as labels.

NEURAL NETWORK A highly abstract and simplified model of the human brain used in machine learning. A set of units takes parts of an input (for example pixels in a photo), performs simple calculations on them and passes them to the next unit level. The final layer represents the answer.

NEUROMORPHIC CHIP A computer chip designed to act as a neural network. It can be analog, digital, or a combination.

REINFORCEMENT LEARNING A type of machine learning in which the algorithm learns by acting towards an abstract goal, such as 'earning a high score in video games' or 'running a factory efficiently.' Each effort is evaluated based on its contribution.

SUPERVISED LEARNING A type of machine learning in which the algorithm compares its outputs with the correct outputs during training. In unsupervised learning, the algorithm merely looks for patterns in a set of data.

STRONG AI As intelligent and complete as a human being. Some say it is impossible. Current AI is weak or restricted. He can play chess or drive, but not both, and he lacks common sense.

TENSORFLOW A collection of software tools developed by Google for use in 'deep learning'. It is open source, which means anyone can use or improve it. Similar projects include Torch and Theano.

TRANSFER LEARNING A technique in machine learning in which an algorithm learns to perform one task, such as recognizing cars, and builds on that knowledge when learning a different but related task, such as recognizing cats.

TURING TEST A test of the AI's ability to be recognized as human. In Alan Turing's original conception, an artificial intelligence would be judged by its ability to converse through written text.

AI IN GASTROENTEROLOGY

Substantial progress has been made in AI and its application to medicine since 2010. AI has been tested in gastroenterology for endoscopic lesion analysis, cancer detection, and to facilitate the analysis of inflammatory lesions or gastrointestinal bleeding during video capsule endoscopy. AI has also been tested to evaluate for liver fibrosis and to differentiate patients with pancreatic cancer from those with pancreatitis. AI could also be used to establish patient prognoses or predict their response to treatments, based on multiple factors.

In healthcare, AI has begun to make a real impact by interpreting images quickly and accurately, improving workflow and reducing medical errors. There is a notable growing interest in the ability of AI to increase the performance characteristics of image processing modes in endoscopy and allow the achievement of certain diagnostic thresholds, especially in non-expert operators. The two areas of gastroenterological endoscopy in which AI has so far found the greatest application are computer-assisted detection (e.g., polyp detection), and computer-assisted diagnosis (e.g., distinguishing adenomatous from hyperplastic polyps). Artificial intelligence systems designed to improve the quality of colonoscopy by decreasing variations in the detection rate of adenomas have attracted great interest. Indeed, artificial intelligence systems distinguish between hyperplastic and neoplastic polyps. New guidelines highlighting the use of artificial intelligence suggest that for AI systems to integrate effectively into the clinical workflow, they must be packaged in an 'all-in-one' solution. For colonoscopy, this means that artificial intelligence systems should have the ability to detect and characterize polyps and label polyps. Another very important field of application of AI in gastroenterology is the early diagnosis of oesophageal and gastric tumours. Adequate surveillance of Barrett's oesophagus and eradication of associated dysplasia is key to preventing transformation into oesophageal adenocarcinoma. Dysplasia can be difficult to localize, resulting in low sensitivity of biopsy specimens despite standardized protocols. Artificial intelligence systems can correctly identify oesophageal squamous cell carcinoma even at an early stage (T1), as well as oesophageal adenocarcinoma. Artificial intelligence systems diagnose gastric cancer with high accuracy, even smaller than 5mm. Assessment of the depth of gastric cancer invasion is also important for management strategies (endoscopic submucosal dissection versus surgery). Artificial intelligence systems can differentiate lesions that invade 500 mm or more into the submucosa from more superficial ones. Also with regard to chronic inflammatory bowel diseases (IBD), AI has been applied to endoscopic evaluation. Indeed, endoscopic assessment of IBD can be subjective and variations in the assessment of disease severity can lead to different management strategies and patient outcomes. AI can help improve biopsy sampling and identify dysplastic areas. A recent work published in the prestigious journal Gastroenterology by Catherine Le Berre and others has the merit of making a systematic review of the studies that have used AI in the gastroenterology and hepatology fields, and of clearly identifying the main research gaps in the field of applied AI. to gastroenterology and hepatology. These gaps are variations in AI performance levels due to lack of high quality datasets, wide variety of statistical tests to evaluate performance (sensitivity, specificity, diagnostic accuracy etc.), lack of validation techniques in many studies, lack of randomized controlled trials comparing AI-assisted approaches with current non-AI-based approaches, the adoption of 'black-box models' that prevent physicians from finding potential confounders, ethical issues, inherent bias, and lack of studies outside the field of diagnosis and prognostic care gastroenterolology.

RADIOMICS IN GASTROENTEROLOGY

Radiomics is an emerging field of radiology focused on the relationships between imaging phenotypes and molecular markers. In radiomics, digitally encrypted images that contain information relating to the physiopathology of the tumour are transformed into extractable data. The process used in radiomics involves the identification of vast sets of quantitative characteristics within digital images, the storage of such data in databases and the subsequent mining of the data for the extraction and application of knowledge. The steps of radiomics in general include: image acquisition, identification of the region of interest (VOI) (through machine-learning or expert radiologist), segmentation of the region of interest (through automatic, semi-automatic or manual design), the extraction of imaging features and data extraction. Using this method, it is possible to retrospectively analyze the archived images (both CT and MRI) leading to the creation of a predictive radiomic model, whose accuracy is directly proportional to the amount of clinical, radiological and biochemical 'information' available. However, variability in image quality and technical parameters for image acquisition can affect image characteristics and therefore the results of predictive models. Radiomic characteristics (such as intensity, shape, texture or wavelet) provide information on the cancer phenotype and tumour microenvironment when combined with other data (such as clinical, treatment-related or genomic), can therefore constitute accurate decision support systems and robust evidence-based, therefore representing a powerful tool in modern medicine. Radiomics has been applied in hepatology, in particular to the diagnostics and prognostic characterization of primary liver tumours. Cholangiocarcinoma (CCA) has offered researchers an extremely interesting field of study due to the possibility of conducting correlation studies between radiomics and histological and/or demonstrated the validity of a normogram, developed using radiomics and clinical characteristics, in predicting the early recurrence of CCA after surgical resection, or have developed a combined model of qualitative and quantitative radiological data in relation to the expression of VEGFR accurate in predicting the occurrence of CCA. Recently, the diagnostic accuracy of a radiomics-based approach for the classification of histological subtypes of intrahepatic cholangiocarcinoma (iCCA) (small bile ducts vs large bile ducts) has been evaluated using computed tomography (CT) images (56 patients). The approach based on radiomics for the definition of iCCA of the small bile ducts vs that of the large bile ducts has shown that an algorithm called Relief and that the use of a specific classifier (SVM) is able to ensure a maximum accuracy of 69.67%, while the combination of the PCA and Relief algorithms allow to improve accuracy up to 88.89% (through the combined use of the classifiers called k-NN and SVM).

Radiomics is an emerging field of radiology focused on the relationships between imaging phenotypes and molecular markers. In radiomics, digitally encrypted images that contain information relating to the physiopathology of the tumour are transformed into extractable data. The process used in radiomics involves the identification of vast sets of quantitative characteristics within digital images, the storage of such data in databases and the subsequent mining of the data for the extraction and application of knowledge. The steps of radiomics in general include: image acquisition, identification of the region of interest (VOI) (through machine-learning or expert radiologist), segmentation of the region of interest (through automatic, semi-automatic or manual design), the extraction of imaging features and data extraction. Using this method, it is possible to retrospectively analyze the archived images (both CT and MRI) leading to the creation of a predictive radiomic model, whose accuracy is directly proportional to the amount of clinical, radiological and biochemical 'information' available. However, variability in image quality and technical parameters for image acquisition can affect image characteristics and therefore the results of predictive models. Radiomic characteristics (such as intensity, shape, texture or wavelet) provide information on the cancer phenotype and tumour microenvironment when combined with other data (such as clinical, treatment-related or genomic), can therefore constitute accurate decision support systems and robust evidence-based, therefore representing a powerful tool in modern medicine. Radiomics has been applied in hepatology, in particular to the diagnostics and prognostic characterization of primary liver tumours. Cholangiocarcinoma (CCA) has offered researchers an extremely interesting field of study due to the possibility of conducting correlation studies between radiomics and histological and/or molecular characteristics. The application of radiomics in the CCA is still in a preliminary phase. Studies published so far have limitations related to small patient populations and none of these are randomized multicentre. It has been developed a model based on the combination of radiomic data and the values of Ca 19.9 to discriminate the CCA metastasis. Finally, other studies have demonstrated the validity of a normogram, developed using radiomics and clinical characteristics, in predicting the early recurrence of CCA after surgical resection, or have developed a combined model of qualitative and quantitative radiological data in relation to the expression of VEGFR accurate in predicting the occurrence of CCA. Recently, the diagnostic accuracy of a radiomics-based approach for the classification of histological subtypes of intrahepatic cholangiocarcinoma (iCCA) (small bile ducts vs large bile ducts) has been evaluated using computed tomography (CT) images (56 patients). The approach based on radiomics for the definition of iCCA of the small bile ducts vs that of the large bile ducts has shown that an algorithm called Relief and that the use of a specific classifier (SVM) is able to ensure a maximum accuracy of 69.67%, while the combination of the PCA and Relief algorithms allow to improve accuracy up to 88.89% (through the combined use of the classifiers called k-NN and SVM) (**Figure 4.2**).

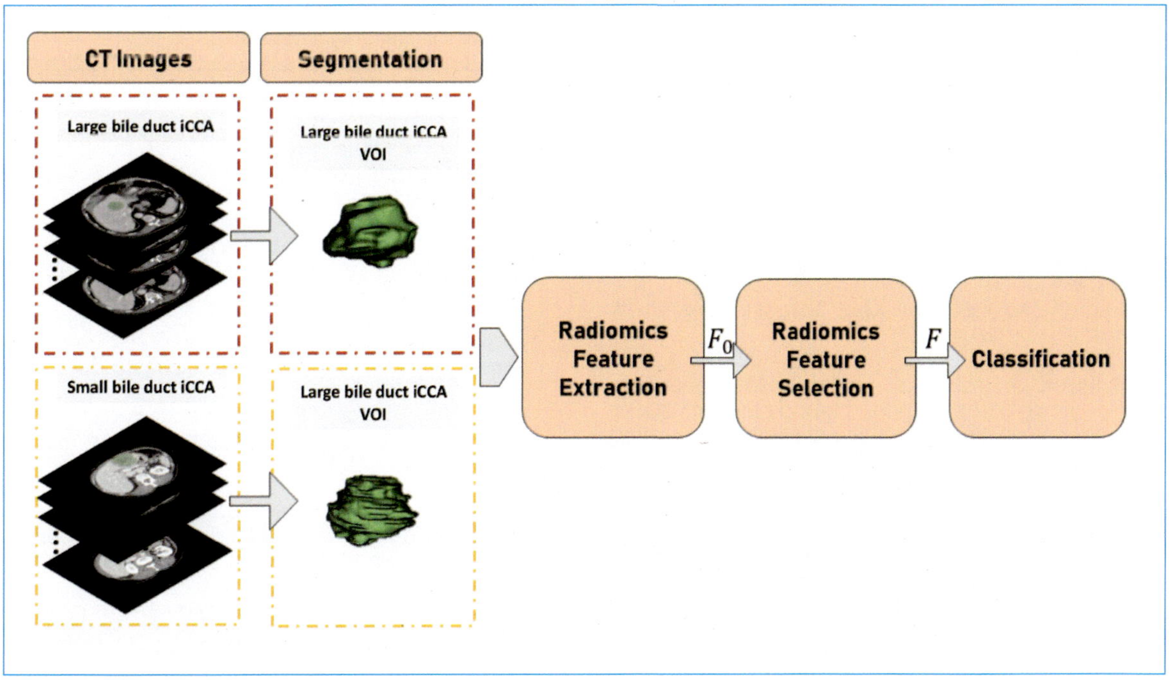

Figure 4.2 Diagram of the algorithm for the extraction of radiomics features from Computed Tomography (CT) images of the histological subtypes of intrahepatic cholangiocarcinoma (iCCA). VOI: volume of interest (region of interest).

NETWORK MEDICINE

Given the functional interdependencies between molecular components in a human cell, a disease is rarely a consequence of an abnormality in a single gene, but reflects the perturbations of the complex intracellular and intercellular network that connects tissues and organ systems. Emerging network medicine tools offer a platform to systematically explore not only the molecular complexity of a particular disease, leading to the identification of disease modules and pathways, but also the molecular relationships between seemingly distinct (pathways) phenotypes. Advances in this direction are essential for identifying novel genes involved in the pathogenesis of various diseases, for discovering the biological significance of disease-associated mutations identified by 'genome-wide association studies', by sequencing the entire human genome or microbiota, and from multiomics studies (transcriptomics, proteomics, metabolomics) and to identify pharmacological targets and biomarkers for complex diseases.

CONCLUSIONS

Contrary to what is reported by anecdotes circulating in the media, European medical students are not at all worried by the idea that AI will replace doctors, and are aware of the possible applications and implications of AI in medicine. Another reason why AI and digital health should be included among the teachings for medical students.

KEY CONCEPTS

- Have an integrated vision of traditional medicine and digital health, and consider the possibility that there may be a systemic approach to health and research, which has the same objectives of the traditional medicine and public health, but which complements the traditional tools (visit, hospitalization, diagnosis etc.) and the tools of digital health, AI, data science etc.
- Digital health is an emerging field of study at the intersection of healthcare, medicine, biomedical research and digital technologies.
- Telemedicine seen as a means of remote interaction aimed at maintaining health, to be implemented in society needs the complementary approach of health education aimed at patients, the general population, and caregivers (telehealth).
- AI has been tested in gastroenterology for endoscopic lesion analysis, cancer detection and to facilitate the analysis of inflammatory lesions or gastrointestinal bleeding during video capsule endoscopy. AI has also been tested to evaluate for liver fibrosis and to differentiate patients with pancreatic cancer from those with pancreatitis.

BIBLIOGRAFIA ESSENZIALE

- Barabási AL, Gulbahce N, Loscalzo J. Network medicine: a network-based approach to human disease. Nat Rev Genet. 2011 Jan;12(1):56-68.
- "Benefits of TED Talks" (https://www.ncbi.nlm.nih.gov/pmc/articles/ PMC4264800). Canadian Family Physician. 60(12):1080.
- Capone A, Cicchetti A, Mennini FS, Marcellusi A, Baio G, Favato G. Health Data Entanglement and artificial intelligence-based analysis: a brand new methodology to improve the effectiveness of healthcare services. Clin Ter. 2016;167(5):e102-e111.
- Chiara Losquadro. Small and Large Bile Ducts Intrahepatic Cholangiocarcinoma Classification: A Preliminary Feature-Based Study. International Conference on Computer Analysis of Images and Patterns, 237-244.
- Fatehi F, Samadbeik M, Kazemi A. What is Digital Health? Review of Definitions. Stud Health Technol Inform. 2020;275:67-71.
- Goyal H, Sherazi SAA, Mann R, Gandhi Z, Perisetti A, Aziz M, Chandan S, Kopel J, Tharian B, Sharma N, Thosani N. Scope of Artificial Intelligence in Gastrointestinal Oncology. Cancers (Basel). 2021;13(21):5494.
- http://www.salute.gov.it/imgs/C_17_pubblicazioni_2129_allegato.pdf
- Hutson M. AI Glossary: Artificial intelligence, in so many words. Science. 2017 Jul 7;357(6346):19.
- Iyawa GE, Herselman M, Botha A. Digital health innovation ecosystems: From systematic literature review to conceptual framework. 2016.
- Ji G-W, Zhu F-P, Zhang Y-D, et al. A radiomics approach to predict lymph node metastasis and clinical outcome of intrahepatic cholangiocarcinoma. Eur Radiol. 2019;29(7):3725-35.
- Lambin P, Leijenaar TH R, Deist TM et al. Radiomics: the bridge between medical imaging and personalized medicine. Nat Rev Clin Oncol. 2017;14(12):749-62.
- Le Berre C, Sandborn WJ, Aridhi S, Devignes MD, Fournier L, Smaïl-Tabbone M, Danese S, Peyrin-Biroulet L. Application of Artificial Intelligence to Gastroenterology and Hepatology. Gastroenterology. 2020;158 (1):76-94.e2.
- Liang W, Xu L, Yang P, et al. Nomogram for Preoperative Prediction of Early Recurrence in Intrahepatic Cholangiocarcinoma. Front Oncol. 2018 Sep 4;8:360.
- Miller EA. Solving the disjuncture between research and practice: telehealth trends in the 21st century". Health Policy. 2007;82(2):133-41.

- Mosconi C, Cucchetti A, Bruno A, et al. Radiomics of cholangiocarcinoma on pretreatment CT can identify patients who would best respond to radioembolisation. Eur Radiol. 2020;30(8):4534-44.
- O'Reilly KB. Digital health funding hits $8.1 billion. How to spend it wisely [Internet]. 2019 [cited 12 Sep 2020]. Available from: https://www.ama-assn.org/practice-management/digital/digital-healthfunding- hits-81-billion-how-spend-it-wisely.
- OMS fact-sheets on noncommunicable diseases. https://www.who.int/news-room/fact
- Pinto Dos Santos D, Giese D, Brodehl S, Chon SH, Staab W, Kleinert R, Maintz D, Baeßler B. Medical students' attitude towards artificial intelligence: a multicentre survey. Eur Radiol. 2019;29(4):1640-46.
- Rowlands D. What is digital health? And why does it matter? [White paper]. Health Informatics Society of Australia 2020. Available from: https://www.hisa.org.au/wpcontent/
- Sadot E, Simpson AL, Do RK et al. Cholangiocarcinoma: Correlation between Molecular Profiling and Imaging Phenotypes. PLoS One. 2015;10(7):e0132953.
- Saini A, Breen I, Pershad Y et al, Radiogenomics and Radiomics in Liver Cancers. Diagnostics (Basel). 2018;9(1):4.
- Shaw DK (June 2009). "Overview of telehealth and its application to cardiopulmonary physical therapy". Cardiopulmonary Physical Therapy Journal. 2(2):13-8.
- "TeleHealth" (http://www.hrsa.gov/rural-health/telehealth/index.html). The Health Resources and Services Administration. 2017-04-28.
- US Food and Drug Administration (FDA). Digital health innovation action plan [Internet]. 2019. Available from: https://www.fda.gov/medical-devices/digital-health.
- What is Telehealth?" (http://cchpca.org/what-is-telehealth.). The Center for Connected Health Policy.
- World Health Organization. Digital Health [Internet]. 2020 [cited 12 Sep 2020]. Available from: https://www.who.int/health-topics/digital-health
- Xu L, Yang P, Liang W et al. A radiomics approach based on support vector machine using MR images for preoperative lymph node status evaluation in intrahepatic cholangiocarcinoma. T. Theranostics. 2019;9(18):5374-85.
- Zhao L, Ma X, Liang M et al. Prediction for early recurrence of intrahepatic mass-forming cholangiocarcinoma: quantitative magnetic resonance imaging combined with prognostic immunohistochemical markers. Cancer Imaging. 2019;19(1):49.

CHAPTER 5

OESOPHAGEAL PATHOPHYSIOLOGY AND RELATED SYMPTOMS

Santino Marchi, Elisa Marabotto

LEARNING OBJECTIVES

- To know the basic concepts of the oesophageal functional anatomy.
- To know the basic concepts of oesophageal motor activity and sensitivity.
- To know the concept of oesophageal mucosal barrier and salivary clearance.
- To know the most important oesophageal symptoms.

The oesophagus allows bolus transit from pharynx to stomach. Anatomically and functionally, it is divided into three parts: the upper oesophageal sphincter (UES), the oesophageal body and the oesophago-gastric junction (EGJ). The EGJ is a complex valvular structure, consisting of the lower oesophageal sphincter (LES) and the crural diaphragm (CD).

ESOPHAGEAL ANATOMY

Upper Oesophageal Sphincter

The UES is a high-pressure area that extends for about 2-4 cm below the pharynx; in the upper two thirds it consists of distal striated fibers of the pharynx's lower constrictor muscle and in the lower third it consists of the crico-pharyngeal muscle. The crico-pharyngeal muscle is innervated by the pharyngeal plexus in the upper part and by the recurrent laryngeal nerve in the lower; the sphincter maintains a closed resting tone and responds quickly to swallowing, vomiting and belching.

The Oesophageal Body

The oesophagus is a tubular muscular organ about 18-26 cm in length in adults. In resting condition, it is a virtual cavity. Structurally, the oesophageal wall is composed of four layers: innermost mucosa, submucosa, muscularis propria and adventitia. Furthermore, unlike other portions of the gastrointestinal tract, the oesophagus has no serosa, and its outer wall is bounded by a thin layer of connective tissue. This fact explains the early spread of malignant tumours. The mucosa of the oesophageal body consists of a stratified non-keratinized squamous epithelium. The oesophageal submucosa contains mucipar glands, while the muscularis propria is composed of two layers: an inner circular muscle and a longitudinal muscular layer. The proximal oesophagus (cervical oesophagus) consists of striated muscle, while the distal two thirds of the oesophagus (thoracic oesophagus) consist of smooth muscle. The transition from striated to smooth muscle is gradual. The segment (4-6 cm) contains both types of striated and smooth muscle and is usually located at the aortic arch level. It is visualized as a low-pressure area - transition zone - at high-resolution oesophageal manometry (HRM). In physiological conditions, the oesophagus is anchored to the diaphragm, but is not hermetically wrapped around the hiatus as it needs to expand to accommodate the luminal content.

The Oesophago-gastric Junction

The EGJ is a complex valvular structure, the functional balance between LES and CD controls trans-sphincteric transit (**Figure 5.1**).
The length of the LES is 2-4 cm, it is composed of thicker muscle tissue than that in the remaining part of the oesophagus. It appears as a non-circular axial orifice at rest, while it assumes an almost circular shape during swallowing. The EGJ is an important barrier for gastro-oesophageal reflux (GER) and its morphology has been shown to be an important determinant of EGJ barrier function. The HRM allows to identify the dynamic nature of EGJ, the correct position of LES and CD and their relationship.

ESOPHAGEAL NEURAL CONTROL

The oesophagus has a parasympathetic and sympathetic innervation. Parasympathetic innervation is mediated by the ambiguous nucleus and

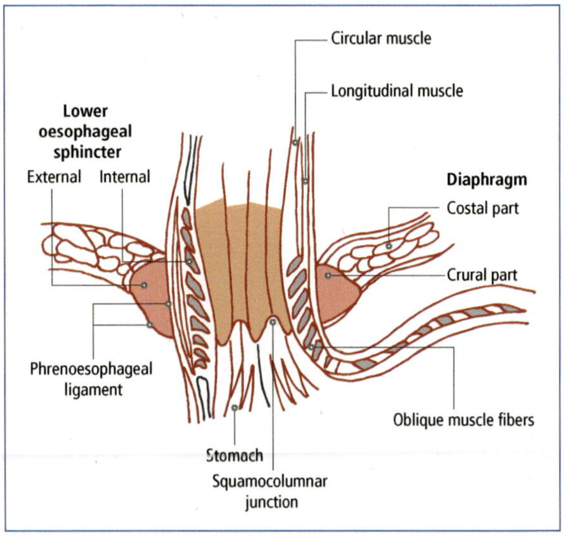

Figure 5.1 Diagram of the gastro-oesophageal junction. Yazaki E, Sifrim D. Dis Oesophagus. 2012; 25:292-8

the dorsal motor nucleus of the vagus (DMV) and provides motor innervation to the muscles and secretory-motor of the glands. Sympathetic innervation is mediated by the intermediate-lateral T1-T10 spine and regulates blood vessel contractions (blood supply), oesophageal sphincter tone, relaxation of the muscular wall, and glandular function. Motor innervation occurs mainly through the vagus nerves. Regarding the smooth muscle, the motor nerve fibers originate from the DMV. There are two types of preganglionic neurons: the one (fast twitch fibers) in the caudal part of the DMV, with synapses on post-ganglia inhibitory neurons in the myenteric plexus (of Auerbach), and the other (slow-twitch fibers) in the rostral part of the DMV, with synapses on post-cholinergic exciters neurons in the myenteric plexus.

SENSORY PHYSIOLOGY

The vagal afferents that emerge from the oesophageal smooth muscle layer and from the serosa are sensitive to muscle stretching. The afferent fibers of the vagus in the mucosa are sensitive to chemical (acid), thermal (cold or hot), and mechanic stimuli and mainly act as nociceptors. Changes in oesophageal sensitivity can occur at the peripheral and/or central level (neurons in the spinal cord and brain). The development of visceral hypersensitivity is now a recognized mechanism in oesophageal symptoms. In fact, peripheral sensitization has been implicated in the "up-regulation" of receptors responsible for perception of acid. Changes in mucosal permeability, activation of the immune system and cortical (central) processing of pain perception are mechanisms involved in the development of visceral hypersensitivity in GER disease (GERD).

MOTILITY PHYSIOLOGY

Swallowing

Swallowing is a complex act. It occurs through the control of the swallowing center, which is present in both cerebral hemispheres at the level of the motor cortex, by the activity of cranial nerves V, VII, and IX. The swallow in humans is classically described as a four-stage sequential model. The pre-oral phase, preparatory phase, includes the posture taken for swallowing, the movements to transport food to the mouth, together with stimulations from the sight smell, and touch of food or drink. The oral phase, almost completely voluntary, is characterized by formation of the food bolus through chewing. Subsequently, there are the pharyngeal and oesophageal phase.

Primary Peristalsis

Swallow-induced peristalsis is called primary peristalsis. Once the pharyngeal contraction wave has moved the bolus through the relaxed UES, a wave of contraction of the circular musculature of the oesophagus originates at the upper oesophagus and proceeds along the oesophagus to push the bolus through the relaxed LES. Primary peristalsis usually moves most of the oesophageal contents into the stomach; a correct amplitude pressures of the contraction waves, a normal duration of the wave and a determinate peristaltic velocity are necessary.

Contraction of the Longitudinal Musculature – Shortening of the Oesophagus

Contraction of the longitudinal smooth muscle shortens the oesophageal wall during peristalsis, but its role in oesophageal physiology has not yet been fully elucidated. It has been suggested that the synchrony between the contraction of the circular and the longitudinal muscles is essential to move the bolus effectively along the oesophagus. Moreover, shortening of the oesophagus due to contraction of the longitudinal musculature also seems to play a very important role in promoting axial movement and opening of the LES during swallowing and during GER.

Secondary Peristalsis

Secondary peristalsis is initiated by distention of the mechanoreceptors in the oesophageal wall secondary to the presence of food residues or to episodes of GER. It occurs through a reflex mechanism that can cross the intrinsic and the extrinsic nerve pathways, and is not matched by pharyngeal contraction or relaxation of the UES. In the secondary peristalsis, amplitude and velocity of the waves are similar to those of primary peristalsis (**Figure 5.2**).

Control of Oesophageal Peristalsis

The peristalsis in the oesophageal striated muscle is entirely dependent on the central vagal pathways. The control of peristalsis in the smooth muscle part is more complicated. In fact, the peristalsis of the thoracic oesophagus is mediated by both central and peripheral mechanisms. The pre-programmed intramural mechanisms, which control the inhibitory (non-cholinergic) and excitatory (cholinergic) activity of neurons, cooperate in the control of peristalsis in the oesophageal smooth muscle. There is also a myogenic control system that helps to regulate the contraction of smooth gastrointestinal muscle tissue. Finally, there is a central mechanism for supervising the peristalsis of the oesophageal smooth muscle. The neurotransmitters of the excitatory nerves consist essentially of acetylcholine and substance P, while nitric oxide (NO) and vasoactive intestinal peptide (VIP) have an inhibitor function.

PHYSIOLOGY OF THE GASTRO-OESOPHAGEAL JUNCTION

The LES maintains a tonic resting contraction in the absence of exogenous control. The origin of the basal tone of the LES is mainly myogenic, while the cellular mechanisms of its control are multiple and not completely understood. Excitatory and inhibitory neural activity influences the LES resting tone, modifying its myogenic tone. The excitatory neurons of the myenteric plexus release acetylcholine and substance P in order to increase the LES pressure. The inhibitory neurons reduce the pressure by the release of NO; NO is the most important inhibitory neurotransmitter involved in the post swallow LES relaxation. In humans, the vagus nerve exerts a tonic inhibitory effect. As a consequence, vagotomy can result in contraction of the LES, while vagal stimulation can result in its release.

Motility Physiology

The LES relaxation, in response to swallowing, starts 2 second after pharyngeal swallowing and is followed by a rebound contraction when the peristaltic wave reaches the distal oesophagus. It allows the bolus transit into the stomach and it is mediated by the vagal inhibitory pathway through the release of NO by the postganglionic neurons located at the myenteric plexus. The presence of the bolus in the oesophagus prolongs LES relaxation. The LES relaxation is often associated

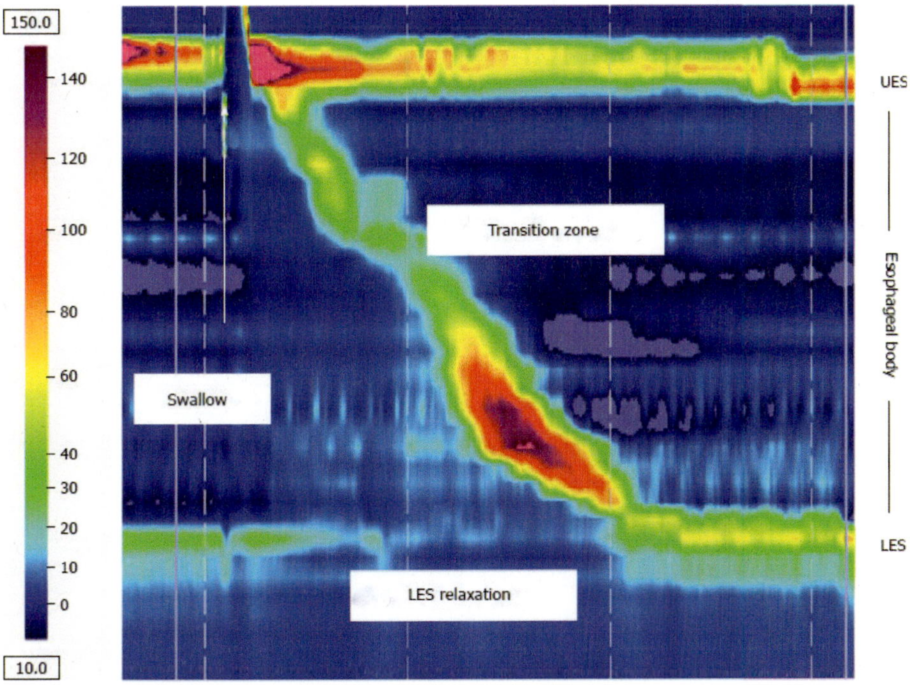

Figure 5.2 Portion of a high resolution oesophageal manometry tracing acquired with a 36-channel solid-state probe that visualizes the different phases of swallowing: opening of the upper oesophageal sphincter, activation and progression of the peristaltic wave along the oesophagus and opening and closing of the gastro-oesophageal junction. Nicola de Bortoli, Irene Martinucci, Lorenzo Bertani, et al. World J Gastrointest Pathophysiol 2016; 15: 72-85

with shortening of the distal oesophagus causing consequent EGJ excursion. This transient hernia facilitates opening of the LES and the bolus transit into the stomach.
The transient LES relaxations play an important role in the pathogenesis of GERD. They may persist for up to 30 and are generally evoked by gastric distension through mechanosensitive vagal afferent pathways terminating in the central nucleus of the solitary tract. The signal is then transmitted to the dorsal motor nucleus of the vagus where vagal efferent depart and reach inhibitory synapses on the myenteric plexus neurons, which, in turn, induce NO release, with an abrupt decrease of the LES pressure. During transient LES relaxations, the cyclical contractility of the CD is also inhibited, thus effectively disrupting the barrier to GER. The LES pressure can be influenced by other factors, as shown in **Table 5.1**.

PHYSIOLOGY OF THE MUCOSAL BARRIER AND SALIVARY CLEARANCE

GERD is a condition that occurs when stomach contents flow back into the oesophagus causing symptoms and/or complications. The aetiology is multifactorial and the main cause is the association between an altered mucosal permeability and the impairment of EGJ because of a hiatal hernia, a reduced LES pressure or presence of transient LES relaxation.
Mucosal damage results from an imbalance between aggressive factors (mainly acid and pepsin, with a certain contribution from the harmful potential of bile acids) and protective factors.
The oesophageal mucosal barrier contributes to the prevention of epithelial damage, promotes healing of epithelial cells and could help prevent the potential development of intestinal metaplasia, dysplasia or oesophageal adenocarcinoma. The secretions of the oesophageal submucosal glands and salivary glands constitute a pre-epithelial protective mechanism and are fundamental both in the luminal mechanical clearance of gastro-oesophageal reflux and in the neutralization of the acid and proteolytic activity of pepsins. Water, bicarbonate, mucus, mucins, epidermal growth factor and prostaglandins lead to the formation of a protective layer, approximately 95 µm thick, with a visco-elastic consistency, that can buffer and defend the oesophageal mucosa from gastric reflux. Key components of the oesophageal mucosal barrier are the tight junctions, such as claudins, occludins and junctional adhesion molecules.

Table 5.1 Factors that influence lower oesophageal sphincter pressure.

	Increase	Decrease
Hormones	Gastrin Motilin Substance P Somatostatin	Secretin Cholecystokinin Vasoactive intestinal polypeptide
Neurotransmitters	Alpha-adrenergic agonists Beta-adrenergic antagonists Cholinergic agonists	Beta-adrenergic agonists Alpha-adrenergic antagonists Cholinergic antagonists
Food	Proteic meals	Fatty meals Chocolate Alcohol Peppermint
Others	Histamine Antacids Metoclopramide Domperidone Coffee Migrating Motor Complex Increased abdominal pressure	Nitric oxide Theophylline Caffeine Acid Smoke Pregnancy Morphine Dopamine Calcium channel blockers Diazepam Obesity

The harmful effects of gastric acid and pepsins are implicated in the pathogenesis of oesophagitis and their oesophageal exposure time, that can be affected by impaired oesophageal motility, is directly correlated with the severity of the disease. Furthermore, acid reflux, bile salts and trypsin are able to modulate the expression of tight junctions, helping to interrupt mucosal integrity.
An impaired oesophageal mucosal integrity, a dilation of the intercellular spaces (DIS) and/or an increase in the flow of electrolytes through the intercellular spaces lead to an increase in the oesophageal current flow (i.e. to a decrease in the oesophageal mucosal impedance) and therefore they can be easily and indirectly measured.
Esophageal impedance pH monitoring measures the mucosal impedance through pairs of electrodes near the mucosa. It evaluates the permeability of the oesophageal mucosa and in particular, lower values suggest an alteration of the mucosal barrier integrity. The introduction of two new impedance parameters, namely MNBI (mean nocturnal baseline impedance) and the PSPW index (post-reflux swallow-induced peristaltic wave index), allows us to accurately evaluate mucosal integrity and oesophageal chemical clearance. They can be easily calculated and used in clinical practice.
The MNBI is assessed from the most distal impedance channel during nighttime recumbent period, without reflux, pH drops or swallowing. Three 10-min time periods (around 1.00 am, 2.00 am, and 3.00 am) are selected and the software computes the mean baseline for each and then the mean of the three measurements is manually calculated to obtain the MNBI.
The PSPW is defined as an antegrade 50% drop in impedance relative to the pre-swallow baseline that originates in the most proximal measurement site and reaches the distal site within 30 seconds after the end of a reflux episode, followed by a rise of at least 50%. The PSPW index is evaluated as the ratio between the total number of refluxes followed in the next 30 seconds by a PSPW and the total number of refluxes.
The PSPW index reflects the integrity of oesophageal peristalsis stimulated by reflux episodes and is an expression of the chemical clearance resulting from the presence of salivary bicarbonates. Impaired clearance is more frequently associated with a severe gastro-oesophageal reflux disease and the resulting mucosal damage (**Figure 5.3**).
Currently, these two parameters efficiently distinguish patients with non-erosive reflux disease and hypersensitive oesophagus from patients with functional heartburn, patients with proton pump inhibitors (PPI)-refractory reflux-related heartburn, and patients with eosinophilic oesophagitis non responding to PPI therapy. Furthermore, they can be helpful in selecting patients for anti-reflux surgery.

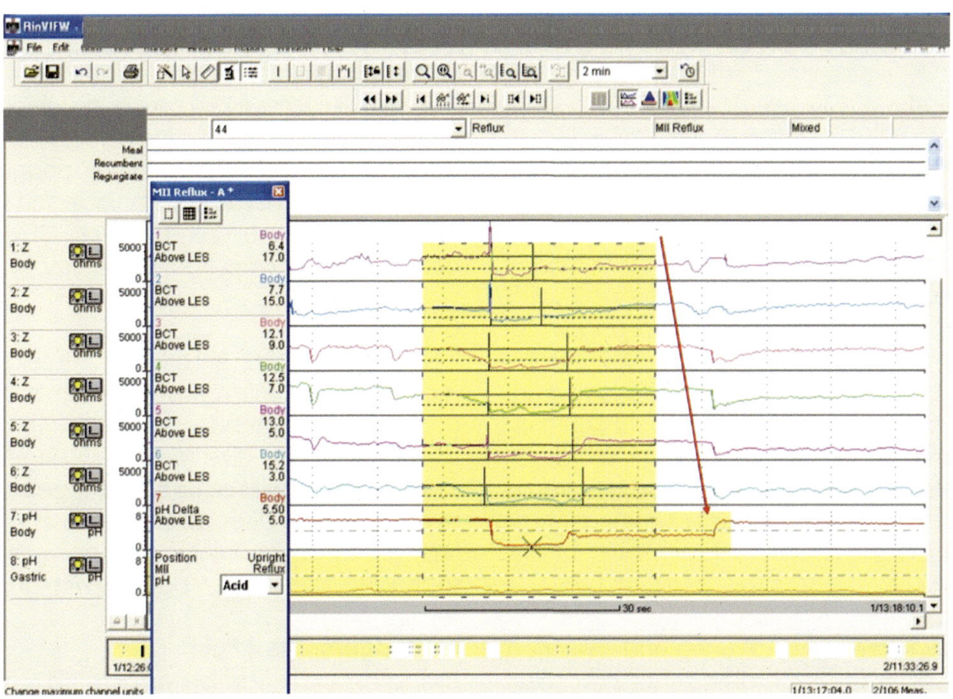

Figure 5.3 Example of PSPW measurement on a pH-Impedance tracing.

ESOPHAGEAL SYMPTOMS

The main symptoms are due to oesophageal motor disorders or GERD. It is crucial, to optimize clinical management, to obtain a detailed medical history that must include the presence of alarm signs or symptoms. Some symptoms present a high sensitivity and specificity for diagnosing certain diseases.

Heartburn

Heartburn or the sensation of retrosternal burning, is the most frequent symptom in the Western population. The burning can reach the neck and occasionally the back, it is intermittent and often triggered by meals (foods high in lipids, alcohol), the supine body position and sudden increases in intra-abdominal pressure. Heartburn can be frequent and significantly interfere with normal activities or sleep. It can be associated with regurgitation, chest pain and belching. Although reflux of gastric contents in the oesophagus is commonly associated with heartburn, the exact pathogenetic mechanism of this symptom is not entirely clear. Recent studies have demonstrated that disruption of tight junction barrier function in the oesophageal epithelium, dilation of intercellular spaces and the subsequent penetration of H+ ions into the deeper mucosa layers (the site of chemo-receptive nerve endings), may constitute the responsible mechanism independently by presence or absence of mucosal damage endoscopically visible (see Chapter on GERD).

Regurgitation

The term regurgitation refers to the perception of spontaneous or provoked flow of contents from the stomach to the oesophagus and oropharynx, occurring in the absence of extrinsic muscular phenomena of vomiting. Frequently, it occurs in supine position and during anteflexion of the body. It is generally not associated with nausea or abdominal contractions. It is often present in GERD, it can be acid, weakly acid or nonacid. Regurgitation can indicate the proximal flow of oesophageal contents; it is one of the most important symptoms of achalasia. For this reason, it is important evaluate correctly the patients in order to avoid incorrect diagnosis or important diagnostic delay.

Dysphagia

Dysphagia is related to swallowing and is referred as the sensation of arrest, difficulty or slowing of bolus transit from the mouth to the stomach. The correlation with swallowing distinguishes this symptom from the pharyngeal globus (see below). Dysphagia is classically defined as oropharyngeal when the striated, proximal, oesophageal muscle is involved and oesophageal when the smooth muscle of the oesophageal body and/or the LES is involved. When the symptom appears within few seconds (1-3) after ingestion of the bolus, followed by immediate regurgitation, even nasal, coughing or a sense of suffocation, is strongly indicative of altered pharyngeal motor function. Failure to start swallowing due to a defective oral phase will result in patency of the nasopharynx with consequent nasal regurgitation and aspiration in the airways. Dysphagia may be caused by a mechanical obstruction or neuromuscular changes. A mechanical dysphagia is usually chronic or progressive and starts with solid foods, while dysphagia due to neuromuscular disorders can be intermittent and there are no differences related to the meal consistency. Anamnestic data can guide the origin of dysphagia and help the choice of diagnostic tests. Dysphagia represents an important alarm symptom. Oesophago-gastro-duodenoscopy is mandatory if the symptom is continuous or progressive, in order to accurately assess and diagnose organic lesions - including oesophageal and cardias tumours. Dynamic radiological study with fluoroscopy is the test of choice in case of oro-pharyngeal dysphagia. Oesophageal manometry, if possible, with high-resolution technology, is the test of choice in oesophageal dysphagia when motor disorders are suspected.

Odynophagia

The term indicates a dull pain or an intense pain radiating to the back occurring during swallowing. It is the most frequent symptom in oesophageal inflammations caused by infections, ingestion of caustic substances or more rarely by severe GERD or carcinoma of the proximal tract of the oesophagus.

Globus

It is the continuous sensation of a foreign body in the throat, regardless of swallowing. It usually occurs away from meals, and swallowing of liquid or solid boluses can give temporary benefit. It is often associated with other oesophageal symptoms in patients with diseases of the oesophagus and may be a feature of increased perception of oesophageal distention in patients with anxiety.

Esophageal Chest Pain

The chest pain can be associated with various diseases and, generally, is considered a medical-surgical emergency for its possible cardiac origin. Patients with chest pain should initially be evaluated by a cardiologist in order to exclude a cardiologic origin. Oesophageal, musculoskeletal, respiratory and psychiatric causes are frequently associated with non-cardiac chest pain (from 70 to 80% of patients that go to an emergency department). Non-cardiac chest pain is very common in the general population (average prevalence 23%) and has a strong negative impact on quality of life. The pathophysiology of oesophageal chest pain is not entirely clear because of the coexistence, in the oesophageal wall, of two afferent nerve pathways, responsible for regulation of reflexes induced by chemical and mechanical (vagal) stimuli and for transmission of visceral pain (spinal), both controlled by the central nervous system. Intra-esophageal perfusion of acidic solutions and balloon oesophageal distension are known to cause thoracic pain in healthy subjects and the threshold of perception is significantly lowered in some categories of patients. The most common aetiological factors include GERD (60% of cases of non-cardiac thoracic pain), disorders of oesophageal motility (15%), visceral hyper-sensitivity (esophageal) and/or alterations in the central processing of intra-esophageal stimuli (8-10%).

Reflux-related Cough

The cough is a symptom that results from a sudden reflex or voluntary exhalation to free the airways, it is a physiological defense mechanism and can be consequent to various aetiologies. It is also an atypical symptom of GERD and therefore an initial accurate differential diagnosis is essential. The mechanism by which GERD can cause cough is not yet fully understood, but the two most accredited pathophysiological mechanisms are represented by:

- A possible micro-aspiration of refluxed gastric material which stimulates the cough reflex through direct irritation of the respiratory tract structures;
- A stimulation mediated by the vagus nerve.

Reflux-related cough usually occurs chronically, may not be associated with typical reflux symptoms and must be investigated with pH-impedance measurement to better set up the subsequent therapeutic process.

Asthma

The American Thoracic Society (ATS) defines asthma as a condition characterized by episodes in which the patient experiences wheezing, cough, or dyspnea and an increase in forced expiratory volume in one second (FEV1) of 20% compared to baseline after administration of bronchodilators or 20% decrease in FEV1 after methacholine challenge test. The two main pathophysiological mechanisms suggested to explain the possible association between asthma and reflux are the same two theories previously described for the reflux-related cough.

Reflux Associated Laryngitis

Reflux associated laryngitis, inflammation of the laryngeal mucosa and vocal cords following episodes of laryngopharyngeal reflux, causes dysphonia, need to clear the throat, sore throat, foreign body sensation or cough. Often these symptoms are not accompanied by typical reflux symptoms and must be investigated with pH-impedance analysis.

KEY CONCEPTS

- Anatomically and functionally, the oesophagus is divided into three parts: the upper oesophageal sphincter (UES), the oesophageal body and the oesophago-gastric junction (EGJ), consisting of the lower oesophageal sphincter (LES) and the crural diaphragm.
- The coordinated functions of these structures, together with activity of the oropharynx and the stomach, regulate the bolus transit from the pharynx to the stomach, prevent the gastro-esophageal reflux, and allow belching and vomiting.
- Various mechanisms control the motor activity of the sphincters and the oesophageal body. They are situated in the central nervous, in the peripheral nervous system and in intramural muscles. In the oesophagus the voluntary and involuntary control mechanisms cooperate in a coordinated manner to allow the activity of both types of muscles.
- The voluntary act of swallowing is the primary input for oesophageal activity, but also other stimuli such as distension of the oesophagus or stomach can trigger motor activity of the oesophagus and oesophageal sphincters.
- The oesophageal mucosal integrity is due to a balance between aggressive and protective agents and can be evaluated by the new pH-impedance parameters.
- The most common oesophageal symptoms are the result of motor disorders and GERD.

REFERENCES

- azaki E, Sifrim D. Anatomy and physiology of the esophageal body. Dis Esophagus. 2012 May;25(4):292-8.
- Broers C, Tack J, Pauwels A. Review article: gastro-oesophageal reflux disease in asthma and chronic obstructive pulmonary disease. Aliment Pharmacol Ther.2018;47:176-191.
- Savarino E, Frazzoni M, Marabotto E et al. A SIGE-SINGEM-AIGO technical review on the clinical use of esophageal reflux monitoring. Digestive and Liver Disease 52 (2020) 966–980.
- Herregods TVK, Pauwels A, Jafari J et al. Determinants of reflusx-induced chronic cough. Gut 2017 Dec; 66(12):2057-2062.

CHAPTER 6

OESOPHAGEAL MOTOR DISORDERS

Roberto Penagini, Nicola de Bortoli

LEARNING OBJECTIVES

- To accurately define the main disorders of oesophageal motility and their clinical presentation.
- To know high-resolution oesophageal manometry and other diagnostic techniques.
- To know the Chicago Classification.

HIGH-RESOLUTION OESOPHAGEAL MANOMETRY

Patients with oesophageal symptoms potentially associated to oesophageal motor disorders such as dysphagia, chest pain, heartburn and regurgitation, represent one of the most frequent reasons for referral to gastroenterological evaluation. The utility of oesophageal manometry in clinical practice is: to accurately define oesophageal motor function; to identify abnormal motor function; to establish a treatment plan based on motor abnormalities.

This chapter is focused on briefly summarizing the main oesophageal motor disorders.

Esophageal high-resolution manometry (HRM) is considered the gold standard for diagnosing oesophageal motor disorders. It is depicted with a color pressure topography and allowed a revolution in categorizing these motor abnormalities in a hierarchical classification (Chicago Classification) formulated firstly in 2009 (first version) and available in its fourth reviewed version (2020-2021) by the effort of a group of international researchers (International HRM Working Group).

Esophageal motor disorders may be due to an abnormal function of the upper oesophageal sphincter (UES) and/or the cervical oesophageal region which is provided with striated muscle (3-5 cm of proximal oesophagus); abnormal function of the mid and distal oesophageal body which contain smooth muscle; abnormal function of the lower oesophageal sphincter (LES) or the oesophago-gastric junction (EGJ) obtained by interaction of the two contractile elements, the LES and the crural diaphragm (CD).

The main disorders of UES are due to abnormalities of the striated muscle or to the extrinsic neurologic compound. The abnormalities of this region cause oro-pharyngeal dysphagia and may be due to abnormal relaxation of UES or the tongue base region.

The main causes of oro-pharyngeal dysphagia are classified in:

- *Central nervous system diseases*: Parkinson disease; TIA or Ictus; amyotrophic lateral sclerosis; Huntington disease;
- *Encephalic nerve diseases*: paralysis of the recurrent laryngeal nerve; Diphtheria disease; lead poisoning;
- *Skeletal muscle disease*: inflammatory myopathy; polymyositis; myasthenia gravis; myotonic dystrophy; muscular dystrophy.

Esophageal motor function and bolus movement may be evaluated with different tests: barium X ray, scintigraphy and more recently with intraluminal impedance.

HRM is actually considered the 'gold standard' in order to evaluate oesophageal motor activity.

Solid-state oesophageal HRM is characterized by a high number of pressure sensors (up to 36 sensors) spaced closely. HRM has some advantages in clinical practice: in contrast to conventional manometry the pull-through for detecting sphincters is not required and shifts of position do not affect the reliability and reproducibility of pressure recordings. Moreover, in order to better visualize the data, a process of interpolation between sensors has been incorporated in order to display the information in the form of seamless isobaric color regions on oesophageal pressure topography plots (EPT) which represent oesophageal motility and sphincter functions on color-coded, pressure-space-time plots. Both upper and lower oesophageal sphincters may be immediately visualized as two high-pressure zone area.

Patients should fast for a minimum of 6 h for solids and 2 h for liquids prior to the procedure which consist in observing for a few minutes resting EGJ and than recording motor activity following 10 swallows of 5 ml of water separated by 30 sec (**Figure 6.1**). This standard protocol has been recently updated in the Chicago Classification (CC) version 4.0. In **Table 6.1** is detailed the protocol sug-

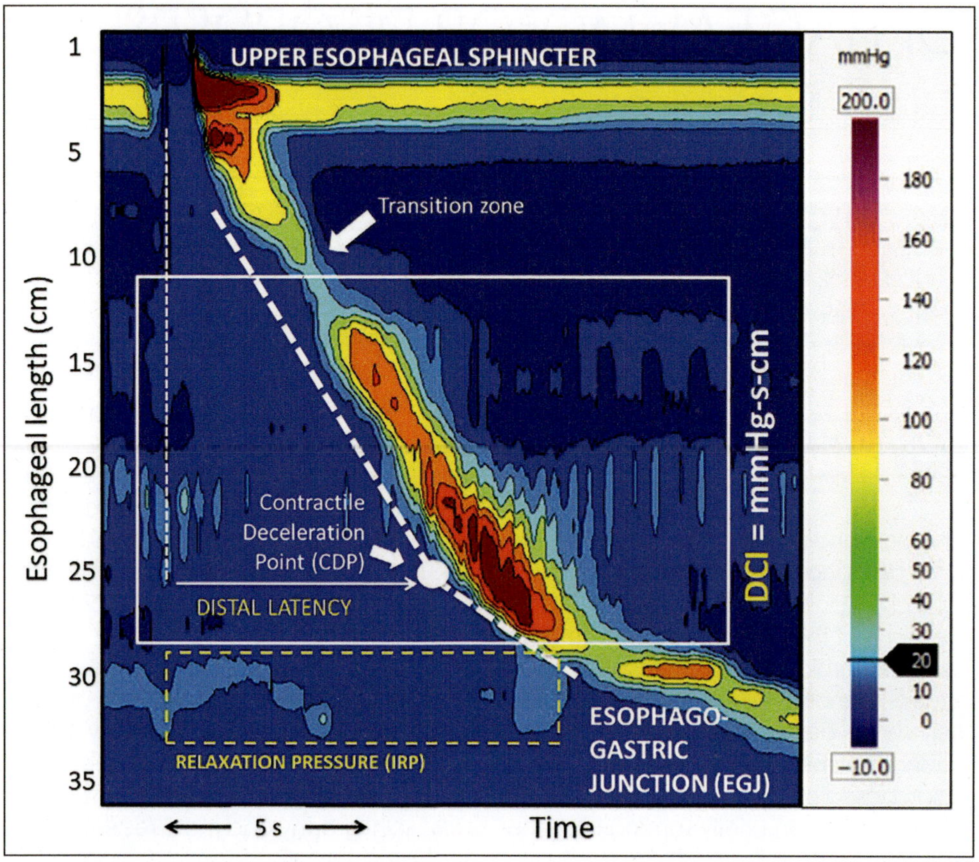

Figure 6.1 Metric of high-resolution manometry (HRM). Two high pressure zones are present: upper and lower oesophageal sphincters (the latter included into the EGJ). The white squared area refers to DCI calculation by means of 20 mmHg isobaric contour. The contractile deceleration point (CDP) is easily identifiable; it allows the calculation of distal latency (DL).

Table 6.1 Oesophageal HRM standard protocol according to the Chicago Classification 4.0.

Supine Position	
Resting Pressure	A baseline period of at least 30s is captured to enable identification of anatomic landmarks including the upper oesophageal sphincter (UES) and lower oesophageal sphincter (LES)
Esophageal peristalsis evaluation	Ten 5ml wet swallow with water or saline (when using impedance) spaced 20-30 s apart
Multiple Rapid Swallow (MRS)	Five 2 mL wet swallow 2 s apart (within 10 s)
Orthostatic Position	
Resting pressure	A baseline period of at least 30 s is captured to enable identification of anatomic landmarks including the upper oesophageal sphincter (UES) and lower oesophageal sphincter (LES)
Oesophageal peristalsis evaluation	Ten 5ml wet swallow with water or saline (when using impedance) spaced 20-30 s apart. In upright position the integrated relaxation pressure value of LES/EGJ (IRP) is normal when <12 mmHg
Rapid Drinking Challenge (200 mL)	200 mL water, ingested as fast as possible through a straw

gested for doing oesophageal HRM according to the CC 4.0. Any type of drug that potentially might influence oesophageal motility, if possible, should be discontinued some days before the test.

Oesophago-Gastric Junction (EGJ) Morphology

Two different constituents compose the EGJ: the lower oesophageal sphincter (LES) and the crural diaphragm (CD). The EGJ morphology is simply classified into three types: type I, where there is a complete overlap of CD and LES with no spatial separation on the Clouse plot; type II, where LES and CD are partially separated (< 2cm); type III, where LES and CD are clearly separated (>2cm). Different EGJ characteristics (type, resting pressure, contractile integral) were recently correlated with GERD. During swallowing, EGJ relaxation is evaluated using the integrated relaxation pressure (IRP). This is defined as the mean of the 4 s (contiguous or non-contiguous) of maximal deglutitive relaxation in the10 s window beginning at deglutitive UES relaxation. The 4-s IRP using a cutoff of 15 mmHg performs optimally with 98% sensitivity and 96% specificity in the detection of achalasia.

EPT Metrics to Score Individual Swallows

The main HRM deglutitive peristaltic metrics used to evaluate oesophageal contractile function are the distal contractile integral (DCI) and the distal latency (DL). The DCI represents the contractile vigor of the oesophageal contraction. It was introduced with the Chicago Classification (CC) and represents the amplitude × duration × length (mmHg-s-cm) of the distal oesophagus contraction with an isobaric contour of 20 mmHg from proximal to distal pressure troughs. The DL represents the interval between UES-relaxation and the inflection point along the 30mmHg isobaric contour where propagation velocity slows demarcating the tubular oesophagus from the phrenic ampulla (contractile deceleration point, CDP). The DL represents an indirect measurement of deglutitive inhibition and thus of normal peristalsis when its value is >4.5 s. On the other hands a value lower than 4.5 s defines a premature contraction. The characteristics of peristaltic wave (contraction vigor and contraction pattern) are reported in **Table 6.2**.
The following sections of this chapter are dedicated to describing the main oesophageal motor disorders diagnosed by means of HRM. The currently classification of oesophageal motor disorders is the Chicago Classification version 4.0 (2021) (**Table 6.3**). The first version of the classification was described in 2009 after an international meeting of gastroenterology – Digestive Disease Week – in San Diego in May 2008. The second version was

Table 6.2 Parameters of high-resolution manometry.

Parameter	Definition	Values
IRP (Integrated Relaxation Pressure)	Mean/median of 4 s of maximal deglutitive relaxation in the 10-s window beginning at UES relaxation	<15 mmHg complete >15 mmHg incomplete
DCI (Distal Contractile Integral)	Represents the vigor of contraction: amplitude x duration x length (mmHg-s-cm) of the distal oesophageal contraction exceeding 20 mmHg from the transition zone to the proximal margin of the LES	<100 failed 100-450 weak 450-8000 normal >8000 hypercontractile
DL (distal latency)	Interval between UES relaxation and the CDP (vn ≥4.5 s). It represents the oesophageal relaxation that precede the contractile wave	>4.5 s normal <4.5 s premature
CDP (Contractile deceleration point)	Inflection point along the 30 mmHg isobaric contour at which propagation velocity slows demarcating the tubular oesophagus from the phrenic ampulla	
Panesophageal pressurizzation	Uniform pressurization extending from the UES to the EGJ with 30 mmHg isobaric contour	
Fragmented wave	It is a peristaltic wave (DCI >450) with a large break (>5 cm) along the 20 mmHg isobaric contour	

Table 6.3 The Chicago Classification of oesophageal motor disorders. Version 4.0.

IRP >15 mmHg	**Disorders of Oesophago-Gastric Junction**
Achalasia type 1	100% failed contractions
Achalasia type 2	100% failed contractions with panesophageal pressurization occurring with at least 20% of swallows
Achalasia type 3	No normal peristalsis; there are some residual motor activity in the distal oesophagus with at least 20% premature contractions, defined as DL <4.5 s
EGJ-outflow obstruction (EGJOO)	A manometric diagnosis of EGJOO is always considered clinically inconclusive. It is defined as an elevated median IRP in the primary (IRP< 15 mmHg) and secondary position (IRP >12 mmHg) and ≥ 20% swallows with elevated intrabolus pressure in the supine position, with evidence of peristalsis. Conclusive diagnosis of EGJOO requires clinically relevant symptoms with supportive investigations supporting obstruction (TBE, time barium oesophagogram)
IRP <15 mmHg	**Disorders of Peristalsis**
Aperistalsis	100% of failed contraction (DCI <100 mmHg-s-cm)
Distal oesophageal spasm	100% normal contraction with at least 20% or more premature contraction defined as a distal latency (DL <4.5 s)
Hypercontractile oesophagus	Normal peristalsis with occurrence of ≥20% of swallows with a DCI >8,000 mmHg-s-cm and normal latency
Ineffective oesophageal motility (IEM)	50% or more failed peristalsis (DCI <100 mmHg-s-cm) More than 70% ineffective swallow. Ineffective swallow may be failed or weak (DCI 100-450 mmHg-s-cm). More than 70% fragmented waves (DCI >450 mmHg-s-cm) with large break (>5 cm).
	Normal
Normal	Achieving none of the above diagnostic criteria

described in 2012 after the International High Resolution Manometry Working Group in Ascona, Switzerland in April 2011. The present version has been processed during the international COVID lockdown by means of virtual meetings throughout 2020.

MAJOR DISORDERS OF OESOPHAGEAL MOTILITY

Oesophageal Achalasia

Definition
Achalasia is defined by oesophageal outflow obstruction because of abnormal relaxation of the lower oesophageal sphincter (LES) due to deranged inhibitory control, associated with an impaired oesophageal peristalsis.

Epidemiology
Achalasia occurs with an annual incidence of 1 in 100,000 and prevalence of 10 in 100,000. There is no racial or gender preference, and although the onset of symptoms can occur at any age, they most commonly manifest between the ages of 30 and 60 years.

Aetiology
Achalasia is an idiopathic disease with unknown aetiology, only few cases *expecially* in South-*america* are due to a *Tripanosoma cruzii* infection (Chagas disease).
Achalasia results from the degeneration of neurons in the oesophageal wall. Histologic examination reveals decreased numbers of neurons (ganglion cells) in the myenteric plexuses. Some inflammatory degeneration is reported, and it preferentially involves the nitric oxide-producing,

inhibitory neurons that effect the relaxation of oesophageal smooth muscle; the cholinergic neurons that contribute to LES tone by causing smooth muscle contraction may be relatively spared. This reaction maybe due to the T-lymphocyte immune mediated host reaction based on a genetic predisposition (HLA locus). It has been hypnotized that a virus infection maybe involved in this process.
However, the disordered motility that characterizes achalasia appears to result primarily from the loss of inhibitory neurons within the wall of the oesophagus itself. Loss of inhibitory innervation in the LES causes the basal sphincter pressure to rise and renders the sphincter muscle incapable of normal relaxation. In the smooth muscle portion of the oesophageal body, the loss of inhibitory neurons results in aperistalsis.

Clinical Presentation

The primary presenting symptom is dysphagia (reported in 90% of patients) for both solids and liquids that may continuous or intermittent early in the disease. Patients learn to adapt to the condition and often describe themselves as "slow eaters." Dysphagia in achalasia differs from that attributable to mechanical causes, because it is often accompanied by regurgitation of undigested food and saliva minutes or even hours after the meal. The regurgitation can occur at night, and patients sometimes compensate by elevating their head or even sitting upright to sleep. Regurgitation in achalasia (reported in 60-70% of patients) can be distinguished from reflux-related regurgitation by its bland taste, which is devoid of gastric acid or bile. Few patients may experience *ab-ingestis polmonitis.*
However, patients sometimes also experience chest pain or heartburn (less than 30%) that should be distinguished from those having gastro-oesophageal reflux disease.
Weight loss is unusual until late in the disease.

Diagnosis

Achalasia should be diagnosed with HRM. The HRM test should be required after endoscopy and a barium X ray that firstly should be performed to explore dysphagia and exclude organic diseases. Barium X-ray typically, reveals a dilated, aperistaltic oesophagus with bird-beak narrowing at the EGJ because of functional obstruction caused by non-relaxation of the LES. Upper endoscopy should be performed to exclude neoplastic lesion at EGJ that clinically may be similar to achalasia presentation. If no abnormalities and no dilation are detected during upper endoscopy, biopsy samples should be collected from oesophageal mucosa to exclude eosinophilic oesophagitis.
The HRM is determinant to split the achalasia diagnosis in three different sub-type. Firstly, IRP (median value) should be higher than 15 mmHg:
Type I: absent oesophageal body smooth muscle contractility. This likely represents late-stage achalasia with loss of muscle tone and dilation of the oesophageal body. Alternatively, even if some contractility is retained, the oesophagus may be too dilated for contraction to generate recordable pressure events (**Figure 6.2 A**).
Type II: panesophageal compartmentalization of intrabolus pressure in at least 20% of sequences. The smooth muscle oesophagus retains its tone and biophysical properties, and swallows generate panesophageal isobaric pressure increases which help emptying the oesophagus (**Figure 6.2 B**).
Type III: premature sequences in at least 20% of sequences with shortened distal latency. Timing of oesophageal body peristalsis is deranged; therefore, sequences arrive in the distal oesophagus earlier than expected and are not peristaltic.
The utility to distinguish three different sub-type of achalasia is due to the different therapeutic options (**Figure 6.2 C**).

Therapy

The aim of the treatment is to palliate the symptoms and to reduce complications. The main therapeutic options are:

- Pharmacologic therapy (calcium channel blockers or nitrates) is not particularly successful in short- or long-term symptom resolution. While oral smooth muscle relaxants can be attempted, durable benefit cannot be expected, and side effects can be limiting. It may be used as "bridge to therapy" approach.
- Pneumatic dilation (PD) involves forceful dilation of the LES to 2–4 cm using a hydrostatic balloon. The risk of perforation is lower if a graded dilation approach is used, starting with a 3-cm balloon. This approach maybe successfully used especially in type I (70%) and type II (90%) of symptom improvement.
- An alternative to PD is laparoscopic myotomy of the LES (Heller myotomy, HM). A concurrent antireflux surgical procedure, typically an anterior Dor fundoplication, can reduce the likelihood of GERD from LES disruption. Subtyping of achalasia has facilitated tailoring of management. Both procedure PD and HM are effective in treatment of achalasia. Residual symptoms are reportedly highest with type 3, where HM is favored over PD.

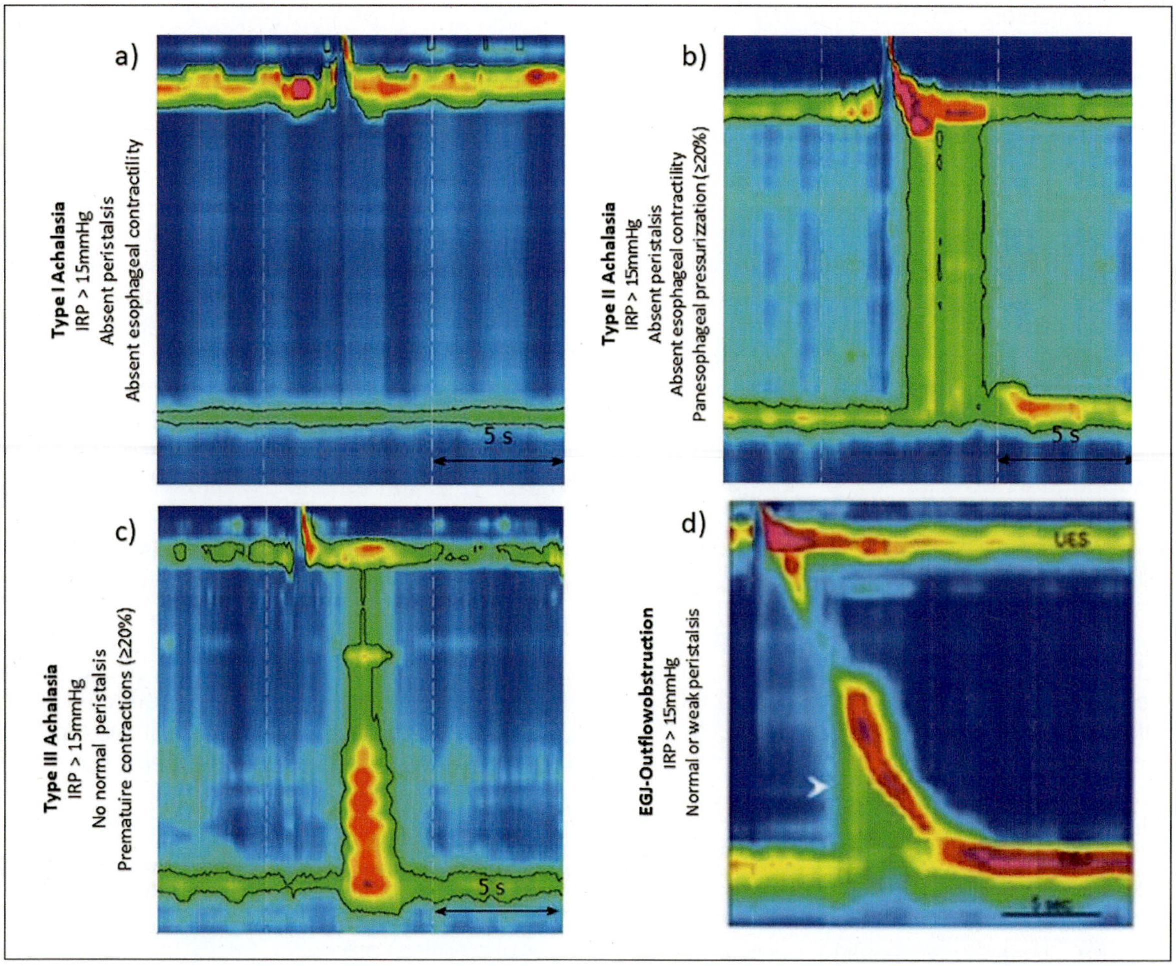

Figure 6.2 Distinct patter of achalasia: type I (a) is characterized by IRP> 15 mmHg no peristalsis or oesophageal contraction; type II (b) is characterized by IRP > 15 mmHg and panesophageal pressurization (30 mmHg isobaric contour); type III (c) is characterized by IRP > 15 mmHg, no normal peristalsis and at least 20% or more spastic contraction (DL< 4.5 s); EGJ-OO (d) is characterized by IRP> 15 mmHg (IRP >12mmHg in upright position) and normal or weak peristalsis and increased intrabolus pressure in 20% of supine swallow.

- Per oral endoscopic myotomy (POEM) is a new natural orifice approach to myotomy performed using an endoscope through a submucosal tunnel created in the oesophagus extending to the EGJ and beyond. Endoscopic cutting tools are then utilized to disrupt the circular muscle fibers of the LES, extending into the proximal stomach distally and the oesophageal body proximally. POEM does carry a higher risk of GERD compared to HM or PD. POEM is suggested when PD or HM failed in reducing symptoms.

GEJ Outflow Obstruction

Definition

Oesophagogastric junction outflow obstruction (EGJOO) definition changed in the last version of CC 4.0 and manometric finding of elevated relaxation pressure (IRP >15 mmHg) in combination with intact or weak peristalsis should not be considered conclusive (**Figure 6.2 D**).

Clinical presentation should report obstructive symptoms (dysphagia and non-cardiac chest pain), elevated relaxation pressure (IRP >15 mmHg) in supine position should be confirmed in upright position (IRP >12 mmHg) and ≥20% swallows with elevated intrabolus pressure (IBP).

A clinically relevant conclusive diagnosis of EGJOO requires a manometric diagnosis of EGJOO and clinically relevant symptoms with at least one of the following supportive investigations supporting obstruction (TBE, i.e. time barium swallow and/or FLIP, i.e. functional lumen imaging probe).

Following introduction of EGJOO as a motility disorder, nearly 10% of patients undergoing HRM were identified to have an EGJOO motility pattern.

While a proportion of EGJOO may evolve toward achalasia or represent a variant of achalasia, more than one-third of cases may be clinically irrelevant and related to benign aetiologies including mechanical effects, opioid use, and artifact as detailed in the subsequent EGJOO technical review. To avoid unnecessary treatments and to optimize outcomes, there is a critical need to clarify which patients with manometric EGJOO have obstructive physiology causing symptoms and requiring intervention.

The aetiology remains uncertain and there is a lack of consensus regarding treatment.

Before diagnosing EGJOO upper endoscopy and biopsies should be performed to exclude eosinophilic oesophagitis. Primary EGJOO may be treated with calcium channel blockers or nitrates. Some reports have described treatment of EGJOO with pneumatic dilatation as it is done with achalasia, with good outcome results. Recently, an Italian paper described first case series of patients with EGJOO treated with Heller-Dor myotomy.

DISORDERS OF PERISTALSIS

Aperistalsis

Aperistalsis (or absent peristalsis) is defined as normal relaxation of EGJ (IRP <15 mmHg) and failed oesophageal contraction (100% with DCI <100 mmHg-s-cm) (**Figure 6.3 A**)

Frequently aperistalsis is a manifestation of systemic disease—for example, scleroderma, a connective tissue disorder (Systemic Lupus Erythematosus and Polymyositis) often involving the smooth muscle of the oesophagus and EGJ. Contrast radiography visualizes a partially dilated aperistaltic oesophagus, with partial barium retention, and some retrograde movement of the bolus. Patients frequently refer with heartburn or regurgitation and may be diagnosed as having GERD. Systemic lupus erythematosus and polymyositis also may manifest with smooth muscle oesophageal motility disorders. A differential diagnosis with type I achalasia should be evaluated (considering clinical presentation, endoscopy

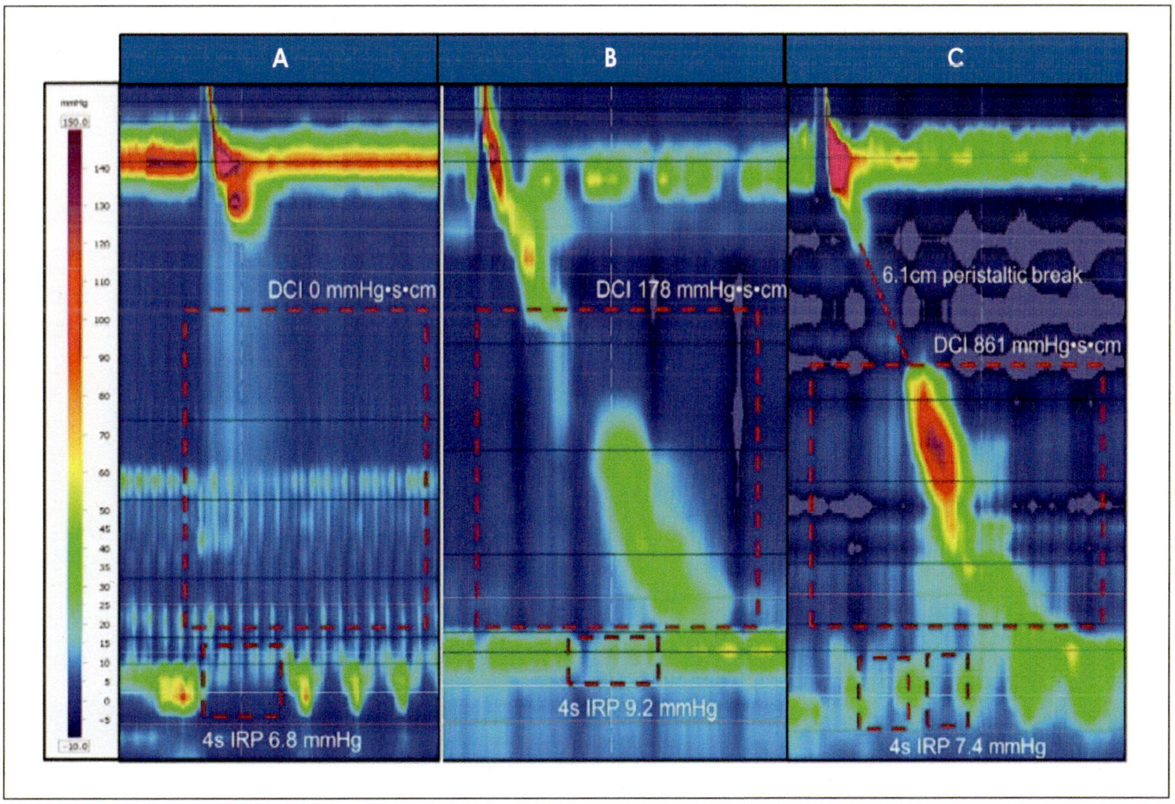

Figure 6.3 Disorders of Peristalsis with Reduced Contractile Vigor or Integrity of Peristalsis. These include absent contractility or ineffective oesophageal motility (either related to reduced contractile vigor or fragmented peristalsis). When DCI is <100 mmHg-s-cm (failed contraction; a) in 100% of wet swallow it is diagnostic for Absent Contractility. IEM is characterized by ≥ 50% of failed peristalsis or >70% of weak peristalsis (b) with a normal IRP. In the third example of IEM (c), the DCI is normal with a fragmentation in peristalsis of >5 cm in the setting of a normal IRP.

and barium X-ray) as some cases of type 1 achalasia with IRP<15mmHg have been reported. Multiple clinical tests are recommended before considering the diagnosis of aperistalsis.

Ineffective Oesophageal Motility

Prior iterations of Chicago Classification categorized ineffective oesophageal motility (IEM) and fragmented peristalsis as minor motility disorders. In CCv4.0, fragmented peristalsis is included under the definition of IEM. Further, the diagnostic criteria for IEM have been made more stringent, commensurate with emerging data. As a result of these changes to IEM and fragmented peristalsis, CCv4.0 does not distinguish between major or minor disorders.

A conclusive diagnosis of IEM requires more than 70% ineffective swallows (weak or failed) or at least 50% failed peristalsis. An ineffective swallow includes failed peristalsis (DCI <100 mmHg-s-cm), (see Figure 6.3 A) and/or weak contraction (DCI ≥ 100 mmHg-s-cm and <450 mmHg-s-cm), (**Figure 6.3 B**) or a fragmented swallow (**Figure 6.3 C**). A fragmented peristalsis is defined by the presence of normal DCI (>450 mmHg-s-cm) with large breaks (>5 cm) along a 20mmHg isobaric contour.

IEM is the most common abnormality observed in routine oesophageal manometry, with an estimated prevalence of 20-30%. It has been reported a prevalence of 51% in patients with oesophageal dysphagia.

IEM is present in 50% of patients with GERD where it is associated with higher acid exposure time during 24-h pH monitoring tests, especially in recumbent position, presumably because of reduced oesophageal clearing.

IEM is frequently associated with Barrett oesophagus, diabetic neuropathy, acute alcohol abuse, eosinophilic oesophagitis and rheumatic autoimmune diseases (i.e. scleroderma).

No effective treatment option is currently available in order to improve oesophageal motility (buspirone and itiopride have recently been evaluated in clinical trials and may prove useful, however they are not available in Italy). Large clinical trials are needed in order to better define the pathophysiology and the impact of minor oesophageal peristaltic disorders on patients' symptoms.

Distal Oesophageal Spasm

Distal oesophageal spasm (DES) is diagnosed with HRM when IRP <15 mmHg and at least 20% or more premature contractions (DL <4.5 s) are described during 10 wet swallows (**Figure 6.4 A**).

DES is an uncommon oesophageal motility disorder. Several adult studies from referral centers have reported prevalence rates ranging from 3 to

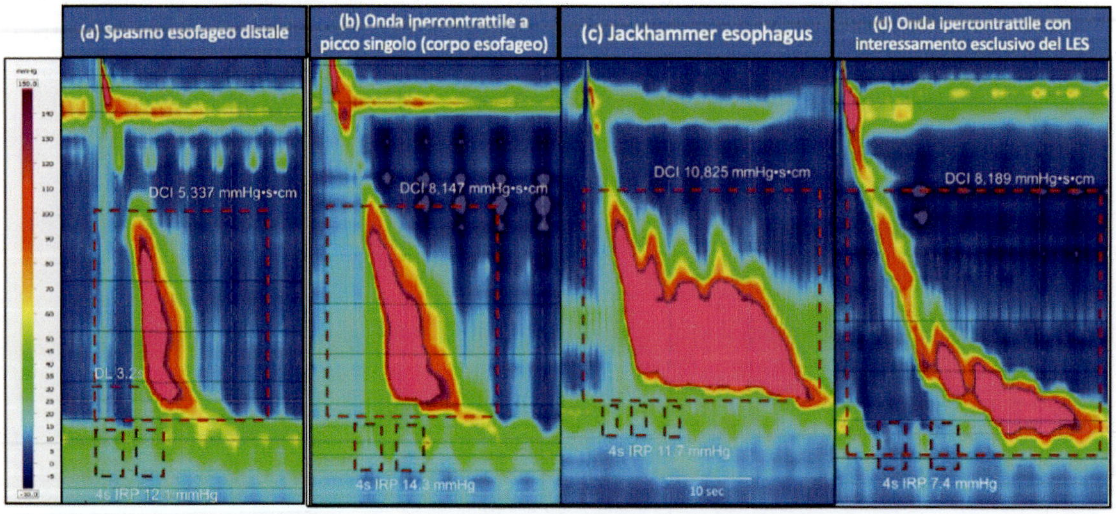

Figure 6.4 Disorders of Peristalsis with Oesophageal Spasticity or Hypercontractility. These include distal oesophageal spasm or hypercontractile oesophagus. In this example of Distal Oesophageal Spasm (a), the DCI is normal with a reduced distal latency (DL< 4.5 s) and normal IRP. Hypercontractile oesophagus includes sub-groups: Single peak hypercontractile swallow (b), hypercontractile with jackhammer oesophagus (c) characterized by caotic propagation of the wave and repetitive contraction, and hypercontractile with LES after contraction (d).

9% in large series of patients undergoing oesophageal motility testing. Mean age is around 60 years and there is a bit higher prevalence female (55%). The cause of DES remains incompletely understood and its clinical presentation is characterized by dysphagia and chest pain.

Some of the patients with DES have been shown to have a characteristic "cork-screw" appearance at barium X-ray.

There is lack of histo-pathological information, since patients with this condition rarely come to autopsy. Studies have suggested that DES represents a disorder of loss of neural inhibition. Experimental work in both animal and human studies have found that blocking nitric oxide (NO) results in simultaneous contractions in the distal oesophagus, a pattern that characterizes DES, whereas administration of NO reverses the defect. DES has been sometime observed in patients with gastro-oesophageal symptoms.

Hypercontractile Oesophagus

Hypercontractile oesophagus describes a distinct manometric abnormality defined by excessive peristaltic vigor, which may include excessive LES after-contraction, not associated with a mechanical obstruction.

A conclusive manometric diagnosis of hypercontractile oesophagus is defined as 20% or more hypercontractile supine swallows (DCI >8,000 mmHg-s-cm) (**Figure 6.4 B-D**).

There are three general sub-groups of hypercontractile oesophagus: single- peaked hypercontractile swallows, (**Figure 6.4 B**), jackhammer with repetitive prolonged contractions (especially in the post-peak phase), (**Figure 6.4 C**) and hypercontractile swallows with a vigorous LES after contraction (**Figure 6.4 D**).

Multipeaked contractions can be synchronized with respiration or not and are generally located in the distal two thirds of the oesophageal body and occasionally in the LES.

There is lack of histo-pathological information useful to better characterize this oesophageal motor abnormality. The pathophysiology is complex and incompletely understood, but it has been suggested that abnormal oesophageal contraction could be related to an imbalance between excitatory and inhibitory innervation. Spontaneous contractions may occur and be generated by discharges of acetylcholine independently of swallows.

It has subsequently become apparent that hypercontractile oesophagus can occur along with other abnormalities such as EGJOO, gastro-oesophageal reflux disease (GERD), or eosinophilic oesophagitis. The most frequently reported symptom is chest pain and cardiac origin should be excluded. Dysphagia may be reported in 30-60% of patients without any weight loss.

Both for DES and JE there is no consensus on management. In clinical practice slow-releasing nitrates and endoscopic injection of botulinum toxin are firstly chosen. A low dosage of antidepressants may be suggested in tailored patients. Doses can be increased each week to achieve the desired goal. POEM has been proposed for treating patients with hypercontractile oesophageal disorders that are refractory to medical management, especially when the main symptom is dysphagia and successful results have been recently reported, although no data are available regarding long-term outcomes.

KEY CONCEPTS

- The oesophageal HRM is considered the gold-standard test to classify oesophageal motor disorders.
- The major disorders of oesophageal motility are associated to the EGJ abnormalities. The lack of relaxation of the EGJ is associated with outflow-obstruction that is frequently associated with achalasia.
- The HRM allows to classify achalasia in three different sub-types. This sub-classification of achalasia is useful to better drive the different therapeutic options.
- The major disorders of peristalsis are due to absent peristalsis (apreristalsis) or to hyperkinetic motility (distal oesophageal spasm or jackhammer oesophagus).
- The minor disorders of peristalsis represent the more frequent disorder of peristalsis observed in a manometric laboratory. These are frequently associated to a chronic gastro-oesophageal reflux disease: ineffective oesophageal motility or fragmented peristalsis.

REFERENCES

1. Yadlapati R, Kahrilas PJ, Fox MR, Bredenoord AJ, Gyawali CP, Roman S, Babaei A, Mittal RK, Rommel N, Savarino E, Sifrim D, Smout A, Vaezi MF, Zerbib F, Akiyama J, Bhatia S, Bor S, Carlson DA, Chen JW, Cisternas D, Cock C, Coss-Adame E, de Bortoli N, Defilippi C, Fass R, Ghoshal UC, Gonlachanvit C, Hani A, Hebbard GS, Jung KW, Katz P, Katzka DA, Khan A, Kohn GP, Lazarescu A, Lengliner J, Mittal SJ, Omari T, Park MI, Penagini R, Pohl D, Richter JE, Serra J, Sweis R, Tack J, Tatum RP, Tutuian R, Vela MF, Wong RK, Wu JC, Xiao Y, Pandolfino JE. Esophageal motility disorders on high-resolution manometry: Chicago classification version 4.0© Neurogastroenterol Motil. 2021 Jan;33(1):e14058.
2. Savarino EV, de Bortoli N, Bellini M, Galeazzi F, Ribolsi M et al. Practice guidelines on the use of esophageal manometry – A GISMAD-SIGE-AIGO medical position paper. Dig Liv Dis. 2016 Oct;48(10):1124-35
3. Gyawali CP, Roman S, Bredenoord AJ, Fox M, Keller J and International GERD Consensus Working Group. Classification of esophageal motor findings in gastro-esophageal reflux disease: Conclusions from an international consensus group. Neurogastroenterol Motil. 2017 Dec;29(12) (on-line only).
4. Yadlapati R, Pandolfino JE, Fox MR, Bredenoord AJ, Kahrilas PJ. What is new in Chicago Classification version 4.0? Neurogastroenterol Motil. 2021 Jan;33(1):e14053. doi: 10.1111/nmo.14053. Epub 2020 Dec 19.
5. Chen JW, Savarino E, Smout A, Xiao Y, de Bortoli N, Yadlapati R, Cock C. Chicago Classification Update (v4.0): Technical review on diagnostic criteria for hypercontractile esophagus. Neurogastroenterol Motil. 2021 Jun;33(6):e14115.
6. Gyawali CP, Zerbib F, Bhatia S, Cisternas D, Coss-Adame E, Lazarescu A, Pohl D, Yadlapati R, Penagini R, Pandolfino J. Chicago Classification update (V4.0): Technical review on diagnostic criteria for ineffective esophageal motility and absent contractility. Neurogastroenterol Motil. 2021 Aug;33(8):e14134.

CHAPTER 7

GASTRO-OESOPHAGEAL REFLUX DISEASE

Laurino Grossi, Sandro Ardizzone

LEARNING OBJECTIVES

- To define and identify GERD.
- To know its epidemiology and pathophysiology.
- To identify symptoms and clinical features for diagnosis.
- To know the available therapeutic options.

Gastro-oesophageal reflux Disease (GERD) is a clinical condition in which the reflux of gastric content into the oesophagus elicits troublesome symptoms and/or complications (Montreal Classification 2006). Gastro-oesophageal reflux (GER) is a paraphysiological phenomenon that occurs only when the ineffectiveness of the barrier between the stomach and oesophagus facilitates an abnormal reflux of gastric contents, or when hypersensitivity to physiological GER is present. It is a recent opinion that functional heartburn should no longer be considered part of GERD and that efforts should be targeted at better identifying, either clinically or with dedicated procedures, a true GERD condition (Lyon Consensus, 2018). Most patients have no visible mucosal damage at endoscopy, so they are catagorized as having non-erosive reflux disease (NERD). Oesophagitis is present only in 30-35% of patients, mainly consisting of uncomplicated erosions; less frequent is the detection of more severe lesions, such as ulcers, peptic strictures, Barrell's oesophagus or oesophageal adenocarcinoma. An accurate epidemiologic evaluation is not easy because many GERD patients have light symptoms.

What is clear from the published data is the increasing prevalence of the disease in Western countries, although more recent reports suggest a similar trend for Asia. This seems to be attributable to the parallel increase in obesity and unhealthy lifestyles (**Figure 7.1**). Based on the most common symptom of GERD, heartburn, population studies indicate a disease prevalence between 10 and 30%.

Similar data are referable to the Italian population, although precise epidemiological data are lacking. When considering the presence of oesophagitis, the prevalence is about 15-16%, though this analysis does not include asymptomatic or slightly symptomatic patients not undergoing endoscopy.

The natural history of GERD is partially defined, but

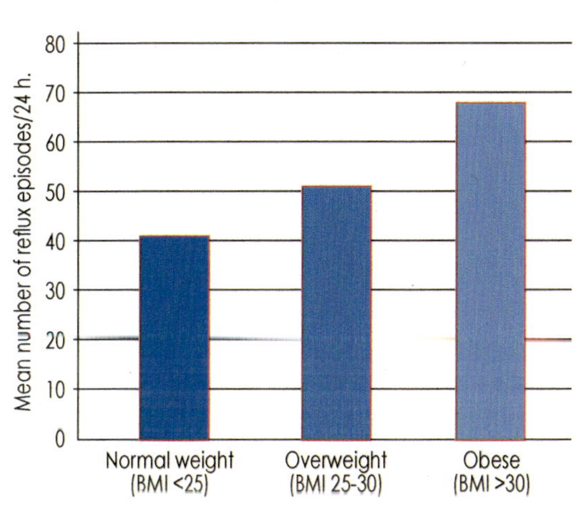

Figure 7.1 Relationship between body-mass index (BMI) and reflux episodes during 24 hours. Reflux episodes are directly correlated with the increase in BMI (adapted, Dig Dis Sci 2012).

it seems that progression from less serious to severe disease is uncommon. NERD or reflux oesophagitis tends to remain unchanged over time, the progression rate from NERD to ERD, from mild to severe ERD and from severe ERD to Barrett's oesophagus is very low (0-30%, 10-22% e 1-13%, respectively). Moreover, in progression from non-erosive to erosive disease, the degree of oesophagitis is usually mild, i.e., grade A or B according the Los Angeles Classification (**Table 7.1**).

CLINICAL FEATURES

GERD may present with typical or atypical extraesophageal symptoms.

Typical Symptoms

Heartburn is the classic symptom of GERD and has high specificity (89-90%), with lower sensitivity (38%)

Table 7.1 Endoscopic classification of oesophagitis according to the Los Angeles scale

Grade A	One or more erosions limited to single folds, <5 mm
Grade B	One or more erosions > 5mm limited to single folds but not bridging the tops of folds
Grade C	Continuous mucosal erosions extending toward the tops of two or more folds, not circumferential
Grade D	Mucosal erosions circumferential

for diagnosis; it also has a low predictive value of the degree of mucosal damage (see chapter on Oesophageal Pathophysiology).

Regurgitation is another typical symptom of GERD. When occurring right after a meal or during clinostatism, it is a clear indicator of disease. Dysphagia is quite common in refluxers (about 30% of patients), less common symptoms are belching, odynophagia, hiccups, nausea or vomiting.

Atypical Extraesophageal Symptoms

GERD may trigger a variety of atypical symptoms: non cardiac chest pain, asthma, posterior laringytis, chronic cough, recurrent pneumonia, dental erosions and sleep disturbances often require accurate differential diagnosis. Some can be present together with typical GERD signs, but most patients are "silent refluxers", which makes diagnosis difficult. Moreover, a direct causal relationship may not be easy to find, as patients can present with two concomitant diseases, even in abnormal pH-monitoring, with no cause-effect link.

GERD PATHOPHYIOLOGY

GERD pathogenesis is multifactorial and generally depends on the imbalance between aggressive and protective factors of the oesophagus. The former are acidity of gastric refluxate, its volume, the harmful action of pepsin, and possible refluxes of duodenal content composed of biliary and pancreatic secretions that are equally harmful toward oesophageal mucosa.

Protective factors include buffering activity of saliva, integrity of epithelium and particularly of the tight junctions, which have been shown to be altered in non-erosive disease and in reflux hypersensitivity, oesophageal peristalsis, competence of lower oesophageal sphincter, and a proper gastric emptying (**Table 7.2**).

Although GERD is an acid-related disease, its main cause is not an increase in acid secretion, which is usually normal, but the impaired function of the natural anti-reflux barrier at the gastro-oesophageal (GE) junction. The GE junction is an anatomically and functionally complex structure that comprises the intrinsic LES and its intraabdominal location, the diaphragmatic crura, the phrenoesophageal ligament, and the acute angle of His. The basal tone of this region separates the gastric cavity from the oesophagus, with relaxation normally occurring only after deglutition.

The main mechanism that lowers the barrier is transient lower oesophageal sphincter relaxation (TLESR), a reflex that occurs independent of swallowing, not accompanied by peristaltic activity, and persisting longer than postdeglutitive LES relaxation.

In normal conditions TLESR is a protective mechanism against gastric overdistention but in GERD TLESR is much more frequent and facilitates long-

Table 7.2 Aggressive and protective factors involved in GERD.

Aggressive Factors	Protective Factors
Acidity of gastric refluxate	Buffering saliva
Volume of refluxate	Mucosal integrity (tight junctions)
Pepsin activity	Oesophageal peristalsis
Biliary secretion in the refluxate	Competence of lower oesophageal sphincter
Pancreatic secretion in the refluxate	Gastric emptying

lasting reflux episodes. Sliding hiatal hernia is a further pathogenetic mechanism in GERD, since it may reduce the competence of the GE junction and facilitate the presence of acid near the diaphragm, inside the thoracic cavity, where the pressure is lower than in abdomen. The so-called "acid pocket" is a zone in the gastric cardia that remains unbuffered after meals.

This pocket is a likely source of acidic refluxate since it has a lower postprandial pH than either the distal oesophagus or the stomach. Although present also in controls, it is more frequent and has a greater proximal extension in GERD patients.

DIAGNOSIS

Although various tests are available to evaluate patients with suspected GERD, such procedures may be unnecessary because the disease can be identified only by classic symptoms, i.e., heartburn and regurgitation. In such cases, an empirical trial of acid suppression with proton pump inhibitors (PPI) can be the first diagnostic step: symptoms responding to PPI in 1-2 weeks ("PPI test") and relapsing after discontinuation allow a diagnosis with a sensitivity of 68%-83%.

When symptoms are more complex and a clinical diagnosis is not possible, it is necessary to perform diagnostic procedures to identify GERD and its complications.

Endoscopy

Upper GI endoscopy is the preferred procedure to diagnose oesophagitis and to rule out other organic conditions potentially linked to symptoms. Oesophagitis is currently classified according to the Los Angeles scale, which describes the extension of mucosal damage longitudinally and circumferentially. It identifies four increasing degrees, from A to D; in severe oesophagitis (grade C-D) it is recommended to repeat the endoscopic exam after adequate anti secretory therapy to better evaluate the possibility of Barrett's oesophagus.

The sensitivity of endoscopy is low, because only 30-35% of patients with GERD present mucosal damage, the majority showing normal mucosa (NERD).

Moreover, no direct correlation exists between symptoms and organic damage, which further limits the role of endoscopy in GERD diagnosis and related therapeutic decisions.

24-Hour Oesophageal pH-Monitoring

This is the gold standard to document a pathological acid exposure of the oesophagus and its correlation with symptoms. The catheter is connected to a portable recorder and placed trans-nasally with the electrode conventionally located 5 cm proximal to the LES. The indications for this procedure are atypical symptoms, in patients with negative endoscopy, or the persistence of symptoms despite antisecretive therapy. Moreover, pH monitoring allows differential diagnosis between "true refluxers", i.e., patients with pathological acid exposure, those with a temporal association between symptoms and physiological reflux episodes (reflux hypersensitivity), and those with "functional heartburn" who have a normal pH profile and a negative association between symptoms and reflux episodes (no GERD) (**Figure 7.2**).

Combined pH Impedance

This technology combines measurement of pH with electrical impedance analysis for investigating the composition of refluxate (liquid, gas or mixed) and its direction inside the oesophageal lumen.

Therefore, pH-metry, will help to diagnose frankly acid reflux (by convention <4), whereas pH impedance can identify weakly acidic refluxes (pH between 4 and 5), as well as the deglutition of acidic substances, which is not detectable with pH monitoring alone.

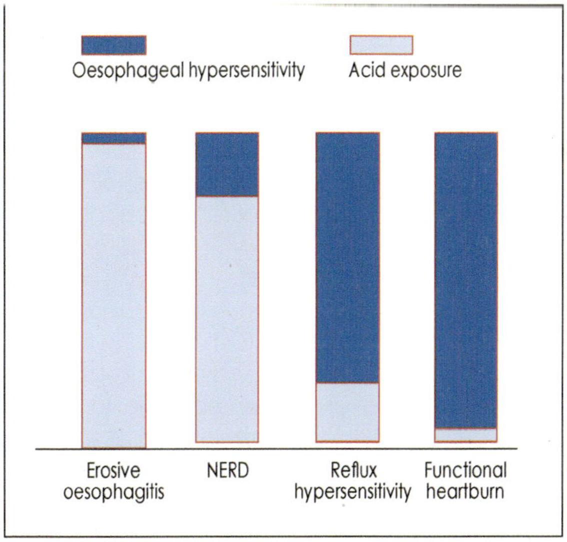

Figure 7.2 Relationship between oesophageal hypersensitivity and acid exposure in the reflux symptom spectrum. Abnormal acid exposure elicits symptoms in erosive oesophagitis, whereas oesophageal hypersensitivity is the main cause of functional heartburn. NERD and reflux hypersensitivity result from a combination of the two factors (modified from Aziz et al. Gastroen-

Oesophageal Manometry

Manometry does not play a key role in GERD diagnosis. This exam is reserved for the study of the oesophageal body and LES motor pattern, especially in patients undergoing surgery to modulate the degree of fundoplication, which has to be adapted to the motor performance of the oesophagus.

Barium Oesophagogram

This procedure no longer plays a pivotal role in GERD diagnosis. Radiologic study can identify anatomical alterations, such as narrowing, the presence and degree of hiatal hernia, rings, and webs. It cannot identify Barrett's oesophagus and the use of radiation limit indication for this exam, which is now less recommended than endoscopy.

THERAPY

The therapeutic goal of GERD treatment is the relief of symptoms, healing oesophagitis in patients with endoscopically found lesions, and therefore maintaining clinical and endoscopic re- sponsibility. Given the various clinical manifestations and pathogenic factors of GERD, the therapeutic options can also be varied and include behavioral aspects, as well as pharmacological treatments.

Lifestyle Changes

These should be explained to the patients, especially those with mild symptoms, and include elevating the head of the bed, reducing consumption of alcohol and smoking, changing eating habits, reducing the intake of fats, carminatives, coffee, citrus fruits, and chocolate. Hyper-caloric meals tend to increase acid secretion, slow gastric emptying, and reduce LES basal tone, all factors facilitating the occurrence of reflux episodes.

Proton Pump Inhibitors (PPIs)

They represent the drug of choice in GERD treatment and have replaced H2-blockers which for decades were the main antisecretory drugs. Many medications are available (omeprazole, lansoprazole, pantoprazole, rabeprazole, and esomeprazole) and all have similar efficacy. PPIs provide an intragastric pH>4 for 10-14 hours, as compared to 6-8 hours obtained with H2-blockers.

The greatest efficacy of PPIs is obtained if assumed in the fasting state, better early in the morning and before breakfast, because the protonic pumps are fully working on an empty stomach and the inhibitory effect on secretion is greater. GERD patients vary in response to PPIs according to the disease phenotype: generally, patients with moderate-severe oesophagitis tend to have better response than NERD patients; similarly PPIs seem to control typical symptoms better than atypical manifestations which usually require longer treatment. In lack of response to PPIs, a brief trial with double dose, with a second dose assumed at night, always before meal may be considered; a switch toward another drug of the same class is a further option.

The wide use of PPIs raised concerns about their safety in the longterm. Fundic gland polyps are the most common findings at endoscopy and prolonged use of PPIs, from 1 to 5 years, is associated with up to a 4-fold increase in risk. This happens because acid suppression elicits hypergastrinic stimulus, leading to hyperplasia of parietal cells. However, these polyps are not real adenoma and do not pose risk of degeneration.

Contrasting data are present about the theoretical risk of developing respiratory or intestinal infections (mainly *Clostridium difficile*) because of reduced acid secretion, whilst prolonged hypochlorhydria generally facilitates iron, B12 vitamin, calcium and magnesium malabsorption. Moreover, some classes of PPIs have potential metabolic interactions with other drugs (warfarin and clopidogrel) due to their action on cytochrome P450, common metabolic site.

H2-Blockers

For years the antisecretory drug of choice before the introduction of PPIs, their use is to date less common and reserved for particular situations. A bedtime single dose is warranted to overcome the so-called "nocturnal breakthrough", a transient increase in acidity occurring during the night. H2 blockers can be used in patients assuming clopidogrel, because of their lower drug interaction, or in non-responders or patients intolerant to PPIs. However, the healing rate in more severe degrees of oesophagitis (C-D on the Los Angeles scale) is significantly lower than with PPIs.

Antacids

They are useful in patients with milder symptoms, sometimes even "on demand". Most antacids temporally neutralize gastric acidity and should be taken in the fasting state. Alginate has a further mechanical effect of blocking the refluxate through a raft effect floating on the gastric pool and displacing the acid pocket below the diaphragm, which is why alginate should be taken after meals.

Prokinectics

Currently, this drug class of drug has demonstrated very limited efficacy in GERD treatment. In the recent past, cisapride, a 5-HT4 agonist was highly effective in reducing reflux episodes. The drug was withdrawn from the market because of serious effects on heart rate. Metoclopramide, domperidone, and levosulpiride have a slight prokinetic action, but their prolonged use is limited by side effects.

Drugs That Reduce LESRS

Regulation of TLESRs is the ideal therapeutical option since it can block the majority of reflux episodes. Currently, the only drug proven effective is baclofen, an agonist of gamma-aminobutyrric acid used to treat spasticity. However, its use ("off-label") is limited by side effects. Similar drugs are under investigation but none has obtained approval.

Surgery

Surgical fundoplication (Nissen 360-degree or partial Toupet procedure) is basically the only approach to reconstitute the gastro-oesophageal barrier. It should be reserved for younger patients showing good response to PPIs.
Since patients not responding to antisecretory drugs could be affected by other diseases (functional heartburn, oesophageal motor diseases, pill-induced oesophagitis), the surgical option needs to be carefully evaluated.
A major limitation of surgical fundoplicatio is the long-term failure of the barrier, leading to the use of PPIs 6 years post-surgery.

Endoscopic Therapies

Endoscopic procedure proposed in the last years still lack convincing long-term efficacy.
The Stretta endoscopic radiofrequency procedure partial fundoplicatio (EsophyX), magnetic LES augmentation (LINX) or electrical stimulation of the junction (Endostim) are still under investigation and none of them has definitively shown efficacy.

KEY CONCEPTS

- GERD is one of the most frequent diseases of the GI tract. Clinical symptoms may be typical, with heartburn and regurgitation or atypical and extraoesophageal. The main mechanism is failure of the gastro-oesophageal junction, particularly transient LES relaxation, associated with an imbalance between the action of gastric acid and oesophageal protective factors.
- Diagnosis is clinical in typical symptoms but requires dedicated procedures in more complex situations. Upper GI endoscopy is mandatory when alarm symptoms occur and helps identify complications of GERD, such as oesophagitis, Barrett's oesophagus or adenocarcinoma.
- The gold standard procedure is oesophageal pH monitoring, recently implemented by combined impedance measurement. This exam is indicated in patients with atypical symptoms, in those not responding to antisecretory drugs or candidate for surgery.
- Mild cases could be managed first with lifestyle changes (elevate the head of the bed, lose weight, avoid supine position after meals, reduce caloric intake). Medical therapy is based on antisecretory drugs, especially PPIs, currently more rapid and effective than H2-blockers.
- Surgical fundoplication is a valid option, usually reserved for younger patients with a definitive diagnosis of GERD. Endoscopic procedures, although promising, are still under investigation.

REFERENCES

- Gyawali CP, Fass R. Management of Gastroesophageal Reflux Disease. Gastroenterology. 2018 Jan;154(2):302-18.
- Hunt R, Armstrong D, Katelaris P, et al. World Gastroenterology Organisation Global Guidelines: GERD Global Perspective on Gastroesophageal Reflux Disease. J Clin Gastroenterol. 2017 Jul;51(6):467-78.
- Iwakiri K, Kinoshita Y, Habu Y, et al. Evidence-based clinical practice guidelines for gastroesophageal reflux disease 2015. J Gastroenterol. 2016;51:751-67.
- Katz PO, Gerson LB, Vela MF. Guidelines for the Diagnosis and Management of Gastroesophageal Reflux Disease. Am J Gastroenterol. 2013; 108:308-28.
- Tack J, Pandolfino JE. Pathophysiology of Gastroesophageal Reflux Disease. Gastroenterology. 2018 Jan;154 (2):277-88.

CHAPTER 8

OESOPHAGITIS NOT ASSOCIATED WITH GASTRO-OESOPHAGEAL REFLUX DISEASE

Chiara Ricci, Edoardo Vincenzo Savarino

LEARNING OBJECTIVES

- To know the main diseases associated with oesophagitis, which are not related to gastro-oesophageal. reflux disease and oesophageal acid exposure, but raise suspicion of the disorder based on clinical and endoscopic findings.
- To identify the major mechanisms involved in the pathogenesis of non-reflux oesophagitis.
- To understand the diagnostic and therapeutic implications of non-reflux oesophagitis, including medical and endoscopic treatment strategies.

Among the forms of oesophagitis not associated with gastro-oesophageal reflux are those of infectious origin, those secondary to use of drugs or prolonged therapeutic cycles (NSAIDs, antibiotics, chemo- and radio-therapy), systemic diseases (Crohn's disease and Behcet's disease) caustic lesions, and eosinophilic oesophagitis.

INFECTIOUS OESOPHAGITIS

Infectious oesophagitis is commonly diagnosed in immunocompromised patients, specifically those with HIV infection or leukemia, lymphoma, or other tumours.
In immunocompetent patients, although less frequent, oesophageal infections are associated with pathophysiological or mechanical factors that predispose to their development (diabetes mellitus, cirrhosis, alcoholism, critical illness, scleroderma, and aging).
Functional or structural anomalies such as oesophageal strictures, pseudodiverticulosis, prior gastro-oesophageal surgery or dysmotility (i.e., achalasia, diffuse oesophageal spasm) may increase risk. Moreover, some medications have been linked to oesophageal candidiasis through challenges to the natural defenses of the mucosa, such as topical or inhaled corticosteroids, or acid-suppressive medications.
Infectious pathogens include fungi (*Candida albicans*, Aspergillus, Blastomyces, Cryptococcus, Histoplasma), viruses (herpes simplex virus – HSV, cytomegalovirus – CMV, varicella zoster virus – VZV, Epstein-Barr virus – EBV, human papillomavirus – HPV, human immunodeficiency virus – HIV), bacteria (*Staphylococcus aureus*, *Streptococcus epidermidis*, and *Bacillus* species).
Symptoms can include dysphagia or odynophagia, heartburn, nausea, chest pain, and, sometimes, haematemesis.

Yeast Oesophagitis

Candida-related oesophagitis is common, especially in HIV-infected patients or in patients with haematologic malignancies.
The main causative organism is *C. albicans*. Pain or difficulty swallowing are the most common complaints by patients with candidal infection of the oesophagus. The diagnosis is usually made through endoscopy with biopsy of white mucosal plaque-like lesions (**Figure 8.1**).
Histology demonstrates the presence of yeasts and pseudohyphae with a culture confirming *Candida*.

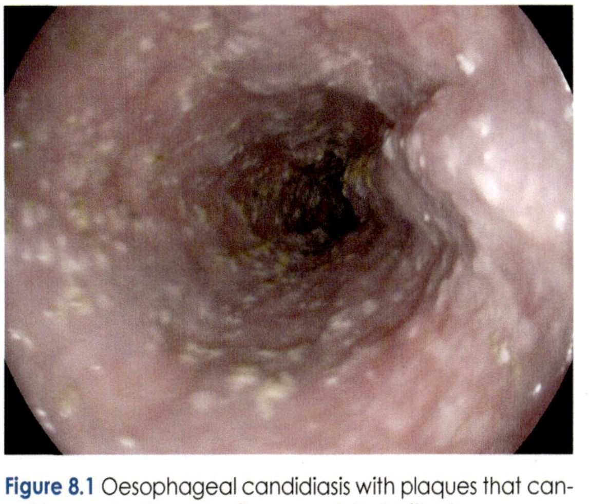

Figure 8.1 Oesophageal candidiasis with plaques that cannot be washed away, often associated with ulcers.

It requires systemic antifungal therapy. The first line therapy is oral or intravenous fluconazole (itraconazole and voriconazole can be used as an alternative).

Viral Oesophagitis

Herpetic oesophagitis is the most common and is typically due to HSV-1. While mostly occuring in HIV-infected individuals, HSV oesophagitis may be associated with recipients of solid organ or bone marrow transplants. Rare but severe organ-specific, CMV oesophagitis has been documented. Acute and severe odynophaghia is reported to be the typical presentation for HSV or VZV oesophagitis, whereas more vague complaints (nausea and vomiting, epigastric discomfort, anorexia, and fevers) are more frequently attributed to CMV oesophagitis.
The endoscopic appearance of HSV oesophagitis ranges from early vesicle formation to non-specific erosive changes up to superficial or deep ulceration, possibly with associated plaques, pseudomembranes, or pale yellow exudates (**Figure 8.2**). Biopsies obtained at ulcer edges have the highest yield for these findings, with multinucleated giant cells and glassy eosinophilic intranuclear inclusions. First-line therapy for HSV oesophagitis consists of oral acyclovir (or intravenous if severe dysphagia or odynophagia). Treatment for CMV oesophagitis involves antiviral therapy (intravenous ganciclovir or foscarnet) or oral valganciclovir.

Rare Infectious Oesophagitis

Tuberculous infection of the oesophagus is quite rare even in endemic areas. Its typical endoscopic appearance involves the formation of superficial gray ulcers with irregular borders. The treatment is 6 to 9 months of multimodal drug therapy.

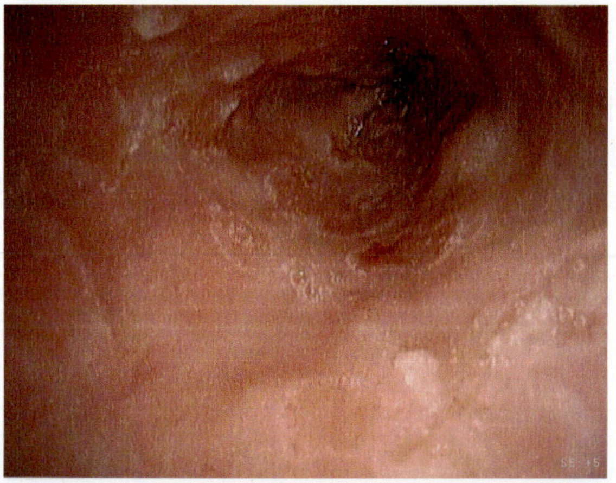

Figure 8.2 Herpetic oesophagitis with erosions/ulcers and vesicles with detected and hyperemic edges.

CAUSTIC OESOPHAGITIS

Ingestion of caustic substances with extremes of pH (less than 2 or greater than 12) is corrosive and can create severe injury and burns, especially in the oesophagus and stomach. The majority (68%) of cases involve children (unintentional, accidental ingestion) but also adults with psychiatric disturbances, after suicide attempts or alcoholics.
The severity of injury depends on the concentration of the substance, amount ingested, length of time of tissue contact, and pH of the agent. Alkaline substances react with proteins and fats, resulting in liquefactive necrosis. Acids ingestion reacts with tissue proteins, converting to acid proteins. The mode of tissue injury is coagulation necrosis. Mucosal injury is characterized by necrosis and haemorragic congestion secondary to the formation of thrombosis in the small vessels.
The most common symptom reported is dysphagia. Short-term complications include perforation and death. Chronic complications of caustic ingestion include stricture, gastric outlet obstruction and malignant transformation.
Upper GI endoscopy is a highly recommended diagnostic tool, especially during the first 12-48 hours after caustic ingestion. Gastric acid suppression and mucosal protection are the main mode of treatment. The primary treatment of caustic oesophageal stricture is endoscopic dilatation. Corrective surgery (partial or total oesophagectomy) for oesophageal strictures from caustic injury is done only in severe cases where endoscopic therapy fails or is harmful.

ACTINIC OESOPHAGITIS

The oesophagus can be exposed to radiation during treatment of cancer of the lung, breast, and oesophagus carcinoma. Patients typically present dysphagia and odynophagia. Endoscopic changes such as erythema and ulceration are nonspecific and nondiagnostic. Histology shows inflammatory cells infiltrate and radiation-related atypia of endothelial and stromal cells. Factors responsible for increased severity of symptoms are: double daily radiation treatment, advanced illness, age, and dose of radiation received. Acute onset of pain is related to early oesophageal mucositis. Although radiation oesophagitis is usually self-limiting, complications, such as ulceration, perforation, and even tracheoesophageal fistula formation, can occur. The most common late complication is fibrosis, leading to stricture, which may appear at least 3 months after treatment.

EOSINOPHILIC OESOPHAGITIS

Eosinophilic oesophagitis (EoE) is a chronic, immune/antigen-mediated disease characterized clinically by symptoms related to oesophageal dysfunction and histologically by eosinophil-predominant inflammation. EoE incidence has dramatically increased in recent years, with a prevalence of around 43–55 per 100,000 inhabitants in Western countries.

A number of potential risk factors have been proposed, including the decreased prevalence of *H. pylori* infection, increased use of proton pump inhibitors (PPIs), and early life exposures to antibiotics.

Eosinophilic oesophagitis seems to be more frequent in young adult males (male/female sex ratio 3:1). Similarly, in Italy a recent prospective study observed that oesophageal eosinophilia is quite commonly encountered in the Gastroenterology Unit, with nearly 12% of patients with dysphagia and/or bolus impaction having ≥15 eosinophils/HPF, and about 9.3% with a definite diagnosis of EoE.

Physiopathology

EoE is characterized by eosinophil infiltration within the oesophageal epithelium, and T-helper 2 (Th2)-type immune responses, which are typical of other atopic conditions. Commonly, patients with EoE have a high incidence of concurrent atopic disease, including asthma and airway hyper-responsiveness, atopic dermatitis, and rhinitis. Moreover, they present sensitization to cutaneous, ingested, and/or inhaled allergens and seasonal allergens may play a role in some patients.

EoE has a strong hereditability pattern, with familial associations having relative risk ratios as high as 64 times amongst siblings. Studies have identified multiple genes that likely contribute to the development of EoE, including thymic stromal lymphopoietin (TSLP), calpain 14 (CAPN14), EMSY, and LRRC32, STAT6, ANKRD27, CCL 26.

The role of Th2 cytokines remains central to our understanding of EoE. In fact, in EoE the oesophageal epithelium is infiltrated not only by eosinophils but also by T-cells, B cells, and mast cells. Moreover, increased levels of cytokines (IL-4, IL-5, IL-9 and IL-13) have been noted in the oesophageal mucosa of patients with EoE. In addition, oesophageal epithelium cells express TNF-α and eotaxin-3, which are responsible for the recruitment of eosinophils in the oesophagus. Finally, eosinophils also produce TSLP, a cytokine promoting Th2 differentiation and tumour growth factor (TGF) β, a cytokine involved in epithelial growth, fibrosis, and tissue re-modeling. The consequent oesophageal inflammatory process results in oesophageal dysfunction. Gastro-oesophageal reflux disease (GERD) may induce microscopic oesophagitis, including dilation of intercellular spaces, and eosinophilic infiltration. Different hypotheses have been raised to explain this phenomenon and understand the interplay between EoE and GERD. For instance, healing of a disrupted epithelial barrier by treating acid refluxate may prevent further histological damage, reduce antigen exposition and thus decrease immune activation. PPI may have some anti-inflammatory properties that reduce the inflammatory burden.

Clinical Presentation

Patients with EoE may present with a wide range of symptoms, including dysphagia, food impaction, heartburn and chest pain. The clinical presentation may differ according to the age at onset. In adults, dysphagia is the most typical symptom of EoE (about 90% of cases) with food impaction the most severe presentation. Indeed, 35–50% of adults experience at least one episode of food impaction requiring endoscopic bolus removal during the natural history of their disease. A minority of patients also complains of retrosternal pain, heartburn, and regurgitation. Other symptoms such as nausea, vomiting or abdominal pain, as well as diarrhoea and weight loss can also occur.

In children younger than 2 years of age, feeding disorders (refusal to eat, chewing problems, choking after liquids or solids ingestion) and failure to thrive are dominant symptoms, while up to the age of 12, vomiting, nausea, abdominal pain, heartburn and regurgitation are the most common symptoms (5-82%). Finally, EoE may be associated with oesophageal complications such as spontaneous perforation.

Diagnosis

Upper endoscopy with oesophageal biopsies is the first step in the diagnostic work up of patients with dysphagia and suspected EoE. A considerable number of endoscopic findings can be observed in EoE (**Figure 8.3**).

They include normal endoscopy, mucosal oedema (decreased vascular markings), exudates (whitish plaques), furrows, rings, stricture, or crêpe paper mucosa (mucosal fragility). These patterns may co-exist in the same patient. However, endoscopic features are neither sensitive nor specific EoE.

In such cases, 6 to 8 biopsies from the distal and mid- and/or proximal oesophagus, obtained during endoscopy, are needed to identify patients with EoE with a high level of sensitivity. Within these biopsies, an eosinophil count >15 per high-power field (HPF) is diagnostic EoE or will define the disease as active. Other histological features are presented in **Table 8.1**.

The disease is limited to the oesophagus and other causes of oesophageal eosinophilia should be excluded (i.e., eosinophilic gastro-enteritis, Crohn's disease, and achalasia). A standardised endoscopic classification is EoE Endoscopic Reference Score (EREFS) (**Table 8.2**). Barium swallow provides data on the length and diameter of oesophageal strictures. Serum IgE and skin-prick testing for aero, and food allergy is warranted to identify comorbid food-induced allergic diseases in EoE patients, although they do no, predict response to allergy-testing based diet.

Table 8.1 Histological features of EoE.

- Eosinophilic infiltration with eosinophil count >15 in a high-power field (HPF)
- Eosinophil microabscesses
- Superficial layering of eosinophils
- Extracellular eosinophil granules
- Increased number of mast cells and lymphocytes
- Basal cell hyperplasia
- Dilated intercellular spaces
- Lamina propria fibrosis

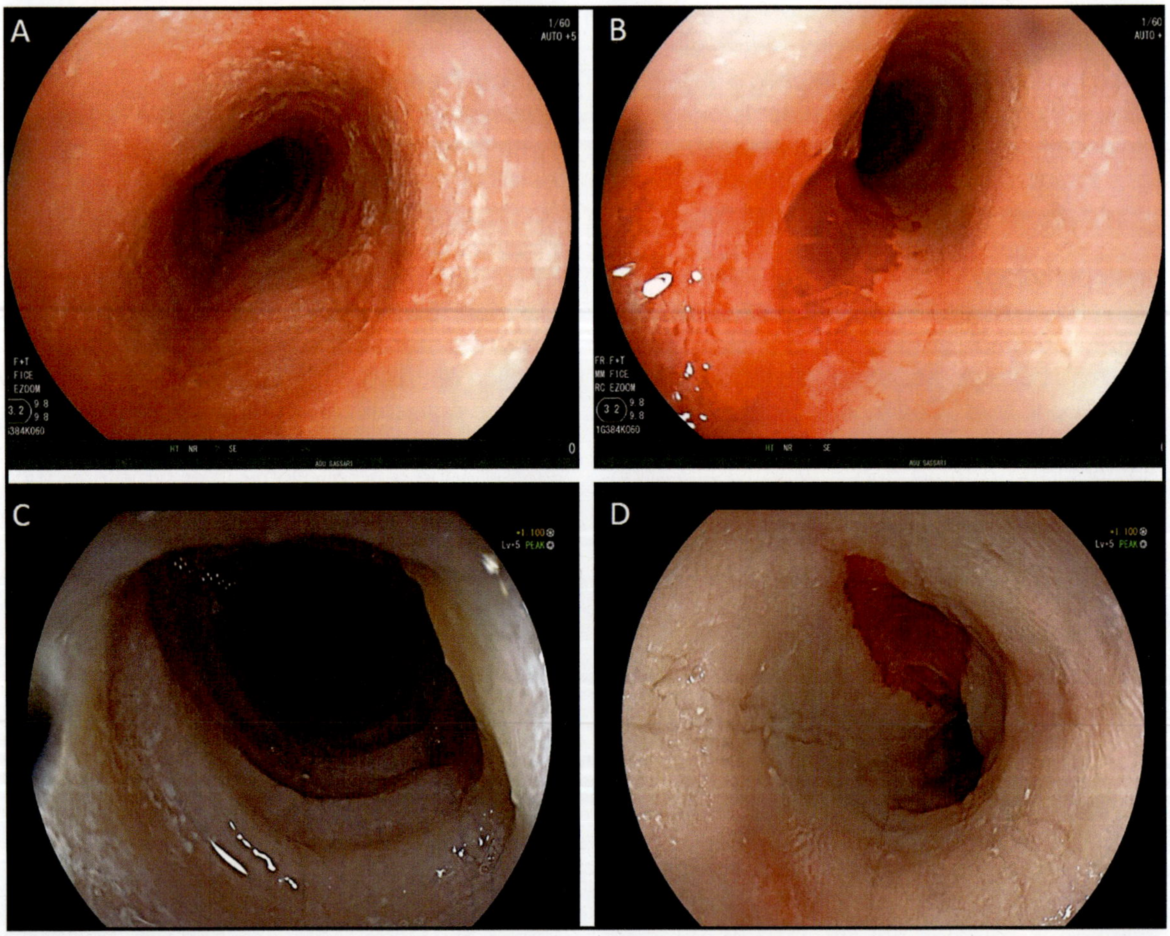

Figure 8.3 Endoscopic images of EoE: white exudates and oesophageal narrowing (A), stricture and tear (B), rings (C), oedema and furrows (D), which are markers of acute inflammation.

Table 8.2 Endoscopic classification for endoscopic assessment of eosinophilic oesophagitis: the Endoscopic Reference Score (EREFS).

Endoscopic Signs	Classification
Rings	Grade 0: absent
	Grade 1: mild (subtle circumferential rings)
	Grade 2: moderate (distinct rings, still passage of diagnostic endoscope)
	Grade 3: severe (distinct rings, no passage of diagnostic endoscope)
White exudates	Grade 0: absent to mild (<10 % of oesophageal surface area)
	Grade 1: severe (>10 % of oesophageal surface area)
Furrows	Grade 0: absent
	Grade 1: present
Oedema	Grade 0: absent to mild (loss of clarity of vascular markings)
	Grade 1: severe (absence of vascular markings)
Stricture	Grade 0: absent
	Grade 1: present
Crepe paper oesophagus	Grade 0: absent
	Grade 1: present

Therapy

There are three treatment approaches to EoE: drugs, diet, and dilation.

Drugs and dietary changes target the inflammation associated with the pathogenesis of EoE, whereas dilation treats oesophageal remodeling and fibrotic complications. Choice of treatment depends on clinical features, patient and provider preferences, local expertise, and costs. As for drugs, the use of PPI is recommended as first therapy. In PPI failure, oral topical corticosteroids, such as budesonide (1 mg), and fluticasone (800 µg), are highly effective in resolving the symptoms and signs of EoE.

EoE is a chronic disease, and symptoms and inflammation generally relapse within few weeks after cessation of topical corticosteroid treatment. Therefore, many patients need long-term therapy. Diet therapy, including the 6-food elimination diet (with elimination of gluten, milk, soy, egg, nuts, and seafood) is an alternative to corticosteroid therapy.

Factors limiting the use of diet therapy for EoE regard restrictions on of life and social activities.

Progressive dilation with bougienage or balloons is the only available endoscopic treatment for EoE. Dilation of oesophageal strictures can lead to long-lasting reduction in dysphagia in adults and children with EoE, with a low risk of complications (perforation in 0.1% to 0.2% of cases). Dilatation should be performed gradually, based on symptoms and initial diameter of the oesophageal lumen.

KEY CONCEPTS

- Oesophagitis not associated with gastro-oesophageal disease may be caused by infectious disease, caustic injury, drugs or therapies (NSAIDs, antibiotics, chemotherapy or radiation), systemic disorders (Crohn's and Behcet's disease) or eosinophilic oesophagitis.
- Infectious oesophagitis is commonly diagnosed in immunocompromised patients, while in immunocompetent patients, it is usually associated with pathophysiological or mechanical factors. Severityof injury from ingestion of caustic substances is related to the type of ingested substance, the amount and the time of tissue exposure.
- Eosinophilic oesophagitis (EoE) is a chronic, immune/antigene-mediated disease characterized clinically by symptoms related to oesophageal dysfunction and histologically by eosinophil-predominant inflammation.
- Diagnosis of eosinophilic oesophagitis requires upper endoscopy with biopsies and presence of an eosinophil count >15 per high-power field (HPF), whereas the therapeutic approach is based on the use of drugs (proton pump inhibitors, topical corticosteroids), diet (6-fod elimination diet), and dilation.

REFERENCES

- Ahuja NK, Clarke JO. Evaluation and Management of Infectious Esophagitis in Immunocompromised and Immunocompetent Individuals. Curr Treat Options Gastroenterol. 2016;14:28-38.
- de Bortoli N, Penagini R, Savarino E, Marchi S. Eosinophilic esophagitis: Update in diagnosis and management. Position paper by the Italian Society of Gastroenterology and Gastrointestinal Endoscopy (SIGE). Dig Liver Dis. 2017 Mar;49(3):254-60.
- De Lusong MA, Timbol AB, Tuazon DJ. Management of esophageal caustic injury. World J Gastrointest Pharmacol Ther. 2017;8:90-8.
- Roman S, Savarino E, Savarino V, Mion F. Eosinophilic oesophagitis: from physiopathology to treatment. Dig Liver Dis. 2013 Nov;45(11):871-8.
- Straumann A, Katzka DA. Diagnosis and Treatment of Eosinophilic Esophagitis. Gastroenterology. 2018 Jan; 154(2):346-59.

CHAPTER 9

OESOPHAGEAL NEOPLASMS AND PRECANCEROUS LESIONS*

Francesco Luzza, Fabiana Zingone

LEARNING OBJECTIVES

- To know the epidemiology and risk factors of common oesophageal neoplasms.
- To recognize symptoms and perform diagnostic and therapeutic procedures.
- To understand the surveillance strategies for precancerous lesions, with special regard to Barrett's oesophagus.

INTRODUCTION

The most common types of oesophageal cancer are adenocarcinoma and squamous cell carcinoma. The first, which is increasing in prevalence over the past decade is primarily localized in the lower oesophagus and results from a metaplastic epithelium, with intestinal or gastric phenotype so called Barrett's oesophagus. Oesophageal malignancies often bear poor outcome. For this reason, in the last year efforts have been focused on the technological advances in early detection, precancerous lesion surveillance scrupulous preoperative staging, and integration of therapeutic approaches.

EPIDEMIOLOGY

Adenocarcinoma and squamous cell carcinoma account for about 95% of oesophageal malignancies, with the remaining 5% comprise small cells, verrucous, mucoepidermoid and adenoid-cystic carcinoma, carcinosarcoma, sarcoma (leiomyosarcoma, fibrosarcoma and gastrointestinal stromal tumours (GIST), melanoma, lymphoma and neuroendocrine tumours (NET). Males have approximately a 3-fold higher risk of oesophageal cancer than females and the highest incidence rate is usually found in adults aged 60 years and over. Geographical distribution is variable. A high-risk area has been recognized, called the oesophageal cancer belt, including parts of Northern Iran, Southern Russia, Middle Asia and Northern China, where squamous cell carcinoma accounts for 90% of cases of oesophageal carcinoma. In these risk areas, oesophageal carcinoma is the fourth leading cause of cancer. In Europe, a significant higher incidence in Normandy, Calvados, and the Triveneto region in Italy has been reported. In Italy, the risk of developing oesophageal carcinoma is 1 in 182 men and 1 in 705 women: in both genders the risk increases with increasing age. Mortality risk is 1 in 198 men and 1 in 874 women, with a 13% 5-year survival. In both sexes the incidence of oesophageal carcinoma is slightly higher in the northern regions than in the central-south regions of the country.

An increased risk is associated with nutritional habits, smoking, and alcohol consumption. There is a tendency to a reduction in incidence and mortality over time, especially in males. The reduction is mainly due to the squamous cell forms; instead, the relevance of adenocarcinomas has increased over time and, at present, an adenocarcinoma is diagnosed for every three squamous cell carcinomas.

RISK FACTORS

The two main histotypes of malignant neoplasia have different risk factors (**Table 9.1**). Gastro-oesophageal reflux disease (GERD), smoking, body-mass index (BMI) and red meat consumption increase the risk for adenocarcinoma, while H. pylori infection, low/moderate consumption of alcohol, physical activity, consumption of fruit, vegetable, folate, fiber, beta-carotene and vitamin C, were found to reduce the risk. Consumption of alco-

*The Authors would like to thank Dr. Rocco Spagnuolo for his assistance.

Table 9.1 Risk factors for oesophageal cancer.

Adenocarcinoma		Squamous Cell Carcinoma	
Oesophageal reflux disease	↑	Alcohol consumption	↑
High body-mass index	↑	Smoking	↑
Smoking	↑	Read meat consumption	↑
Red meat consumption	↑	Ingestion of caustics	↑
Helicobacter pylori infection	⇩	Very hot drinks	↑
Low/moderate alcohol consumption	⇩	Tylosis (hyperkeratosis palmar)	↑
Physical activity	⇩	Achalasia	↑
Consumption of fruit, vegetables, folate, fibre, beta-carotene, vitamin C	⇩	Papilloma virus infection	↑
		Body-mass index	⇩
		Consumption of fruit, vegetables, folate, fibre, beta-carotene, vitamin C	⇩

hol, smoking habits, red meat, feeding, ingestion of caustics, tylosis a genetic syndrome characterized by palmar and plantar hyperparacheratosis and by an overall risk of oesophageal epidermoid cancer of 60 to 70%, achalasia and infection with papilloma virus increase the risk for squamous cell carcinoma, while a low body-mass index, consumption of fruit, vegetables, white meat, folate, and some carotenoids decrease the risk. Cessation of alcohol and smoking significantly reduces the risk of squamous carcinoma.

BARRETT'S OESOPHAGUS

Population studies suggest that about 1.6% of Europeans have Barrett's oesophagus (BE), a condition in which the squamous epithelium in the distal oesophagus, due to the chronic injury from gastro-oesophageal reflux, is transformed in a metaplastic columnar epithelium. The first description dates back to the English surgeon Norman Barrett in 1950. From the 1960s to the mid-1970s, various histological descriptions followed, including subtypes of columnar epithelium: with villi and goblet cells (known as intestinal metaplasia, IM), junctional epithelium and gastric epithelium (gastric metaplasia, GM). Since the early 1980s, the association between BE and adenocarcinoma and the predisposition for MI to develop dysplasia has been confirmed

Diagnostic Criteria for EB

Oesophagogastroduodenoscopy (EGDS) is the gold standard to diagnose BE. During endoscopy, the following must be recognized: 1 diaphragmatic pinch; 2 the gastro-oesophageal junction; 3 the squamo-columnar junction. Diaphragmatic pinch coincides with the passage point of the oesophagus through the diaphragm and, if there are more than 2 cm from the two junctions, it indicates a sliding hiatal hernia. The gastro-oesophageal junction is the apical point of the gastric folds, while the squamo-columnar junction (Z line) is easily recognizable by the pale pink color of the squamous epithelium while the columnar one has a bright light red color. In the normal oesophagus, the gastro-oesophageal junction coincides with the squamo-columnar junction, whereas when the latter is at least 1 cm from the gastro-oesophageal junction, it suggests the presence of BE. At endoscopy, the circumferential extension (C) of the metaplastic epithelium and the maximal extension (M) of the "flames" from the gastro-oesophageal junction are reported in centimeters (Prague classification, **Figure 9.1**) and biopsies are performed at the four quadrants of the oesophagus at 2 cm intervals along the extension of BE, in addition to biopsies of any suspected areas (Seattle protocol). As the number of oesophageal biopsies increases, the diagnostic accuracy for the diagnosis of BE significantly improves (from 4 to 8 to ≥16 biopsies, from 35% to 68% and 100%, respectively). However, to date, the histological criteria for the diagnosis of BE are controversial. While the American College of Gastroenterology requires as a prerequisite the presence of IM, the British Society of Gastroenterology does not, and considers also GM a marker of BE. Furthermore, an important international working group, called BOBOCAT (Benign

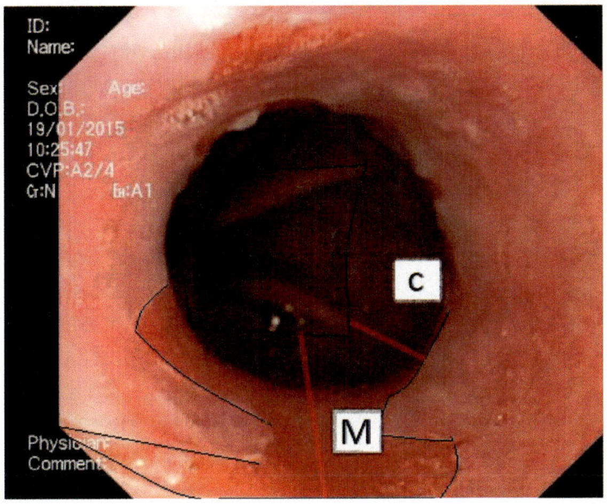

Figure 9.1 Endoscopic image of Barrett's oesophagus. Diaphragmatic pinch, gastro-oesophageal junction, and squamo-columnar junction are shown. The extension of Barrett is denoted with the letters C and M according to Prague classification.

Barrett's and Cancer Taskforce), established that BE is characterized by the presence of columnar epithelium in the oesophagus (including both IM and GM) but that it is important to indicate if IM is present. Indeed, excluding a finding of dysplasia, the two most important risk factors for progression to adenocarcinoma are the length of the affected section and the presence of IM. Since most patients with BE are not diagnosed, techniques have been developed to improve the diagnosis of BE and possibly even the detection of dysplasia. Among these, confocal endomicroscopy with laser beams, endomicroscopy with optical coherence tomography (OCT) and the Cytospongewith subsequent search for trefoil factor-3 (the protein is over-expressed in BE). However, application of these methods is limited to reference centers. The use of intra-vital stains Lugol or Methylene blu) the magnification endoscopy and the virtual chromo-endoscopy as Narrow Banding Imaging (NBI) are more widespread.
The progression of BE to adenocarcinoma is characterized by the appearance, within the metaplastic area, of phenotypiccellular changes in the epithelial layer and defined as high or low grade dysplasia.Given the significant inter-observer variability, concordance between two expert pathologists is recommended before confirming the presence or degree of severity of dysplasia.

Surveillance and Therapy for BE

While screening of persons at greatest risk (e.g., GERD, obesity, smoking) has not proven effective in reducing mortality due to adenocarcinoma, it is generally accepted that endoscopic surveillance of patients with BE can increase survival, providing an early diagnosis of adenocarcinoma. However, data are still insufficient to demonstrate that systematic surveillance of all patients with BE results in decreased mortality due to adenocarcinoma. According to the ESGE guidelines (2017), in absence of dysplasia, the endoscopic surveillance interval depends on the length of the Barrett segment (**Figure 9.2**). A 6-month surveillance interval is recommended for patients with evidence of low grade dysplasia (LGD) confirmed by a second expert pathologist; in absence of dysplasia after 6

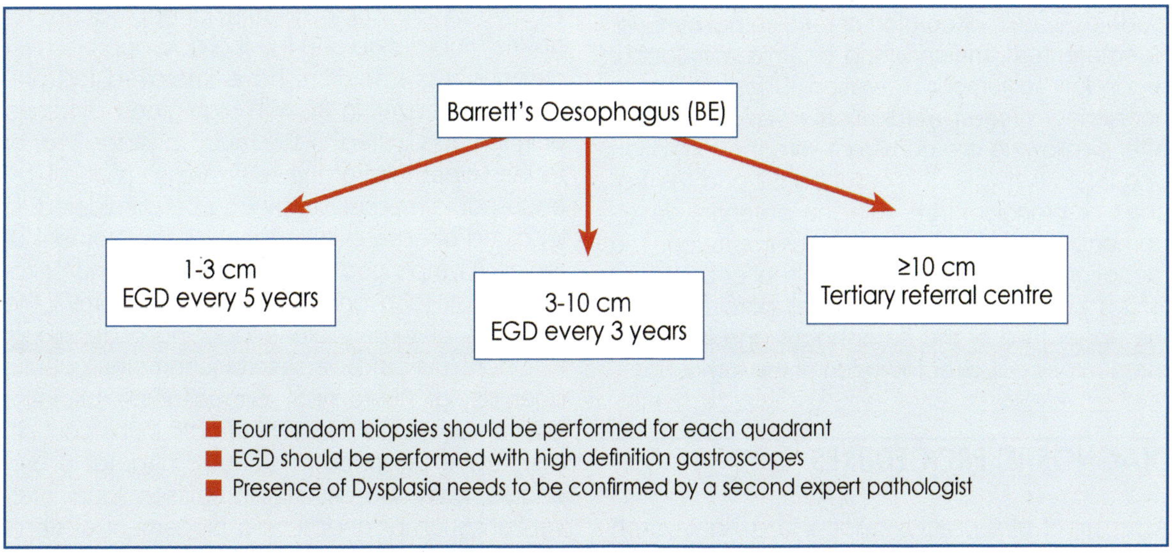

Figure 9.2 Algorithm for the management of Barrett's oesophagus (BE).

months, the surveillance interval can be extended up to 1 year. After 2 consecutive negative controls for dysplasia, the standard endoscopic surveillance for patients with Barrett's oesophagus without dysplasia is indicated. Endoscopic radiofrequency ablation should be proposed if LGD is confirmed in further endoscopic examinations.
Patients with High Grade Dysplasia (HGD) confirmed by a second expert pathologist should be undergone to a further Oesophagogastroduodenoscopy (EGD) performed with High Definition gastroscopes at a referral center: any abnormalities displayed should be removed using endoscopic resection techniques for appropriate histopathological staging. In absence of visible lesions suspected of being dysplasia to a macroscopic assessment, random biopsies should be performed in the four quadrants. If no dysplasia is detected, EGD should be repeated after three months; otherwise in presence of HGD, endoscopic radiofrequency ablation or mucosectomy is recommended. Finally, use of the proton pump inhibitor therapy is recommended in all patients with EB.

CLINICAL CHARACTERISTICS

Small malignancies may be asymptomatic and accidentally discovered during endoscopy performed for other reasons. In advanced stages, in both adenocarcinoma and squamous cell carcinoma, the most frequent clinical presentation is progressive dysphagia for solids due to local progression of the tumour causing obstruction, while dysphagia for liquids may occur later. Dysphagia leads to progressive weight loss, and ultimately to a state of cachexia. Non-specific symptoms may include epigastric discomfort or retrosternal burning. Haematemesis, melena, and anemia may occur secondary to tumour ulceration. Chest pain and hoarseness suggest mediastinal invasion. Coughs after swallowing are consistent with the formation of a fistula between the oesophagus and the trachea or bronchial tree, with the potential development of pneumonia and pleural effusion. The formation of the oesophago-tracheal or bronchial fistulas is typical of squamous cell carcinomas of the upper third of the oesophagus and is the expression of local, direct invasion of the tumour.

DIAGNOSTIC PROCEDURES

Assessment of supraclavicular and axillary lymph node involvement during examination is a crucial goal. Barium oesophagogram could be an option in the initial clinical exam but EGDS with biopsies must be performed for diagnostic confirmation. The execution of multiple biopsies and their large number guarantees a high accuracy of the procedure for histological diagnosis (1 biopsy = 93%, 4 biopsies = 95%, 7 biopsies = 98%).
Computed tomography (CT) of the thorax and abdomen should be performed to evaluate extension of the primary tumour and to look for possible liver metastases and involvement of celiac lymph nodes. However, CT may have some limitations as it is not the method of choice for assessment of intraparietal extension, has a low sensitivity for lymphnode evaluation, and occasionally may underestimate the presence of small metastases, particularly of the peritoneum. Echoendoscopy is the method of choice to assess locoregional extension, with an accuracy of 90% for both oesophageal wall and locoregional lymph node involvement. For the assessment of distant metastases, positron emission tomography (PET/CT) is a valid method

THERAPY

At diagnosis, approximately 40% of patients show distant metastases or invasion of surrounding organs and are judged inoperable. Traditionally, oesophagectomy with mediastinal and upper abdomen lymphadenectomy has long. been the only therapeutic option for high-grade dysplasia and malignant neoplasms of the oesophagus. The surgical procedure is complex and burdened by 2-5% mortality and 30-50% morbidity, particularly due to respiratory complications. Recently, minimally invasive laparoscopic abdominal approaches for gastric mobilization and the thoracic approach for oesophageal resection, have improved the outcome. Moreover, in BE with high-grade dysplasia or in tumours limited to the mucosa (stage T1a) or to the upper third of the sub-mucosa (stage T1b), endoscopic mucosectomy can be considered. In localized disease or when there is involvement of regional lymph nodes, chemotherapy and/or radiotherapy (also concomitant) may improve the outcome of surgery alone inducing a debulking. In distant metastases, several chemotherapeutic agents (e.g., fluorouracil, capecitabine, cisplatin) have shown good palliative effects. In this context, due to the presence of stenosis, intractable dysphagia, pain and difficulty in nutrition, local interventions such as endoscopic placement of stents and/or radiotherapy may be indicated.

KEY CONCEPTS

- Adenocarcinoma and squamous carcinoma account for about 95% of malignant neoplasms of the oesophagus.
- The squamous form and adenocarcinoma have different risk factors, mainly smoking and alcohol consumption for the squamous form and pathological gastro-oesophageal reflux for adenocarcinoma.
- Dysphagia is the first symptom of oesophageal cancer and immediately requires diagnostic investigation by EGDS with biopsies.
- Once a diagnosis has been made, echoendoscopy and a thoracic-abdominal CT scan with contrast will allow correct tumour staging.
- Barrett's oesophagus is a columnar metaplasia of the lower third of the oesophagus, deriving from pathologic gastro-oesophageal reflux. The intestinal type is a risk factor for development of adenocarcinoma and requires endoscopic follow-up.
- If a low-grade dysplasia in Barrett's oesophagus is detected, EGDS will be repeated after 6 months and, if confirmed, endoscopic radiofrequency ablation is indicated.
- Endoscopic mucosectomy and/or radiofrequency endoscopic ablation are recommended in Barrett's oesophagus with high-grade dysplasia or tumours limited to the mucosa (stage T1a) or to the upper third of the submucosa (stage T1b).
- Minimally invasive laparoscopic abdominal approaches for gastric mobilization and the thoracic approach for oesophageal resection have improved clinical outcome.
- In squamous carcinoma, preoperative chemo and radiotherapy facilitate and/or make possible the surgical demolition.

REFERENCES

- Castro C, Peleteiro B, Lunet N. Modifiable Factors and Esophageal Cancer: A Systematic Review of Published Meta-Analyses. J Gastroenterol. 2018;53: 37-51.
- http://www.aiom.it/fondazione-aiom/aiom-airtum-numeri-cancro-2017/1,3021,1 I tumori in Italia rapporto 2017- Aiom/Airtum
- Recio-Boiles A; Babiker HM. Cancer, Esophageal. Stat Pearls Publishing; 2018 Jan- 2017 Oct 22.
- Weusten B, Bisschops R, Coron E et al. Endoscopic management of Barrett's esophagus: European Society of Gastrointestinal Endoscopy (ESGE) Position Statement. Endoscopy. 2017; 49:191-8.

CHAPTER 10

GASTRIC PATHOPHYSIOLOGY

Carola Severi, Marco Montagnani

LEARNING OBJECTIVES

- To know the key concepts of gastric motor activity and how its alteration can affect health and require therapeutic interventions.
- To gain basic knowledge of the role of gastric secretion in macronutrient and mineral digestion and absorption, and to understand the pathophysiology of gastroduodenal diseases.

The stomach performs numerous functions, including food storage, mechanical crushing, and mixing of food with gastric juice, which is rich in acid and enzymes. The stomach is anatomically divided into three regions: the fundus, the corpus, and the antrum. At a functional level it is divided into two regions, proximal and distal, with their respective extensions differing in motor activity and secretion: the gastric corpus motor function, similar to the antrum, while its secretory function is similar to the gastric fundus.

GASTRIC MOTILITY

Concerning motor activity, the stomach is divided into a proximal portion, which includes the fundus and the upper part of the corpus, and a distal portion that includes the remaining part of the corpus and the antrum. The proximal part provides tonic contractions and food storage. The distal part is characterized by peristaltic propulsive activity with low frequency circular contractions. Two completely different motor patterns can be identified: the interdigestive (fasting) motor pattern and the post-prandial motor pattern.

Interdigestive Motor Pattern

During the interdigestive phase, the proximal portion of the stomach maintains a high muscular tone, while the distal portion displays recurrent contractions, migrant motor complexes (MMC). This typical contractile pattern occurs after gastric emptying and originates from a pacemaker area located on the greater curvature, between the fundus and the corpus (**Figure 10.1**), consisting

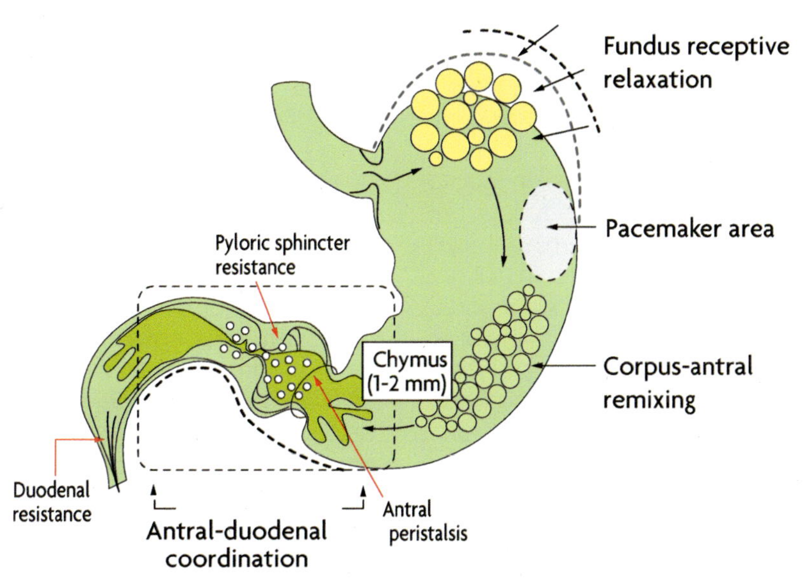

Figure 10.1 Postprandial gastric activity (solid food), modified from Manuale UNIGASTRO 2010-2012.

of the interstitial cells of Cajal. These cells, which act as an interface between enteric nerves and smooth muscle cells, spontaneously generate electric slow waves (3/min) that propagate to the surrounding musculature, maintaining it in a latent activation state and regulating the contractile rhythm.

MMCs are characterized by various phases. Phase I is a protract period of quiescence without motor activity; phase II consists of irregular and random, low amplitude contractions; phase III is characterized by short contractile cycles with high amplitude. Phase III contractions consist of groups of contractile waves that migrate through the small intestine to the terminal ileum at regular intervals during the fasting periods.

Half of the phase III waves originate from the stomach, the other half from the duodenum. The function of phase III contractions is to ensure a pulsatile flow that keeps the stomach and the small intestine free from secretions, food residues, and microorganisms during fasting, and to prepare the stomach to receive the next meal. Phase IV to follow begins with a progressive reduction in motor activity which ends with the recovery of phase I.

The regulation of gastric MMCs is still debated and seems partly due to the central nervous system. The beginning of phase III is regulated by enteric hormones, such as somatostatin (duodenum) and motilin (stomach).

Postprandial Motor Pattern

During the ingestion of food, the motor pattern changes dramatically. The proximal part of the stomach (fundus and proximal corpus) relaxes, functioning initially as a reservoir. This receptive relaxation, without changes in muscle tone (compliance), is mediated by parasympathetic reflexes that reduce cholinergic input and activate the release of nitric oxide, while maintaining low intragastric pressure during food ingestion. Subsequently, the tonic contraction of the fundus and corpus wall moves the food distally, while the contractions of the distal corpus and antrum mix and fragment the food through regular and vigorous contractile circular waves that start from the proximal antrum and proceed towards the pylorus at a frequency of 3 waves per minute. The postprandial motor pattern has three mechanical functions: a reservoir of the proximal part that allows the ingestion of large amounts of food; fragmentation scrambling and crushing of food into smaller particles to be later processed in the intestine; constant and controlled emptying of food into the duodenum (see Figure 10.1).

Gastric motility plays a key role in the regulation of hunger, given that stomach distension activates wall mechanoreceptors which, through the vagus and the splanchnic nerves, transmit neural inputs to the central nervous system, in particular to the nucleus of the solitary tract of the encephalic trunk. Post-prandial fullness seems partly regulated by hormones such as cholecystokinin (CCK) and type 1 glucagon-like peptide (GLP-1), whereas a minor role is ascribed to nutrients (lipids, carbohydrates or proteins). In altered gastric accommodation, e.g., after vagotomy, in Chagas disease (a tropical parasitic disease characterized by extensive myenteric plexus injury) or in patients with functional dyspepsia, the rapid increase in intragastric pressure during food ingestion induces early satiety. Bariatric surgery (e.g., gastric banding) reduces the size of the proximal stomach, thus inducing a sense of early satiety and favoring weight loss.

Gastric emptying of a solid meal typically displays a biphasic pattern: a first phase of redistribution, which can last up to 30-60 minutes, during which the solid food is distributed in the stomach and fragmented into minute particles to allow their successive passage through the pylorus during the second phase of gastric emptying.

The speed of gastric emptying is not influenced by the food (lipids, carbohydrates or proteins) but rather negatively correlates with the acidity, osmolarity, and viscosity of the ingested food and the caloric content of the nutrients, through a duodenal-gastric feedback mechanism mediated by vagus and some hormones (e.g., GLP-1, PYY, and CCK).

The main clinical condition associated to impaired gastric emptying is gastroparesis (**Figure 10.2**). This chronic condition is characterized by symptoms associated to significantly delayed gastric emptying (GE) rate in the absence of any mechanical obstruction. Cardinal symptoms are nausea (95%) and vomiting, that have to occur in a time frame of at least 3 months. Nausea and vomiting may be associated to variable range of functional dyspepsia-related symptoms (early satiation, postprandial fullness, epigastric distention). Mandatory for diagnosis are the absence of a mechanical obstruction and an objective demonstration of delayed GE using a 99mTechnetium-labeled solid meal or 13C- breath test.

The epidemiology of gastroparesis is not established. The idiopathic subgroup is the largest. Principal causes of the secondary subgroup are diabetes (more frequently type 1), surgery (partial gastric resection/vagotomy, bariatric surgery, an-

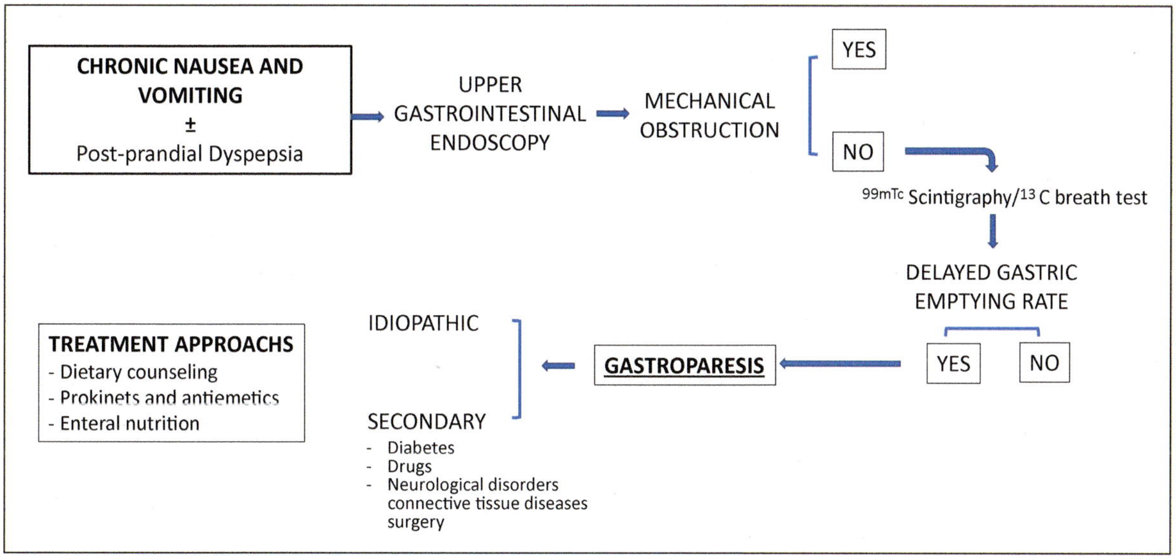

Figure 10.2 Gastroparesis: diagnostic and therapeutic flowchart.

tireflux surgery), some neurological disorders (e.g., Parkinson's disease, multiple sclerosis), some connective tissue diseases and some drugs (e.g., opioids). Minor risks factors are acute gastrointestinal infections and hypothyroidism.
Gastroparesis is associated with a significant decrease in quality of life and is an important source of loss of work productivity. This condition is associated with psychosocial comorbidities, such as anxiety and depression and, in the last years, it proved to be a major source of healthcare costs. As a diagnosis of gastroparesis requires an objective demonstration of delayed gastric emptying, no population-based studies have addressed its prevalence, even if a female predominance has been demonstrated.
Pathophysiology of gastroparesis is not completely clarified since the relationship between symptom severity and emptying delay remains poor. Impaired gastric accommodation to meal and, likely, hypersensitivity to gastric distention contribute to symptom generation while the role of primary neuromuscular alterations remains to be verified. In turn, altered gastric acid secretion, Helicobacter pylori infection, duodenal mucosal or microbiota alterations seem not to be involved in gastroparesis pathophysiology.
Treatment approach is based on the use of prokinetics (5-HT4 receptor agonists) and antiemetics (Dopamine-2 antagonists). A small particle size diet is a useful approach, and a nutritional support in the form of enteral nutrition might be necessary in the more severe forms.

GASTRIC SECRETION

The gastric mucosa has both exocrine and endocrine secretory functions; it can be classified into two anatomic regions: the oxyntic region, which includes the proximal two-thirds of the stomach (fundus and corpus) with predominant exocrine secretion, and the antropyloric region with predominant endocrine secretion.
The gastric mucosa is covered by a surface epithelium distributed on the entire organ composed of mucus and bicarbonates secreting cells, which sinks into the gastric pits (or foveolae) that provide the gastric glands access to the stomach lumen. The gastric gland epithelium varies by gastric region (**Figure 10.3**). The oxyntic mucosa glands are composed of parietal cells that secrete hydrochloric acid and intrinsic factor, chief cells that produce pepsinogens and lipase, and the enterochromaffin-like (ECL) cells producing histamine. In the antral mucosa, the epithelium is predominantly composed of endocrine cells that produce gastrin and somatostatin. Multipotent cells are located in the isthmus of the gastric glands.
The multipotent cells can transform into mucus-secreting cells that migrate to the foveolar zone, or into glandular cells, that migrate towards the bottom of the gland.

Exocrine Secretion

Hydrochloric Acid and Intrinsic Factor
The main product of gastric exocrine secretion is

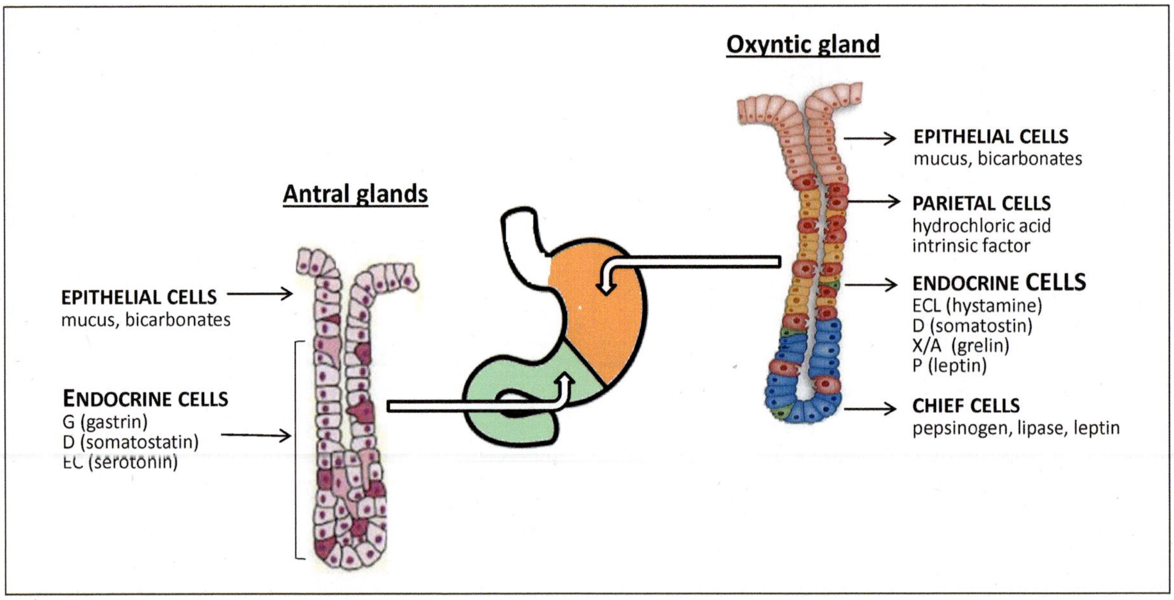

Figure 10.3 Gastric glands.

hydrochloric acid (HCl) produced by the proton pumps (H^+/K^+ ATPase) of the parietal cells in the oxyntic mucosa. The H^+/K^+ ATPase releases hydrogen ions at high concentration (0.16M) first in the glandular lumen that flow in the gastric lumen. The secretion of chloride is activated on the apical membrane. These pumps are contained in cytoplasmic vesicles inside the cells and translocate to the apical membrane only in the presence of a secretory stimulus. HCl production is regulated via nervous, paracrine, and endocrine stimuli (see the section on acid-peptic secretion regulation). The main secretory stimulants are acetylcholine, histamine, and gastrin. Acetylcholine, released by the postganglionic intramural vagal neurons, directly activates muscarinic receptors (subtype M_3). Histamine, produced by ECL cells, activates via the paracrine pathway H_2 receptors. Muscarinic and histaminic receptors are located on the basolateral membrane of the parietal cells. Gastrin, an endocrine hormone secreted by the G cells in the antrum, stimulates the ECL cells to secrete histamine and, to a lesser extent, parietal cells directly by interacting with CCK-2 receptors expressed on the basolateral membrane (**Figure 10.4**).

Gastric acid secretion can be inhibited by the administration of drugs such as proton pump inhibitors (e.g., omeprazole and derivatives) and/or selective H_2 receptor antagonists (e.g., famotidine, ranitidine). Selective antagonists of M3 receptors are not available.

Parietal cells produce the intrinsic factor necessary

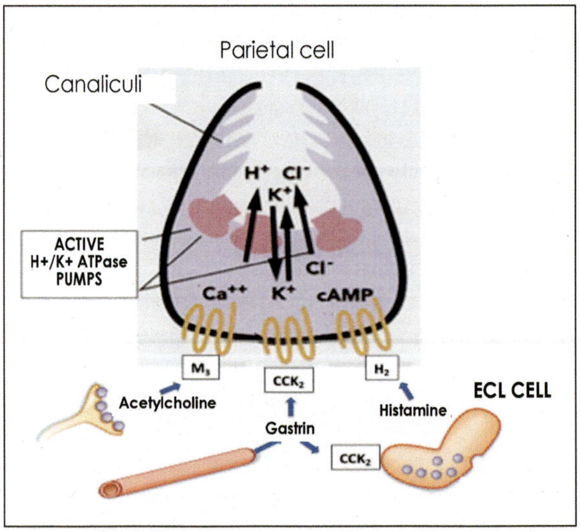

Figure 10.4 Stimulation of gastric parietal cells.

for vitamin B12 absorption. Its secretion is stimulated by the same receptors that activate the secretion of HCl. Therefore, intrinsic factor secretion is inhibited by H_2 antagonists and by vagotomy, but, unlike the acid secretion, not by proton pump inhibitors.

Hydrochloric acid has multiple functions, including antimicrobial activity and promotion of trace minerals absorption. It inhibits microbial growth and protects the intestine from possible colonization by environmental pathogens. Hydrochloric acid promotes the dissociation of insoluble calcium salts and the formation of calcium chloride, whic is very water soluble and easily absorbed at the duodenojejunal level. Moreover, hydrochloric acid is necessary for the dissociation of inorganic (non-heme) iron contained in vegetables and the reduction from its ferric (Fe^{3+}) to ferrous (Fe^{2+}) form which is more soluble. This reaction is facilitated by the presence in gastric juice of ascorbic acid, which binds and maintains in solution the Fe^{2+} ion, allowing its successive absorption by duodenojejunal enterocytes. Hydrochloric acid is also necessary to dissociate the vitamin B12 contained in foods. In the gastric lumen, vitamin B12 is bound by salivary proteins (R proteins). The complex is then hydrolyzed by pancreatic enzymes in the duodenum, where the newly released vitamin B12 is bound by the intrinsic factor (produced by the gastric parietal cells) and transported to the terminal ileum, where it is finally absorbed. A deficient production of hydrochloric acid can lead to iron and vitamin B12 deficiency, i.e., microcytic and hypochromic sideropenic anemia or macrocytic pernicious anemia. Hydrochloric acidic environment of the stomach is also necessary for the absorption of drugs such as thyroxine, L-dopa, and ketoconazole.

Pepsinogens

Another product of gastric secretion is pepsinogen, a pro-enzyme synthesized in the chiet cells ot the oxyntic mucosa that in lthe uminal acid environment is transformed into pepsin, its active form. Pepsin hydrolyses proteins and plays a bactericidal function. The gastric mucosa produces 2 types of pepsinogen.

Type I pepsinogen is produced by the glands of the oxyntic mucosa, while type II pepsinogen is produced by the oxyntic and pyloric mucosa and also by Brunner's duodenal glands. Pepsinogen secretion is controlled by the neuroendocrine mediators that modulate parietal cell secretion. The different production sites of the two types of pepsinogen are explored, in non-invasive diagnostic, to indirectly monitor gastric secretory function. For example, low serum Pepsinogen I levels are indicative of oximetry mucosal atrophy.

Bicarbonates

Other products of exocrine gastric secretion are bicarbonates and mucus, both involved in mucosal protection against the acid-peptic environment. Bicarbonate ions are secreted by the superficial epithelial cells and the parietal cells, concurrently with the secretion of hydrogen ions. In the parietal cells, carbonic anhydrase catalyzes the hydrolysis of carbonic acid (H_2CO_3) into hydrogen ions and bicarbonate ions ($H_2CO_3 \rightarrow H+$ and HCO_3-). While hydrogen ions are secreted by proton pumps into thc glandular lumcn, bicarbonatc ions cross thc cellular basolateral membrane and reach the luminal mucosal surface through mucosal microcirculation, constituted by vessels running along the longitudinal axis of the gastric glands (**Figure 10.5**). This "alkaline tide" creates a pre-epithelial alkaline layer that protects the underlying mucosa from the luminal acid-peptic environment, preventing self-digestion. Mucosal vascular flow is modulated by prostaglandins.

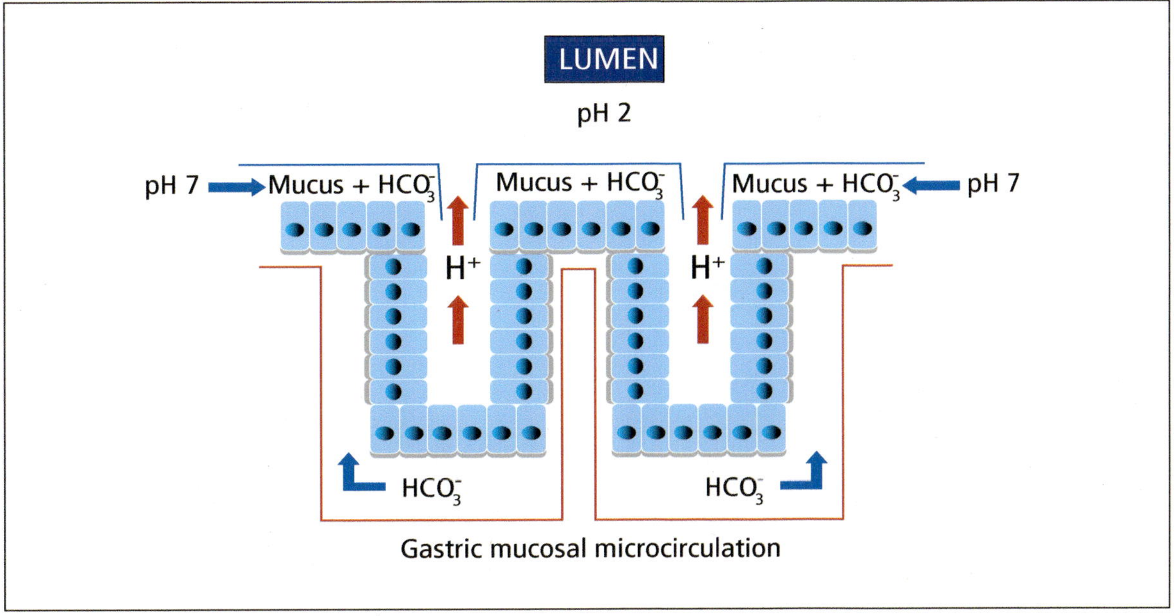

Figure 10.5 The gastric mucosal barrier.

Mucus

The surface epithelial cells of gastric mucosa secrete mucus, whose function is to separate the epithelium from the luminal environment. The mucus is composed of high – molecular – weight glycoproteins, with particular peptide bonds that prevent pepsin digestion. The mucus physical barrier prevents the back diffusion of hydrogen ions and helps maintain an almost neutral pH at the epithelial surface. Besides mucus, the epithelial cells also secrete pepsin-resistant, low – molecular – weight proteins, called trefoil factor.

These proteins have an anti-inflammatory activity and stabilize the mucous gel by increasing its viscosity. Mucus and bicarbonates secretion is stimulated by prostaglandins.

Any condition disrupting these protective mechanisms, such as colonization by *H. pylori* (which enters the mucus and adheres to the epithelial surface) or non-steroidal anti-inflammatory drugs (NSAIDs which reduce the production of prostaglandins) can facilitate the back-diffusion of hydrogen ions and tissue damage and eventually a mucosal lesion.

Endocrine Secretion

Gastric endocrine secretion varies by distribution of endocrine cells in the gastric glands (see Figure 10.3). Gastrin, a key hormone in the control of acid secretion, is produced by gastrin cells (G cells), located in the antral mucosa. Somatostatin, a hormone with inhibitory paracrine action, is produced by D cells located in all gastric glands. In the antral mucosa, somatostatin inhibits gastrin secretion, while in the oxyntic mucosa it inhibits acid secretion by combined modulation of the parietal and the ECL cells. The apical membrane of G and D cells is in contact with the gastric lumen (open cells), so that the pH of the luminal content can modulate their activation.

In the glands of the oxyntic mucosa, ECL cells produce histamine, the main stimulus to induce acid secretion.

Additional endocrine cells producing ghrelin and leptin are located in the oxyntic glands. Ghrelin and leptin are involved in hunger regulation and in body weight control. These two hormones also regulate digestive functions. Ghrelin, an orexigenic hormone produced by X/A cells, stimulates histamine release and acid secretion via a vagal-dependent mechanism. Moreover, modulates gastric motility by inducing gastric emptying and the migrating motor complex.

Leptin is an anorexigenic hormone that regulates the sensation of satiety, slows gastric emptying, and reduces endocrine gastro-intestinal-pancreatic secretions. It is secreted by the P cells located in the deep part of oxyntic glands. Leptin granules have been found within the chief cells, suggesting that leptin might have both endocrine and exocrine functions.

Regulation of Gastric Acid and Peptic Secretion

The regulation of gastric secretion occurs through a series of steps (**Figure 10.6**).

In the initial phase (cephalic phase), gastric stimu-

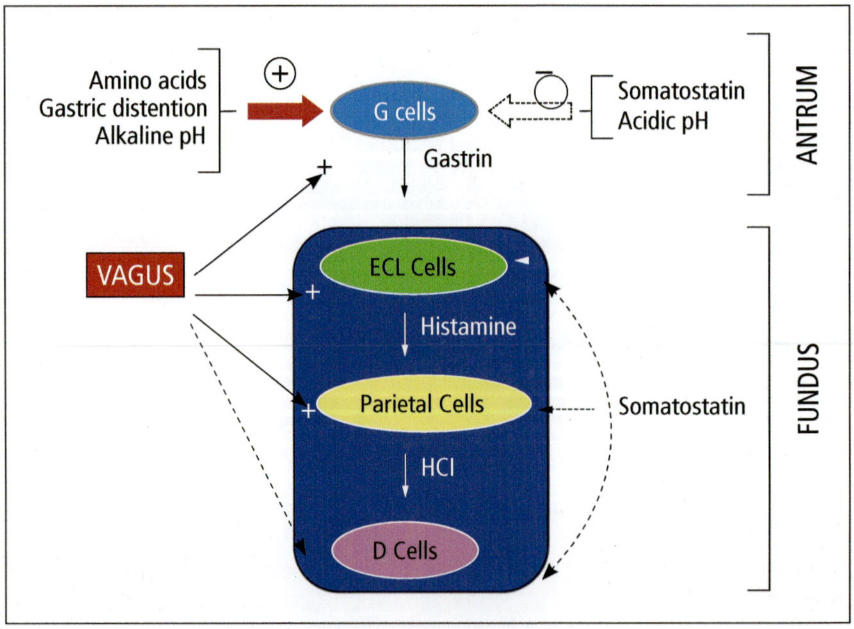

Figure 10.6 Neuroendocrine regulation of the gastric acid secretion.

lation is predominantly vagal. Both the sight of food and gastric distension following food ingestion result in the release of acetylcholine from vagal terminations. Acetylcholine release, in turn, stimulates gastrin production by G cells, histamine production by ECL cells, and direct acid secretion by parietal cells. These mechanisms are further amplified by the inhibitory effect that acetylcholine exerts on somatostatin secretion by D-cells in the antral and the oxyntic glands. In this way, the somatostatin inhibitory effect on G, ECL, and parietal cells is lacking. The next step after vagal stimulation is the gastric phase. Alkalinization due to the presence of food and proteins in the stomach stimulates gastrin secretion, followed byt histamine production by ECL cells, and finally hydrochloric acid secretion by parietal cells. The consequent lowering of luminal pH, in turn, stimulates the production of somatostatin, which starts a new inhibitory feedback on both the G cells and the oxyntic cells.

KEY CONCEPTS

- The main functions of the stomach are motor activity and secretion, both under neuro-endocrine control.
- Motor activity differs between the proximal (fundus) and the distal (corpus/antrum) part. The proximal part acts as a reservoir, while the distal part has a mixing and propulsive activity. The function is to receive and store food, then to mix it with gastric secretions, reducing the solid components into minute particles and promoting the progression of chyme. Disruption of gastric fundus accommodation and gastroparesis are pathophysiological conditions that can contribute to dyspeptic symptoms.
- Secretory activity is both exocrine and endocrine. Exocrine secretion consists of hydrochloric acid, pepsin, and intrinsic factor necessary for food digestion, antimicrobial activity, and absorption of iron, calcium, and vitamin B12. Further secretory products are mucus and bicarbonates, both necessary for mucosal protection against the aggressive action of acid-peptic secretion. Endocrine secretion (gastrin, somatostatin, leptin and ghrelin) plays a regulatory role in exocrine secretion, motor activity, and control of satiety and hunger. Imbalance between aggressive factors (acid, pepsin) and defensive factors (bicarbonates, mucus) of exocrine secretion play an important role in the pathogenesis of peptic disease.

REFERENCES

- Engevik AC, Kaji I, Goldenring JR. The Physiology of the Gastric Parietal Cell. Physiol Rev. 2020;100(2):573-602.
- Hunt RH, Camilleri M, Crowe SE, et al. The stomach in health and disease. Gut. 2015;64(10):1650-68.
- Schol J, Wauters L, Dickman R, et al. United European Gastroenterology (UEG) and European Society for Neurogastroenterology and Motility (ESNM) consensus on gastroparesis. Neurogastroenterol Motil. 2021;33(8):e14237.
- Schubert ML, Rehfeld JF. Gastric Peptides-Gastrin and Somatostatin. Compr Physiol. 2019 Dec 18;10(1):197-228. doi: 10.1002/cphy.c180035. PMID: 31853955.
- Yandrapu H, Sarosiek J. Protective Factors of the Gastric and Duodenal Mucosa: An Overview. Curr Gastroenterol Rep. 2015 Jun;17(6):24.

CHAPTER 11

DYSPEPSIA

Bruno Annibale, Gabrio Bassotti

LEARNING OBJECTIVES

- To know the definition, epidemiology, and classification of dyspepsia.
- To understand the pathophysiological mechanisms of functional dyspepsia.
- To understand the diagnostic path of the patient with dyspeptic symptoms and basic therapeutic concepts.

DEFINITION AND CLASSIFICATION

The term dyspepsia refers to a clinical syndrome characterized by chronic or recurrent symptoms affecting the epigastric region: epigastric pain and/or burning, post-prandial fullness, bloating, early satiety, nausea, and vomiting. Their presence does not predict a specific underlying pathologic condition nor an abnormal gastroduodenal function.

Studies involving large cohorts of dyspeptic patients undergoing upper GI endoscopy, imaging, and laboratory evaluations have identified, two forms of dyspepsia:

- Organic dyspepsia: gastroduodenal mucosal lesions, bilio-pancreatic abnormalities, and/or biochemical abnormalities that correlate with the symptoms (**Table 11.1**);
- Functional dyspepsia structural and/or biochemical abnormalities do not corrrelate with symptoms, even though it is possible to identify microscopic abnormalities of the gastro-duodenal mucosa in subgroups of these patients.

An organic cause of the dyspeptic symptoms is identified in only a minority of patients (Table 11.1), whereas the cause for the complaints remains unknown in most of them. To identify the possible pathophysiological mechanisms underlying the genesis of symptoms, patients with functional dyspepsia (FD) have been catagorized based on the association or the predominance of symptoms suggesting motor abnormalities or gastroduodenal sensitivity. This approach, however, proved ineffective in identifying therapeutic strategies, due to the wide overlap and time variability of dyspeptic symptoms and the frequent association with other gastrointestinal symptoms, such as those related to irritable bowel syndrome (IBS) and gastro-oesophageal reflux disease (GERD).

According to the recent Rome IV criteria, published in 2016, functional dyspepsia, characterized by postprandial fullness, early satiety, epigastric pain, epigastric burning, all symptoms defined as "bothersome" (i.e., severe enough to influence normal daily activities) and in the absence of structural abnormalities, has been subdivided in two forms:

- post-prandial distress syndrome characterized by bothersome symptoms on at least 3 days per week, consisting in post-prandial fullness and/or early satiety (defined as inability to complete a normocaloric meal); as accompanying symptoms epigastric pain or burning may be present;
- epigastric pain syndrome characterized by the bothersome presence on at least 1 day per week of epigastric pain or burning; the pain may be induced or relieved by meal ingestion or appear during fasting, and accompanied by nausea, bloating, or post-prandial belching (**Table 11.2**).

These symptoms must be present in the last three months, must have begun at least six months before, and can co-exist with IBS or GERD. In addition, in both subgroups of FD patients vomiting or pain relieved by bowel movements should direct the clinician toward a different diagnosis.

Table 11.1 Main causes of organic dyspepsia.

- Peptic ulcer with or without *H. pylori*
- Gastro-oesophageal cancer
- Biliary lithiasis
- Drugs (NSAIDs, calcium antagonists, iron supplements, angiotensin-converting enzyme inhibitors, methylxanthines, glucocorticoids)
- Chronic pancreatitis or pancreatic cancer
- Parasitic infections (*Giardia lambia*, strongyloides, anysakis)
- Infiltrative disease (eosinophilic gastroenteritis, sarcoidosis)
- Endocrine-metabolic diseases (diabetes, thyroid diseases)

EPIDEMIOLOGY

Dyspepsia is frequently observed in daily clinical practice. Since symptoms are often mild or of short duration, they are usually self managed and only when they become chronic and/or recurrent is a physician consulted. In Western countries the prevalence of dyspepsia is around 15-30%, with an incidence (new cases/year) of 1-2% mainly among adults aged 40-50 years, without gender predilection.
From an epidemiological point of view it is important to differentiate between dyspeptic patients without previous diagnostic evaluations to exclude organic diseases and those who have undergone such evaluations; the prevalence (50-60%) of FD is greater in these latter patients than in those with organic abnormalities, whose main causes are reported in Table 7.1. For the prevalence of these causes see specific chapters elsewhere in this book.
It is still difficult to estimate the prevalence of FD since, like other "functional" conditions, it is basically a diagnosis of exclusion, which requires invasive and expensive investigations. To further complicate the picture, FD patients are often noted to have a symptom overlap with other functional gastrointestinal conditions, such as IBS (about 30%) and GERD (about 40%).
Concerning the natural history of dyspepsia, prospective epidemiological investigations revealed that, time, about 50% of patients become asymptomatic, whereas about 25% develop symptoms compatible with IBS or GERD. Factors associated with persistence of dyspeptic symptoms or development of lower abdominal symptoms are female gender and high somatization levels.

PATHOPHYSIOLOGY

If it is possible to identify an organic cause (e.g., gastric cancer), the therapeutic approach will be obviously targeted to the specific underlying condition. In functional dyspepsia the pathophysiological mechanisms underlying the onset of symptoms are various and poorly known. Among the mechanisms more extensively investigated are alterations in gastric motility, particularly meal-induced fundic reflex of gastric accommodation, velocity of gastric emptying, abnormal gastroduodenal perception, and concomitant presence of psychological abnormalities (**Table 11.3**).
About 25-40% of FD patients have abnormal gastric emptying after ingestion of a caloric meal, as shown by scintigraphy, octanoic acid breath test, or ultrasound evaluation of gastric emptying. Delayed or accelerated gastric emptying may be associated with post-prandial fullness, bloating, early satiety, nausea, and vomiting. In about 40% of patients, an altered gastric fundus accommodation after meal ingestion may be documented. This increases intragastric pressure, tension of the gastric wall, and activation of specific mechanoreceptors, causing early satiety and post-prandial fullness.
Failure to relax the gastric fundus appropriately also causes antral distension, associated with epigastric distension and, in a subgroup of patients, post-prandial drowsiness.
Dyspeptic symptoms without meal ingestion may be reported by patients: the main complaint is epigastric pain and/or burning. Such patients present visceral hypersensitivity, with a decreased threshold of activation of gastric mechanoreceptors to pressure stimuli. In addition, recent studies have

Table 11.2 Rome IV Diagnostic criteria for diagnosis of functional dyspepsia.

- Postprandial distress syndrome (PDS): bothersome postprandial fullness and/or early satiety severe enough to impact on usual activities or finishing a regular size meal on at least 3 days a week. Other gastrointestinal symptoms may coexist with PDS.
- Epigastric pain syndrome (EPS): bothersome epigastric pain and/or burning severe enough to impact on usual activities at least once a week. Other gastrointestinal symptoms may coexist with EPS.*

Functional dyspepsia is diagnosed if a patient reports having ≥1 of these symptoms for the past 3 months with onset at least 6 months before diagnosis, without evidence of organic disease that is likely to explain the symptoms.

*PDS and EPS may coexist.

Table 11.3 Pathophysiology of functional dyspepsia: mechanisms and symptoms.

Mechanism	Associated Symptoms
	Delayed gastric emptying
Post-prandial fullness, epigastric bloating, nausea,	
	vomiting, weight loss
Visceral hypersensitivity to gastric distention	Epigastric pain
Abnormal gastric accommodation	Early satiety, weight loss
Acid and/or lipid duodenal hypersensitivity	Epigastric pain, nausea

highlighted the possible pathophysiologic role of gastric chemical receptors, particularly toward acidic solutions and/or fatty substances.

Although often classified as having "functional" dyspepsia, some FD patients actually display microscopic organic abnormalities, as demonstrated by low-grade inflammation with increased number of macrophages and eosinophils within the duodenal mucosa. This kind of inflammation might be one of the pathophysiological mechanisms responsible for chemical stimuli hypersensitivity. It is likely associated with increased mucosal permeability that allows, direct stimulation of nerve fibers by the acid load in the duodenum. Supporting such hypothesis is the clinical observation that drugs inhibiting acid secretion (H2 antagonists or proton pump inhibitors) reduce the severity of symptoms in more than 35% of dyspeptic patients. However, notwithstanding the evidence for altered visceral perception the basic mechanisms causing abnormal processing of visceral stimuli by the central nervous system are still unclear.

The importance of psychosocial factors in FD patients is confirmed by the clinical observation that they often complain of symptom worsening during "stressful" episodes, from positive response to reassurance after excluding organic conditions, and by the clinical benefit deriving from antidepressants administration and/or psychological therapies.

The role of *H. pylori* infection in the pathogenesis of symptoms in FD is still under debate. In fact, although the infection is almost always associated with active chronic gastritis, there is no firm evidence that this histopathological finding causes dyspeptic symptoms or motor or perceptive abnormalities of the stomach. In addition, eradication of the pathogen does not significantly relieve symptoms in the long term.

Just as observed in post-infectious IBS, so too for FD it has been hypothesized that a previous episode of acute gastroenteritis (bacterial, viral, protozoan infestation) might be a risk factor to develop, even after years, dyspeptic symptoms. Some prospective cohort studies seem to confirm this hypothesis, with additional risk factors including female gender, cigarette smoking, and previous presence of IBS symptoms.

Hence, it is quite clear that FD is a multifactorial condition, whose aetiology is still unknown; though the pathophysiological mechanisms may contribute to explain some symptoms, often there is no significant association between these mechanisms and specific symptoms.

CLINICAL APPROACH TO THE DYSPEPTIC PATIENT

The management of dyspepsia starts with the differentiation between organic and functional dyspepsia (**Figure 11.1**).

Like other pathological conditions, accurate history taking is of paramount importance to gain information for a correct diagnostic and therapeutic approach, carefully looking for possible alarm signs and/or symptoms also by means of blood chemistry and upper abdominal ultrasound scans (**Table 7.4**) suggestive of an organic condition and orienting toward more invasive diagnostic approaches. To date, the clinical dogma that a patient with alarm symptoms needs upper endoscopy to exclude malignancies of the upper gut still holds, although in Western countries, including Italy, the prevalence of oesophagogastric malignancies is relatively low.

Based on findings from accurate history and physical examination, in the absence of sign/symptoms of alarm, after having excluded organic or secondary causes for the onset of symptoms (see Table 11.1) and the concomitant presence of symptoms attributable to IBS or GERD, the diagnostic and therapeutic options (**Figure 11.1**), are:

- Empirical medical therapy for 2-4 weeks with antacids or gastric acid secretion inhibitors,

with endoscopic evaluation therapeutic failure;
- Upper endoscopy and specific therapy (e.g., finding a gastric ulcer);
- Non-invasive testing for *H. pylori* infection and eradicating therapy in positive cases.

Since the likelihood to encounter in clinical practice a FD patient is about 50-60%, the decision to perform an early upper endoscopy depends on the costs and the availability of the technique.

In countries like Italy, where the prevalence of *H. pylori* infection is about 20%, and that of gastric cancer is relatively low (<2%), the best cost-benefit option in patients aged <50 years seems to be *H. pylori* testing and eradicating therapy in positive cases. In fact, this approach will successfully treat patients with ulcers associated with *H. pylori* infection, presumably responsible for dyspeptic symptoms, and also a small subgroup of FD patients.

THERAPY

The reader is referred to the relative chapters discussing the organic causes of dyspepsia. Concerning FD, as in other functional gastrointestinal disorders, the magnitude of symptoms strongly depends on the psycho-emotional status of the patient, with symptoms often apparently not having any causal explanation. Therefore, the therapeutic response may be favorably influenced by a correct diagnostic and therapeutic methodological approach, as shown by the high placebo response rate.

For these above reasons, it is of paramount importance to identity the beliefs often accompanying the patient's history with the use of simple and understandable explanation for the genesis of symptoms, and assessing each time the patient's capacity to understand. Once the diagnosis is made,

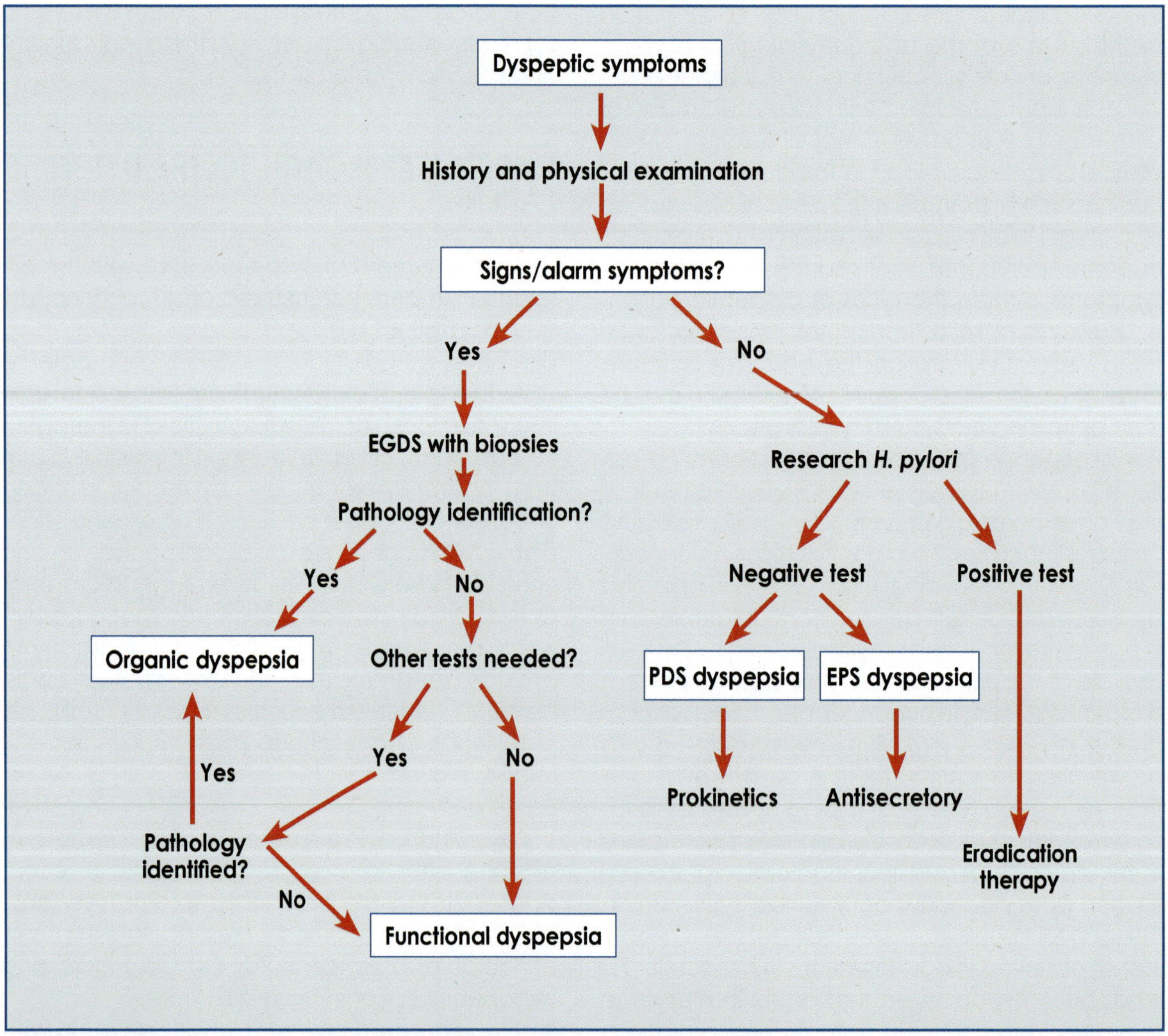

Figure 11.1 Diagnostic-therapeutic algorithm in patients with dyspeptic symptoms.

Table 11.4 Alarm symptoms in dyspeptic patients imposing performance of gastroscopy.

Alarm Symptoms in Dyspeptic Patients Requiring Gastroscopy
New-onset dyspepsia at age >55 years
Dysphagia and/or odynophagia
Persistent vomiting
Unintentional weight loss
Iron-deficiency anemia
Signs or Clinical Conditions Requiring Upper Gastrointestinal Endoscopy
Family history of gastric or oesophageal cancer
Palpable abdominal mass or adenopathy

there is the need to reassure the patient by focusing on the main worries and allaying their fears.
The pharmacologic approach is multifaceted, due to the uncertain pathogenesis and the mechanisms possibly involved.
Among commercially available drugs, the most widely used are, alone or in combination: gastric acid secretion inhibitors; prokinetics; also acting drugs on gastric fundus accommodation; antidepressants.
Whatever the therapeutic choice guided by the symptomatic classification of FD, it is always wise to follow the symptoms over time course and, not continuous, to prefer brief treatments repeated several times in patients with frequent symptom relapse.

KEY CONCEPTS

- Dyspepsia is frequently observed (15-40%) in the general population. In most cases it is functional since no organic or biochemistry abnormalities responsible for symptom onset be detected.
- There is considerable overlap between functional dyspepsia and other functional gastrointestinal disorders, such as irritable bowel syndrome and gastro-oesophageal reflux disease.
- The clinical approach to the dyspeptic patient includes careful search possible alarm symptoms suggesting organic disease and needing specific procedures such as upper endoscopy.

REFERENCES

- Du L, Chen B, Kim JJ, et al. Micro-inflammation in functional dyspepsia: a systematic review and meta-analysis. Neurogastroenterol Motil. 2018;30:e13304.
- Enck P, Azpiroz F, Boeckxstaens G, et al. Functional dyspepsia. Nat Rev Dis Primers. 2017;3:17081.
- Koduru P, Irani M, Quigley EMM. Definition, pathogenesis, and management of that cursed dyspepsia. Clin Gastroenterol Hepatol. 2018;16:467-79.
- Stanghellini V, Chan FK, Hasler WL, et al. Gastroduodenal Disorders. Gastroenterology. 2016;150:1380-92.
- Yamawaki H, Futagami S, Wakabayashi M, et al. Management of functional dyspepsia: state of the art and emerging therapies. Ther Adv Chronic Dis. 2018;9:23-32.

CHAPTER 12

HELICOBACTER PYLORI INFECTION AND RELATED DISEASES

Rocco Maurizio Zagari, Marco Romano

LEARNING OBJECTIVES

- To understand the epidemiology of *Helicobacter pylori* infection.
- To understand the role of *H. pylori* in the aetiopathogenesis, of digestive and extra-digestive diseases.
- To understand the epidemiology, aetiopathogenesis, clinical features, diagnosis and therapy of peptic ulcer.
- To understand the diagnostic tests and treatment for *H. pylori* infection.

INTRODUCTION

In 1982, two Australian researchers, Warren and Marshall, identified a bacterium, first called Campylobacter and then, due to its spiral shape, *Helicobacter (H) pylori*, in the stomach of a patient with chronic gastritis.
H. pylori infection causes chronic gastritis of varying severity in all infected patients. In a subgroup of patients, *H. pylori* also causes other digestive diseases, such as peptic ulcer, gastric malignancies, and extra-digestive diseases.
The consequences of *H. pylori* infection depend on the interaction between the virulence of the bacterial strain, the environmental factors, and the genetic predisposition of the subject.
These factors play an important role in the outcome of the infection, being able to determine the location and severity of the gastric inflammation, and also its clinical evolution (peptic ulcer, stomach tumours).

EPIDEMIOLOGY AND TRANSMISSION PATHWAYS OF *H. PYLORI*

H. pylori infection is one of the most diffuse in the world, with a prevalence, that varies in different populations and is inversely related to socio-economic conditions.
Though the prevalence of *H. pylori* infection has declined over recent decades due to improved socio-economic conditions, it still affects approximately 30-40% of the general population in Italy and Europe. The infection is usually acquired early, in infancy, via ingestion of the bacterium and then tends to persist for life. The transmission pathways are still unclear, but inter-human fecal-oral and/or oral-oral transmission is the most plausible pathway.

PATHOGENIC MECHANISMS OF *H. PYLORI*-INDUCED DAMAGE

H. pylori is a gram-negative spiral-shaped, micro-anaerobic bacterium that is able to survive in the acidic environment of the stomach, where it penetrates into the mucus layer and reaches the gastric epithelium, aided by three colonization factors: urease, flagella, and adhesins. Urease is an enzyme that hydrolyses the urea in the gastric lumen, generating ammonia and bicarbonate. These neutralize intragastric acidity, creating an alkaline, protective environment around the bacterium. The flagella provides for mobility, while the adhesins on the bacterial surface allow it to adhere to the gastric epithelium.
H. pylori is almost always localized in the mucus-bicarbonate layer lining the gastric epithelium.
H. pylori exerts its pathogenic effect on the mucosa by means of two mechanisms: inducing an inflammatory response and releasing enzymes and toxins.
The inflammatory response of the gastric mucosa is induced by numerous antigenic substances, such as urease and lipopolysaccharides, which activate T lymphocytes and macrophages, with the consequent release of pro-inflammatory cytokines, such as Interleukin 1 (IL-1), 6 (IL-6) and 8 (IL-8). Furthermore, *H. pylori* produces toxins that alter the mucus layer and damage the gastric mucosa. Approximately 60% of *H. pylori* strains produce

cytotoxin-associated gene A (CagA), encoded by the cagA gene and the vacuolating cytotoxin A (VacA) encoded by the vacA gene.

In particular, by means of the type IV secretion system, which is one of the products of the cag pathogenicity island (*cagPAI*), a 30-gene DNA insert, the bacterium inoculates inside the epithelial cell the cytotoxin CagA, which induces the production of a large quantity of IL-8 by the epithelial cell. Moreover, CagA induces a modification of the cytoskeleton of the epithelial cell and plays an important role in gastric carcinogenesis, stimulating cell proliferation and favoring epithelial-mesenchymal transition. Another important virulence factor is VacA, a protein that induces the formation of vacuoles in epithelial cells. VacA plays an important role in the survival of the bacterium, increasing the permeability of the gastric epithelium, thus facilitating the acquisition of substances needed for its survival. Among the CagA and VacA positive *H. pylori* strains, those which express the genotype of vacA s1m1 cause a more intense inflammation and more severe damage to the gastric mucosa, with a consequently greater risk of developing gastric cancer.

CHRONIC GASTRITIS

H. pylori infection causes acute gastritis that subsequently, due to the persistence of the bacterium, becomes chronic.

In fact, the bacterium is capable of eluding the immune response of the host, probably by stimulating the production of factors that inhibit T lymphocyte activity.

Chronic gastritis from *H. pylori* usually affects the antrum; however, in a subgroup of patients, it can also extend to the entire stomach (pangastritis). *H. pylori* always causes active chronic gastritis, which is characterized by the presence of neutrophil granulocytes in the lamina propria in addition to chronic inflammatory cells, such as lymphocytes and plasma cells.

In the majority of patients, chronic gastritis from *H. pylori* is asymptomatic, without developing symptoms, digestive or extra-digestive diseases.

In a subgroup of patients, *H. pylori*-related chronic gastritis causes dyspeptic symptoms. It has been estimated that *H. pylori* gastritis is the cause of dyspeptic symptoms, such as epigastric pain, post-prandial fullness, and early satiety in approximately 10% of patients with endoscopically-negative dyspepsia.

The fact that gastritis from *H. pylori* can be a cause of dyspepsia has led to a change in the diagnosis of functional dyspepsia, which is currently not only based on the endoscopic exclusion of organic lesions of the upper digestive tract (ulcers, neoplasias, etc.) but also on the exclusion of *H. pylori* infection or, in patients with *H. pylori* gastritis, on the persistence of symptoms after eradication of the infection.

The eradication of *H. pylori* is associated with regression of gastritis, with disappearance of neutrophils and a marked reduction in lymphocytes and plasma cells in the gastric mucosa. Thus, the patient goes from active chronic gastritis to a so-called quiescent chronic gastritis and, over time, can also have complete restitutio ad integrum of the mucosa. The eradication of *H. pylori* also brings a reduced risk of dyspepsia and *H. pylori*-related diseases if they have not already developed.

PEPTIC ULCER

Definition

Peptic ulcer is a lesion of the mucosa and submucosa that sometimes also reaches the muscolaris propria. In recent decades, in parallel with the reduced prevalence of *H. pylori* infection, the incidence of peptic ulcer has drastically decreased and is diagnosed in only approximately 5-9% of patients with dyspepsia.

Aetiopathogenesis

Peptic ulcer has a multifactorial aetiopathogenesis, but it is always the result of an imbalance between aggressive factors (hydrochloric acid and pepsin) and defensive factors (mucus and bicarbonates) of the gastroduodenal mucosa.

H. pylori is the most frequent cause of peptic ulcer, being responsible for approximately 80% of gastric and duodenal ulcers.

Another frequent cause of peptic ulcer is the use of non-steroidal anti-inflammatory drugs (NSAIDs), including low-dose aspirin (see the chapter "Chronic gastritis and gastropathy caused by drugs").

In approximately 3-5% of the cases peptic ulcer is caused by pathological conditions associated with an increase in acid secretion, such as Zollinger-Ellison syndrome and antral G-cell hyperplasia, or from surgical stress.

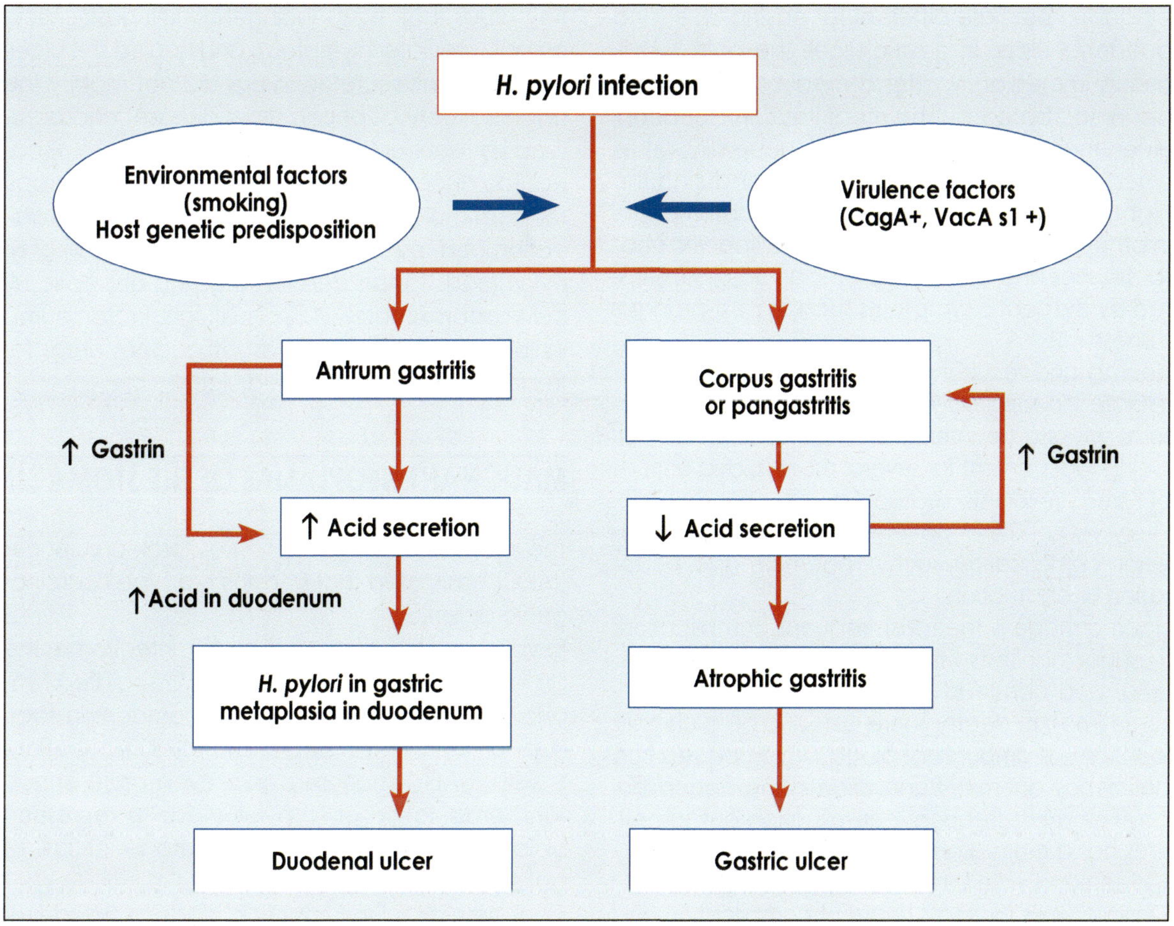

Figure 12.1 The role of *H. pylori* in the pathogenesis of gastric and duodenal ulcers.

The pathogenetic mechanisms by which *H. pylori* causes peptic ulcer are still not clear, even if the pathogenic process underlying the development of duodenal ulcer seems to differ from that which leads to gastric ulcer ((**Figure 12.1**).

In general, duodenal ulcer is associated with chronic antral gastritis and acid hypersecretion, which is a consequence of an increased production of gastrin.

Hypergastrinemia can be due to various factors linked to *H. pylori*, including inhibition of somatostatin secretion, a hormone produced by D cells that, inhibits the liberation of gastrin by G cells.

However, gastrin hypersecretion is associated with acid hypersecretion in only 10% of patients with antral gastritis from *H. pylori*. These patients likely have either an increased number of parietal cells or parietal cells that respond in an exaggerated manner to gastrin.

Acidic hypersecretion can contribute to the development of areas of gastric metaplasia in the duodenal bulb as a response to the increased duodenal acid load. These areas may then be colonized by *H. pylori*, with the consequent development of duodenitis and, ultimately, peptic ulcer.

Unlike duodenal ulcer, gastric ulcer is associated with chronic atrophic gastritis which affects the entire stomach (pangastritis) with reduced acid secretion.

The pathogenesis of gastric ulcer is likely consequent to a reduction in the defense mechanisms of the mucosa to peptic-acid attack. It is the consequence of chronic inflammation and of the damage to the mucosa by *H. pylori*.

Clinical Features

Although peptic ulcer can be asymptomatic and may appear with a complications, such as haemorrhage, in the majority of cases it causes epigastric pain. Classically, the characteristics of epigastric pain are different for gastric ulcer and duodenal ulcer. In gastric ulcer, the pain is dull, arising immediately after a meal or it can even be exacerbated by the meal itself. In duodenal ulcer the pain is burning and generally arises when fasting, 2-3 hours after meals or during the night, and it is attenuated by food consumption. In other cases, the pain presents less specific characteristics and can be accompanied or substituted by dyspeptic symptoms such as post-prandial fullness.

Healing and recurrences characterize an *H. pylori*-related peptic ulcer, and, consequently, symptoms will also be intermittent, with periods of wellbeing that can last for several months, and periods of flares, prevalently seasonal in spring and autumn. Every year, 1-2% of patients with peptic ulcer develop complication, such as haemorrhage, perforation or obstruction.

Haemorrhage is the most frequent complication; it usually manifests with haematemesis and/or melena, and can lead to hypovolemic shock and, sometimes, to death. There can also be a chronic loss of small amounts of blood, which causes iron deficiency anemia. Perforation in the abdominal cavity is a less frequent complication but sometimes has a more dramatic onset characterized by sudden and violent abdominal pain.

Obstruction is the least frequent complication and is usually due to pyloric sub-stenosis or stenosis caused by fibrosis and/or scar-induced deformation of the pyloric channel. The typical symptoms of obstruction are nausea and postprandial vomiting.

Diagnosis

Although a classic clinical presentation may allow a clinical diagnosis, a definitive diagnosis of peptice ulcer is based on oesophagogastroduodenoscopy.

Upper endoscopy has a sensitivity of 95-100% and allows biopsies of the gastric mucosa for the diagnosis of *H. pylori* infection by means of a rapid urease test and/or histological examination. In patients with gastric ulcer, histological examination also permits differential diagnosis between benign gastric ulcer and a neoplastic ulcer. Radiological examination with barium meal is less sensitive and should be reserved for rare cases of contra-indication to endoscopic examination.

Therapy

Before the discovery of *H. pylori*, the therapy for peptic ulcer was exclusively based on anti-secretory drugs that, by reducing the intra-gastric acid output, alleviated symptoms and healed the ulcer. However, anti-secretory drugs did not modify the natural history of peptic ulcer disease, characterized by recurrences within one year in 80% of cases. The discovery of *H. pylori* modified the therapy for peptic ulcer that currently relies on the eradication of *H. pylori* infection. The eradication of *H. pylori* leads to the definitive healing of peptic ulcer in approximately 90% of patients. Proton pump inhibitors (PPIs) are the most efficacious drugs for treating non-H.pylori-related ulcers.

MALIGNANT NEOPLASIAS OF THE STOMACH

The International Agency for Research on Cancer (IARC) has stated that *H. pylori* is a Type I carcinogenic agent.

Beyond gastric cancer, *H. pylori* infection is the principal cause of MALT (mucosa-associated lymphoid tissue) lymphoma of the stomach. In fact, *H. pylori* is present in approximately 80% of patients with MALT lymphoma and, even more important, eradication of *H. pylori* leads to regression of low-grade malignant lymphoma in 70-80% of patients.

Over time, *H. pylori* infection leads to the development of lymphatic follicles from the aggregation of T and B lymphocytes in the gastric mucosa, which are the necessary prerequisite for the development of lymphoma. However, only rarely does lymphoid tissue undergo genetic and phenotypic transformations leading to the development of lymphoma.

H. pylori is the most important risk factor for intestinal-type gastric adenocarcinoma. A meta-analysis of randomized clinical trials showed that the eradication of *H. pylori* significantly reduced the risk of developing gastric cancer.

H. pylori exerts its carcinogenic activity by three different mechanisms:

- inducing chronic inflammation of the gastric mucosa (chronic gastritis);
- causing an increase in oxidative stress;
- causing genetic and epigenetic mutations with activation of oncogenes and/or inactivation of tumour suppressor genes.

There is no doubt that chronic inflammation is the principal carcinogenic mechanism. *H. pylori* causes chronic gastritis which, in some patients, can evolve into atrophic gastritis and intestinal metaplasia, pre-cancerous conditions that predispose to the development of dysplasia and cancer. Infection with *H. pylori* CagA positive strains is associated with greater alterations in gastric epithelial cells and mucosal inflammation, consequently, with a greater risk of developing precancerous conditions and gastric cancer. In addition to the virulence factors of the bacterium, other co-factors in the gastric carcinogenic process are, however, necessary, such as genetic predisposition of the infected patient and environmental factors, such as smoking and diet. In fact, a diet rich in salt activates genes that encode other membrane proteins involved in adhesion of the bacterium to the host cell, whereas a diet rich in vegetables and antioxidants prevents oxidative damage to DNA.

The prophylactic eradication of *H. pylori* is currently recommended in patients at high risk for stomach cancer, such as those with prior gastric cancer (to reduce the risk of metachronous cancer) and first-degree relatives of patients with gastric cancer.

EXTRA-DIGESTIVE DISEASES

H. pylori has been implicated in the aetiopathogenesis of a number of extra-digestive diseases. Currently, *H. pylori* is clearly involved in the pathogenesis of the following extra-digestive diseases:

- idiopathic iron deficiency anemia;
- idiopathic thrombocytopenic purpura;
- vitamin B12 deficiency.

The association between *H. pylori*-related chronic gastritis and idiopathic iron deficiency anemia has been demonstrated in both adults and children. Two recent meta-analyses showed that the eradication of *H. pylori* improves anemia and haemoglobin levels in patients with moderate-severe iron deficiency anemia not otherwise explained.

Chronic atrophic gastritis induced by *H. pylori* in the body of the stomach can lead to a reduction in hydrochloric acid secretion (hypochloridia), followed by malabsorption of the ferric iron "Fe+++" introduced with foods, which is not converted, or is only partially converted into absorbable ferrous iron "Fe++".

Recent studies have reported an improvement in platelet count in patients with idiopathic thrombocytopenic purpura after the eradication of *H. pylori* infection. For example, one study reported an approximately 50% increase in platelets in patients in whom *H. pylori* infection was eradicated and 9% increase in those with idiopathic thrombocytopenic purpura in whom *H. pylori* infection was not eradicated.

Regarding the association between *H. pylori* and malabsorption of vitamin B12, one meta-analysis has shown that among patients with an unexplained vitamin B12 deficiency, the haematic levels of vitamin B12 were lower in those with *H. pylori* infection. The eradication of *H. pylori* in these patients led to an increase in the hematic levels of vitamin B12.

As for iron deficiency anemia, malabsorption of vitamin B12 is likely associated with the development of atrophic gastritis of the body of the stomach, with impaired production of the intrinsic factor by the parietal cells.

Guidelines recommend testing for *H. pylori*, and eradicating the infection if presentin, patients with iron deficiency anemia or vitamin B12 deficiency that cannot be attributed to other causes, and those with idiopathic thrombocytopenic purpura.

DIAGNOSIS OF *H. PYLORI* INFECTION

Diagnostic tests for *H. pylori* infection are classified as "invasive", i.e., those carried out on bioptic specimens of the gastric mucosa obtained by endoscopic examination, and "non-invasive".

Invasive tests are:

- rapid urease test;
- histological examination;
- culture.

The rapid urease test is carried out by introducing a gastric biopsy into a solution containing urea and an indicator of pH, phenol red. The urease of *H. pylori* hydrolyses the urea, producing ammonia and bicarbonate, thus increasing the pH and turning the color from yellow to red. The rapid urease test is highly accurate in diagnosing *H. pylori* infection, with a sensitivity and specificity of 90% and 95%, respectively.

Histological examination with Giemsa staining or silver impregnation (Wartin-Starry) has a sensitivity and a specificity of up to 99%. Since *H. pylori* has a patchy distribution in the gastric mucosa, the histological examination is carried out on at least two biopsies of the gastric mucosa collected from both the antrum and the body of the stomach.

Culture is complex and costly and, as such, is rarely used. However, culture permits testing the sensitivity of the bacterium to antimicrobials and it is recommended after at least two therapeutic failures or to monitor the development of resistance in various geographic areas.
Invasive tests lose sensitivity if carried out during or shortly after therapy with antibiotics or PPIs. Antibiotics and PPIs should be stopped at least 4 and 2 weeks, respectively, before administering the test. Antibiotics and PPIs reduce the bacterial load of *H. pylori* and transform *H. pylori* from the bacillary to the coccoid form, which is difficult to identify at histological examination; in addition, since the coccoid form does not produce urea, a false negative results on the rapid urease test.
Non-invasive tests are:

- ^{13}C-urea breath test (^{13}C-UBT);
- stool antigen test;
- serology.

The ^{13}C-UBT is a simple and highly accurate test, having a sensitivity and specificity > 95%, both before and after antibiotic therapy. A small quantity of urea labelled with carbon 13 (^{13}C-urea) is administered to the patient orally and two breath samples are taken, before and 30 minutes after administration of urea.
An increase in $^{13}CO_2$ in the breath sample taken after the intake of ^{13}C-urea indicates the presence of *H. pylori* infection.
The stool antigen test is based on an immune-enzymatic method with the use of antibodies that demonstrate *H. pylori* antigens in the stools.
The monoclonal stool test has a high accuracy similar to that of the ^{13}C-UBT in the initial diagnosis and after antibiotic treatment. The limitations of the ^{13}C-UBT and of the stool antigen test are the same as those described for invasive tests: they should not be carried out during treatment with PPIs or antibiotics but rather two (PPIs) or four (antibiotics) weeks after discontinuation of these drugs, respectively.
Serology consists of the detection of immunoglobulin G (IgG) antibodies in the serum against antigens of *H. pylori* by means of the enzyme-linked immunosorbent assay (ELISA).
Serology is less expensive but it cannot differentiate a previous infection from an ongoing one since the IgG antibodies often persist in the blood for years after eradication of the bacterium.
Serology is less accurate test for diagnosing active *H. pylori* infection, and its use in clinical practice should be discouraged. The anti-*H. pylori* IgG test, is not influenced by the assumption of PPIs and antibiotics, and can be used in patients who cannot suspend treatment with these drugs.

THERAPY FOR *H. PYLORI* INFECTION

In the past decade, the increase in the prevalence of *H. pylori* strains resistant to antibiotics has made its eradication more difficult. The most recent guidelines recommend using one of the following therapeutic regimens.
Quadruple therapy without bismuth, also called concomitant, (PPI + clarithromycin 500mg + amoxicillin 1000 mg + metronidazole 500mg twice a day) for 10-14 days or quadruple therapy with bismuth for 10 days. Bismuth quadruple therapy is available in Italy in the so-called "3-in-1 pill" formulation in which three antimicrobials (tetracycline 125 mg, metronidazole 125 mg, and bismuth sub-citrate 140 mg) are contained in one capsule. The therapy consists in three capsules four times a day, taken after meals and at bedtime in combination with a PPI administered twice a day.
Triple therapy with clarithromycin (PPI + clarithromycin 500 mg + metronidazole 500 mg or amoxicillin 1000 twice a day) for 14 days is indicated in areas with a low prevalence of *H. pylori* strains resistant to clarithromycin and in patients who had never taken this antibiotic before.
In failure, a second line therapy with bismuth quadruple therapy, if not already used, or triple therapy with levofloxacin (PPI + levofloxacin 250 mg + amoxicillin 1000 mg twice a day) for 10 days are the recommended regimens. In additional failure, culture followed by an antimicrobial susceptibility test should guide the therapy, based on the susceptibility of *H. pylori* to antibiotics (**Figure 12.2**).
If an antimicrobial susceptibility test is not available, one of the previous empirical therapies could be prescribed, if not previously used.

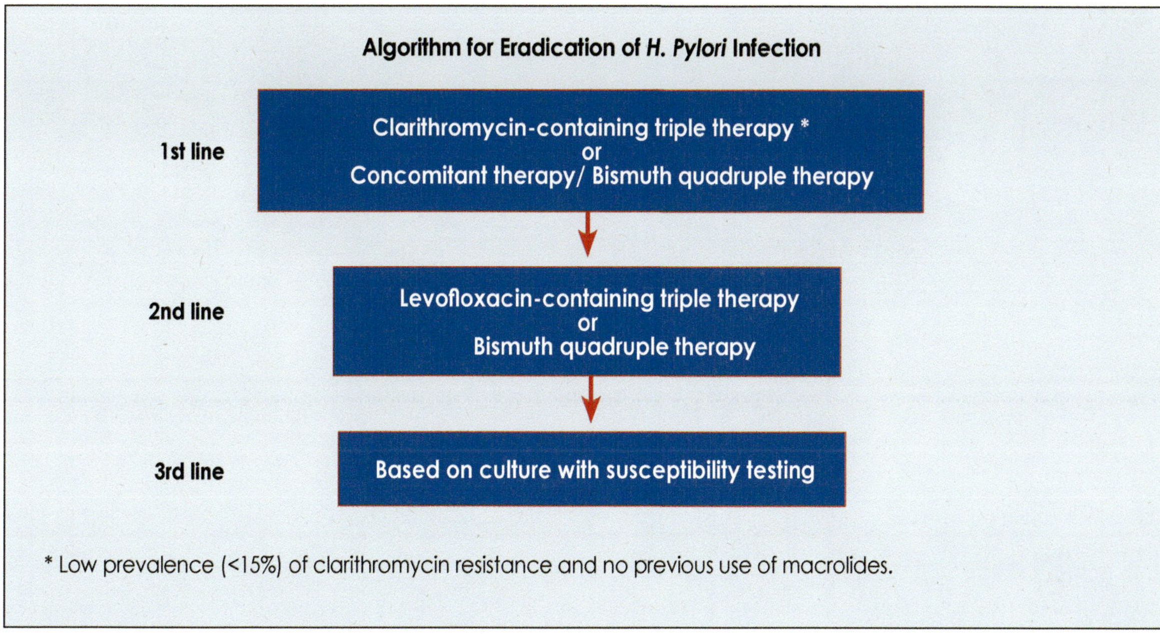

Figure 12.2 Algorithm for the treatment of *H. pylori* infection. (Zagari et al., 2018)

KEY CONCEPTS

- First line therapy for H. pylori eradication should be single capsule bismuth quadruple therapy or non bismuth quadruple therapy (i.e. concomitant). Clarithromycin-containing triple therapy for 14 days can be used only in areas with a prevalence of clarithromycin resistance <15%.
- Although the prevalence of *H. pylori* infection has declined in recent decades, it still affects at least 30% of the general population in Italy and Europe. The infection is usually acquired early, in infancy, by ingestion of the bacterium.
- *H. pylori* infection causes active chronic gastritis of varying severity in patients infected. In a subgroup of patients, it also causes dyspeptic symptoms, digestive diseases, such as peptic ulcer, malignant neoplasia of the stomach, and extra-digestive diseases.
- *H. pylori*-related peptic ulcer is a chronic disease: natural history is characterized by successive recurrences and sometimes fatal complications, such as haemorrhage and perforation. Epigastric pain is the most frequent symptom.
- The diagnosis of *H. pylori* infection can be based on findings from non-invasive tests, such as the 13C-UBT and the stool antigen test, or with invasive tests, such as the rapid urease test and histology. The therapy for *H. pylori*-positive peptic ulcer is based on the eradication of *H. pylori*. The first-line therapy can be triple therapy with clarithromycin or quadruple therapy with or without bismuth.

REFERENCES

- Gravina AG, Priadko K, Ciamarra P, et al. Extragastric Manifestations of Helicobacter Pylori Infection. J Clin Med. 2020;9(12):3887.
- Lanas A, Chan FKL. Peptic ulcer disease. Lancet. 2017; 390;613-24.
- Malfertheiner P, Megraud F, O'Morain CA, et al. Management of Helicobacter pylori infection. The Maastricht V/Florence Consensus Report. Gut. 2017;66:6-30.
- Zagari RM, Rabitti S, Eusebi LH, Bazzoli F. Treatment of Helicobacter pylori infection: a clinical practice update. Eur J Clin Invest. 2018;48:e12857.
- Zagari RM, Romano M, Ojetti V et al. Guidelines for the management of Helicobacter pylori infection in Italy. The III Working Group Report 2015. Dig Liver Dis. 2015;47:903-12.
- Zamani M, Ebrahimtabatar F, Zamani V, et al. Systematic review with meta-analysis: the worldwide prevalence of Helicobacter pylori infection. Aliment Pharmacol Ther. 2018;47:868-76.

CHAPTER 13

CHRONIC GASTRITIS AND GASTROPATHIES FROM DRUGS

Leonardo Henry Umberto Eusebi, Lorenzo Fuccio

LEARNING OBJECTIVES
- To know the potentially harmful drugs for gastric mucosa and their mechanism of injury.
- To identify endoscopic features and evaluate bleeding risk.
- To know the classification.
- To know the pathophisiology of damage.
- To evaluate neoplastic risk.
- To know the special types of gastritis.

Some medications can induce gastric damage, causing acute inflammation of the gastric mucosa (gastritis), which can be complicated by erosions or ulcers or sometimes dangerous bleeding among their side effects.

The main gastro-damaging drugs are:
- non-steroidal anti-inflammatory drugs (NSAIDs), including aspirin or acetylsalicylic acid;
- steroidal anti-inflammatory drugs (corticosteroids);
- bisphosphonates or anti-osteoporotic drugs;
- anticoagulants (heparin, warfarin);
- selective serotonin reuptake inhibitors (SSRIs);
- antineoplastic drugs.

The pathogenesis of gastric damage depends on the type of drug but it will always include an alteration of the gastric mucosal barrier.

The gastric epithelial barrier is a dynamic entity, consisting of various elements: a thick layer of mucus and bicarbonate produced by superficial columnar cells, rapid cell turnover, efficient blood microcirculation, and dense innervation. Every minute, 500,000 cells are lost and replaced and every 5 days the gastric cellular haeritage is completely renewed. This complex mechanism is mainly regulated by prostaglandins (PG), growth factors, and capsacino-sensitive neurons.

Here we will discuss the main classes of gastro-damaging drugs, frequently used in clinical practice.

NON-STEROIDAL ANTI-INFLAMMATORY DRUGS

NSAIDs, as reported by the World Health Organization, are amongst the most widely used drugs in the world, but also the most gastro damaging agents. Every day, more than 30 million people in the world take NSAIDs for several reasons: joint pain, menstrual pain, headache, and inflammatory processes of various origin and nature.

NSAIDs extensive use is also partly due to their availability as over-the-counter drugs, which facilitates self-medication, and their purchase without a prescription. Furthermore, 20-30% of people aged over 60 years assume aspirin daily, for the primary or secondary prevention of cardiovascular accidents.

Although there is a reliable estimate of their large consumption, data on the true incidence of NSAID-related gastric damage are poorly defined. Generally, the use of NSAIDs is associated with abdominal pain, dyspepsia, nausea, epigastric burning, and hyperacidity. Often such episodes spontaneously regress or disappear using antacids without requiring endoscopic investigations. However, in some cases the use of NSAIDs can be associated with the appearance of erosions and ulcers, sometimes complicated by haemorrhagic episodes.

NSAID haemorrhage is one of the most frequent causes of emergency hospitalization, with more than 100,000 hospitalizations/year and about 16,500 deaths/year.

The relative risk of bleeding episodes is 5-6 times greater in patients taking NSAIDs than in the general population. A large American population study (ARTHIS, a database of 14,000 patients with rheumatoid arthritis and osteoarthritis treated with NSAIDs and followed for more than 20 years) identified and catalogued a number of risk factors for gastric damage. Among the were patient age history of peptic disease, chronic use, combination of several NSAIDs or simultaneous use of steroids or other gastro-intestinal agents. The results of these studies published at the beginning of the 1980s were confirmed in 2005.

The pathogenesis of NSAID damage is twofold, recognizing both a topical and a systemic mechanism (**Figure 13.1**).

At the topical level, NSAIDs, by binding to surface phospholipids, the main constituents of gastric mucus, damage the mucosal barrier, increasing its permeability and favoring the back diffusion of hydrogen ions (H+) responsible for gastric mucosal damage.

Systemic action results from the inhibition of cyclo-oxygenases (COX), enzymes responsible for the synthesis, starting from arachidonic acid, of prostaglandins (PG). There are two main isoforms of these enzymes: COX-1 and COX-2. The first is the constitutive form responsible for the synthesis of PGs which have a protective effect on the gastric mucosa. PGs, in fact, stimulate the production of mucus and bicarbonates, ensure adequate mucosal blood flow, and regulate the epithelium re-

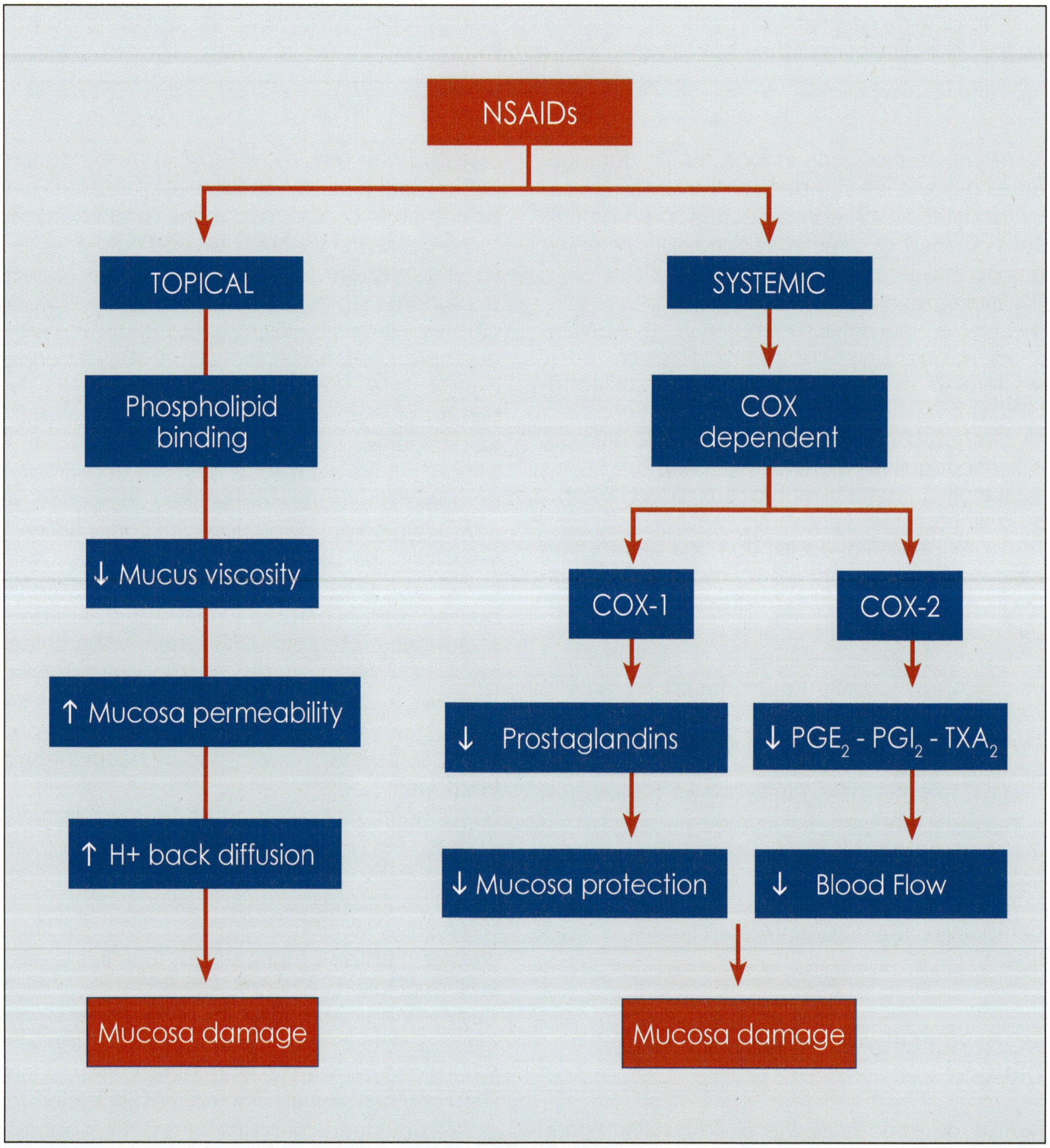

Figure 13.1 Pathogenetic mechanisms underlying NSAIDs damage to gastric mucosa.

pair and cell turnover systems. COX-1 also plays an important role in modulating renal flow and maintaining normal platelet function.
COX-2 is largely inducible by inflammation and is believed to stimulate the production of prostaglandins and thromboxanes (PGE, PGI, TXA), responsible for reducing pain and inflammation but also for the control of blood flow.
NSAIDs, by their non-selective inhibition of both these enzymes, relieve painful symptoms but damage gastric mucosa, with the formation of erosions or ulcers that sometimes are complicated by micro- or macroscopic bleeding. The severity of the damage depends on the degree of cyclo-oxygenase inhibition and varies from drug to drug (**Table 13.1**, **Figure 13.2**).
The use of NSAIDs that selectively inhibit pro-inflammatory COX-2, both first generation (celecoxib and rofecoxib) and second generation (etoricoxib, valdecoxib, parecoxib and lumiracoxib), carries a lower risk of gastric damage.
Macroscopically, on endoscopic examination, the mucosa appears inflamed with multiple punctiform (2-3 mm) immaturc crosions, somctimcs covered with hematin (an indirect sign of recent bleeding), often located at the antral level.
Macroscopically, there is oedema, vasodilation, hyperplasia of the foveolar cells, in the absence of inflammatory cells. The presence of muscle fibers in the lamina propria is a typical finding.
Prevention of gastric damage is suggested in patients requiring long-term NSAID therapy. To this end there are two options: one is the use of selec-

Table 13.1 Selectivity for COX-2 of main NSAIDs.

Drug	COX-2 Selectivity
Ketoprofen	0.1
Aspirin	0.3
Ibuprofen	0.6
Indomethacin	0.7
Naproxen	1.0
Piroxicam	1.3
Ketorolac	1.5
Nabumetone	1.6
Acetaminophen	4.0
Celecoxib	9.2
Mefenamlc acld	12.1
Nimesulide	58.3

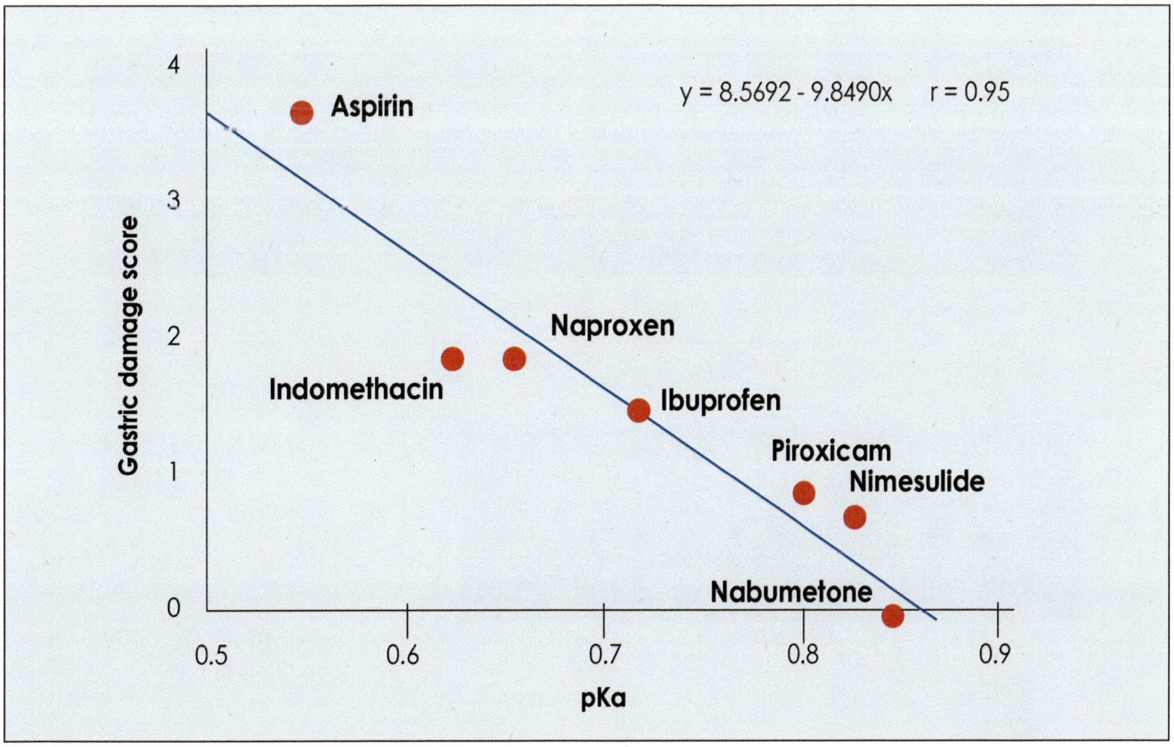

Figure 13.2 Gastric damage caused by major NSAIDs in relation to their intrisic chemical characteristics (pKa dissociation constant).

tive COX-2 inhibitors; the other is the simultaneous administration of NSAIDs with proton pump inhibitors.
Both options were found to be effective in reducing mucosal damage and hospitalization rates for acute events such as haemorrhage or perforation.

Aspirin

Among NSAIDs, aspirin or acetylsalicylic acid, which is the founder of this drug class, deserves special attention because of its particular aspects. Aspirin inhibits COX in a non-selective way, but it also damages gastric mucosa due to its chemical characteristics. Having a low pK in the stomach, were the pH is significantly acid, it is present in dissociated form and promotes the back diffusion of H+ ions.
Consequently, it can damage the gastric mucosa even at low doses (10 mg). Its prolonged use at a dosage lower than 150 mg/day increases the risk of gastrointestinal complications by about 1.5-3 times compared to untreated controls. The risk further increases (up to 5 times), if it is given in combination with a non-selective NSAID.
In patients on chronic therapy with aspirin (100 mg/die) in the prevention of cardiovascular diseases, it is better to combine it with an antisecretory agent in patients with higher risk of bleeding (**Figure 13.3**). This combined therapy seems to be safe, reducing the risk of gastric damage and potential haemorrhagic complications.
However, the increase in gastric pH protects the gastric mucosa from the damaging action of aspirin and promotes healing processes, but it also reduces its absorption and, consequently, its effectiveness.

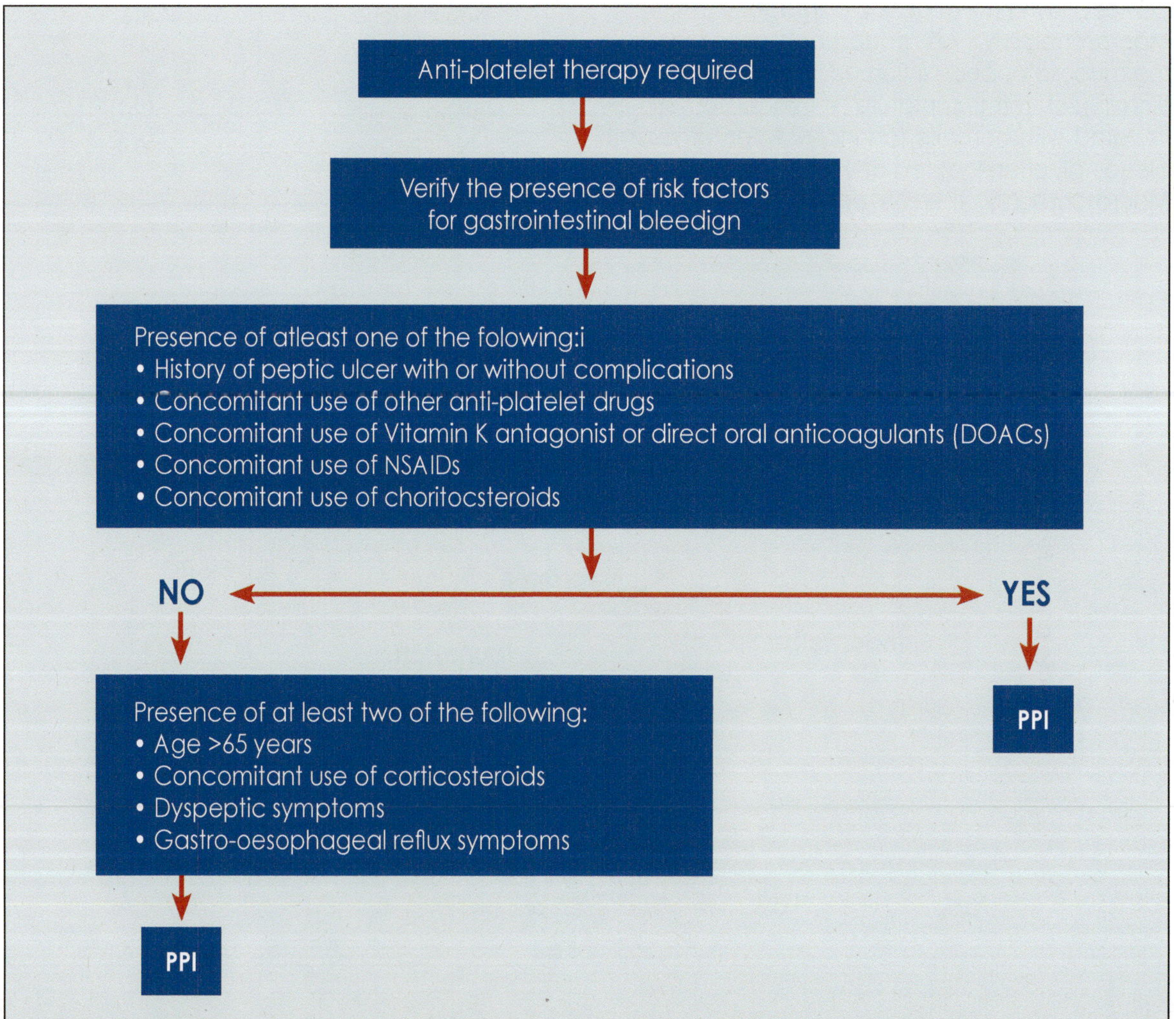

Figure 13.3 Indications for PPI prophylaxis for patients on chronic aspirin therapy.

This effect is mainly described for the combined use of aspirin and PPI (protonic pump inhibitors), at present the most powerful inhibitors of gastric secretion available. An increase cardiovascular risk in cardiopathic patients taking PPI and Aspirin has been reported; nevertheless, data are not definitive and further studies are necessary.

NSAIDs and *H. Pylori*

The high prevalence of *H. pylori* (30 to 65% among European adults, and the use of NSAIDs, suggest that potential interferences between the two may exist. Gastric infection by *H. pylori* increases the risk of gastric damage, doubling the probability to develop a duodenal ulcerous lesion.
Guidelines in gastroenterology currently suggest to search and treat the *H. pylori* infection in patients that require long-term NSAIDs administration.

Steroids

Steroids have both anti-inflammatory and immunosuppressant effects and are widely employed in treating diseases.
Chronic steroids use increases the risk of upper gastrointestinal complications like haemorrhages, perforations, and delayed healing of erosive lesions, but the effective capability to cause erosive and ulcerative damage has not been confirmed yet.
A meta-analysis of prospective clinical trials reports a similar risk of gastric damage between steroids and placebo, while observational studies suggest that gastric risk is low if steroids are taken alone (relative risk (RR)1.1 with a 95% confidence interval (CI): 0.5. 2.1), but that it significantly increases if steroids are taken with NSAIDs (RR 146 with 95% CI 6.7, 3.0).
Pathogenic mechanisms underlying gastric damage include:

- inhibition of the synthesis and secretion of mucus and bicarbonate;
- increase in the mass of parietal cells and in gastrin;
- hydrochloric acid secretion, inhibition of arachidonic acid metabolism and of the synthesis of prostaglandins.

The risk of gastric damage from steroids, unlike that from NSAIDs, varies depending on route of administration. It is higher if steroids are administered orally, lower if by aerosol and parentally.
As a general rule, it is advisable to use monotherapy drugs, but, if NSAIDs are necessary, it is important to pay utmost attention and practice gastroprotective therapy (with PPI).

N-Bisphosphonates

Oral therapy with N-bisphosphonates like alendronate and palendronate is prescribed for the prevention of osteoporosis/osteopenia due to hormonal deficiencies (estrogen in women in physiological and/or surgical menopause) and in other conditions associated with osteoporosis, such as chronic use of corticosteroids.
The use of N-bisphosphonates is linked with evidence of inflammation, erosions, and ulcers in gastric and oesophageal mucosa, and of a lengthening of the healing processes of the lesions present before their use.
The gastric effect, unlike that of NSAIDs, is topical and dose-dependent.
In a study of an ex-vivo model of gastric mucosa, administration of 20-30 mg/ml of these drugs on the mucosal surface caused epithelial damage (superficial necrosis of the foveolae, sometimes extending to glands), while a concentration lower than 3 mg /ml did not cause substantial alterations.
The same study clarified that the pathogenesis of mucosal damage by N-bisphosphonates was independent of the effects that these drugs have on microcirculation.
To date, there is no evidence that N-bisphosphonates inhibit COX and interact with PG synthesis and secretion.

Other Drugs

Potential indirect gastro-damaging effects should be recognized for those drugs that interfere with coagulation (heparin, dicumaroles, and warfarin), with platelet aggregation (acetyl salicylic acid, Clopidogrel, Ticlopidine) and with platelet function (serotonin reuptake inhibitors, Fluoxetine).
These drugs, including recent anticoagulants such as dabigatran and rivaroxaban, facilitate bleeding of pre-existing lesion, but they are not capable of inducing it, and raise the risk in patients assuming NSAIDs. Finally, there is the gastric damage potential of antineoplastic drugs which, by blocking cell proliferation, can damage organs and tissues characterised by a high index of cell replication, such as the stomach.

REACTIVE GASTROPATIES

The epithelial cells of the gastric mucosa can be damaged by a variety of mechanisms that do not produce a significant inflammatory infiltrate. This damage results in rapid epithelial replacement

and cell regeneration with foveolar hyperplasia. This condition is more properly defined as reactive gastropathy, although it is not uncommon to use of the old terminology 'acute erosive gastritis'.
Reactive gastropathy is found in approximately 15% of endoscopic biopsies of the gastric mucosa, and its incidence increases with age and with the co-presence of other inflammatory conditions of the gastrointestinal tract. From an endoscopic point of view, the gastric mucosa appears hyperaemic with subepithelial bleedings, and with multiple erosions or acute ulcers, covered with dark brown hematin due to the exposure of haemoglobin to the gastric juice.
The most frequent causes are the use of drugs, the abuse of toxic substances (**Table 13.2**) and bile reflux, whereas less frequent causes are stress conditions (i.e. physical and thermal trauma, shock, sepsis or head trauma), exposure to ionizing radiation and as consequence of allogeneic organ transplants.

Biliary Reflux

Biliary reflux is extremely common after gastric surgery for peptic disease, cancer and obesity; moreover, it can also occur following cholecystectomy and biliary sphincterotomy, procedures that expose the duodenum to chronic exposure of bile and, therefore, to the risk of duodenal-gastric reflux. This condition can also occur in adults and children who have not undergone surgical or endoscopic treatments.
The diagnosis can be challenging and generally requires a combination of clinical, endoscopic and histological evaluations, although there are no defined and universally accepted diagnostic criteria. Clinically, the patient may report dyspeptic symptoms, vomiting, nausea, heartburn and regurgitation. From an endoscopic point of view, in addition to the general picture of reactive gastropathies described above, it is not uncommon to directly visualise bile in the gastric cavity. Histologically, a foveolar hyperplasia with cystic glandular dilation and few acute and chronic inflammatory elements can be observed; it is also possible to observe the presence of intestinal metaplasia and also mucosal atrophy, conditions that increase the risk of developing gastric cancer.
The treatment can be complex and the scientific literature is based on few controlled clinical studies. Proton pump inhibitors (e.g., rabeprazole 20 mg/day), antacids, the use of ursodeoxycholic acid and cholestyramine have shown some efficacy. Surgery (e.g., Roux-style biliary diversion) may be considered for severe cases refractory to medical therapy.

Radiations

Gastric damage from external ionizing radiation can be classified as acute (<6 months) or chronic (>12 months). The gastric tolerance level is approximately 4500 cGy; with exposures above 5500 cGy, most patients develop gastropathy and/or ulcers. Exposure to Yttrium-90 microspheres, selectively infused through the hepatic artery for the treatment of hepatocarcinoma, can also lead to reactive gastropathy.
Radiation ulcers are usually located in the gastric antrum (**Figure 13.4**) and can be associated with massive bleedings.

Graft-Versus-Host Disease (GVHD)

Post-transplant rejection disease (Graft-Versus-Host Disease, GVHD) occurs more frequently after allogeneic bone marrow transplant, and less frequently after solid organ transplant. The acute disease typically occurs between 21 and 100 days after transplant, while the chronic disease after 100 days. The gastrointestinal tract, especially the intestine, is affected by the acute form.
The main symptoms of the gastric localization include nausea, vomiting, epigastric abdominal

Table 13.2 Drugs, toxic, and illicit substances that cause reactive gastropathy.

Drugs	Toxic Substance
Aspirin, NSAIDs, and COX-1 inhibitors	Corrosive and caustic agents
Bisphosphonates (e.g., alendronate)	Cocaine
Bromazepam	Alcohol
Chemotherapy drugs for cancer treatment	Metals (e.g., mercury sulphate)
Oral iron supplementation	Ketamine
Sodium phosphate (bowel preparation)	Selenium

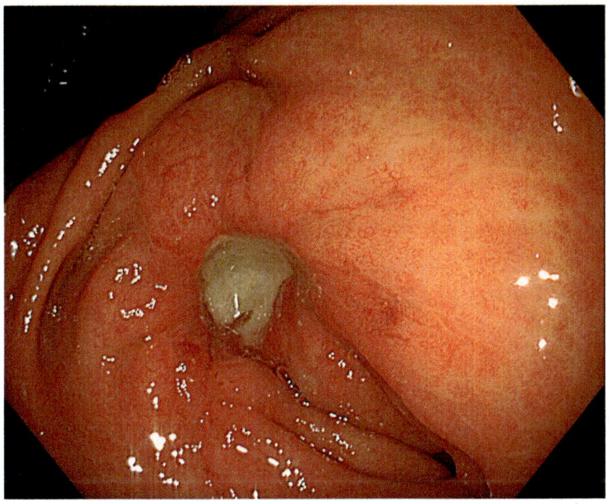

Figure 13.4 Sub-angular gastric ulcer in a patient irradiated for pancreatic cancer, developed 5 months after the treatment.

pain without diarrhoea. Moreover, the presence of diarrhoea is associated with an enteric localization. The diagnosis based on the histology examination, with the presence of apoptotic bodies.

CHRONIC GASTRITIS

Gastritis is defined as chronic when the inflammatory process of the gastric mucosa persists beyond two weeks. It is thexquisitely a pathological entity. In the past, different classifications, often burdened by repetitive and confusing synonyms and on which there was no general consensus, have been coined. In order to standardize the terminology and formulate a globally shared classification, several Consensus meetings were held (Sydney 1990, Houston 1994, Operative Link on Gastritis Assessment - OLGA 2005), with the contribution of expert pathologists from different geographical areas.
These experts identified parameters such as the histologic features (inflammatory infiltrate, atrophy, and metaplasia), topography of lesions (antrum, body, fundus) and aetiology (*H. pylori*), which must be evaluated and/or graded in the description of the histological preparation. Based on these parameters, chronic gastritis is classified:

- non-atrophic gastritis from *H. pylori;*
- atrophic gastritis (multifocal from *H. pylori*);
- autoimmune atrophic gastritis of the body;
- rare forms of gastritis (lymphocytic, granulomatous, and hypertrophic).

Chronic gastritis secondary to *H. pylori* infection are discussed in Chapter 7. Below we will therefore, focus on autoimmune gastritis and the rare forms of gastritis.

Autoimmune Atrophic Gastritis of the Corpus (or Type A)

Autoimmune atrophic gastritis (AAG) is a hereditary form of gastritis (autosomic dominant), mainly present in Northern Europe and in females (F/M 3:1).
An association between AAG and some histocompatibility antigens (HLA-DR4 e HLA-DR4/DR5) has been reported.
AAG is a rare condition (1-3% of chronic atrophic gastritis), though the prevalence of the disease is probably underestimated since it is often asymptomatic or presents with limited symptoms. A recent epidemiological study on 10,000 subjects showed a prevalence of 20% of anti-parietal cell antibodies, the marker of the disease, in the 50-74 age range, but with only 2% of the subjects affected by the disease.
The pathogenesis of AAG is related to the presence of anti-parietal gastric cells and anti-Castle intrinsic factor antibodies. The immune-target is an exchange protein, the ATP-dependent H+/K+ pump (the main functional component of gastric parietal cells, the so-called proton pump). The immune reaction is a Th1 type, summoned by a CD4+ clone in genetically predisposed subjects. A relevant feature is that 20/30% of patients infected with *H. pylori*, develops anti-gastric parietal cell antibodies, while in some studies 75% of AAG patients, show anti-*H. pylori* serum antibodies. These data suggest a pathogenetic correlation between H. pylori and the development of AAG. There are two main hypotheses for the pathogenesis of AAG: the one regards a described molecular mimicry between *H. pylori* and the exchange protein H+/K+ in gastric parietal cells; the second hypothesis is based on the fact that the T cell-mediated immune reaction can trigger aggression even towards the parietal gastric cells themselves. Therefore, it is firmly recommended to search for anti-*H. pylori* antibodies in serum and, if positive, to treat the infection with eradication therapy.
AAG is localised in the gastric corpus/fundus, macroscopically the gastric mucosa appears pale, thin, with highly evident submucosal vessels. Microscopically (it is recommended to take at least 4 biopsies of the antrum and 4 of the corpus/

fundus) , a lymphocytic infiltrate and atrophy in the corpus can be detected, together with depletion of glandular cells, both parietal and principal celles, and pseudo-pyloric and intestinal metaplasia. In almost half of patients, hyperplasia of the enterochromaffin cells (ECL) can be detected as linear (40% of cases) or as micronodular/nodular (25% of cases).

Diagnosis is confirmed by the presence of anti-parietal gastric cell serum antibodies (positivity in 55-90% of cases) and anti-Castle intrinsic factor antibodies (positivity in 39-70% of cases).

The loss of parietal gastric cells is responsible for the progressive and relevant hypochlorhydria, while Castle intrinsic factor blockage is associated with vitamin B12 malabsorption. Hypo-achlorhydria can be measured by means of a laboratory surrogate test such as serum pepsinogen I (sPGI), being the principal or oxyntic cell, that produce it, adjoining parietal cells secreting hydrochloric acid, so both are involved in gastric damage.

Due to the physiologic negative feedback between hydrochloric acid and gastrin, the AAG laboratory phenotype is characterized by low levels of sPGI and high levels of gastrin 17 (the isoform of the gastrin secreted in the gastric antrum) or of total gastrin (less specific).

Usually, patients present with a dyspeptic syndrome characterised by difficult and slow digestion. The anemia could be related to the depletion of vitamin B12 (macrocytic anemia or pernicious anemia, less frequent) as well as to iron malabsorption (gastric hypochlorhydria prevents the conversion of the non-absorbable iron Fe+++ to the absorbable one Fe++). Symptoms related to vitamin B12 malabsorption (fatigue, paraesthesia, palpitations, and neuropsychiatric alterations) are late and associated with the most severe cases.

AAG is associated with others immune disorders such as type I diabetes, Hashimoto's thyroiditis, vitiligo, and celiac disease. In patients with I type diabetes and/or with autoimmune thyroiditis, the prevalence of AAG is 5 to 10 times higher than in the general population.

The relative risk of developing gastric cancer in these subjects is almost 3 times higher than in the general population (as reported by a population study on 4.5 million of American male subjects). The risk is correlated to changes in the gastric microenvironment (decreased production of HCl and increased production of pH) that facilitates the conversion of alimentary nitrate into nitrite and the subsequent formation of nitrosamine and nitroamide, with potential mutagenic effects. Even higher is the risk of developing a benign form of neuroendocrine tumour (NET), the so-called type I carcinoid, due to the continuous stimulation exerted by the high levels of gastrin, probably in predisposed patients. These small and slow-growing tumours are to be managed endoscopically.

Rare Forms of Chronic Gastritis

Lymphocytic Gastritis

It is characterised by abundant infiltrate of T lymphocytes (CD8+) in the superficial and foveolar epithelium (normally less than 10% of epithelial cells), associated with a chronic inflammatory infiltrate in the lamina propria. It can be detected during the healing, post eradication phase of *H. pylori* infection and in 1/3 of cases of celiac disease.

Eosinophilic Gastritis

This rare condition is characterised by a huge infiltration of eosinophilic cells, organised in compacted clusters, dislocated in every layer of the gastric wall. The entire alimentary tract can be involved though the stomach is the preferential site. A history of allergic diathesis and a peripheral hypereosinophilia can often be identified in affected individuals.

Granulomatous Gastritis

This condition is characterised by the presence, in the gastric mucosa, of epithelial granulomas, an expression of a defensive response of the reticulo-endothelial system to pathogens. The disorder can be primary or secondary to infectious (tuberculosis) and non-infective diseases (sarcoidosis, Crohn's disease).

Hypertrophic Gastritis

This condition is characterised by oedema of the mucosa, with giant and elevated folds, that create a brain-like macroscopic pattern in the stomach. Currently, three forms are distinguished:

- hyperplasia of epithelial foveolar cells with atrophic or normal oxyntic glands (Mènètrier type);
- increase in parietal cells with conservation of mucus-secreting cells (Zollinger-Ellison);
- mixed type with hyperplasia of parietal mucus-secreting cells.

Mènètrier disease is a rare condition, first described in 1888, which develops after age 50, with diffuse oedema and significant general decay. It is characterised by macroscopic thickening of the mucosa, with giant folds of the gastric corpus/fundus, and foveolar hyperplasia, glandular atrophy, and pseudo-pyloric metaplasia.

The patient reports dyspeptic symptoms such as nausea and anorexia; there are clinical and laboratory signs of hypo-proteinaemia, due to protein loss caused by obstruction of the lymphatic ducts and altered capillary permeability. The course of the disease is progressive and total gastrectomy provides the only solution.

KEY CONCEPTS

- In a patient with epigastric pain and anemia, or haematemesis and/or melena it's important to perform a careful pharmacological history and record information about the assumption of drugs that could damage the stomach.
- The drugs that generally lead to a gastric damage are NSAIDs: their side effects are independent of the dose and the route of administration.
- Prophylactic treatment with PPI and eradication of *H. pylori*, if present, should be perforrmed in patients on chronic NSAIDs therapy.
- Bisphosphonates, steroids, anticoagulant drugs, antidepressant, and antineoplastic drugs are all potential pathogenetic factors of new gastric damage or complications of pre-existent lesions. It is recommended to prescribe prophylactic treatment with PPI which, however, is to be evaluated for eventual interactions in the absorption and/or action of the drug that caused the damage.

REFERENCES

- Almazar AE, Penfield JD, Saito YA, Talley NJ. Survival Times of Patients With Menetrier's Disease and Risk of Gastric Cancer. Clin Gastroenterol Hepatol. 2021 Apr;19(4):707-12.
- Fuccio L, Eusebi LH, Bazzoli F. Gastric cancer, Helicobacter pylori infection and other risk factors. World J Gastrointest Oncol. 2010;2(9):342-7.
- Lahner E, Zagari RM, Zullo A, Di Sabatino A, Meggio A, Cesaro P, Lenti MV, Annibale B, Corazza GR. Chronic atrophic gastritis: Natural history, diagnosis and therapeutic management. A position paper by the Italian Society of Hospital Gastroenterologists and Digestive Endoscopists [AIGO], the Italian Society of Digestive Endoscopy [SIED], the Italian Society of Gastroenterology [SIGE], and the Italian Society of Internal Medicine [SIMI]. Dig Liver Dis. 2019;51(12):1621-32.
- Malfertheiner P, Megraud F, O'Morain CA, Gisbert JP, Kuipers EJ, Axon AT, Bazzoli F, Gasbarrini A, Atherton J, Graham DY, Hunt R, Moayyedi P, Rokkas T, Rugge M, Selgrad M, Suerbaum S, Sugano K, El-Omar EM; European Helicobacter and Microbiota Study Group and Consensus panel. Management of Helicobacter pylori infection-the Maastricht V/Florence Consensus Report. Gut. 2017;66(1):6-30.
- Pimentel-Nunes P, Libânio D, Marcos-Pinto R, Areia M, Leja M, Esposito G, Garrido M, Kikuste I, Megraud F, Matysiak-Budnik T, Annibale B, Dumonceau JM, Barros R, Fléjou JF, Carneiro F, van Hooft JE, Kuipers EJ, Dinis-Ribeiro M. Management of epithelial precancerous conditions and lesions in the stomach (MAPS II): European Society of Gastrointestinal Endoscopy (ESGE), European Helicobacter and Microbiota Study Group (EHMSG), European Society of Pathology (ESP), and Sociedade Portuguesa de Endoscopia Digestiva (SPED) guideline update 2019. Endoscopy. 2019;51(4):365-88.
- Shah SC, Piazuelo MB, Kuipers EJ, Li D. AGA Clinical Practice Update on the Diagnosis and Management of Atrophic Gastritis: Expert Review. Gastroenterology. 2021;161(4):1325-1332.e7.

CHAPTER 14

PRECANCEROUS LESIONS AND CANCER OF THE STOMACH

Gerardo Antonio Pio Nardone, Antonietta Gerarda Gravina

LEARNING OBJECTIVES

- To understand the epidemiological burden of gastric cancers.
- To identify the main risk factors of gastric cancer.
- To classify gastric cancer in relation to histological, endoscopic, and prognostic criteria.
- To analyze the multistep process of gastric carcinogenesis.
- To define clinical presentation, diagnosis, staging, surveillance, and therapy of gastric cancers.

Based on cell origin, gastric tumours may be classified in epithelial and non-epithelial cancer, or as benign or malignant according to their biological behavior (**Table 14.1**). The most frequent stomach tumour in the stomach is adenocarcinoma (90%), which is historically classified in intestinal and diffuse histotype according to Lauren's criteria, 1965. Although this classification has been recently substituted by that introduced by the WHO, it is quoted here for the frequent recall throughout the text.

ADENOCARCINOMA

Epidemiology and Aetiology

In spite of its progressive decrease in the last century, gastric adenocarcinoma (GA) continues to be one of the most frequent (1,000,000 new cases per year) and lethal (800,000 deaths per year) cancer worldwide with a 5-year survival rate of 30-35%. It affects often white males (M/F = 2/1) older than 60 years, while it is rare before age 50. The standard incidence in people 50-70 years old is about 49% and 20% in males and females, respectively. In 2006, in Italy 62,225 cases of GA were recorded. Overall GA is the fifth most common malignancy and the third neoplasia for cancer related deaths. The worldwide distribution of GA is variable, with countries with high prevalence, such as East Asia, East Europe, and South America, and other countries with low prevalence such as North Africa, North America, South Asia, and Australia. In Italy the prevalence of GA is low in the southern and high in the Centre-North. The varying distribution suggests that environmental factors rather than genetic ones, play a key pathogenetic role. In the early 19th century, Virchow hypothesized that cancer should be considered an adaptive response to an adverse environment. In support of this theory, analysis of people migration has shown that Japanese people migrated to the United States have the same risk as the Japanese

Table 14.1 WHO classification of gastric tumours.

	Benign	Malignant
Epithelial	Adenoma	Adenocarcinoma Carcinoid
Non-Epithelial	Leiomyoma Lipoma Fibroma Schwannoma Neurofibroma Haemangioma GIST	Leiomyosarcoma Liposarcoma Fibrosarcoma Schwannosarcoma Neurofibrosarcoma Haemangiosarcoma Sarcoma Kaposi GIST Lymphomas

living in Japan, whereas Japanese children born in the United States, have the same risk as other Americans. Not too long ago, diet was considered the most important environmental factor involved in the pathogenesis of GA. A diet rich in fruit and vegetables lowers the risk due to its anti-oxidant properties while a diet rich in salt, nitrate, smoked food, and cured meat increases the risk. Salt, due its osmotic properties, increases the amount of intracellular water and induces cell death which in turn triggers cell proliferation, the first step carcinogenesis. Nitrates, commonly used as food additives, in a low-acidic gastric environment, i.e., – that of chronic atrophic gastritis, are transformed in nitrites, which in turn react with alimentary amines to generate nitrosamines, well known mutagenic agents. The progressive decrease in GA prevalence is largely related to the use of food refrigeration, for food storage without salts and nitrates. Cigarette smoking and alcoholic beverages are also recognized as environmental factors. However, while a direct relationship between cigarette smoking and GA is well documented, with a relative risk 1.5.2-fold higher in smokers than in non-smokers, no clear evidence exists that alcohol drinkers have an increased risk of GA. Currently, it is universally recognized, that the main environmental factor involved in the pathogenesis of GA is *Helicobacter pylori* (*H.p.*) infections, one of the most frequent infections worldwide. In 1982, Barry Marshall and Robin Warren first described H.p. in the stomach but some years later, in 1994, the International Agency for Research on Cancer (IARC) and the WHO classified H.p. as a class I carcinogen, as is smoking for lung cancer. The relationship between GA and infection is prevalently based on epidemiological data.

A large meta-analysis of case control studies showed that the risk of GA is 3-fold higher in patients with infection than those with- out infection. In addition, the risk of GA increases up to 6 fold if Hp infection persists for more than ten years and up to 7 folds if patients were infected before the age of 50. Taken together, these data suggest that the earlier the infection, the greater the risk. Amongst the possible infectious agents of GA, Epstein Barr virus (EBV) and the overexpression of its related genes has been detected at the tissue level in a subgroup of patients with GA. Genetic alterations also contribute to increasing the risk. Of note, genetic alterations are prevalently associated with diffuse histotype, whereas environmental factors are prevalently associated with intestinal histotype. A family history of GA is reported in 10% of cases, while patients with hereditary diffuse histotype account for 1-3% of GA cases. Hereditary diffuse GA is characterized by a germ-line mutation of the CDH1, gene encoding the E-cadherin protein that regulates cell adhesion. The first cluster of hereditary GA is that of Napoleon Bonaparte. The Emperor, his brother, two sisters, his father, grandfather, and uncle all died of GA. The relatives of patients with GA carrying the same E-cadherin mutation have a 70% probability to develop GA. Thus, prophylactic gastrectomy is recommended in these patients. Single nucleotide polymorphisms of interleukins IL-1, TNF-α, IL-10, or toll-like receptor4 gene have also been described in GA, playing a facilitating but not a causative role. Patients carrying these polymorphisms show an increased incidence of GA in the presence of infection. In patients with hereditary tumour syndromes such as FAP, HNPCC, and juvenile polyposis, GA has been reported in 10-20% of cases. Finally, 8-10% of patients with a diffuse GA histotype have a somatic mutation of the ARID1A gene, involved in DNA repair, and in more than 70% of cases associated with EBV infection.

Pathogenesis

According to P. Correa, GA may be considered a multistep process, starting from chronic gastritis and progressing to cancer through atrophy, intestinal metaplasia, and dysplasia. This multistep process is triggered by H.p. infection and takes several decades. However, only 1% of patients with infection develops GA and only the H.p. strain presenting the pathogenicity island, which are CagA-positive, are involved in gastric carcinogenesis. Once in the stomach (most likely by orofecal transmission), H.p. through the urease enzyme, produces ammonia that neutralizes the gastric acid. Thus, it escapes acid elimination, penetrates the mucus layer using its flagellin and motilin, colonizes the epithelium, and triggers a complex inflammatory response that damages the gastric mucosa. In the first phase, H.p. related inflammatory response is restricted to the antrum and associated with increased acid secretion and peptic ulcer risk. With time, but not always, the inflammatory response involves the gastric body and disrupts the parietal cells that are substituted by fibrotic tissue or metaplastic, not appropriate glands. This condition, i.e., atrophic gastritis, through decreased acid secretion, modifies the gastric microenvironment and allows the development of nitrous compounds potentially exerting a mutagen activity. The modified gastric microenvironment and the presence of mutagenic agents, promote the transition of mucosal cells from secretory to absorptive, with progressive development of intestinal metaplasia, and of cell atypias, i.e., dysplasia. Atrophic gastritis, intestinal metaplasia, and dysplasia may progress in time to GA and are defined as precancerous lesions. Unlike the intestinal type, diffuse type GA develops directly from inflamed mucosa. Although they develop through different pathogenetic pathways, H.p. is a crucial aetiologic agent for both histotypes (**Figure 14.1**). Even in the absence of the bacterium in tumour and peritumour tissues, it may be detected in more than 70% of cases by serum test (IgG anti-Hp).

GASTRIC PRECANCEROUS LESIONS AND CONDITIONS

Gastric precancerous changes include histological lesions and pathological conditions linked to an increased risk of GA.

Chronic Atrophic Gastritis

It is characterised by the substitution of gastric glandular cells with fibrotic tissue or inappropriate glands and it is closely linked to H.p.-related chronic inflammation. According to the Operative Link on Gastritis Assessment (OLGA) system

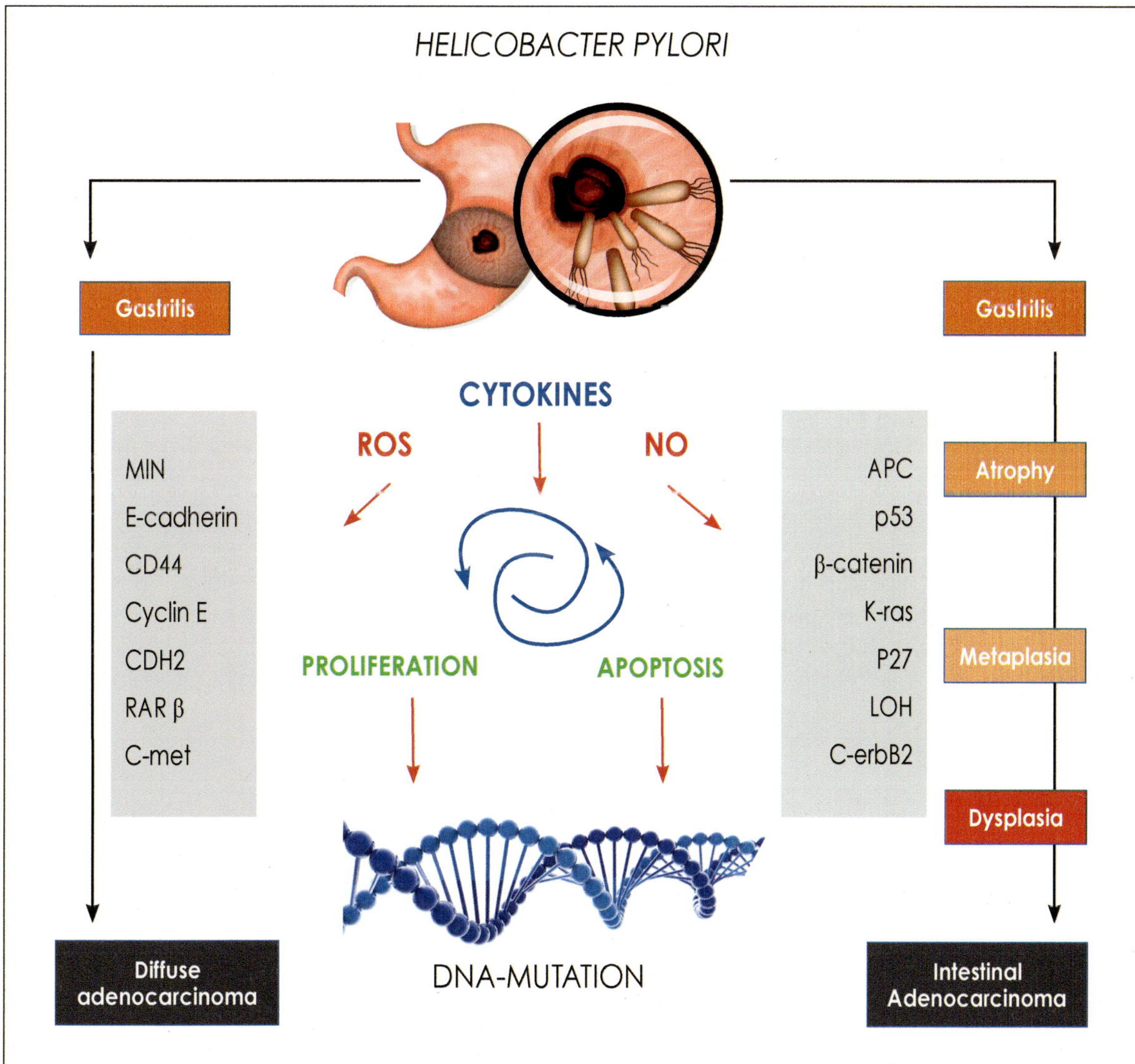

Figure 14.1 *H. pylori*-related gastric carcinogenesis. Phenotypic alterations that underlie gastric cancer development are the consequence of epigenetic and genetic alterations that, although differing by histotype, are triggered by *H. pylori* related inflammatory response.

gastric atrophy is classified in five stages for antrum and body, respectively (**Figure 14.2**). This system, recently validated, shows that the risk of GA is closely related to the extension and score of atrophy (and is basically limited to stage III and IV). Gastric atrophy may be also detected by a serum test measuring PGI and PGII levels, secreted by the corpus and the antrum, respectively, and the PGI/PGII ratio, the lower the two parameters the higher being the stage of atrophy and therefore the risk of GA.

Intestinal Metaplasia

This condition is characterized by the substitution of gastric glandular cells by specific cells generally found outside of this specific district. This condition, termed intestinal metaplasia (IM), has a spotty distribution. According to Jass and Felipe, it may be classified in three subtypes: 1) Complete, small bowel-like; 2) incomplete, goblet cells like; 3) incomplete, colonic cells like, which is at greater risk of neoplastic transformation. This classification is based on the staining for sialomucins (type I) and solphomucins (types II and III) at immune histochemistry. A new type of metaplasia, Spasmolytic Polypeptide-Expressing Metaplasia (SPEM), has been recently described. It is characterized by the substitution of gastric glandular cells with intestinal-like cells expressing the trefoil peptide (TFF). In respect to IM, SPEM is diffuse and, reportedly, holds a relatively high risk of GA.

Dysplasia

Chronic inflammation of gastric mucosa and the modified microenvironment allow the development of *atypias* in glandular cells, i.e., dysplasia. Dysplasia does not infiltrate the epithelial basal membrane or adjacent tissues being more recently denominated intraepithelial neoplasia, due to its genotypic and phenotypic similarities with cancer), and may be classified in low and high grade. High grade dysplasia was previously denominated "in situ" carcinoma. In a recent population study involving 407.152 subjects, followed for about 30 years, the risk for developing GA at 20 years was 1/50, 1/39, and 1/19 for atrophy, IM, and dysplasia, respectively, while it was 1/250 for healthy controls. These evidences suggest that patients with precancerous gastric lesions need close endoscopic and histological surveillance, even after H.p. eradication, as reported in **Table 14.2** according to MAPS II guidelines (Management of epithelial precancerous conditions and lesions in the stomach),. In fact, the risk of neo- plastic progression of precancerous lesions, even if reduced, persists after the eradication of the bacterium. Furthermore, high grade dysplastic lesions can and must be treated endoscopically (see above EMR) when diagnosed on endoscopically recognizable lesions. SPEM which is at medium-high risk of neoplastic transformation, needs an endoscopic surveillance every 3 years even if, the MAPS II guidelines do not give indications on this topic.

Gastric Ulcer

Gastric ulcer may progress to GA in 0.5 to 6% of cases. However, gastric ulcer generally develops in a setting of chronic atrophic gastritis and IM and GA may resemble an ulcer (type II or III according to Bormann classification). Therefore, it is mandatory for correct diagnosis, to perform at endoscopy multiple mucosal biopsies (≥8 from the base and edges), at baseline and two months after diagnosis.

Atrophy Score		Corpus			
		No Atrophy (score 0)	Mild Atrophy (score 1)	Mild Atrophy (score 2)	Severe Atrophy (score 3)
ANTRUM	No Atrophy (score 0) (including *incisura angularis*)	Stage 0	Stage I	Stage II	Stage II
	Mild Atrophy (score 1) (including *incisura angularis*)	Stage I	Stage I	Stage II	Stage III
	Moderate Atrophy (score 2) (including *incisura angularis*)	Stage II	Stage II	Stage III	Stage IV
	Severe Atrophy (score 3) (including *incisura angularis*)	Stage III	Stage III	Stage IV	Stage IV

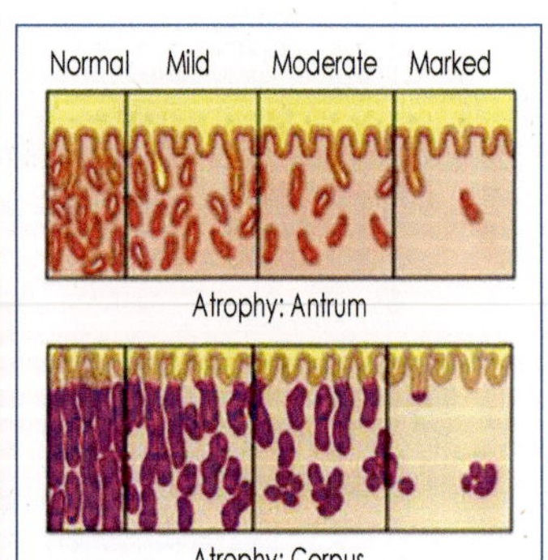

Figure 14.2 Staging of chronic atrophic gastritis according to the Operative Link for Gastritis Assessment (OLGA) system (Rugge et al., 2005). A classification of the histological phenotypes of gastritis along a scale of progressively increasing gastric cancer risk, from the lowest (stage 0) to the highest (stage IV).

Table 14.2 Cancer risk of precancerous gastric lesions and timing of endoscopic surveillance.

Precancerous Lesion	Cancer Risk	Endoscopy Timing
Antral Atrophy	Low	Not required
Body Atrophy	Moderate-High	3 years
Complete Metaplasia type I	Low	Not required
Incomplete Metaplasia types II-III	Moderate-High	3 years
SPEM*	Moderate-High	3 years
Low grade dysplasia	High	12 months
High grade dysplasia	Very High	6 months

*Spasmolytic Polypeptide Expressing Metaplasia

Autoimmune Gastritis

This is a relatively rare disease, but recent epidemiologic data have indicated that is more frequent that previously estimated. It is caused by antibodies against parietal cells and, less frequently, against Castle's intrinsic factor. The loss of parietal cells induces a progressive failure of gastric function, with severe hypoacidity that corresponds to body fundic gastric atrophy. In patients with autoimmune gastritis, the risk of GA is 3-fold higher than in the general population according to a large study on 4.5 million subjects, but the affected patients, mostly females with concurrent autoimmune diseases, presented a relatively high risk of developing gastric carcinoids (NET, Neuro-Endocrine Tumours, see below). These patients may develop macrocytic anemia and neurological disorders due to the chronic lack of vitamin B12 absorption.

Gastric Polyps

The frequency of gastric polyps in the general population ranges between 0,8-2.4%. Polyps are classified in fundic (50%), hyperplastic (40%), and adenomatous (10%). Fundic polyps are generally cystic, benign, secondary to chronic proton pump inhibitors (PPI) use. The risk of GC is quite low, apparently depending on polyp size (>1cm) and coexistence of FAP. Hyperplastic polyps, generally benign, are detected in a setting of gastric atrophy, IM and H.p. infection. The eradication of infection may induce regression of hyperplastic polyps. The risk of GA depends on the presence of dysplasia, that is an infrequent finding. Adenomatous polyps are quite rare and may progress to cancer in 10% of cases in 4 years. Endoscopic polypectomy should be performed, to eradicate infection if present.

Gastrectomy

Before the introduction of antisecretory drugs and the discovery of H.p. infection, patients with peptic disease frequently underwent gastrectomy. They were at increased risk to develop GC, starting 20 years after surgery and particularly if surgery was performed before age 50 years. Patients who undergo Billroth II gastrectomy have a four-fold increased risk of GA compared with those who undergo Billroth I gastrectomy. Tumour develops on the gastric side of anastomosis; atrophy of gastric remnant, hypochlorhydria, bile and pancreatic enzymes reflux and bacterial overgrowth account for the increased risk. Currently, because surgery is rarely performed for peptic disease, the related risk for GA is negligible.

Hypertrophic Gastritis or Menetrier's Disease

This rare condition is characterized by hypertrophy of gastric folds and foveolar cells. Being a rare condition, often treated by gastrectomy due to the lack of effective drugs, it is impossible to establish the risk for GA. In a revision of clinical cases, 15% of patients with Menetrier's disease had GA.

CLASSIFICATION

Based on histological findings, GA has been historically classified in intestinal and diffuse type according to Lauren's criteria and subsequently in expanding and infiltrating according to Ming's classification. Finally, GA was classified in well differentiated (tubular, papillary and mucinous) and poorly differentiated (including signet ring cells), according to WHO criteria. The well differentiated GA, according to the WHO classification, corresponds to the intestinal type by Lauren and to the expanding growth pattern by Ming. This tumour is typically associated with H.p. infection and precancerous lesions, has a glandular structure, occurs at older age, and carries a better prognosis. The poorly differentiated GA by the WHO classification corresponds to the diffuse type by Lauren and to the infiltrating growth pattern by Ming. This tumour is not associated to with H.p. infection, may be hereditary, occurs at younger age, is prevalently constituted by scattered glandular cells, does not have precancerous lesions, and carries a poor prognosis. Recently, a new classification of GA, based on molecular alterations, has been introduced: Epstein Barr Virus (EBV)-positive, with microsatellite instability, genetically stable and with chromosomal instability. This classification must be increasingly used in clinical practice for therapeutic implications and the calculation of prognostic risk.

CLINICAL MANAGMENT

Symptoms

The lack of specific symptoms is one of the reasons for the poor prognosis of GA. In its early stages, GA may manifest with an unspecific or ulcer like dyspeptic syndrome while in advanced stages patients complain of nausea, anorexia, early satiety, and weight loss. Epigastric pain, usually not improving with PPI, is a late symptom, suggestive of neoplastic infiltration of gastric nerve terminations. Other late symptoms include dysphagia, which occurs when there is neoplastic infiltration of the cardia, and food vomiting, when there is neoplastic infiltration of the antropyloric region. GA is rarely (2-3% of cases) a cause of haematemesis or melena, but frequently of chronic anemia. Palpable abdominal mass, liver enlargement, and ascites are late symptoms that suggest peritoneal or liver metastasis. Infrequently, gastric tumoural cells that have "fallen" into the pelvic cavity may colonize the ovary (Krukenberg's tumour) or invade the supraclavicular lymph nodes (Virchow-Troisier node).

Diagnosis

Altered blood tests, including haemoglobin levels and inflammation markers, are unspecific and very late. The carcinoembryonic antigen (CEA) is elevated in 30-40% of case, but it is poorly sensitive and unspecific, being increased in several tumours (lung, pancreas, ovarian, colon etc.). If CEA is increased at baseline, its measurement over time may help to evaluate the efficacy of therapy or suggest the recurrence of neoplasia.

Upper endoscopy is the gold standard diagnostic test that should be performed in each patient with alarm symptoms (anemia, weight loss, food vomiting, nausea, and epigastric pain) and in dyspeptic patients with a relative diagnosed with GA or older than 50 years. Gastric adenocarcinoma is confined to the gastric corpus in 40% of cases, to the antrum in 35%, to the cardias region in 20%, and is diffuse in the remaining 5%. Early gastric cancer (cancer beyond the basal membrane but limited to the mucosal or submucosal layers, ECG) may be classified in three subtypes: protruded (0-1); elevated, flat, depressed (2 a,b,c) and excavated (3); while advanced gastric cancer may be classified according to Bormann in four types: type I polypoid; type II ulcerated; Type III ulcerated and infiltrating; type IV diffusely infiltrating 'linitis plastica'. Upper endoscopy allows the detect lesions and to perform mucosal biopsies (at least 8-10 samples from the center and edges of ulcerated, de- pressed, protruding or infiltrating lesions). Diagnostic accuracy depends on the number of biopsies (3, 6 or 8-10 biopsies match a diagnostic accuracy of 60, 80, and 100% respectively). Currently, the endoscopist, during oesophagogastroduodenoscopy, may use coloring and image magnification techniques, such as chromoendoscopy with magnification and use of vital dyes, virtual chromoendoscopy (e.g., Narrow Band Imaging), autofluorescence and confocal microendoscopy. These techniques make it possible to identify, at an early stage, lesions that can escape traditional endoscopy and allow targeted biopsy sampling.

Primary Prevention

The aim is to correct dietary habits starting at an early age (high intake of fruits and vegetables and low intake of smoked foods, cured meat, salt and nitrates) and to test and treat H.p. infection in areas at high incidence of GA and in first degree relatives of GA patients. Doubts exist on the possibility of a generalized policy of screening for H.p. or with PGI determination.

Secondary Prevention

This entails seeking and eradicating H.p. in patients with precancerous lesions that must in any case be rechecked at a distance from eradication and which, if the lesions persist after eradication, must continue to be monitored carefully (endoscopic and biopsy surveillance).

Staging

Contrast enhanced computed tomography allows to define local extension and lymph node involvement and to disclose the presence of metastases. Endoscopic ultrasounds allow to define the depth of gastric wall invasion and the involvement of loco regional lymph nodes. It is used particularly in suspicion of EGC. Finally, the TNM staging system (T = size and extension of the tumour; N = regional lymph node involvement; M = distant metastases) is generally used in clinical practice to predict the prognosis.

Therapy

Since GA is radio and chemotherapy resistant, surgery is the therapy of choice, however, an advanced stage at diagnosis makes surgery a palliative procedure in most cases. Total gastrectomy is performed for cardia GA, while partial gastrectomy (antrectomy) is indicated for non-cardia GA. Extended lymphadenectomy is mandatory in both cardia and non-cardia GA. Adjuvant chemotherapy is prescribed in patients with locally advanced stage at surgery. Finally, neoadjuvant radio and chemotherapy alone or in combination are a promising option.

In a subgroup (20-25%) of GA expressing HER-2 receptor (of the growth factor receptors family) the combination of conventional chemotherapy (5-Fluorouracile) with the monoclonal anti body Trastuzumab has shown beneficial effect. Endoscopic therapy, based on two techniques: endoscopic mucosal resection (EMR) and endoscopic submucosal dissection (ESD), the latter being more aggressive, is indicated for early GA, with tumour involving only the mucosal and submucosal layers. These procedures are routinely performed in countries where incidence is high and screening programs have been adopted. These procedures are available at selected Italian centers. Prognosis depends on histological subtype and TNM staging. Overall, the 5-year survival rate is high (80-90%) for EGC and low (30-35%) for advanced GA.

Carcinoids

Neuroendocrine tumours are rare in the stomach (0.3% of gastric tumours; 3% of gastrointestinal neuroendocrine tumours) in spite of its richness in endocrine cells like (ECL). They are generally (90% of cases) well differentiated, localized in the body fundic area, and their growth is stimulated by the presence of high gastrin levels. Carcinoid syndrome (flushing, hypotension, sweating, diarrhoea, and broncho constriction) occurs only when vasoactive hormones including histamine, serotonin, and kallikrein are secreted by tumour metastases. Three main subtypes have been reported. Type 1, the most frequent one (80%) is generally diagnosed in advanced age (>60 years), predilects female sex (75%), and is associated with chronic autoimmune atrophic gastritis and hypergastrinemia. It is more commonly multifocal, of small size (<1 cm) and very rarely displays malignant behavior. Type 2, less frequent (6%), develops in middle aged adults of both sexes and is generally associated with hypergastrinemia or Zollinger-Ellison syndrome (MEN 1). It is more commonly multifocal, of small size (<1.5 cm), confined to mucosa or submucosa, and generally has benign behavior. Type 3 14% of cases, affects more often males, is generally diagnosed at 50-60 years, develops on non-atrophic gastric mucosa and is never associated with hypergastrinemia. It is more commonly monofocal, of small size (≥1 cm), with loco regional metastases in 75% of the cases and a mortality rate of 25%. Surgery, when feasible, remains the cornerstone of treatment for type III and provides the only chance of a cure. If metastasis of carcinoid tumour has occurred and surgical excision is not feasible currently recommended treatment is treatment is chemotherapy. Cytostatic agents, such as somatostatin ana- logs and interferon alpha, should be administered in slow growing neoplasms, while combination regimens including cisplatin, etoposide, streptozotocin, and 5-fluorouracil should be reserved for treatment of highly proliferating tumours.

NON-EPITHELIAL NEOPLASIA

Lymphoma

Gastric non Hodgkin lymphoma is the second most frequent gastric neoplasia (5%) and accounts for up to 70% of extranodal lymphomas. The commonest histotype is a low grade lymphoma, known as mucosa associated lymphoma tissue (MALT) associated lymphoma, while the high grade diffuse B large cell lymphoma (DLBCL) is less frequent. The mean age at diagnosis is 50-60 years, with a higher occurrence in males (M/F 2-3/1) and in geographic areas with an increased prevalence of H.p. infection. Helicobacter pylori related inflammatory response is responsible for B lymphocytes recruitment (MALT acquisition). Chronic stimulation for B lymphocytes recruits and activates T lymphocytes. The subsequent occurrence of V gene mutations (IgG variable region) leads to the onset of neoplasia. The commonest symptoms are epigastric pain, nausea, and weight loss, while haematemesis and melena may occur in 10-20% of cases. The gastric antrum is frequently involved (40%), while a multifocal disease is observed in 1/3 of the cases. Three macroscopic subtypes have been described: giant folds (20%), polypoid mass (30%), and infiltrative disease with multiple erosions and ulcers (50%). For prognostic purposes, echoendoscopic staging is useful form to limited the mucosa and to the submucosa because they regress with medical therapy and H.p. eradication, while the forms involving the muscle layer and the serosa involving the muscle and the serosa layers are burdened by a high rate of failure. The diagnosis is histological and is performed on biopsy samples taken during endoscopy. The therapy consists in the eradication of the infection from H.p., which leads to a remission of the neoplasm in 75-80% of cases. H.p. eradication leads to disease remission but fails in presence of translocation t (11;18); in these cases, local radiotherapy (30-50 gy) or chemotherapy (rituximab + fludarabine) achieve disease remission in 85-100% of cases. Surgery is indicated in the presence of complications or when chemo and radiotherapy are contraindicated. In patients who respond to therapy endoscopic and histological surveillance is mandatory at three months and then every six months for two years.

Stromal Tumours

Stromal tumours are rare and generally have benign behavior (lipoma, schwannoma, leiomyoma). They are often asymptomatic and rarely cause upper gastrointestinal bleeding. The malignant variant leiomyosarcoma is a rare disease (<1%) that only in advanced stage may be associated with nausea, vomiting and, sometimes, gastric haemorrhage. Surgery, when feasible, is the therapy of choice, but prognosis is poor when the diagnosis is at an advanced stage (5-year survival rate 25-30%). Gastrointestinal stromal tumour (GIST) is a rare (0,1-2%) tumour, with gastric localization in more than 50% of cases. The male sex is more frequently affected (M/F 1.5/1) and the mean age at diagnosis is 50-60 years. GIST arises from the Cajal cells of the myoenteric plexus, expresses the KII protein, and harbors the mutation of a gene that encodes a type III receptor tyrosine kinase involved in cell cycle. Mutations in the kit receptor make it chronically active, independent of ligand binding. GISTs are generally capsulated with a low potential for growth and invasion. Symptoms are aspecific and more often absent; in advanced stages, bleeding episodes may occur. The biological behavior is variable and depends on size and proliferation index. Surgery is the therapy of choice; if surgery is unfeasible or in metastatic disease, therapy with Imatinib, a kit receptor antagonist, is recommended.

KEY CONCEPTS

- In spite of its progressive decrease, gastric cancer continues to be one of the most frequent and lethal cancers worldwide and carries a poor prognosis.
- Gastric adenocarcinoma is the most frequent (>90%) malignant tumour and H.p.is the main aetiologic agent.
- The main precancerous lesions are: chronic atrophic gastritis, intestinal metaplasia, and dysplasia.
- The gold standard diagnostic test is upper endoscopy with bioptic sampling; it that is recommended in patients with alarm symptoms (bleeding, anemia, food vomiting, weight loss), and in dyspeptic adults older than 50 years.
- Primary prevention aims to correct dietary habit starting from early age (high intake of fruits and vegetables and low intake of smoked foods, cured meat, salt, and nitrates) and to test and treat H.p. infection in areas at high incidence of gastric cancer and in first-degree relatives of gastric cancer patients.
- Primary and secondary prevention consist in testing and treating H.p. infection in patients with a family history of gastric cancer or gastric precancerous lesions or with dyspepsia less than 50 years of age, performing endoscopy in dyspeptic patients over 50, and plan endoscopic surveillance of precancerous lesions after eradication of H.p. infection.

REFERENCES

1. Cancer Genome Atlas Research Network. Comprehensive molecular characterization of gastric adenocarcinoma. Nature. 2014;513(7517):202-9.
2. Machlowska J, Baj J, Sitarz M, Maciejewski R et al. Gastric Cancer: Epidemiology, Risk Factors, Classification, Genomic Characteristics and Treatment Strategies. Int J Mol Sci. 2020; 21:4012.
3. Rugge M, Meggio A, Pravadelli C, et al. Gastritis staging in the endoscopic follow-up for the secondary prevention of gastric cancer: a 5-year prospective study of 1755 patients. Gut 2019; 68: 11-17
4. Song H, Ekheden IG, Zheng Z, et al. Incidence of gastric cancer among patients with gastric precancerous lesions: observational cohort study in a low risk Western population. BMJ. 2015;351:h3867.
5. Pimentel-Nunes P, Libânio D, Marcos-Pinto R et al Management of epithelial precancerous conditions and lesions in the stomach (MAPS II): European Society of Gastrointestinal Endoscopy (ESGE), European Helicobacter and Microbiota Study Group (EHMSG), European Society of Pathology (ESP), and Sociedade Portuguesa de Endoscopia Digestiva (SPED) guideline update 2019. Endoscopy. 2019; 51:365-88.

CHAPTER 15

INTESTINAL PATHOPHYSIOLOGY

Pierluigi Consolo, Federico Biagi

LEARNING OBJECTIVES

- To understand mechanisms of altered intestinal transit.
- To know when to suspect malabsorption.
- To recognize clinical features of a patient with malabsorption.
- To learn dynamics of fluids in order to understand the various forms of diarrhoea.

The small intestine, consisting of the duodenum, jejunum and ileum, is the organ in which the digestion and absorption of nutrients occurs. The colon forms faeces by absorbing about 90% of the 1,500 mL of fluid received from the ileal effluent, a fluid consisting mainly of water, fibers, mineral salts and bile residues. The transport of food along the alimentary tract is coordinated with the phenomena of secretion and absorption to allow its optimal exposure to digestive enzymes and the right contact of the nutritive principles with the mucosa. Intestinal motility is governed by longitudinal and circular musculature, which moves the contents along shorter or longer segments, or stops and holds them in place. The whole is a complex neuro-endocrine-paracrine-humoral system that governs contractions, distension and basic tone. In this chapter we will mention some elements of the pathophysiology of motility with references to some motor alterations; processes of digestion and absorption of foods with reference to the phenomena of maldigestion and malabsorption; dynamics of intestinal fluids with references to various forms of diarrhoea.

MOTILITY

Motility regulates intestinal transit through peristalsis, segmentation activity and sphincters. Peristalsis is chracterised by a contraction wave preceded by a distension which proceeds in an aboral direction or, more rarely, in the opposite direction. The segmentation activity consists in non-propagating contractions that alternate with distension without significant displacement of the contents, aimed at mixing the food bolus to ensure contact with the digestive enzymes and allow complete absorption. The sphincters are fibers of circular muscle displaying high basal tone that relax at the arrival of the peristaltic wave, separate some compartments and prevent the upstream reflux (**Figure 15.1**).

Muscular contractions are induced by intestinal release of vasoactive intestinal peptide (VIP) and adenosine triphosphate by inhibitory motor neurons. The electrophysiological control of intestinal smooth muscle is given by the interstitial cells of Cajal (CIC) located in the mucosa and in the circular muscular layer. These cells are responsible for slow, phasic depolarizations and action potentials,

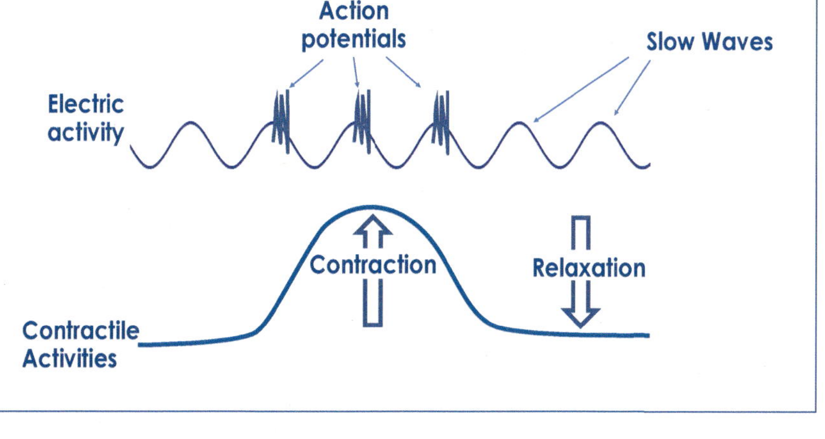

Figure 15.1 Schematic representation of slow waves with sovraimposed action potentials (top) and contractile activity (bottom). Notice how the contraction is related to action potentials.

generally associated with contractions. They represent the pacemaker of intestinal motor activity and are interconnected with each other and with the enteric nervous system (ENS), the so-called digestive brain, which works with a good functional integration also with the central nervous system and peripheral system. In fact, the plexuses of Auerbach and Meissner, autonomously coordinate all the digestive functions from the lower oesophageal sphincter up to the internal anal sphincter, while extrinsic nerves are intimately involved in the control of the skeletal muscle of the proximal portion of the oesophagus and of the external anal sphincter. Furthermore, it should be noted that the extreme parts of the alimentary canal, controlling swallowing function and external anal sphincter controlling defecation, have the possibility to be controlled also by the central nervous system with a voluntary act.

Motor activity is different during fasting and after meals. During fasting, motor activity is characterized by the so-called Interdigestive Migrating Motor Complex (IMMC), consisting of a peristaltic wave which begins in the gastric antrum-body, proceeds in an aboral direction up to the colon in about 2 hours and is repeated every 2-3 hours (**Figure 15.2**). It is preceded by a phase of motor quiescence (phase I) and one of uncoordinated activity (phase II). The peristaltic phase is phase III, characterised by regular propagating contractions that repeat with a frequency equal to the maximum decreasing frequency from the duodenum (11-12/min) to the terminal ileum (8/min). It is also called "activity front" and acts as a "housekeeper" of the enteric tract, since its function is to clean the intestinal lumen from undigested food residues, desquamated cells, bacteria and secretions that would otherwise accumulate during the interdigestive period.

IMMC is integrated with secretory activity. Indeed, the gastric, biliary, and pancreatic juices are secreted in increasing amount during phase II and reach their peak between the end of phase II and the beginning of phase III. Phase III pushes these secretions in the aboral direction, with the result that the intraluminal concentrations decrease rapidly returning to baseline values with the new phase I. All these mechanisms are under neurogenic control with a fine regulation between ENS and extrinsic innervation. Phase I is an expression of muscle bioelectrical activity and CIC.

Meals interrupt the IMMC and the small bowel alternates between periods of segmentation with slow transit and short peristaltic waves to mix and

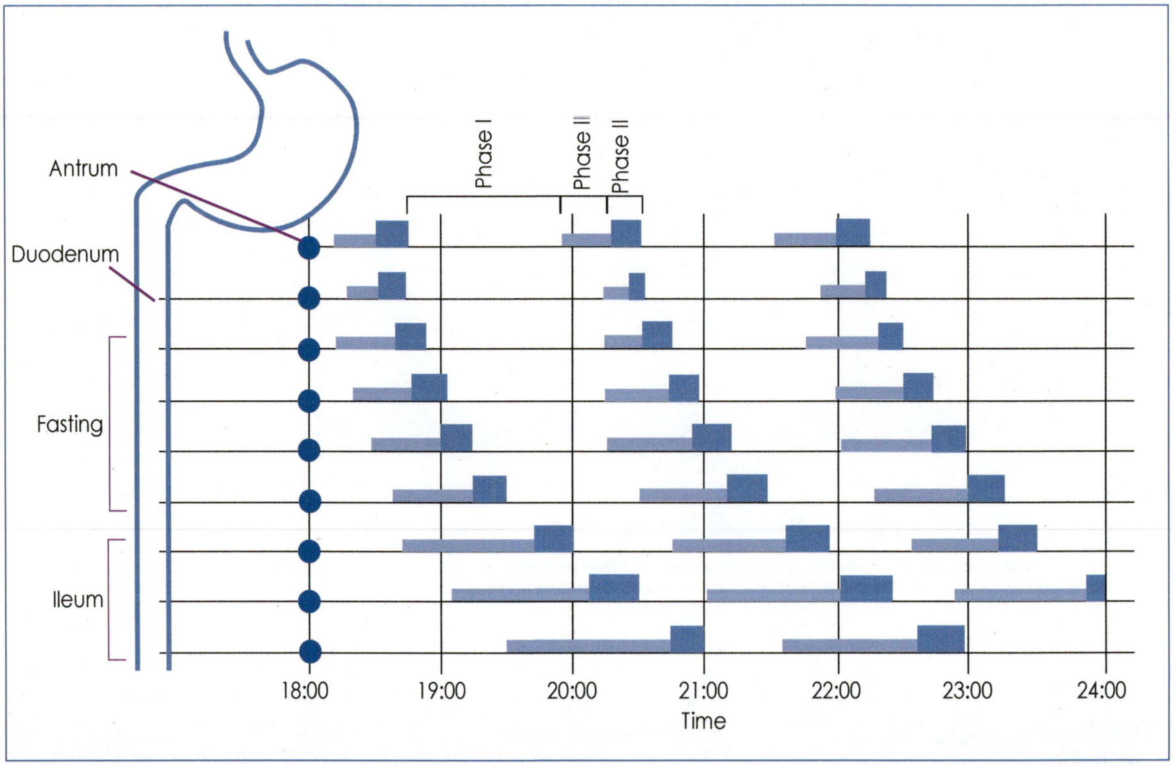

Figure 15.2 Schematic representation of the three phases of CMMI and its aboral progression. Further details in the text.

absorb chime. This process is aided by the muscularis mucosae which provides motility to microvilli, favouring surface contact with luminal contents. In the small bowel the luminal contents are propelled towards the colon by contraction of upstream intestinal segments combined with relaxation of those downstream.

The ileocecal valve acts as a sphincter which regulates flow from the ileum to the cecum and prevents retrograde flow from the cecum to the ileum. The ileocecal valve opens when peristaltic waves produce a sufficient pressure to overcome its resistance. Excessive distension of an intestinal segment induces relaxation of the remaining other intestinal segments (intestino-intestinal reflex). Activity of the terminal ileum may also be increased by gastric motor and secretory activity (gastro-ileal reflex).

Transit in the colon is much slower than in the small bowel. Two forms of motor activity occur, segmental and peristaltic. The motor activity of the colon is 80% segmental, aimed at allowing the absorption of fluids and the formation of faeces. Peristaltic movements can be of low and high amplitude (50 and 100 mmHg respectively). The former move liquid and gas for short tracts, the latter move solid material for longer segments.

Segmental activity is characterised by phasic non-propagated annular contractions lasting 4-6 seconds (repeating 3-6 cycles/minute). Its function is to mix intestinal contents, especially in the transverse and descending colon. Propulsive activity is characterised by annular monophasic contractions, propagates at different speeds (4-9 cm/sec), usually for short tracts, in aboral direction. Generally such propulsive activity may be regulated by excitatory oral reflexes (mediated by release of acetylcholine, substance P, neurokinin A) and inhibitory anal reflexes (mediated by release of VIP and nitric oxide). The main physiological stimuli for peristaltic activity are meals (gastrocolic reflex) and awakening.

The anal canal is about 2.5 cm long and is normally closed by the internal and external anal sphincters. When colonic material reaches the rectum evokes the need to evacuate. The internal anal sphincter relaxes and its receptors distinguish gas and solid or liquid faeces. Depending on the possibilities, the subject can decide whether or not to release the external sphincter to evacuate or postpone rectal emptying. The decision to postpone the evacuation is generally followed by the disappearance of the stimulous and the permanence of the faeces in the rectum until the arrival of a new peristaltic activity which is infrequent in the colon. This is one of the causes of constipation that more commonly is reported in clinic.

Alterations of segmental activity, peristalsis, sensitivity of the rectum and of the sphincter mechanisms, can provoke constipation or diarrhoea. Abnormalities of CICs, plexuses, neurons or ganglia may reduce or increase the strength and frequency of peristaltic waves (atonic constipation, irritable bowel syndrome, postprandial diarrhoea), increase or decrease rectal sensitivity (anorectal dissynergia, megarectum). Systemic neurological, endocrinological, or infectious conditions or pharmacological interventions may also alter the motility of the colon, but also of all the other intestinal tracts.

The intestinal content, therefore, is constantly moved by pressure gradients generated by coordinated contraction and relaxation. Uncoordinated contractions do not allow transit and lead to distension of the colon. This produces classic colic pain, which becomes more and more intense in the presence of a real obstacle (intestinal obstruction).

Sensory stimuli start from nerve endings located at various levels in the intestinal wall and form both sympathetic and parasympathetic neural pathways. Sensory neurones are pesudounipolar and their axon divides into central and peripheral branches. The central projections of spinal sensory neurons take synaptic relationship with neurons on which the somatic afferents responsible for the so-called "referred pain" also converge.

Alterations of the structure and function of the sensory nerve pathways, of the central and/or peripheral areas of sensory innervation, can cause visceral hypersensitivity phenomena known as hyperalgesia, an exaggerated painful response to a mild nociceptive stimulous, and allodynia, i.e., pain in response to a physiologic, not normally painful stimulous.

PATHOPHYSIOLOGY OF FLUID DYNAMICS

During the 24 hours, the digestive tract manages about 10 liters of fluid that are almost completely absorbed. About 1500 cc of this fluid arrive to the colon, but only 200 cc of them are expelled with the faeces. The colon, moreover, has a so-called functional reserve that allows it to increase its resorption capacity up to 3-4 times (**Figure 15.3 A**). Further details on the absorption mechanisms are given in **Figure 15.3 B**.

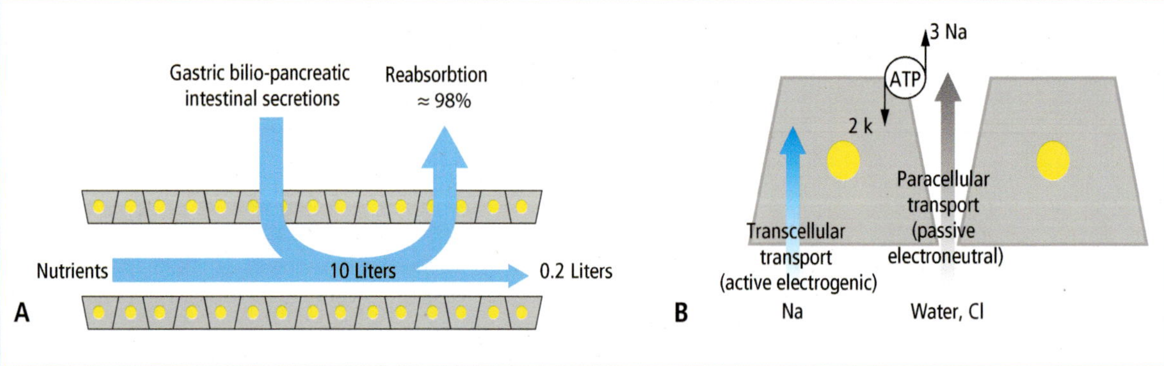

Figure 15.3 A) Schematic representation of the dynamics of intestinal fluids. The highest percentage of fluids is absorbed in the jejunum and in the ileum. The colon absorbs about 1500 cc of fluid even if it can triple its absorbing capacity. Further details in the text. B. Absorption and secretion of fluids occur through intestinal epithelial membranes (active, electro-diffusive, and facilitated trans-cellular transport) or through intercellular junctions (passive or intercellular paracellular transport). The absorption takes place in the cells of villi of the small intestine and in superficial cells of the colon while the secretion takes place in the glandular crypts of the small intestine and the colon. The absorption of electrolytes is an eminently active process generated by the sodium pump (ATP) that by extruding 3 sodium ions against 2 potassium ions generates both a negative electrical gradient within the cell which is favourable for sodium absorption and a concentration gradient in the intercellular space, favourable to the passive absorption of water. The final product is a net absorption of sodium, chloride and water. In the small intestine the presence of glucose and amino acids enhances the electrogenic absorption of sodium while in the colon is the presence of short chain fatty acids to enhance the electroneutral absorption of Na^+ in exchange with H^+.

An increase in secretion, a reduction in absorption and an increased luminal osmotic load can alter these exchanges.

Increased Secretion

Infections, hormones, pro-inflammatory cytokines and other inflammatory mediators can stimulate enterocytes to actively secrete a large amount of chloride that passively drags electrolytes and water into the intestinal lumen producing an abundant diarrhoea with watery stools (>1000 ml/24 h), rich in Cl^-, Na^+ and HCO_3^-. The clinical consequences are dehydration, metabolic acidosis and negative response to the fasting test (**Figure 15.4 A**).

Reduced Absorption

Reduced absorption can occur when intestinal mucosal is damaged, in the presence of an accelerated intestinal transit or after surgical resections. When mucosa is damaged by inflammation, a loss of epithelial cells occurs with consequent reduction of the absorbent surface. In addition, lost epithelial cells are replaced with immature cells that have lower absorptive capacity. These cells are generated by a compensatory increase in the proliferative activity of the crypts. Similarly to food, fluids need an adequate contact time with the intestinal epithelium to be absorbed. Therefore, all the conditions that determine an increase in the transit speed are responsible for their reduced absorption (**Figure 15.4 B**).

It may happen when damage to the ENS occurs (diabetes), in case of hormonal hyper-stimulation (hyperthyroidism) or when the volume of intestinal fluids (hypersecretion) is increased. Nevertheless, even a reduced motility can indirectly generate diarrhoea, favouring an increased intestinal bacterial colonization (scleroderma and, more rarely, diabetes). Intestinal resections can also decrease the absorption of fluids by reduction of the mucosal surface. Usually, this is a transitory problem because, some adaptive phenomena intervene over time that are able to compensate the reduced surface and allow an adequate absorption. When unabsorbed solutes are present in the intestinal lumen, a net secretion of water is produced. When this amount is superior to the opposite movement linked to sodium absorption, a net loss of fluids occur (Figure 15.4 a,b). Finally, it must be underlined that increased secretion and reduced absorption are never isolated phenomena. All these alterations represent the physiopathological basis of the diarrhoea.

Physiology of Intestinal Absorption

The small bowel consists of the duodenum, jejunum and ileum and it is an organ that digests and absorbs the nutrients ingested with diet. A digestive phase occurs in the oral cavity and in the stomach, by salivary amylase and gastric pepsin, respectively. In the duodenum nutrients are finally processed into absorbable molecules by the ac-

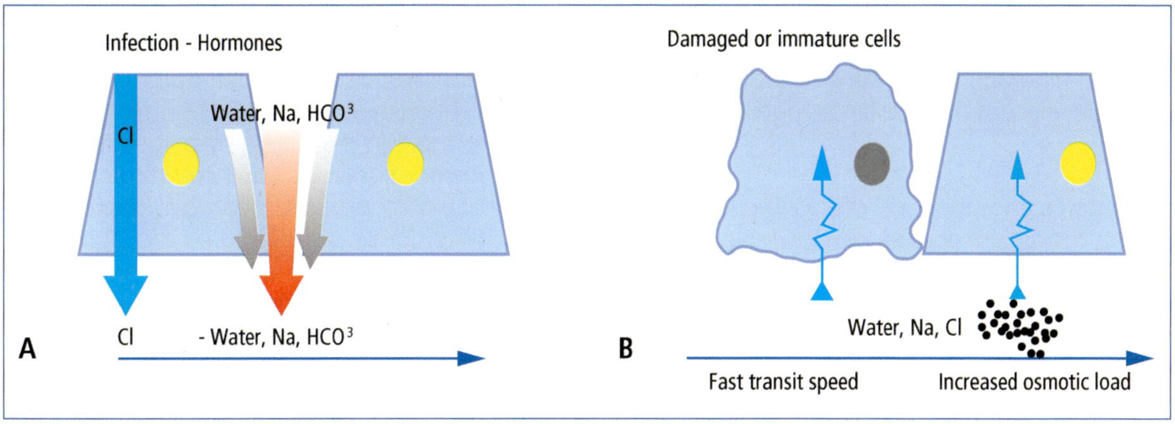

Figure 15.4 Pathophysiology of secretion (A) and absorption (B). See the text for details.

tion of pancreatic enzymes and bile. Cholecystokinin is an enzyme secreted by enterochromaffin cells of the duodenal mucosa, that triggers the secretion of pancreatic enzymes and bile upon contact with the acidic chyme coming from the stomach. Nutrients, once digested, are then absorbed in more distal segments of the small intestine i.e. jejunum and ileum.

The small bowel has functional and anatomical features that promote nutrient absorption by allowing their contact with the intestinal mucosa for an appropriate amount of time and modulating the intestinal flora. It is important to highlight the fact that the majority of nutrients can be absorbed all along the small bowel, while the absorption of some others is limited to specific areas. This is the case of iron, which is absorbed only in the proximal part of the duodenum, above the papilla of Vater; calcium and folic acid are absorbed only in proximal jejunum, while the vitamin B12 complexed with the intrinsic factor (produced by the gastric mucosa) is absorbed in terminal ileum.

The mucosal extension itself and the motor activities of the small bowel are the key elements that allow an adequate contact between nutrients and enteric mucosa. Circular folds (valves of Kerckring), intestinal villi and enteric microvilli create an absorption surface of approximately 200m2. The small bowel also possesses a finely tuned motor activity, which modulates the passage of nutrients along the intestine and facilitates the contact with the absorbing surface. This tightly regulated motor activity is provided partly by the macro motility of muscular layer, which determines the mixing and the movement of the luminal contents and, partly, by the micro motility of microvilli on enterocytes.

Finally, the gastric secretions, the pylorus, the peristalsis and the ileocecal valve, along with the mucosal immune system, modulate the microbiota composition. Additionally, gastric secretions and pyloric control of stomach emptying dramatically reduce the small bowel bacterial load; intestinal peristalsis avoids stagnation and hence, proliferation of bacterial flora; the ileocecal valve prevents the backflow of the colonic flora into the small bowel.

In conclusion, the pillars of physiological nutrients absorption are surface area of absorption, intestinal motility, and modulation of microbiota.

NUTRIENT DIGESTION

Carbohydrates

Dietary carbohydrates, mainly starch, lactose and sucrose, provide about 50% of daily calories. Starch digestion begins in the oral cavity under the action of salivary amylase and it is completed by pancreatic amylase in the duodenum and proximal jejunum. Pancreatic amylase cleavage produces oligo-disaccharides, which are digested together with other dietary disaccharides (lactose and sucrose) by the brush border enzymes into glucose, galactose and fructose. Specific active transporters control the absorption of glucose and galactose, while fructose is absorbed via facilitated diffusion.

Proteins

Protein digestion begins in the stomach under the action of both acidity and pepsin, while further breakdown is completed in the small intestine by trypsin and chymotrypsin, as well as by luminal exo- and endo-peptidase; the final products are oligopeptides, dipeptides and amino acids. Oligopeptides and dipeptides are further digested into amino acids by brush border peptidase and then absorbed by specific carriers in enterocytes.

Very small amounts of intact proteins are able to cross the intestinal epithelium via endocytosis, allowing an interaction with the immune system in order to develop an immune or tolerogenic response.

Lipids

Cholesterol, phospholipids, and long chain triglycerides provide 30% of average daily caloric intake. Lipid digestion occurs to a limited extent in the mouth and in the stomach under the action of salivary and gastric lipase, but it predominantly occurs in the duodenum by the action of biliary salts and pancreatic juices. Biliary salts and lectin emulsify lipids, so that pancreatic lipase can digest phospholipids into free fatty acids, monoglycerides and lysophospholipids. These are collected into very small structures called micelles, together with cholesterol and biliary salts. Micelles are free to diffuse across enterocytes.

Biliary salts are secreted into the bile once conjugated with taurine and glycine in the liver. In the last intestinal loop, biliary salts are reabsorbed with an active mechanism in order to establish the recycling pathway known as enterohepatic circulation. A small amount of biliary salts escapes the recycling pathway, enters the colon, where they are deconjugated by the intestinal flora and eliminated through the faeces. About 200-600 mg/die of bile salts are lost into the faeces and roughly the same amount is newly produced by the liver. Dietary lipophilic vitamins (A, D, E, K) are digested by the same processes and absorbed at the terminal ileum.

Water, Electrolytes, and Micronutrients

Water and ions are absorbed by means of pumps and carrier proteins, both via a paracellular route through tight junctions and a paracellular route through enterocytes themselves. Among the water-soluble vitamins, thiamin (vitamin B1) is absorbed via passive diffusion together with water. Thiamine deficiency, occurring almost always due to insufficient dietary intake, leads to beri-beri, a pathogical condition characterised by neurosensory deficits with difficulty in walking (dry beri-beri) and/or heart failure with oedema (wet beri-beri). Riboflavin (vitamin B2) is absorbed via a saturable mechanism. Niacin, also known as nicotinic acid, vitamin PP (Pellagra Preventis), or vitamin B3, is absorbed via a specific transporter. Dietary deficiency of this vitamin, classically in northern Italy because of a diet constituted almost exclusively by foods lacking this vitamin, such as corn polenta and chestnuts, leads to the development of pellagra within a few months. Pellagra has been defined as the syndrome of the four Ds: dermatitis (photosensitive), diarrhoea, dementia, and death. The absorption of ascorbic acid (vitamin C) occurs via a mechanism mediated by a specific carrier and localised at the apex of the enterocyte. Deficiency of this vitamin, almost always due to insufficient dietary intake, leads to the development of scurvy, a haemorrhagic syndrome which begins with gingival haemorrhage and slowed wound healing. Folic acid (vitamin B9) is absorbed after hydrolysis by a specific carrier. Deficiency of folic acid manifests initially as macrocytic anaemia. Vitamin B12 (cobalamin or cobalaminic acid) binds first to gastric intrinsic factor produced by parietal cells, then is led along the small bowel until reaching the last ileal loop where it is absorbed via a specific receptor for intrinsic factor. Chronic atrophic gastritis, gastrectomy, and diseases of the last ileal loop (Crohn's disease in particular) and right colectomy are all conditions which may lead to a deficiency of vitamin B12 which manifests initially with macrocytic anaemia but which may progress up to irreversible neurological deficits.

MALABSORPTION

Definition

Before beginning to discuss the pathophysiology of intestinal malabsorption it is very important to precisely define the meaning of malabsorption, malabsorption syndrome and enteropathy. These are in fact terms, which despite having a very precise meaning, in clinical practice are used in a interchangeable manner. Malabsorption refers to the defective passage across the small intestinal mucosa of the products of normal digestion. It is therefore a distinct mechanism from maldigestion, which refers, instead, to the lack of nutrient demolition and therefore to the impossibility for the healthy small intestine to absorb them. Malabsorption syndrome instead refers to the collection of symptoms and signs that develop due to malabsorption. Finally, enteropathy refers to the pathologic process causing malabsorption.

Pathophysiology

As mentioned in the initial paragraph, the extent of the absorbent surface, intestinal motility and control of bacterial flora are the three pillars which permit the physiological absorption of nutrients. These three pillars are however strictly connected to each another and therefore the pathological

alteration of one of these leads to corresponding secondary alterations in the other two, which, in theory, will have a compensatory effect. A typical example is the well-known increase of the length of villi in the residual intestine in patients affected by short bowel syndrome. Another example is the so-called "ileal brake". This is a compensatory mechanism triggered by the presence of malabsorbed lipids reaching the terminal ileum and mediated by PYY, a neuroenteric hormone that slows gastric emptying and intestinal transit. Its function is to increase the contact time between the intestinal mucosa and nutrients, and hence to favour their absorption. It should not be forgotten, however, that the same malabsorbed lipids which trigger the ileal brake may also stimulate a secretory diarrhoea. Furthermore, if the enteropathic process leads to malabsorption of lipids, it is very likely that sugars will also be malabsorbed, which may contribute to the development of an osmotic diarrhoea with a reduction of intestinal transit time. The slowing of intestinal transit which by increasing the contact time between mucosa and nutrients compensates for malabsorption may however in turn aggravate it if, becoming excessive, it favours bacterial proliferation and therefore bacterial overgrowth.
All these secondary alterations may therefore have double meaning: on the one hand, they may act opposing the primary alteration and therefore try to compensate for malabsorption, and on the other, they may act in concordance with the primary alteration, and therefore aggravate it. It is understandable therefore how the final result is extremely complex and depends on the algebraic sum of all these elements. In trying to summarise these pathophysiological concepts we may conclude by saying that enteropathy causes malabsorption, which manifests as a clinically evident malabsorption syndrome when the compensatory capabilities of the unaffected intestine are breached or when an intestinal tract with specific absorptive functions, which cannot be supplied by other districts, is involved.

Clinical Picture

Once the compensatory capacity of the unaffected portion of the small intestine is overwhelmed, a malabsorptive syndrome develops, whose severity depends mainly on the extension and location of the affected portion. In the case of an enteropathy affecting a limited portion of the small bowel, but which is responsible for the absorption of a specific nutrient, the patient will develop a selective malabsorption syndrome. In particular, involvement of the first part of the duodenum leads to a malabsorption of iron and hence the development of iron-deficiency anaemia. Involvement of the first part of the jejunum may lead to malabsorption of folates with consequent development of megaloblastic anaemia or to malabsorption of calcium and consequent osteoporosis. Involvement of the terminal ileum impedes the absorption of vitamin B12 and therefore leads to megaloblastic anaemia and, in those severe cases, to severe central and peripheral neuropathies which may begin as vague sensory abnormalities and progress up to spastic paresis.
If the enteropathy involves most of the mucosal surface, it is very likely that the patient may develop a global malabsorptive syndrome with symptoms and signs originating from both the lack of nutrient utilization and the persistence of the unabsorbed nutrients within the intestinal lumen. Among the symptoms caused by the loss of nutrient utilization, we recall asthenia and weight loss which are due to malabsorption of nutrients in general, oedema due to protein malabsorption, and several specific nutritional deficiencies. Deficiency of vitamin K leads to a lack of hepatic synthesis of vitamin K-dependant coagulation factors, particularly of factor VII, with consequent haemorrhagic manifestations. Malabsorption of vitamin D leads to rickets in children and osteomalacia in adults. Deficiency of vitamin A leads to glossitis, aphthous ulcers of the oral cavity, cutaneous dystrophies characterised by loss of skin elasticity with the end result that the skin may be lifted and even modelled into folds which maintain the form given to them. Furthermore, vitamin A deficiency may be responsible for a rare but characteristic eyesight abnormality, called night blindness. Patients affected by this symptom refer normal vision in well-lighted environments but a much longer adaptation period to darkness than normal. Deficiency of vitamin E seems to be responsible for central and peripheral neuropathies. The symptoms which are due to the persistence of nutrients within the intestinal lumen are obviously bloating, abdominal pain, diarrhoea and steatorrhoea. It should however be very clear to the student that the development of a global malabsorptive syndrome with the presence of all the aforementioned symptoms is rare and that even the presence of only one of these symptoms is absolutely not a good reason to exclude a malabsorptive syndrome. Likewise, the presence of a symptom differing from those previously men-

tioned is not a good reason to rule out the diagnosis. For example, the finding of faeces with characteristics of steatorrhoea is without a doubt suggestive of malabsorption but its absence is absolutely not a reason to rule out this possibility when the clinical picture is suggestive of malabsorption for other reasons. Even the presence of obesity is insufficient to exclude a diagnosis of enteropathy causing malabsorption.

Diagnosis

On the basis of what has previously been mentioned, it should therefore be clear that in clinical practice it is very frequent to encounter patients affected by an enteropathy causing malabsorption, whose clinical manifestation is a malabsorptive syndrome, but which may be modest and misleading. Keeping this in mind, it becomes clear that the classical diagnostic approach directed to first confirm the presence of malabsorption via tests which explore global absorptive function such as measuring stool fat and the xylose absorption test, and then, should these be positive, proceed to search for the causative enteropathy, is now considered outdated. Currently, it is thought that once malabsorption is suspected based on the clinical picture, the physician should directly search for the causative enteropathy.

The diagnosis of the conditions causing malabsorption shall be explained in detail in the following chapters. At this point, we may summarise briefly some key concepts: duodenal biopsy will be performed in the suspicion of diffuse enteropathies and intestinal lymphangiectasia, small bowel enema and videocapsule endoscopy will be used to exclude focal enteropathies, stool studies will be performed in the suspicion of parasitic infection and a detailed history taking will be very useful in the suspicion of small bowel bacterial overgrowth, short bowel syndrome and actinic enteritis.

KEY CONCEPTS

- Motility governs the path of the food bolus along the entire intestine to allow an adequate mixture with digestive enzymes and complete absorption.
- Malabsorption determines the presence in the colon of undigested nutrients with subsequent fermentation by the intestinal flora and the recall of water that, in turn, cause meteorism and diarrhoea.
- Malabsorption can be selective, as in the case of lactase deficiency, or total, as in the case of coeliac disease (the Italian version lacks this sentence).
- The dynamics of intestinal fluids can be altered by increased secretion, reduced absorption and increased osmotic load. All these mechanisms, once exceeded the capacity of colonic compensation, produce diarrhoea.

REFERENCES

- Goldstein AM, Thapar N, Karunaratne TB, De Giorgio R. Clinical aspects of neurointestinal disease: Pathophysiology, diagnosis, and treatment. Dev Biol 2016; 417:217-28
- Bassotti G, de Roberto G, Castellani D, Sediari L, Morelli A. Normal aspects of colorectal motility and abnormalities in slow transit constipation. World J Gastroenterol 2005;11:2691-6
- Abumrad NA, Nassir F, Marcus A. Digestion and absorption of dietary fat, carbohydrate, and protein. In: Feldman M, Friedman LS, Brandt LJ, editors. Sleisenger and Fordtran's Gastrointestinal and Liver Disease. Pathophysiology, diagnosis, management. 10th ed. Philadelphia: Elsevier Saunders; 2016. p. 1736-64
- Said HM, Trebble TM. Intestinal digestion and absorption of micronutrients. In: Feldman M, Friedman LS, Brandt LJ, editors. Sleisenger and Fordtran's Gastrointestinal and Liver Disease. Pathophysiology, diagnosis, management. 10th ed. Philadelphia: Elsevier Saunders; 2016. p. 1765-87
- Högenauer C, Hammer HF. Maldigestion and malabsorption. In: Feldman M, Friedman LS, Brandt LJ, editors. Sleisenger and Fordtran's Gastrointestinal and Liver Disease. Pathophysiology, diagnosis, management. 10th ed. Philadelphia: Elsevier Saunders; 2016. p. 1788-1823
- Leiper JB. Fate of ingested fluids: factors affecting gastric emptying and intestinal absorption of beverages in humans. Nutr Rev 2015;73 Suppl 2:57-72.
- Fagerberg JH, Bergström CA. Intestinal solubility and absorption of poorly water soluble compounds: predictions, challenges and solutions. Ther Deliv 2015;6:935-59.

CHAPTER 16

IRRITABLE BOWEL SYNDROME

Michele Pierluca Guarino, Paola Iovino

LEARNING OBJECTIVES

- To clarify the definition of irritable bowel syndrome, in the light of the new diagnostic criteria, as well as the epidemiology of this disorder.
- To describe the pathophysiological mechanisms underlying symptoms.
- To provide a reasoned approach to the main clinical features, the diagnosis, and the differential diagnosis.
- To describe the main therapeutic approaches, both non-pharmacological and pharmacological according to symptom type and severity.

DEFINITION

Irritable bowel syndrome (IBS), according to the latest Roma IV criteria published in 2016, is defined as a disorder of the brain-gut axis, characterized by abdominal pain, associated with a change in bowel habits after exclusion of biochemical or organic causes (**Figure 16.1**). One of the novelties introduced by the Rome IV Criteria is the recognition of a spectrum of intestinal functional disorders with the transition over time from one form to another. IBS is further classified according to the characteristics of abnormal bowel movements in IBS-D (diarrhoea predominant >25% 6-7 according to Bristol Stool Form Scale (BSFS)), IBS-C (constipation predominant, >25% 1-2 according to Bristol Stool Form Scale (BSFS)), IBS-M (mixed diarrhoea and constipation); IBS-U (unclassified; the symptoms cannot be categorized into one of the above three subtypes).

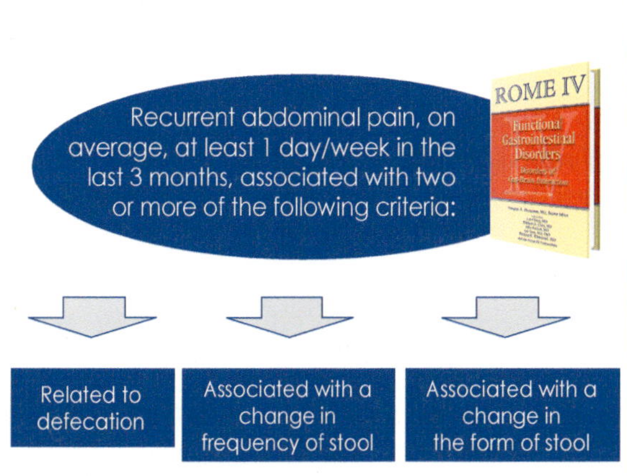

Figure 16.1 Rome IV criteria for the diagnosis of irritable bowel syndrome.

EPIDEMIOLOGY

The world prevalence of IBS is widely heterogenous. The prevalence of IBS is lower according to the recent Rome IV criteria that consider the presence of abdominal pain alone without abdominal discomfort. Moreover, between the second and the fourth decade of life, with predominance of the female sex (F:M ratio 2:1).

PATHOGENESIS

Although the aetiology of IBS remains largely undetermined, our understanding of the potential mechanisms involved in intestinal dysfunction, visceral sensation, and symptom generation is rapidly advancing. IBS is a multifactorial syndrome; its pathogenesis involves pathophysiological mechanisms: increase in the perceptions of stimuli from the intestinal tract (or visceral hypersensitivity); changes in gastrointestinal motor activity; psychological disturbances.
Recent studies have also identified the involvement of cellular and molecular mechanisms.
These mechanisms concern genetic factors and genetic polymorphisms (mainly the regulatory mechanisms of serotonin and inflammatory cytokines), alterations in gastrointestinal neurotransmitters, intestinal microbiota, intestinal permeability, and mucosal immune system.

Alteration in Visceral Sensitivity

The threshold of pain during rectal balloon distention is lower in IBS patients than in healthy volunteers. This alteration is named visceral hypersensitivity and has been shown at the ileum, the recto-sigmoid and the anorectal region. However, recent data indicate that only a percentage of patients (20 and 70%), with IBS present visceral hypersensitivity. This finding suggests that this pathophysiological mechanism is not enough to explain the genesis of symptoms in all patients.

Gastrointestinal Motility Dysfunction

Several changes in colonic motor function have been observed, including an increase in colonic contractions due to psychological and physical stress and an increase in colonic postprandial contractions. Impairment of motility has also been shown in the small bowel, thus explaining the more recently accepted definition of "Irritable bowel" as opposed to the more restrictive term "irritable colon". However, results of myoelectric, motility, and transit studies in both the colon and small intestine are inconsistent.

Psychological Factors

Studies have reported the presence of psychological disorders such as anxiety, hostility, phobia, paranoia, somatization, alcohol and drug abuse in patients with IBS.

The brain, the gut, its microbiota, and the immune system are inter connected. The brain, through the autonomic nervous system, can influence intestinal motility, fluid secretion, intestinal epithelial permeability, immune function, and intestinal microbial composition; recent evidence has also shown that gastrointestinal symptoms can induce psychological disorders.

Endoluminal Factors and Intestinal Microbiota

Potential endoluminal factors include dietary factors, biochemical components of digestive secretions (such as bile acids), gas, and intestinal microbiota.

There is growing evidence for the altered composition of the intestinal microbiota in the pathophysiology of IBS, but its aetiologic role remains uncertain. Experiments with animal models have shown that colonization of germ-free animals with microbiota of patients with IBS can induce visceral hypersensitivity, alter intestinal permeability and gastrointestinal transit time, indicating the importance and the possible aetiological role of the microbiota in the IBS. In support of a relationship between microbiota and IBS there is evidence from microbiological studies on fecal material of a reduction in lactobacilli and bifidobacteria and an increase in streptococci and *Escherichia coli*. More recent studies using molecular biology techniques have found significant differences in bacterial families. Furthermore, in support of a role of the microbiota in the genesis of IBS, there is evidence that infectious gastroenteritis is the only recognized aetiological factor.

Persistent digestive symptoms compatible with a diagnosis of IBS are present in 7 to 31% following an acute infectious event.

Bile acid malabsorption is another endoluminal factor in patients with a diarrhoeal predominant IBS. An increase in intestinal bile salt concentration can irritate the intestinal mucosa, and contribute to the pathogenesis of diarrhoea in this subgroup of patients.

Alterations in the Serotoninergic System

Serotonin (5-hydroxytryptamine, 5-HT) is a monoamine: 5% in the central nervous system and 95% in the gastrointestinal tract (90% in enterochromaffin cells and 10% in enteric neurons).

Serotonin receptors are strategically located on intrinsic nerve pathways (enteric nervous system) involved in the control of gastrointestinal motor activity, and on primary afferent nerve fibers, implicated in the transmission of visceral sensory stimuli. Studies have shown the presence of alterations in the release of 5-HT from the intestinal mucosa and in the number of enterochromaffin cells.

An increase in the number of enterochromaffin cells has been documented in the rectal and colonic mucosal biopsies of patients with IBS and confirmed in patients with post-infectious IBS and in larger series of patients with IBS. Other studies have shown that the postprandial plasma concentration of 5-HT is reduced in IBS-C and increased in IBS-D, while a recent study demonstrated an increased spontaneous release of 5-HT from colic mucosal biopsies regardless of the characteristics of the patients examined. These observations support the use of 5-HT receptor modulator drugs.

Role of the Mucosal Barrier and of the Immune Activation/Intestinal Inflammation

Recent studies have shown that altered permeability of the intestinal barrier can contribute to the pathophysiology of IBS, playing a key role in the relationship between the host and the external environment. In particular, in vivo studies have shown an increased permeability of the small intestine in some subgroups of patients, such as those with post-infectious IBS or with predominantly diarrhoeal IBS.

In recent years, focus has been directed to the role of mast cells and their mediators, which seem

to be involved in the sensory-motor dysfunction present in IBS.
A greater number of mast cells has been found in the colonic mucosa and the small intestine of some subgroups of patients with IBS.
In the human intestine, mast cells are close to gut mucosal innervation. Once activated, the mast cells of the colonic mucosa release mediators that cause abnormalities of gastrointestinal motor functions and visceral hypersensitivity.
Clinical trials have partly demonstrated the efficacy of mast cell stabilizing drugs in some subgroups of patients with IBS.

DIAGNOSIS

The cardinal symptom of IBS is recurrent abdominal pain.
Although present in all abdominal quadrants, it is mainly evoked by palpation along the colic frame and is associated with defecation or change in bowel habits. Stool consistency can be assessed using the Bristol stool form scale on days when patients have abnormal bowel habits. Associated symptoms that support the diagnosis are urgency, feeling of incomplete evacuation, and mucus in feces.
Bloating is also a common symptom. IBS is frequently associated with other functional digestive disorders, such as dyspepsia (between 40 and 87%), and with extra-digestive disorders, such as fibromyalgia (between 20 and 50%), headache, chronic fatigue syndrome, interstitial cystitis, and temporomandibular joint disorders. In women, worsening of symptoms during menstruation and dyspareunia can frequently be observed. These comorbidities strengthen the diagnosis of IBS, but they can also increase the severity, worsen the quality of life, and are associated with psychiatric or psychological factors.
According to the main guidelines, the diagnosis of IBS is based on a careful medical history, a complete physical and anorectal examination, symptoms that meet the Rome IV criteria, together with a limited battery of tests (complete blood count, C-reactive protein and faecal calprotectin in patients with diarrhoea to exclude IBD), and the exclusion of alarm symptoms/signs such as age over 50, a positive family history of colorectal cancer, inflammatory bowel disease (IBD) or celiac disease, fever, blood in the stools, sideropenic anemia without apparent cause, sudden unintentional weight loss significant change in typical symptomatology or nocturnal symptoms.
The presence of alarm features suggests the likelihood of organic disease and will require additional investigations.
A positive diagnostic strategy that uses a limited number of tests was not inferior to a strategy of exclusion based on a large number of diagnostic tests and had lower direct costs.
Colonoscopy is not indicated in the presence of typical symptoms compatible with the diagnosis of IBS and in the absence of alarm symptoms/signs.
Diagnostic testing for celiac disease should be performed in patients from geographical areas with a high prevalence of this disease. Cost analysis suggests that screening for celiac disease is only indicated in geographic areas where its prevalence in the population is more than 1%.

TREATMENT

Stratification of Patients Based on Type and Severity of Symptoms

Figure 16.2 illustrates the approach to patients with irritable bowel. The choice of treatment depends on severity of symptoms, stool subtype, presence of psychosocial comorbidities, and patient preference (e.g., non-pharmacological vs. medication) and their expectations.
Patients with mild symptomatology often resort to self-medication.
As the degree of illness increases, the family doctor is called upon more frequently. The therapeutic approach involves the establishment of a good doctor-patient relationship that comprises the aspects listed above, and gives a clear explanation of IBS and a reassurance to avoid further unnecessary diagnostic tests. At this stage, the patient is encouraged to modify life style habits and diet, with the eventual use of drugs.
Patients who consult an gastroenterologist a specialist reference center more frequently present abdominal pain or severe abnormalities and associated psychological disorders.

Non-Pharmacological Approach

Patients often report worsening of symptoms after the intake of certain foods, which often leads to self-experimentation with exclusion diets, so the request for dietary advice is very common.
During the visit, the doctor should ask about dietary habits and make sure that the patients follows healthy lifestyle habits.

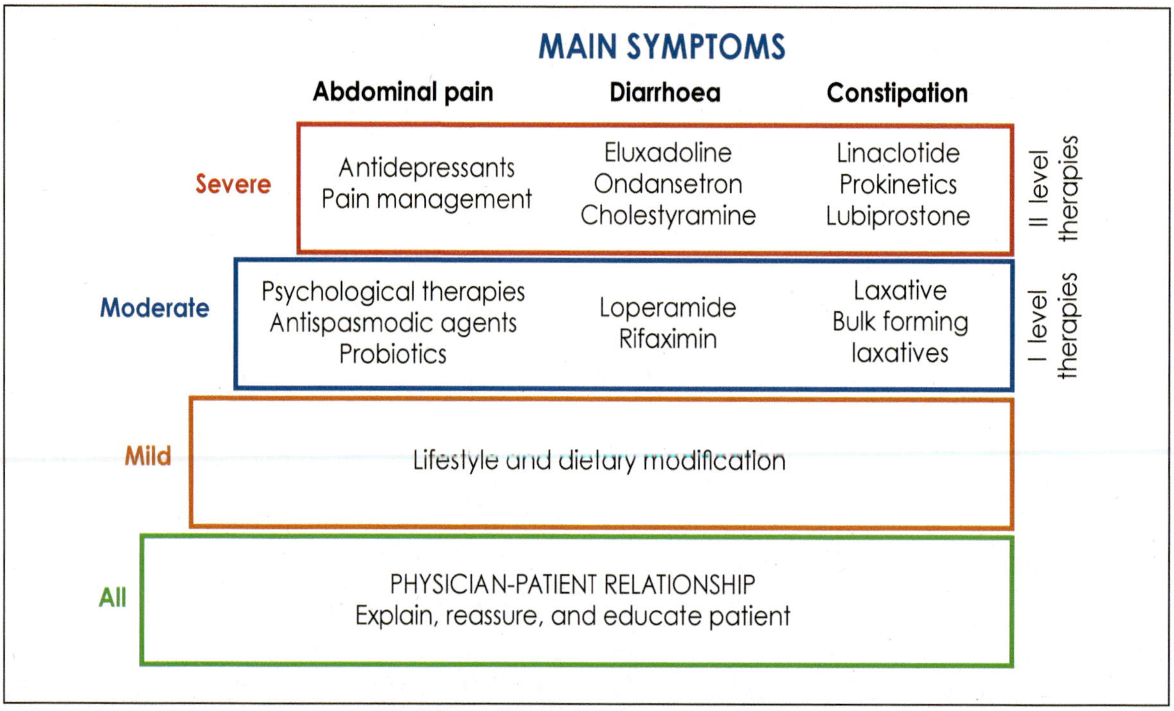

Figure 16.2 Stratification of patients by disease severity and subtypes with related examples of therapeutic strategy.

The addition of fiber in the diet to accelerate transit through the intestine and increase fecal weight in some patients with constipation as the dominant symptom may help to regularize the transit, but it increases the risk of exacerbating abdominal pain. In clinical practice, it is advisable, therefore, to add to the diet 20-30 g of fiber per day or, alternatively, agents to form a mass (derivatives of psyllium, mucilage or glucomannan), which, being soluble, are better tolerated. Many patients are sensitive to certain types of carbohydrates such as fructose, fructans, lactose, and others, i.e., FODMAPs (oligo-, di-, and monosaccharides and fermentable polyols) contained in cereals, vegetables, and fruits. However, long-term exclusion diets should be avoided. The physician's task is to guide the patient through the diagnostic pathway. When necessary a trained dietician should be consulted before adopting an exclusion diet.
Alternative non-pharmacological approaches to abdominal pain in patients with IBS include hypnotherapy, psychotherapy, and acupuncture. Predictors of a favorable response include association with other psychiatric disorders and intermittent pain exacerbated by stress.

Pharmacological Approach

Laxatives. Polyethylene-glycol acts as an osmotic laxative, is effective and well tolerated in chronic constipation, but has not shown a significant effect on abdominal pain or bloating. Laxatives can be considered as a first line strategy given the low cost and the few side effects.
Antidiarrhoeals. Loperamide, a synthesis agonist of μ opioid receptors, is effective in reducing diarrhoea and urgency and in promoting the formation of feces, without appreciable effects on abdominal pain.
Antispasmodics. They are the most common drugs for abdominal pain in IBS. The rationale for their use is based on their property to relax the gut smooth muscle.
A recent meta-analysis showed a global improvement in symptoms in IBS patients. The most common are cimetropium bromide (antimuscarinic compound), pinaverium bromide and otilonium bromide, (quaternary ammonium derivatives with calcium antagonist properties), trimebutine (a weak agonist of μ opioid receptors), and mebeverine (a derivative of βphenyl-ethylamine with anticholinergic activity). Moreover, a recent meta-analysis has shown that also joscina and peppermint oil (another compound with myorelaxant activity) are effective in IBS.
Antidepressants. Antidepressants, both tricyclics (such as amitriptyline, trimipramine, desipramine) and serotonin reuptake inhibitors (such as fluoxetine, sertraline, paroxetine) are frequently used in the treatment of severe and refractory forms of

IBS, both for the treatment of psychological distress, for example, depression, and for the control of abdominal pain.
The latter effect is mainly expressed through an analgesic mechanism on the visceral pain pathways and occurs at lower dosages than those used for the treatment of depression. They are also effective in improving quality of life.
Antibiotics and probiotics. The rationale for the use of poorly-absorbable antibiotics and probiotics is based on the potential alterations in the intestinal microbiota in IBS, from both a qualitative and a quantitative point of view. Rifaximin (a poorly-absorbable derivative of rifampicin) has been shown to be effective in improving overall symptoms in IBS patients with diarrhoea.
Probiotics have numerous properties that are potentially useful in the treatment of IBS, for example, by modulating local and systemic responses of the immune system and barrier functions of the digestive tract. Although widely used in clinical practice, the precise mechanisms of action have not been fully clarified.
Eluxadoline. This new drug recenlly approved in Italy for the treatment of diarrhoea predominant irritable bowel syndrome, is a mu-opioid receptor agonist and delta opioid receptor antagonist that modulates gastrointestinal motility and reduces abdominal pain associated with IBS, but it has been associated with pancreatitis.
Alosetron. This selective 5-HT3 antagonist and it has been shown to be effective in improving abdominal pain and diarrhoea in female patients with diarrhoea predominant IBS. It was withdrawn from the market after reports of adverse events and then reintroduced with considerable restrictions.
Ondansetron, which is used as antiemetic, can also be used to reduce diarrhoea.
Prucalopride. This complete agonist of 5-HT4 receptors, extensively studied in severe chronic constipation and in IBS with constipation as it accelerates the transit of the small intestine and collon, resulting effective and with non-severe adverse events. It is authorized in Italy only for the treatment of chronic constipation in patients who have not responded to common first level therapies.
Lubiprostone. It activates apical type 2 chlorine channels, increasing intestinal water secretion. Lubiprostone accelerates colonic transit, reduces abdominal pain, and improves intestinal function in patients with constipation. It is not currently available in Europe.
Linaclotide. This new guanylate-cyclase-C agonist, a transmembrane protein present at the level of the epithelium of the digestive tract, reduces constipation by increasing fluid secretion and accelerating intestinal transit. It has a modest effect on pain and abdominal bloating, too.
Colestyramine. This a bile acid sequestrant, can be empirically used when other therapies have failed in a minority of patients with diarrhoea predominant IBS.
Other drugs are considered in non-response to second-level drugs, but the scientific evidence is still accumulating on their effectiveness as an anti-inflammatory.
The rationale for the use of anti-inflammatory drugs is based on evidence for immune activation of the intestinal mucosa in a subset of IBS patients. Among anti-inflammatory drugs, for some years now, mast cell membrane stabilizing drugs have been proposed, such as sodium cromoglycate.

KEY CONCEPTS

- Irritable bowel syndrome is a disorder of gut-brain interaction, characterized by abdominal pain, abdominal pain related to disordered bowel function (diarrhoea, constipation or both) for at least 3 months in the absence of evidence of other diseases to explain these symptoms. It is one of the most common clinical problems in Western countries, mainly in females.
- The pathogenesis of irritable bowel syndrome is multifactorial. Three main pathophysiological mechanisms are distinguished: (psychological disorders, gastrointestinal motor activity alterations, and visceral hypersensitivity), together with genetic factors, alterations of gastrointestinal neurotransmitters, intestinal microbiota, intestinal permeability, and the mucosal immune system.
- Diagnosis is essentially clinical and is based on careful history, a physical examination, symptoms (which meet the criteria of Rome IV), exclusion of alarm symptoms/signs and, when necessary, on a limited number of laboratory tests.
- The therapeutic approach can be non-pharmacological and/or pharmacological and is based on stratification of patients by type and severity of symptoms. A good physician-patient relationship will optimize the effectiveness of treatment.

REFERENCES

- Bharucha AE, Wouters MM, Tack J. Existing and emerging therapies for managing constipation and diarrhea. Curr Opin Pharmacol. 2017;37:158-66.
- Drossman DA, Tack J, Ford AC, et al. Neuromodulators for functional gastrointestinal disorders (disorders of gut-brain interaction): A Rome Foundation working team report. Gastroenterology. 2018;154:1140-71.
- Drossman DA. Functional gastrointestinal disorders: history, pathophysiology, clinical features and Rome IV. Gastroenterology. 2016;150:1262-79.
- Lacy BE, Mearin F, Chang L, et al. Bowel disorders. Gastroenterology. 2016:150:1393-407.

CHRONIC CONSTIPATION

Danilo Badiali, Emma Calabrese

LEARNING OBJECTIVES

- To recognize and classify chronic constipation, distinguishing secondary and primitive types.
- To manage a first line diagnostic procedure.
- To prescribe dietary norms and drugs for treatment.
- To recognize when it is necessary addressing the patient to a tertiary centre.

DEFINITION AND EPIDEMIOLOGY

Constipation is a syndrome defined by the presence of multiple and heterogeneous symptoms such as reduced frequency of spontaneous bowel movements (<3 times per week), difficult evacuation, hard stools. These patient-reported symptoms are incorporated in the standardised diagnostic criteria named Rome IV criteria (**Table 17.1**).
Constipation is divided into acute and chronic depending on whether the duration is shorter or longer than 6 months.
Constipation may be due to transient conditions such as bed immobilization, to organic diseases and/or medicine assumption (**Table 17.2**), or more frequently it is primary and defined Functional Constipation (FC) as consequence of neuromuscular dysfunction of the colon or anorectal sensory-motor function, in the absence of any organic disease.
Prevalence of chronic constipation in the general adult population is reported to be 14-20%, but it varies widely according to regions and definition adopted. About 5% of Italians report less than 3 bowel movements per week and 18% at least one defecation disorder. It is more frequent in women than in man (M/F = 1:2–3); its prevalence increases with age and with a low socio-economic status. Insufficient fluid and/or fiber intake or limited exercise alone may not be the only cause of constipation, but correcting these factors can improve symptoms in many patients.
A psychological profile with high levels of hypochondria, anxiety, depression has been described in patients with FC; eating disorders and somatoform disorders have also been reported.
Chronic constipation has a close relationship with the quality of life, and with consumption of health resources; the considerable prevalence in the general population requires that general practitioners can usually manage these patients, reserving the most severe cases to reference centers for an adequate pathophysiological evaluation.

PATHOPHYSIOLOGY AND CLASSIFICATION

The FC is commonly classified into 3 types according with the underlying pathophysiologic mechanism: (1) normal transit constipation, (2) slow transit

Table 17.1 Rome IV Criteria for the Diagnosis of Functional Constipation.

Criteria fulfilled for the last 3 month with symptom onset at least 6 months prior to diagnosis	
1. Must include two or more of the following:	
- Straining during more than one fourth	in ≥25% of defecations
- Lumpy or hard stools (BSFS 1-2)	in ≥25% of defecations
- Sensation of incomplete evacuation	in ≥25% of defecations
- Sensation of anorectal obstruction/blockage	in ≥25% of defecations
- Manual manoeuvers to facilitate (e.g., digital evacuation, support of the pelvic floor)	in ≥25% of defecations
- Fewer than 3 spontaneous bowel movements per week	in ≥25% of defecations
2. Loose stools are rarely present without the use of laxatives	
3. Insufficient criteria for IBS-C	

BSFS: Bristol Stool Form Scale; IBS-C: Irritable Bowel Syndrome with Constipation.

(B.E. Lacy et al., 2016)

Table 17.2 Causes of Secondary Constipation.

Bowel Diseases	Systemic Diseases
• **Anatomical alterations**: stenosis (cancer, ischaemic colitis, diverticular disease), outcomes of surgery, anal disease. • **Alterations of the enteric nervous system**: Hirschsprung's disease, neuronal dysplasia.	• **Endocrine-metabolic diseases**: diabetes, hypothyroidism, hyperparathyroidism, chronic renal failure. • **Electrolyte disorders:** hypercalcemia, hypokalemia, hypermagnesemia. • **Neuromuscular diseases**: Parkinson's disease, multiple sclerosis, autonomic neuropathy, spinal cord injuries, systemic sclerosis, muscular dystrophies. • **Psychiatric disorders**: dementia, depression, eating disorders, somatoform disorders.
Medications	
• **Physician prescription**: opioids, anticholinergics, diuretics, antipsychotics, Ca-antagonists, tricyclic antidepressants, antiparkinsonian, sympathetic mimetics, cholestyramine. • **Self-prescription**: antihistamines, iron supplements, calcium supplements, anti-diarrhoeal agents, NSAIDs, antiacids with calcium and aluminum, analgesics.	

constipation (STC), (3) constipation with outlet disorder, but the mechanism generating the symptoms may exist in the same subject and the symptoms can be similar or overlap regardless of the pathogenetic mechanism.

Normal Transit Constipation

It is the most common form of FC, and it is often associated with asthenia, abdominal pain or bloating; this form is hardly distinguishable from the Irritable Bowel Syndrome with Constipation with the pain being more prevalent in the last one. These conditions are currently interpreted as a spectrum of the same pathophysiological condition with overlapping symptoms and interchangeable diagnoses over time. The pathophysiology of these syndromes involves visceral hypersensitivity, alterations of the enteric nervous system and / or of the gut-brain axis.

Slow Transit Constipation

In these patients, the motor response to meal is compromised, with reduction of the propagated waves transporting the contents from the right colon to the rectum, and an increase of non-propagated and/or retrograde contractions. STC can be caused by neuromuscular dysfunctions of the colon wall, in the absence of systemic neuromuscular diseases. A reduced number of intrinsic nerves and of the interstitial cells of Cajal have been described in these patients. The composition of the microbiota can also affect the bowel transit: the prevalence of methane producer bacteria is significantly higher in patients with delayed colon transit than in normal transit. Prolonged transit in the colon causes reabsorption of water with the production of hard lump faeces, inducing decreased urge to defecate, and difficult evacuation.

Outlet Disorders

Defecation can be defective due to functional causes or anatomical alterations, although the two conditions frequently coexist. In the pelvic dyssynergia the puborectal muscle and/or the anal sphincter do not release in synergy with the abdominal effort so that defecation is difficult and with straining; on the other hand, evacuation may be ineffective due to insufficient pushing associated or not with normal anal relaxation. During the expulsive phase, the rectal mucosa can fold into the rectum or into the anal canal, hindering the passage of faeces or a large rectocele can form collecting faeces that are not evacuated, worsening the evacuation itself.

Constipation in the Elderly

In elderly, there is no clear evidence of slow transit and constipation seems frequently due to defecation disorders. The treatment involves dietary adjustments with optimization of the fiber/liquid ratio intake, however it is to be avoided administrating large amount of fibers due to the risk of forming fecalomas: Whenever possible, drugs inducing constipation should be removed; when a laxative is administered, it is necessary to pay attention that it does not interfere with any other drugs. Pelvic abnormalities such as rectocele, descending pelvic floor syndrome, and mucosal prolapse are common in the elderly population.

Opioid Induced Constipation

It is a progressively frequent condition as a secondary form due to disorders of the mechanisms underlying bowel motor function. Opioid receptors μ and δ are located in the myenteric and submucosal plexuses of the enteric nervous system. Their activation by opioids used for pain management causes decrease in the propulsive motor activity of the colon, inhibition of secretion, and increase in the perception threshold of rectal distension and of the rectal-anal inhibitory reflex.

Refractory Constipation

When a satisfactory remission of symptoms is not achieved with the lifestyle, diet and use of osmotic laxatives, it is useful to perform a diagnostic work up investigating the pathogenetic mechanisms causing the disorder. About 50% of patients asking a visit to a reference center for chronic constipation, display slow bowel transit, and in over 50% it is possible to detect associations between transit disorders, defecation disorders, and pelvic alterations. This condition may require integrated management between specialists of different disciplines for assessing medical needs, psychotherapy, and eventual surgical procedures.

DIAGNOSTIC WORK-UP

The approach to chronic constipation includes the prescription of osmotic laxative as part of the diagnostic work-up, reserving specific diagnostic tests in presence of alarm features and in non-responder subjects (**Figure 17.1**).

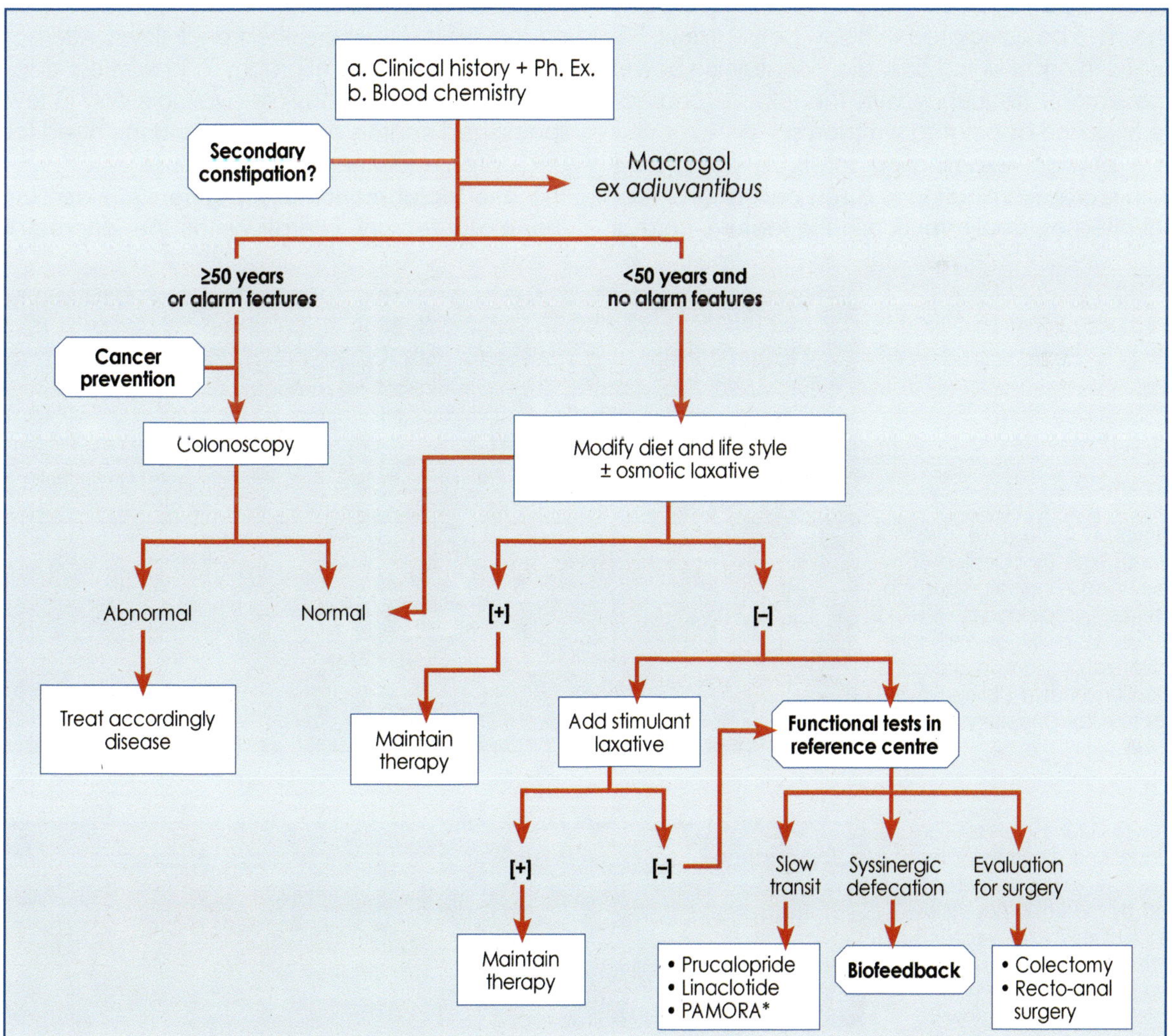

Figure 17.1 Diagnostic algorithm for chronic constipation.
Ph.Ex: Physical Examination; PAMORA: Peripherally-Acting Mu-Opioid Receptor Antagonists; (*) addressed to opioid induced constipation.

During the diagnostic work-up, prescription of macrogol, except in cases of suspected bowel perforation or occlusion, is useful to relieve symptoms and facilitate intestinal preparation in view of a possible colonoscopy.

Clinical History and Physical Examination. The clinical history and physical examination should be aimed to investigate symptoms of organic diseases. It is necessary to evaluate hygienic-dietary habits, presence of systemic diseases, use of laxatives, and drugs inducing constipation (Table 17.2). The characteristic of constipation can be investigated showing the Bristol Stool Form Scale (BSFS) with images of stools of different consistency in relation to the water content, that is inversely proportional to the time spent in the colon. The BSFS classifies the human faeces into seven categories ranging from hard dry goat stools (type I) to watery stools (type VII); stools of type I and II have been shown to be associated with slow bowel transit. It is useful to ask to fill in a daily diary containing bowel movements frequency with the relative characteristics and associated symptoms.

The physical examination must be completed with rectal examination to assess anal and/or rectal diseases, stool retention in the rectum, normal anal relaxation during the evacuation strain.

Blood tests are useful for a metabolic evaluation and for detecting alarm features such as anaemia, hypothyroidism, and electrolyte abnormalities. Colonoscopy or, in some cases, virtual colonoscopy, is required in individuals older than 50 years of age for cancer screening or in presence of alarming symptoms and findings.

Functional Evaluation

Patients who do not respond to first-line therapy, need to be evaluated in tertiary centers to investigate bowel transit and functional and/or structural alteration of defecation.

Bowel Transit can be evaluated upon the ingestion of radiopaque markers with abdominal X-ray to detect their localization along the colorecum (**Figure 17.2**) until their elimination, so obtaining information on the transit time (vn <96 hours) and on the segment where the transit slows. Alternative methods are scintigraphy and wireless capsule, but these methods are available only in few specialized centers due to costs and the need for dedicated equipment and personnel.

The **ano-rectal manometry** (**Figure 17.3**) detects the motor-sensory alterations of the anorectal

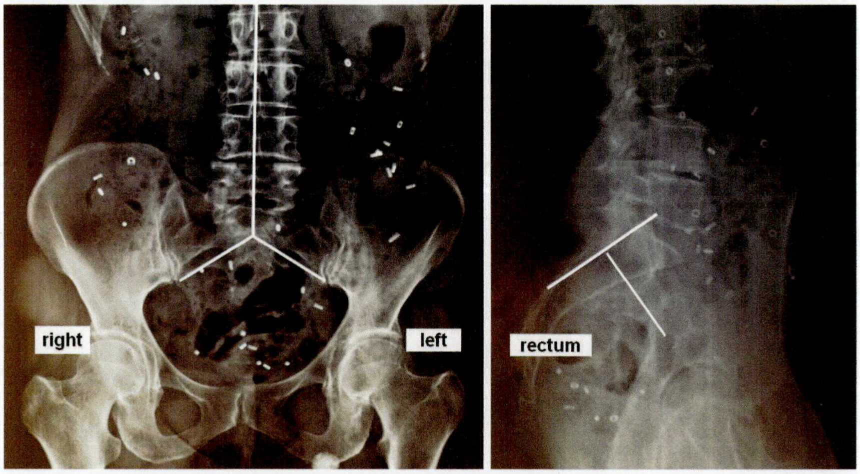

Figure 17.2 Study of intestinal transit time by ingestion of radio-opaque indicators and subsequent radiological checks in antero-posterior and lateral-lateral positions, to check the position and to distinguish the rectum from the sigma, respectively.

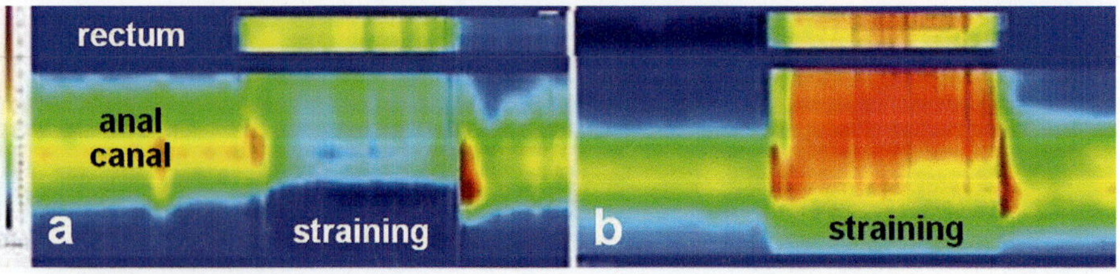

Figure 17.3 High-resolution rectal-anal manometry: the pressure values are indicated by the color that varies from blue (0) to brown (>150 mmHg). (a) normal anal relaxation during straining: the color turns from yellow to light blue in the anal canal and from blue to green/yellow in the rectum indicating that the increase of pelvic pressure is associated with anal opening allowing the passage of the faeces;.(b) pelvic dyssynergia with anal paradoxical contraction during straining: both in the rectum and anal canal the color turns orange to brown to indicate a synchronous increase in pressure at both levels.

complex and dyssinergic behaviour during abdominal strain, to identify and describe patients who can benefit from a re-educational treatment with biofeedback. The manometry can be accompanied by the balloon expulsion test reaching a high sensitivity in identifying constipation due to dyssinergic evacuation.
Functional and morphological aspects of defecation can be explored with Rx-**defecography** or by **defecation-MRI**. These tests can detect the dyssinergic behaviour due to the failure to open the anal canal and/or the lack of relaxation of the puborectal muscle during evacuation, they can measure the effectiveness of rectal emptying and they also can describe the formation, during strain, of rectocele, intra-rectal or anal intussusception and possibly obstacles by neighboring viscera.
Lastly, in patients with severe STC, who are candidates to colectomy, it may be useful to perform, in specialized centers, a colon manometry to assess the severe deficit of bowel motor activity.

TREATMENT

Medical Therapy

Self-medication is the most common practice and although the osmotic laxatives are recommended by the clinical guidelines, market data indicate that stimulant laxatives, including herbal teas, are the most used. However, patients are poorly satisfied about their management of the bowel habit, probably due to the inappropriate use of laxatives.
In the first line approach to SF, it is important to correct dietary and behavioural habits by prescribing a diet with adequate fluid (1.5L/day) and fiber intake, suggesting aerobic physical activity and trying evacuation, even in the absence of stimulous, after a meal and in quiet conditions.
Supplements can be introduced preferring soluble fibers (e.g., psyllium, pectin, glucomannan) to insoluble fibers (e.g., bran, cellulose) which more frequently can cause bloating, distension, and abdominal pain. However, fiber must be incremented gradually to prevent disturbs.
In intolerant or non-responder patients, it is necessary to add a laxative, preferring an osmotic one: the macrogol or the non-absorbable disaccharides (lactulose), taken daily, improves the frequency of the evacuations, reduces the stool consistency and the evacuative strain. Currently, macrogol is preferred to bulk laxatives as first step in the management of chronic constipation; it has been proved to be more effective and faster than psyllium and with fewer undesirable effects in comparison with disaccharides.
Macrogol is an inert polymer of polyethylene glycol (PEG), which permanently binds the hydrogen of water molecules; it is not absorbed and neither fermented. Macrogol is administered in adequate daily doses, and volume is modulated according to the therapeutic response; it can also be used while awaiting an aetiological definition or in organic constipation; it is effective in about 80% of constipated patients maintaining the effect in both the short and medium term.
Contact laxatives (senna and anthraquinones, bisacodyl, sodium pycosulphate) stimulate the propulsive motor activity of the colon, reduce the absorption and/or induce the secretion of water. They act quickly: upon evening intake, they usually induce the evacuation in the following morning, it is recommendable their use 2-3 times per week also in association with the macrogol, when this is ineffective. However, they can cause abdominal pain and a reduced efficacy is observed in prolonged administration.
When the threshold of urge to defecate is increased, evacuation can be induced at regular intervals using rectal stimuli such as suppositories or small volume enemas of glycerol or sorbitol, or contact laxatives (bisacodyl).
In refractory constipation, enterokinetics, active on serotonin receptors, or pro-secretory activators of chlorine channels can be used.
Prucalopride is a high affinity serotonin-4 (5-HT4) receptor agonist; it acts on the motor interneuron of the enteric plexus enhancing the reflex inducing the propagated motor activity. It should be used above all in slow transit constipation. The main side effects are headache, limited to the first days of assumption, abdominal pain, and diarrhoea.
Linaclotide (the only pro-secretory laxative available in Italy) is an intestinal agonist of guanyl cyclase, that activates chlorine channels resulting in endoluminal secretion of chloride and bicarbonate inducing increase in intestinal fluid and acceleration of bowel transit. Furthermore, in the extracellular space it reduces the activity of the nociceptive nerve afferents and therefore ameliorate pain. Linaclotide is particularly indicated in the Irritable Bowel Syndrome with Constipation; the main side effect is diarrhoea with the risk of dehydration and electrolyte imbalances.
In opioid-induced constipation, refractory to the usual laxatives, it is possible to use the Peripherally-Acting Mu-Opioid Receptor Antagonists

(PAMORA) which hinder the constipating effect of opioids without interfering with the analgesic action or cause withdrawal syndrome; among these, naloxegon and naldemedine have the advantage of oral administration.

Biofeedback

The dyssinergic defecation benefits from the rehabilitation of the pelvic floor associated with biofeedback: 4-6 sessions of electromyographyc or manometric biofeedback, obtain benefit in 70-80% of dyssinergic patients. In presence of hard stool, it is useful to soften it with osmotic laxatives. The motivation of the patient, the support of the therapist, the frequency and intensity of the retraining program, and the involvement of behavioral psychologists and/or dieticians, when necessary, are likely to contribute to the chances of success.

Surgery

Surgery with constipation as primary indication is divided into colectomy for STC and procedures of anatomical correction (rectocele, prolapse) in defecation disorders. In both situations surgery must be considered when every type of conservative treatment has proved to be ineffective, the symptoms negatively impact on daily activities and after a careful morphological and functional study addressed at describing the pathophysiological mechanism of the symptoms.

Constipation in Pregnancy

Constipation during pregnancy is due to the inhibitory effect of progesterone on smooth muscle, to the reduction of physical activity, to diet and to weight gain, to compression of the pregnant uterus on the rectal-sigmoid tract. About 11-38% of pregnant women complains constipation and requires medical treatment. In these cases, macrogol should be the first-choice laxative because its pharmacokinetic characteristics does not induce risks for the foetus and for the pregnancy itself.

Megarectum

The presence of megarectum with faecal impact can cause a constant anal relaxation with consequent incontinence to liquid stool (overflow incontinence). This condition is common in children, in elderly especially when bedridden, in neurological patients, in subjects with dementia. The treatment requires the preliminary removal of faeces with enemas which can be medicated with emollient or lubricating agents, later provoking scheduled evacuations using osmotic and/or contact laxatives.

KEY CONCEPTS

- Chronic Constipation can occur with a reduced bowel frequency and/or with defecation disorders: it can be primitive or secondary to organic diseases.
- Three forms are recognised: 1. Constipation with normal bowel transit overlapping with the irritable bowel syndrome with constipation; 2. Constipation with slowed colonic transit; 3. Constipation with altered mechanisms of defecation.
- Colonoscopy is indicated in subjects aged >50 or with alarm features; functional tests are useful in case of failure to respond to usual therapies.
- Treatment involves amelioration of the lifestyle, dietary modification, and administration of laxatives in a step-by step way; macrogol is the first choice, it can be used in organic forms and also during the diagnostic procedure.
- Surgical therapies are indicated in the absence of adequate response to conservative therapy and after a careful pathophysiological evaluation.

REFERENCES

- Chey SW, Chey WD, Jackson K, Eswaran S. Exploratory Comparative Effectiveness Trial of Green Kiwifruit, Psyllium, or Prunes in US Patients with Chronic Constipation. Am J Gastroenterol. 2021;116:1304-12.
- Corsetti M, Brown S, Chiarioni G, et al. Chronic constipation in adults: Contemporary perspectives and clinical challenges. 2: Conservative, behavioural, medical and surgical treatment. Neurogastroenterol Motil. 2021;33:e14070.
- Rossi M, Casale G, Badiali D, et al. Opioid-induced bowel dysfunction: suggestions from a multidisciplinary expert Board. Support Care Cancer. 2019;27:4083-90.
- Sharma A, Rao SSC, Kearns K, et al. Review article: diagnosis, management and patient perspectives of the spectrum of constipation disorders. Aliment Pharmacol Ther. 2021;53:1250-67.
- Tanner S, Chaudhry A, Goraya N, et al. Prevalence and Clinical Characteristics of Dyssynergic Defecation and Slow Transit Constipation in Patients with Chronic Constipation. J. Clin. Med. 2021;10:2027.

CHAPTER 18

DIARRHOEA

Flavio Andrea Caprioli, Nadia Pallotta

LEARNING OBJECTIVES

- To understand the correct definition of diarrhoea.
- To understand the main pathophysiological mechanisms of diarrhoea.
- To understand the main aetiologies responsible for the different forms of diarrhoea.
- To appraise the initial clinical framing of the patient with diarrhoea.

DEFINITION AND EPIDEMIOLOGY

Diarrhoea refers to an increase in daily fecal weight above 250-300 g, given that the daily average weight stool of adults on a Mediterranean diet does not usually exceed 200 g/day. This value varies in relation to diet. If it is rich in fruit, vegetables, and whole products and high fiber content, a fecal weight equal to or greater than 300 grams is normal.

The increase in fecal weight is generally associated with a decrease in fecal consistency in relation to greater water content and with an increase in the number of evacuations. In the absence of increased fecal weight, neither a reduction in the consistency nor a simple increase in the number of evacuations can be defined as diarrhoea. About its duration, diarrhoea is defined as acute if it lasts less than 2 weeks from the onset of symptoms, persistent if it lasts between 2 and 4 weeks, and chronic if it lasts longer than 4 weeks.

a useful classification, particularly relevant for its diagnostic-therapeutic implications, is the aetiological one. Four main types of diarrhoea are distinguished: secretory, osmotic, inflammatory, and secondary to altered motility.

Diarrhoea is a symptom and not a disease, and therefore should not be treated as a first intention, apart from the need for urgent rehydration and an electrolytic rebalancing, as it may occur the most severe forms.

Epidemiology

Diarrhoea, especially the acute form, is one of the main causes of morbidity in the world, and it is burdened with high mortality, particularly in children, and in developing countries: despite a clear improvement in prognosis, in relation to the spread of appropriate rehydration strategies and the reduction of deaths by 90% in the past twenty years, the estimated mortality rate is 500,000 patients/year, 50% of which in children below 5 years of age. In the industrialized countries, mortality is low, but acute diarrhoea is one of the most common causes of hospitalization in children. Chronic diarrhoea is much rarer but is responsible for 1.5% of the causes of hospitalization in adults.

PATHOPHYSIOLOGICAL MECHANISMS

Every day about ten litres of fluids enter the gut, either ingested with diet (2500 mL) or by secretions (saliva, gastric juice, pancreatic juice, bile, enteric juice, for a total of about 7500 mL). In the small intestine and the colon, the fluids are bidirectional, and losses result from the net balance between secretion and absorption.

The greatest part of the absorption of water and solutes occurs in the small intestine (8000-8500 mL), while 1500 mL are reabsorbed in the colon. Thus, only 100-150 mL of water are lost with feces.

The colon is the tract of the digestive system where fecal water undergoes the main changes in electrolytic content, leading to the reabsorption of 98% of the sodium present in the ileal effluent and 96% of chlorine. In contrast with these ions, under physiological conditions the total content of potassium does not vary to a significant extent because absorption is very limited, and its concentration increases while water is reabsorbed. Under homeostatic conditions, potassium is the main fecal cation. Any mechanism that increases secretion or reduces absorption causes an increase in fecal loss of fluids, with the consequent onset of diarrhoea.

The anatomical site (ileum or colon) and the mechanisms underlying these alterations strongly influence the volume of fecal losses and the relevant effects on the quantity and quality of electrolyte leakage.

The main mechanisms of diarrhoea can be traced to four different pathophysiological mechanisms (Table 18.1):

- secretory diarrhoea;
- diarrhoea from increased osmotic load;
- inflammatory diarrhoea;
- diarrhoea due to altered motility.

A good knowledge of these mechanisms is of relevance and has profound therapeutic implications since they lead to forms of diarrhoea that differ in terms of clinical picture and severity. However, it should be underlined that in the pathogenesis of most of the pathologies that manifest themselves with the symptom diarrhoea, two or more of the pathophysiological mechanisms listed above are habitually involved, although with different relevance.

Secretory Diarrhoea

Secretory diarrhoea is characterized by net anion secretion (chlorine or bicarbonate) due to the activation of chlorine channels and inhibition of net sodium absorption.

The most common cause of secretory diarrhoea is pathogens secreting secretory toxins. Among these, the best-known example is the Subunit A of the cholera toxin. In addition to viruses and bacterial toxins (enterotoxins), this mechanism is also shared by hormones (such as VIP), drugs, neurotransmitters, prostaglandins, and bile acids, as well as irritant laxatives like bisacodyl and anthraquinones.

Activation of enzymes such as adenylate cyclase, guanylate cyclase, and phospholipase C leads to the production of high amounts of second intracellular messengers: cAMP, cGMP, and calcium, which, through cascade activation of specific protein kinases, increase the conductance of the apical membrane to chlorine and basolateral conductance to potassium. This is the central element of secretory diarrhoea, characteristic of the small intestine. The clinical effect of this hypersecretion is a form of diarrhoea that may be particularly severe. In addition to stimulation of secretions, the blockade of specific absorption mechanisms is involved, with inhibition of sodium-hydrogen exchange in the small intestine and the colon. A large amount of water and electrolytes is thus lost with stools. In addition, there is severe fecal loss of

Table 18.1 Diarrhoea according to pathophyisiological mechanisms.

Secretory Diarrhoea	
Exosogenous secretagogues	Bacterial Toxins (*Cholera, enterotoxigenic Escherichia coli*)
Endogenous secretagogues	Neuroendocrine tumours (VIP, carcinoids, gastrinoma, medullary thyroid tumours)
Congenital Chloridorrehoea	
Drugs (anti-neoplastic, anti-arrhythmic, anti-hypertensive, anti-infiammatory, PPI, laxatives)	
Osmotic Diarrhoea	
Global malabsorption	Mucosal damage (celiac disease) Infectious/parasitic (Giardia, Whipple disease) Maldigestion (exocrine pancreatic insufficiency) Short bowel syndrome Small bowel bacterial overgrowth
Selective malabsorption	Disaccaridase deficiencies (lactase)
Scarcely absorbable substances (Mg salts, lactulose, sorbitol)	
Inflammatory Diarrhoea	
Infectious (*Shigella, enteropathogenic Escherichia coli, Clostridium difficile, Entameba histolitica*)	
Inflammatory bowel diseases	
Ischaemic damage	
Radiation damage	
Motor Diarrhoea	
Functional bowel disorders (irritable bowel syndrome)	
Diabetic neuropathy	
Hyperthyroidism	
Laxatives	

chlorine, sodium, bicarbonate and water, and to a lesser degree of potassium, and an increase in the pH of feces. In cholera, the losses can also exceed 20L/24 hours hours and quickly lead to death in the absence of adequate rehydration therapy. A very serious metabolic acidosis may occur deriving from both fecal electrolyte leakage, particularly rich in sodium and bicarbonate chlorine, and acute prerenal failure. Other forms of secretory diarrhoea are usually less relevant, rarely is exceeding 1000 mL/24 hours. Secretory diarrhoea is not affected by the fasting test of which is a useful and simple diagnostic test.

Osmotic Diarrhoea

The intestinal mucosa acts as a semi-permeable membrane that allows bidirectional flows of fluids; its magnitude varies in different segments in relation to the polarity of epithelial cells, the transepithelial potential difference, and the degree of permeability of the tight junctions (relatively permeable in the small intestine and poorly permeable in the colon). These differences are reflected by the efficiency of the barrier function and exchange of epithelia in the intestinal tracts.
The presence of osmotically active substances, not absorbed or not absorbable, when the gradient is high, tends to recall water from the intestinal wall to the lumen, especially in the small intestine. In the colon the presence of osmotically active substances is opposed by efficient reabsorption of water and salts, in particular, sodium and chlorine. The flow of water quickly tends to reach a balance, with osmolarity values on two mucosal sides equaling the osmolarity of blood (340 mOsm).
Prototypic forms of osmotic diarrhoea are secondary to selective malabsorption of carbohydrates, such as congenital or acquired lactase deficiency, and those resulting from malabsorption/maldigestion involving macronutrients (carbohydrates, fats and proteins).
Causes of global malabsorption are the widespread damage of the absorbent surface (celiac disease), a deficiency in pancreatic enzymes (chronic pancreatitis) or bile salts, to such an extent as to interfere with the digestion of fats and proteins. The stool is lumpy, foul smelling, and greasy, characterized by an increased concentration of lipids and proteins (steatorrhoea). The reduction in the absorpitive surface, as in extended intestinal resection, may cause osmotic diarrhoea that is transient in most cases, due to activation of compensatory mechanisms leading to increased villi and absorptive surface. Exceptions include severe cases of short intestine, with less than 60-100 cm of residual small intestine and loss of the ileocaecal valve, in which the adaptatory mechanisms, although present, are not adequate.
An osmotic type of diarrhoea may be caused by laxatives (polyethylene glycol, magnesium salts, sulphate and phosphate) and from poorly absorbed carbohydrate intake (such as sorbitol) or not absorbable as lactulose.
In relation to the mechanisms involved, osmotic diarrhoea can be aqueous (disaccharidase deficiency, osmotic laxatives) or with lumpy and greasy stools. This diarrhoea tends to be less conspicuous than secretory diarrhoea (500-1000 mL/24 hours) and is not accompanied by major electrolyte changes and acid-base balance disruptions. Electrolytic concentrations in feces, regardless of volume and osmolarity, are, in fact, lower than normal or in secretory diarrhoea, due to the presence of "other" solutes contributing to the osmotic load. It should be noted that fecal osmolarity is usually normal, provided that transit of the contents is not so fast as to prevent complete transmucosal equilibrium of water and solutes.
Characteristically, osmotic diarrhoea resolves quickly with fasting or reduction of causing agents.

Inflammatory Diarrhoea (with Altered Electrolyte Absorption)

This form of diarrhoea occurs when the intestinal epithelium, especially the colon, is involved by acute or chronic inflammatory processes. The resulting loss of function is substantially the same regardless the origin, either idiopathic (ulcerative colitis), bacterial (*Shigella*), ischaemic, autoimmune (graft versus host disease), drug or radiation-induced, and leads to relevant modifications of transmucosal exchange and of the fecal electrolyte concentration.
Accelerated cell turnover can lead to compensatory hyperplasia of crypts and a higher proportion of relatively immature absorbing cells. Much more important, however, is the infiltration by lymphocytes, plasma cells, macrophages, neutrophils, eosinophils, and mast cells, which release cytokines, eicosanoids, and agents (free radicals, nitric oxide, histamine) that may stimulate intestinal secretion and modulate electrolytic exchange. A typical example of inflammatory diarrhoea is ulcerative colitis, in which the stools are characterized by a high concentrations of sodium and chlorine. In severe cases, these may approach those of the ileal effluent and reflect the inefficiency of the colonic mucosa to limit fecal losses of these ions.

Inflammatory diarrhoea, particularly when the colon is affected, is characterized by fecal loss of blood, which is associated with fecal volume that rarely exceeds 500-700 ml. In extensive and serious damage, the ileal effluent is partially reduced by volume. The effect on electrolytic exchanges is severe, with significant sodium losses (which becomes the main fecal cation), chlorine, and only to a lesser extent potassium.

Alterations in the base-acid equilibrium, if present, result in metabolic alkalosis and depend on the duration of diarrhoea. Alkalosis is a consequence of renal homeostatic mechanisms that maintain plasmatic volume and circulating sodium concentrations. The fasting test is not associated with changes in fecal losses.

Functional Diarrhoea

This is a heterogeneous group of conditions that, operating through heterogeneous mechanisms, accelerate intestinal transit time, particularly in the colon. The contact time between intestinal and mucosal content can be inadequate for optimal water absorption. This mechanism of diarrhoea is exemplified by irritable bowel syndrome (diarrhoea-predominant), which accounts for more than 60% of chronic diarrhoeas in which an organic cause is not diagnosed. Increased intestinal motility may be present in hyperthyroidism, diabetes mellitus, many forms of visceral neuropathy, and amyloidosis.

Some of these pathologies, diabetes in particular, can involve reduced motor activity. In this case, diarrhoea may be caused by different mechanisms, such as small intestinal bacterial overgrowth and alteration in the absorption of macronutrients and an increase in the osmotic component. In irritable bowel syndrome, the stool is characterized by increased water content, but the volume never exceeds 350-400 mL/24 hours, regardless of the number of evacuations. The electrolytic composition is normal and comparable to that of healthy subjects, characterized by high concentrations of potassium and low sodium and chlorine. Although chronic, motor diarrhoea in irritable bowel syndrome does not cause systemic electrolyte imbalances. If present, systemic electrolytic alterations may exclude this pathogenic mechanism.

In human pathology, one of the above-mentioned pathophysiological mechanisms is predominant but it is often associated with other mechanisms, albeit with clinically less relevant weight. Recognition of the prevalent mechanism can help in the diagnostic process is essential to optimize therapy.

DIAGNOSIS

The diagnostic process varies in relation to the duration of diarrhoea, i.e., if it is acute or chronic. Over two-thirds of the acute cases are of infectious origin (viruses, bacteria, parasites, and fungi) and are to a large extent self-limiting. In case of a diarrhoea duration of more than 5 days or when other symptoms are present, it is advisable to proceed with stool cultures and search for parasites.

In chronic diarrhoea the diagnostic process is basically centered on the need to discriminate between organic and functional forms and on the identification of any alarm symptoms (red flags) such as unintentional weight loss of more than 5% of usual weight, bleeding, fever, abdominal masses, anemia, neutrophil leukocytosis, and an increase in inflammation indexes. This avoids unnecessary diagnostic delays in organic pathologies and limits unnecessary investigations to those of functional origin.

Correct diagnosis relies on accurate history, assessment of the characteristics and volume of stools, and physical examination. Subsequent investigations, blood tests, endoscopy, imaging and functional examinations depend on the findings obtained in the first phase of evaluation.

In instances in which an organic cause of chronic diarrhoea is not identified during the initial diagnostic workup, further causes such as microscopic colitis and surreptitious laxative abuse must be ruled out before classifying diarrhoea as functional.

Microscopic colitis is more often observed in females, the middle-aged, and those on multiple drug therapy. Extensive biopsy sampling along the entire colon is crucial, despite macroscopically normal mucosa, during colonoscopy. Diagnosis of laxative abuse is difficult and requires strict observation in hospitalized patients or complex biochemical procedures in those who are not.

Medical History

Duration (acute or chronic) and onset of diarrhoea (sudden or gradual, associated or not with other symptoms) are the starting point for history taking. The presence of nocturnal symptoms should be specifically identified, because it strongly suggests an organic cause. In acute diarrhoea, possible environmental factors or risky behaviors should be investigated (travel, intake of potentially harmful foods, similar symptoms in other persons, hospitalizations, concomitant medications). In chronic diarrhoea alarm symptoms should be investigated. Familial/hereditary conditions, previous illnesses and surgeries, allergies and intolerances, as well as medications should be recorded.

Characteristics of Stools

Diarrhoea can manifest with frankly liquid, runny or lumpy stools, the shape being in relation to the aqueous component. The appearance and fecal weight of 24 hours may suggest the pathophysiological mechanism that caused the symptom and directs towards the diagnosis.

Watery stool, with >1000 mL/24 hours in volume, is typical of secretory diarrhoea in which the aqueous component can reach 99% of total weight. In osmotic diarrhoea the fecal volume is often elevated but generally less than 1000 mL. The stool can be oily in diseases involving global malabsorption of lipids, but tends to be watery when the osmotically active agent is drugs, laxative salts or carbohydrate malabsorption. The fasting test may discriminate between subtypes, as the fecal weight is reduced drastically in osmotic but not in secretory diarrhoea. Bloody diarrhoea or with mucus-pus is indicative of organic pathology and suggests an inflammatory origin. In contrast, the presence of mucus in the stool (regardless of stool consistency) is often considered alarming in patients with chronic diarrhoea, but it is of scarse relevance, as it is often present in irritable bowel syndrome. The color of stool, more or less dark, is usually of little importance, as this depends to a large extent on diet and the length of the intestinal transit. Exceptions are particularly clear stools (acholic) that suggest steatorrhoea and/or a bile salt deficit.

A particularly acrid smell is characteristic of global malabsorption. A characteristic smell is found in infections with *Clostridium difficile*, and directs the diagnostic process towards the research of toxins A and B of the pathogenic agent.

Physical Examination

In profuse or prolonged diarrhoea, especially in children and the elderly, signs of dehydration must be evaluated, such as hypotension and orthostatic tachycardia, mucosal dryness. The presence of such signs suggests a relevant loss of fluids and the need for immediate rehydration. Physical examination of the abdomen will include the search for masses, tenderness or abdominal distention. A digital rectal exploration should always be performed, as it allows a direct assessment of stools, and rules out anorectal or inflammatory lesions in the elderly, or the presence of stool impaction/fecaloma, which sometimes may cause pseudodiarrhoea. Other objective findings may be sought about the type and duration of diarrhoea and the suspected mechanism.

For example, systemic signs of global malabsorption and micronutrients include fragility of nails and hair, aphthoid lesions of the oral mucosa, and peripheral neuropathy. The presence of a rash may be associated with secretory diarrhoea of hormonal origin (VIP and some forms of carcinoids).

Diagnostic Investigations

Targeted diagnostic algorithms may be used, including blood tests and analysis of organic fluids, instrumental investigations (endoscopy), functional tests (breath tests, pancreatic function tests), and imaging studies (MRI, CT, ultrasound and, occasionally, traditional radiological investigations).

Stool Examination

Stool examination includes microbiological examination, including stool cultures for ova or bacteria. The microbiological/ova examination is directed to the search for viruses, pathogenic bacteria, and parasites. Among the bacteria, *Salmonella* and *Shigella* should be sought, together with *Campylobacter jejuni, Yersinia enterocolitica*. Given its increasing prevalence, *Clostridium difficile* toxins should be sought, particularly in the elderly and in hospitalized or institutionalized individuals, particularly after antibiotic therapy. Pathogenic *E. coli* should be sought in particular cases. *Entamoeba histolytica, Giardia lamblia, and Cryptosporidium parvum* should be searched in particular cases. The search for viruses (rotavirus, Norwalk virus, and cytomegalovirus) are generally limited to tertiary reference centres and epidemiological purposes. Fecal calprotectin, a protein of the S-100 family contained in neutrophilic granulocytes, stable for at least 7 days at room temperature, has replaced traditional microscopic examination of stool for the search for leukocytes and cells, to diagnose inflammatory processes.

It is particularly useful to differentiate organic from functional diarrhoea. A threshold value between 50 and 100 ug/g discriminates between these two situations with very high sensitivity and specificity, between 85 and 95%.

The determination of fecal fats and fecal elastases (for the study of pancreatic function) provides information for fat malabsorption and to evaluate pancreatic function. Other parameters, including osmolarity, fecal electrolytes, bile salts and short-chain fatty acids (SCFA) are not readily available and are mostly used for research purposes.

Blood Test

Blood test examinations should be distinguished in first-level and second-level. The first-level ones (blood count, erythrocyte sedimentation rate, C-reactive protein, electrolytes, blood gases, and creatininemia) are useful to identify inflammatory activity and to quantify the systemic effects of diarrhoea, and to guide supportive measures. Other tests can be used to diagnose specific causes of diarrhoea, including anti-endomysium and anti-transglutaminase antibodies for the diagnosis of celiac disease, thyroid hormones in hyperthyroidism, hormones and gastrointestinal peptides (VIP, chromogranin, neuron-specific enolase - NSE) in secretory diarrhoea from neuroendocrine tumours. Antibody titers or IgE may be useful for infectious diarrhoea.

KEY CONCEPTS

- Diarrhoea, in persons on a Mediterranean diet, is defined as an increase in 24-hr stool weight of over 250-300 g, irrespective of the number of bowel movements.
- Diarrhoea is present in many conditions and results from different pathophysiological mechanisms with qualitative and quantitative differences in intestinal losses.
- The identification of the main pathophysiological mechanism responsible for diarrhoea helps to target diagnostic procedures and therapy. Nonetheless, more than one mechanism often concur are in the genesis of diarrhoea.
- Rehydration and correction of acid-base and electrolyte imbalances are the clinical priority in severe diarrhoea and precede diagnostic workup.

REFERENCES

- Gareau MG, Barrett KE. Fluid and electrolyte secretion in the inflamed gut: nover targets for treatment of inflammation-induced diarrhea. Curr Opin Pharmacol. 2013;13:895-9.
- Kaiser L. Surawicz CM. Infectious causes of chronic diarrhea. Best Practice & Research Clinical Gastroenterology. 2012;26:563-71.
- Keusch GT, Walker CF, Das JK, Horton S, Habte D. Diarrheal Diseases. In: Black RE, Laxminarayan R, Temmerman M, Walker N, editors. SourceReproductive, Maternal, Newborn, and Child Health: Disease Control Priorities: The International Bank for Reconstruction and Development / The World Bank, 2016 Chapter 9.
- Menees SB, Powell C, Kurlander J, Goel A, Chey WD. A meta-analysis of the utility of C-reactive protein, erythrocyte sedimentation rate, fecal calprotectin, and fecal lactoferrin to exclude inflammatory bowel disease in adults with IBS. Am J Gastroenterol. 2015 Mar;110:444-54.

CHAPTER 19

CELIAC DISEASE

Antonio Picarelli, Giovanni Latella

LEARNING OBJECTIVES

- To know the clinical features and the incidence and prevalence of Celiac disease.
- To identify persons with celiac disease.
- To know celiac disease screening and diagnosis.
- To know the correct application of a gluten-free diet.
- To know the complications of celiac disease.

Celiac disease (CD) is a chronic inflammatory bowel disease triggered by the ingestion of gluten and affects genetically susceptible individuals.
The term "gluten" refers to alcohol-soluble proteins containing the immuno-stimulating peptides responsible for the disease: gliadins and glutenins of wheat, secalins of rye, hordeins of barley and avenins of oats. CD is usually characterized by intestinal villous atrophy and its multifaceted clinical presentation can include signs and symptoms of malabsorption. Together with a wheat allergy and the so-called "non-celiac gluten sensitivity", CD falls within the spectrum of gluten related disorders and therefore requires an accurate differential diagnosis.

EPIDEMIOLOGY

CD has an estimated prevalence of about 1% in Western countries; however, the extreme variability of the clinical picture together with the lack of knowledge of this pathology, still makes CD frequently underdiagnosed: for these reasons, CD is usually compared to an iceberg, of which only the tip shows above the water.
On the other hand, the recent increase of CD prevalence in the general population may be attributed not only to greater awareness about CD by clinicians and the use of more reliable diagnostic tools, but also to its probable increased diffusion.
As observed in other autoimmune diseases, CD prevalence is higher in females (F:M >2: 1).

PATHOGENETIC MECHANISMS

CD prevalence is higher in first-degree relatives (about 10%), further increases up to 30% in haploidentical brothers and even reaches 70% in homozygous twins.
This clearly indicates that the susceptibility to develop altered immunological responses to gluten is genetically determined. Thanks to studies by Anne Ferguson and Ludvig Sollid from the 1990s, today we know that the HLA-DQ2 alleles (DQA1*05; DQB1*02) and that the HLA-DQ8 alleles (DQA1*03; DQB1*0302) are the predisposing/causative genes in 92% and 5% of CD patients, respectively. In fact, both haplotypes encode a heterodimer expressed on antigen-presenting cells (APCs), which has a great binding affinity for some epitopes of gliadin, the main component of gluten (**Figure 19.1**).
However, this "genetic predisposition" (or even better "genetic susceptibility") is present in about 30% of the Caucasian population as well, thus conferring a necessary but not sufficient genetic potential to develop CD. Therefore, the use of HLA

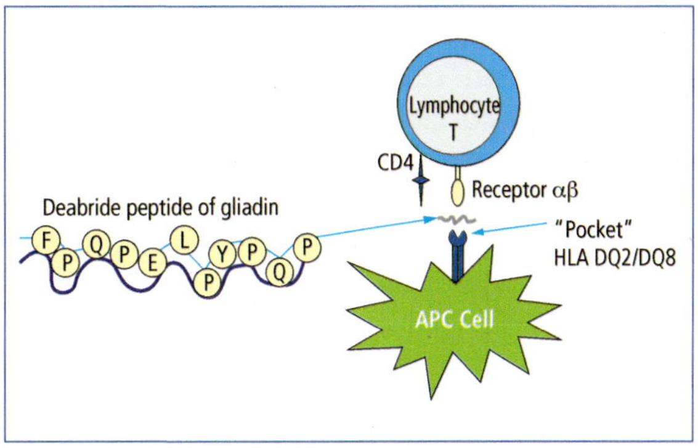

Figure 19.1 Binding of gliadin peptides to the HLA-DQ2 or DQ8 receptor on the antigen presenting cell (APC) the glutamine deamidation is critical for the binding of gliadin peptides to DQ2 or DQ8 molecules, which form a pocket on the APC cell, receive the peptide, and finally engage T lymphocytes.

*The Authors would like to thank Dr. Nicoletta Greco for her assistance.

typing is not indicated for diagnostic or screening purposes and it has only a negative predictive value: the absence of HLA-DQ2 and/or -DQ8 haplotype rules out a diagnosis of CD. On the other hand, the incomplete concordance between homozygous twins suggests that genes not belonging to the HLA complex may also be involved together with extra-genetic factors, such as pregnancy, duration of breastfeeding, nutritional factors, infections, stress, hormonal factors, alteration of intestinal permeability, and gut microbiota.

Amongst environmental factors, the harmful fraction of wheat gluten is gliadins and glutenins, whereas proteases constitute the first line of defense against potentially harmful proteins (including gluten) in the intestinal lumen. However, some fragments are not completely digested due to the lack of endopeptidase. The second line of defence is the intestinal barrier that allows the selective passage of molecules and ions.

Intestinal permeability in CD seems to be primarily altered, with the consequent passage of undigested gliadin peptides directly into the lamina propria, as in the case of 33-mer, a peptide composed of 33 amino acids. Afterwards, the tissue transglutaminase 2 (TG2), a calcium-dependent ubiquitary enzyme that catalyzes post-translational modifications, plays two crucial roles in the pathogenesis of CD: as the autoantigen of anti-endomysial antibodies and responsible for the deamidation of gliadin. The transformation of glutamine residues into glutamic acid stabilizes the binding with the pocket of HLA-DQ2 and/or DQ8 molecules, resulting in a more effective stimulation of T lymphocytes.

Once activated, CD4+ T lymphocytes trigger an inflammatory cascade that leads to characteristic mucosal lesions, such as shortening of the villi, crypt hyperplasia, increased presence of intraepithelial lymphocytes, and expansion of the lamina propria's inflammatory mononuclear infiltrate. In particular, T-helper 1 inflammatory cells produce cytokines, such as interferon-γ, that, in association with CD8+ (cytotoxic) T cells and activated matrix metalloproteinases, increase enterocytic apoptosis and cellular turn-over, with loss of the anatomo-functional integrity of the intestinal mucosa. Other pro-inflammatory cytokines implicated in the pathogenesis of CD are interferon-γ and interleukin (IL)-6, IL-18 and IL-21, whereas tumour necrosis factor (TNF) is not increased. In addition, IL-15 produced directly by epithelial cells is involved in the activation of cytotoxicity of intraepithelial lymphocytes, thus contributing to enterocytic apoptosis, triggering of T-cell clonality, and predispose the patient to refractoriness and lymphomagenesis. Finally, it has also been shown that some gliadin peptides cause direct mucosal damage through an independent pathway of lymphocyte activation (innate response). In this regard, the most studied peptide is the p31-43/49 fragment that stimulates the production of IL-15, which causes epithelial stress and inhibits regulatory T cells. The T-helper 2-type citokine profile (including IL-10 and IL-4) guides the activation and expansion of B cells, with the production of disease-specific antibodies.

DIAGNOSIS

CD diagnosis is based on the correlation of clinical, serological, and histological findings. The diagnostic workup should be performed during a free diet (with gluten), to avoid false negative results. Otherwise, a gluten-containing diet must be started again for a sufficiently long time before starting appropriate diagnostic tests.

Clinical Features

Although in the past diarrhoea, steatorrhea, and weight loss were considered necessary elements for CD diagnosis, nowadays we know that CD has a broad spectrum of presenting features, including extra-intestinal manifestations. Furthermore, oligosymptomatic or even silent cases are not rare. To date, the clinical forms of CD are:

- Classical CD: It manifests with the classic signs of malabsorption, such as weight loss and diarrhoea with steatorrhea and hypocholesterolemia, often associated in children with growth retardation and hypostaturalism, asthenia, and depression. Sometimes abdominal pain and swelling, nausea and anorexia are also evident. The variability of clinical expression is most likely related to: duration of untreated disease; quantity/frequency of gluten intake; subjective reactivity to gluten; extension of intestinal lesions.
- Non-classical CD: Defined as "atypical CD" in the past, today it is the most frequent clinical form of CD. Extra-intestinal signs/symptoms are: sideropenic anemia (more frequent in fertile or pregnant women); vitamin D deficiency, and hypocalcemia with osteopenia/osteoporosis;

vitamin K deficiency with ecchymosis; persistent hypertransaminasemia of unknown origin; paresthesia, muscle cramps, and tetany. In addition, amenorrhea, infertility, recurrent spontaneous abortion, and early menopause are often present.

Finally, CD is frequently associated with other diseases, especially autoimmune disorders, such as Hashimoto's thyroiditis (about 20%), Sjögren's syndrome (4.5-15%), type 1 diabetes mellitus (4-10%), psoriasis, Addison disease, alopecia, neuropathies, cerebellar ataxia, epilepsy with occipital calcifications, rheumatoid arthritis, hepatitis and/or cholangitis, IgA nephropathy, nonischaemic dilated cardiomyopathy. Although genetic relationships are not known, CD is often found in Down syndrome (5-10%). These conditions offer a clear indication to screen for concomitant CD: if CD diagnosis is confirmed, an improvement of the abovementioned diseases can be achieved with an appropriate gluten-free diet.

- Duhring dermatitis herpetiformis (DH). The name "herpetiformis" is used because its typical skin lesions resemble those observable in herpes-related infections. This condition occurs more frequently in Caucasians, with a prevalence of about 1:10,000 and, in contrast to CD, it is more common in men. Duodenal lesions may be minimal or even absent in DH, although IgA deposits directed against epidermal transglutaminase (TG3) can be detected along the dermal-epidermal junction and on top of the dermal papillae by means of direct immunofluorescence analyses of skin biopsies. Its intensely itchy, chronic papulovesicular eruptions are more often evident on extensor surfaces (elbows, knees, buttocks, back of neck) and are symmetrical. Patients suffering from DH present diagnostic serological markers for CD, as well as HLA DQ2/DQ8 genotype, and respond effectively to a gluten-free diet. Once remission has been achieved, persons with CD and DH may report itching and reappearance of skin lesions after exposure to gluten even immediately after contamination or cross-contamination.
- Asymptomatic/silent CD. It is characterised by positive serologic test results and duodenal histopathological alterations, in complete absence of symptoms. This condition is usually found in CD patients involved in family screening for CD; sometimes the term "silent" is improper since a more detailed history will reveal milder symptomatic forms, which disappear with a gluten-free diet.
- Potential/latent CD. Potential CD is characterized by positive serologic tests results but negative histological analysis, whereas the term "latent" is attributed retrospectively to the period between potential CD diagnosis and the first evidence of intestinal lesions. Unfortunately, "potential" and "latent" are often interchanged, resulting in confusion, and even the simple genetic predisposition is incorrectly defined as potential CD.
- Refractory celiac disease (RCD). It consists in the persistence or recurrence of malabsorptive signs and symptoms (especially diarrhoea and weight loss) after at least 12 months from CD diagnosis, despite a very strict gluten-free diet. Histological examination shows persistent duodenal villous atrophy. Type I RCD is characterized by increased aberrant monoclonal intraepithelial lymphocytes, while type II RCD by increased aberrant monoclonal intraepithelial lymphocytes.

Serology

The most common form of CD is characterized by positive serology results (IgA and/or IgG1 class autoantibodies):

- IgA and IgG1 anti-transglutaminase antibodies (anti-tTG). Currently, this is first-line test to diagnose CD. They are autoantibodies directed against tissue transglutaminase 2 (TG2), detected by ELISA. They have sensitivity and specificity estimated up to 98%. Positive anti-tTG results may be also seen in other autoimmune diseases, such as type 1 diabetes, autoimmune liver disease, autoimmune thyroid disease, and inflammatory bowel disease.
- IgA and IgG1 anti-endomysium antibodies (EMA). These second-line tests are used as confirmation test. They have high sensitivity (up to 95%) and specificity (up to 99%). EMA assays are performed by indirect immunofluorescence, thus are operator-dependent.
- IgA and IgG deamidated gliadin peptide antibodies (DGP AGA). These antibodies are raised against the deamidated peptides of gliadin, with less sensitivity (up to 88%) and specificity (up to 98%) than EMA and anti-tTG. Their use is recommended especially in children younger than 2 years.

- IgA and IgG anti-gliadin antibodies (AGA). They are no longer considered useful in CD diagnosis because of their low sensitivity and specificity; they should no longer be done.

The specific serological survey (accompanied by total IgA assay) is reserved for persons with suspected clinical presentation, during case-finding, risk-group screening (**Table 19.1**) or family screening.

Organ Culture

Up to 10% of patients may present negative or border-line results on serological investigation, even in the absence of selective IgA deficiency. In such cases, CD diagnosis can be supported by EMA and anti tTG assayed in supernatants of cultured duodenal biopsies, with an increase of up to 100% in sensitivity and specificity (**Figure 19.2**).
Furthermore, organ culture is useful when the villous height/crypt depth ratio and intraepithelial lymphocyte count are not diagnostic for CD on histological examination.

Endoscopy

CD diagnosis is based on histological examination of duodenal biopsies obtained during oesophago-gastroduodenoscopy (EGD). According to recent ESPGHAN guidelines, CD diagnosis can be made without EGD and biopsy in children and adolescents with classical gluten-dependent clinical presentation, EMA positive results, high anti-tTG titers >10 the upper limit of normality, HLA-DQ2 and or DQ8 positive results; the likelihood of villous atrophy in such cases is high. Duodenal endoscopic markers compatible with CD diagnosis are: scalloped folds; mosaic pattern/nodular mucosa; reduction in number and/or height of folds (**Figure 19.3**).
The absence of these signs, however, does not rule out CD, so multiple duodenal biopsies should be performed with one or two taken from the bulb and at least four from the second portion of duodenum. Biopsies should be preferably oriented to obtain correct histological descriptions.
EGD with duodenal biopsies may be repeated only

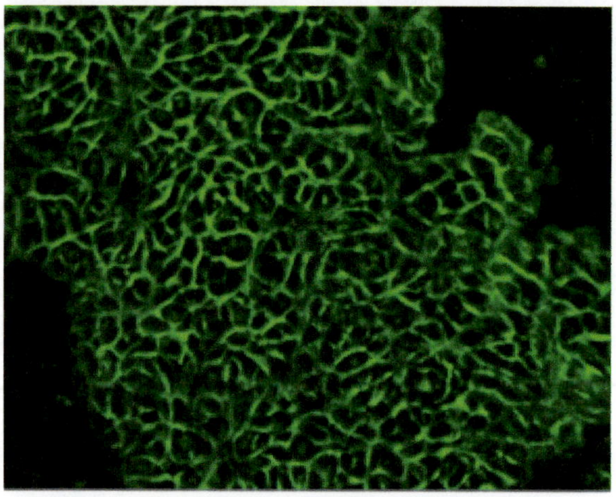

Figure 19.2 Anti-endomysial antibodies (EMA) positive in organ culture (immunofluorescence) in celiac disease.

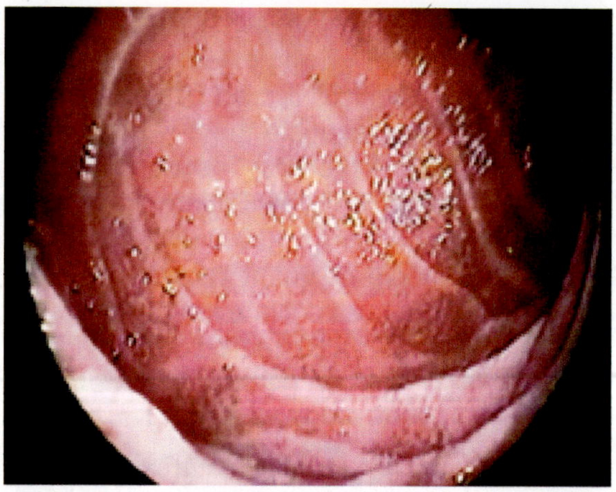

Figure 19.3 Endoscopic aspect of the second duodenal portion in celiac disease.
Possible endoscopic alterations in celiac disease: irregular and hypotrophic folds with "scalloping" of the mucosa in the second duodenal portion.

Table 19.1 Categories in which serological screening for celiac disease is recommended.

First-degree relatives of persons with celiac
Down syndrome, Turner syndrome, Williams syndrome
Autoimmune diseases, diabetes mellitus type 1, sclerosing cholangitis, inflammatory bowel diseases, etc.)
Early osteoporosis
Hypoplasia of dental enamel
History of recurrent abortions, late menarche, early menopause
Neuropathies (deficiencies, cerebellar ataxia, epilepsy)
Iron deficiency anemia, non-virus-related hypertransaminasemia, hypocholesterolemia

in doubtful cases and after an adequate period of having followed gluten-free diet (at least 12-18 months in adults).

Histology

Duodenal gluten-dependent histological alterations can be observed.

The histological description of duodenal mucosa in the suspicion of CD is based on the Marsh-Oberhuber classification, which categorizes the appearance of intestinal villi, as well as the possible presence of intraepithelial lymphocytosis and/or crypt hyperplasia:

- Type 0: normal appearance of mucosa.
- Type I (INFILTRATIVE LESIONS): architecturally normal villi, with normal villo/crypt ratio (3/1); increase in intraepithelial lymphocytes (>25 out of 100 epithelial cells); normal crypts.
- Type II (IPERPLASTIC LESIONS): architecturally normal villi; increase in intraepithelial lymphocytes (>25 out of 100 epithelial cells); hyperplasia of crypts.
- Type III (DISTRUCTIVE LESIONS): atrophy of villi of variable degree (IIIa mild, IIIb moderate, IIIc total); increase in intraepithelial lymphocytes (>25 out of 100 epithelial cells); hyperplasia of crypts.

The alternative classification by Corazza-Villanacci (**Figure 19.4**) contemplates two injury levels:

- GRADE A (NOT ATROPHIC) LESIONS: pathological increase in IELs; possible crypt hyperplasia.
- GRADE B (ATROPHIC) LESIONS subdivided into two groups:
  - B1 (villous height/crypt depth ratio less than 3/1, with still identifiable villi).
  - B2 (villi no longer identifiable).

These findings are characteristic but not specific for CD because they can also be found in other conditions, such as giardiasis, viral enteritis, Whipple's disease, tropical sprue, common variable immunodeficiency, collagenous sprue, use of olmesartan and others medications. Further important confounding elements in the histological diagnosis of CD are: duodenal patchy lesions; variability of histological elements within the same biopsy; biopsy cutting/orientation technique; experience of the histologist.

Given these limitations, histology in CD diagnosis should be supported by specific serological tests (and possibly organ culture), as well as by regression of histological lesions after having followed gluten-free diet.

Endoscopic and histological investigations should be performed during a free (gluten-containing) diet to avoid false negative or border-line test results.

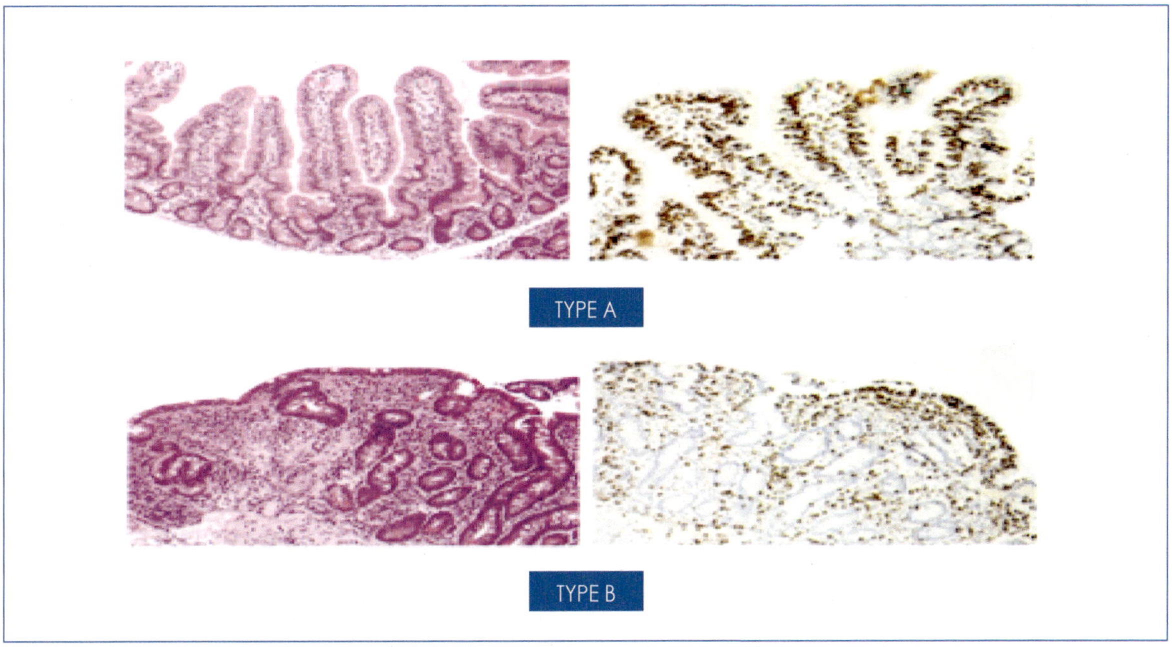

Figure 19.4 Histological classification in celiac disease.
Type A: normal villi but with increase in intraepithelial T lymphocytes (haematoxylin and eosin (H&E) stain H&E left slide; CD3+ right slide 10x)
Type B: villous atrophy (various grades) and increase in intraepithelial T lymphocytes (H&E stain left slide, CD3+ photo right slide 10x).

COMPLICATIONS

The risk of complications is practically absent in CD patients diagnosed in childhood, whereas it is not negligible in cases diagnosed in adulthood: CD patients diagnosed at age >50 have double the burden of mortality compared to the general population.

Enteropathy-associated T-cell lymphoma (EATL) is the leading cause of death. Only in recent years has the pathophysiological relationships between CD and its complications (lymphoma, refractory CD and ulcerative jejunoileitis) been clarified. In the past, they were considered independent conditions, while it is now known that they are three phases of a single evolutionary spectrum.

From the clinical point of view, all three conditions are characterized by persistence or recurrence of a malabsorption syndrome, as well as intestinal lesions after at least 6-12 months of a strict gluten-free diet. However, in most cases the lack of clinical and histological remission is due to voluntary and involuntary dietary transgression. The persistence of intestinal and extra-intestinal symptoms may depend on other conditions frequently associated with CD but not responsive to a gluten-free diet (small intestine bacterial overgrowth, lactase deficiency, microscopic colitis, irritable bowel syndrome, inflammatory bowel diseases, diabetes, thyroid disorders). Therefore, real refractoriness occurs in few patients; such patients should undergo more detailed investigations, such as capsule endoscopy or balloon-assisted enteroscopy.

Ulcerative jejunoileitis is found in 50% of these cases; and it is characterized by deep ulcerations of the intestinal mucosa which result in fibrosis, stenosis and/or perforation. Recent evidence has clarified that most cases of refractory CD and ulcerative jejunoileitis are "cryptic" lymphomas with aberrant intra-epithelial lymphocytes (IELs), even in the absence of neoplasia. These lymphocytes have lost their normal immunophenotypic features and have a monoclonal T-cell receptor rearrangement. The percentage of aberrant IELs can differentiate between refractory CD type 1 and type 2, with type 1 exhibiting <20% aberrant IELs and type 2 >20%. This distinction is essential, since type 2 is burdened by a high risk of developing lymphoma.

Enteropathy-associated T-cell lymphoma (EATL) is subdivided into two variants: the first is characterized by progressive deterioration of general conditions with weight loss, fever, abdominal pain, diarrhoea, and itching. It may emerge in patients already diagnosed with CD and already on a gluten-free diet. The second variant is much more frequent and is characterized by acute abdomen due to intestinal stenosis and/or perforation. CD diagnosis is made after the onset of complications. The prognosis is poor for both EATL variants and one-year mortality is very high.

Diagnostic imaging (ultrasound, MRI, CT, PET-CT) and exploratory laparotomy are indicated in addition to instrumental investigations.

There are no standardized treatment protocols for EATL, but therapy may entail surgical removal of the tumour mass, chemotherapy, and autologous transplantation. Refractory CD and ulcerative jejunoileitis can benefit from corticosteroid, immunosuppressive, and nutritional therapies. Furthermore, recent acquisitions have opened the way to the use of biological drugs, such as anti-CD52 monoclonal antibodies and anti-IL-15 antibodies, as well as cell therapies.

THERAPY: GLUTEN-FREE DIET

The treatment for CD is the same since gluten was identified as the trigger for intestinal lesions in CD patients and it is based on a strict gluten-free diet for a lifetime.

Cereals like wheat, rye, and barley must be completely avoided, while the potential damage from exposure to oats is still debated. Rice, corn, potatoes, quinoa, millet, and sorghum are safe sources of carbohydrates. Legumes (including buckwheat) are additional safe foods for CD patients.

The content of gluten in food is regulated by the Codex Alimentarius (http://www.codexalimentarius.net), which states that gluten-free foods are foods that do not contain wheat, rye, barley, oats, or crossbred varieties of these grains, or foods with a gluten level not exceeding 20 mg/kg (parts per million).

Wheat varieties with low gluten content are currently under study, as well as ways to lower the gluten levels in wheat-based foods (e.g., new techniques modify gliadin peptides): the final aim is to obtain flours with organoleptic properties similar to the original. No alternative to gluten-free diet is currently available for therapeutic use.

Although a gluten-free diet leads to clinical and histological recovery in almost all patients, it impacts on quality of life because it means lifelong duration, strict adherence, and added costs.

FOLLOW-UP

Dietary education, monitoring with regular dietary consultations, and participation in a patient association are essential for achieving adequate compliance.

In patients who respond well to the diet and do not show signs of alarm, periodic clinical and serological controls, usually annual, of anti-tTG IgA should be carried out; negative test results do not rule out nonadherence to the diet. Furthermore, the use of a supplementary martial and/or vitamin therapy should be evaluated on a case-by-case basis. Moreover, among instrumental examinations of follow-up is bone densitometry, which should be performed at diagnosis to document the possible presence of osteopenia/osteoporosis and then repeated after 2 years if present. It should be noted that, in diabetes, thyroid disease or other autoimmune diseases, the specific controls and therapies should be performed.

There is no international agreement between experts on whether or not a second intestinal biopsy should be performed to verify regression of pre-diet lesions.

A good compromise would be to carry out endoscopic and biopsy when the response to diet is uncertain or symptoms appear/worsens. It may also be necessary to reconsider a diagnosis of Crohn's disease. Despite following a strict gluten-free diet and resulting negative for both serology and histology, some patients report the persistence or recrudescence of intestinal and/or extraintestinal symptoms.

In such cases, further differential diagnoses with IBD, IBS and IBS-like syndromes should be considered, such as lactose intolerance, adverse reaction to nickel-containing foods, bacterial overgrowth syndrome, reaction to foods high in fermentable oligo-, di-, mono-saccharides and polyols (FODMAPs) or in enzymatic inhibitors of amylase and trypsin (ATIs).

Finally, with regard to its impact on the quality of life in celiac patients, a strict gluten-free diet seems to improve wellbeing and reduce depression after 12 months.

However, some negative psychological implications have been observed in specific risk categories (women, the elderly and the poorly educated).

NON-CELIAC GLUTEN SENSITIVITY (NCGS)

Some individuals in whom CD has been excluded (negative serology and biopsies on a free diet containing gluten) present with a pleomorphic clinical picture, characterized by intestinal symptoms such as swelling, diarrhoea, dyspepsia, and extraintestinal symptoms such as headache, asthenia, concentration deficit, transient rash, which significantly improves after starting a gluten-free diet. Since there are currently no biological markers confirming "non-celiac gluten sensitivity" (not celiac gluten sensitivity), many questions still persist about the existence and the pathogenic role of gluten or other components of wheat in this condition.

Specifically, patients with suspected NCGS have a histologically normal mucosa or mucosa with slight non-specific alterations (type 0 or I Marsh-Oberhuber classification), although a peculiar distribution of T lymphocytes has recently been observed in small clusters at the surface epithelium or in a linear form above the muscolaris mucosae. An increased number of eosinophilic granulocytes appears (2/3 per 40x field of view) in the lamina propria. It should be emphasized that among persons with NCGS there could be cases of unrecognized CD and in which an appropriate diagnosis could be reached with the support of organ culture (not performed routinely).

Equally numerous are the missed differential diagnoses, primarily those of wheat allergy and/or other cereals.

Adverse reactions to foods with a high content of nickel or fermentable sugars (FODMAPs) should not be overlooked. Finally, the enzymatic inhibitors of amylase and trypsin (amylase trypsin inhibitors, ATIs), make up about 2-4% of the total wheat proteins (compared to about 80-90% of gluten), in plants and pesticides used in cereal crops and can trigger activation of the innate immune response.

For the diagnosis of NCGS a clinical protocol has been proposed with a double blind challenge (gluten versus placebo), better known as The Salerno Experts' Criteria, as well as a patch test of the oral mucosa with gluten. As in CD, clinical remission of disorders should be seen after having followed a gluten-free diet.

KEY CONCEPTS

- Celiac disease has high prevalence in the general population.
- Serological screening is recommended in diseases often associated with celiac disease (e.g., thyroid diseases, autoimmune diseases, hypertransaminasemia, osteoporosis, repeated abortion, Down syndrome, etc.).
- Diagnostic work-up should be carried out on a free (gluten-containing) diet.
- Complications are rare, but possible and fearsome (lymphoma, refractory celiac disease).
- Some people in whom celiac disease has been excluded report improvement of gastrointestinal and extra-intestinal symptoms after a gluten-free diet. This condition, known as non-celiac gluten sensitivity is still debated: gluten or other components of wheat may be involved.

REFERENCES

- Catassi C, Elli L, Bonaz B, et al. Diagnosis of Non-Celiac Gluten Sensitivity (NCGS): The Salerno Experts' Criteria. Nutrients. 2015 Jun 18;7(6):4966-77.
- Ciccocioppo R, Kruzliak P, Cangemi GC, et al. The spectrum of differences between childhood and adulthood celiac disease. Nutrients. 2015 Oct 22;7(10):8733-51.
- Husby S, Koletzko S, Korponay-Szabó IR, et al. European Society for Pediatric Gastroenterology, Hepatology, and Nutrition guidelines for the diagnosis of coeliac disease. J Pediatr Gastroenterol Nutr. 2012 Jan;54(1):136-60.
- Lebwohl B, Sanders DS, Green PHR. Coeliac disease. Lancet. 2018 Jan 6;391(10115):70-81.
- Ludvigsson JF, Bai JC, Biagi F, et al.; BSG Coeliac Disease Guidelines Development Group; British Society of Gastroenterology. Diagnosis and management of adult coeliac disease: guidelines from the British Society of Gastroenterology. Gut. 2014 Aug; 63(8):1210-28.
- Picarelli A, Borghini R, Di Tola M, et al. Intestinal, Systemic, and Oral Gluten-related Alterations in Patients With Nonceliac Gluten Sensitivity. J Clin Gastroenterol. 2016 Nov/Dec;50(10):849-58.
- Picarelli A, Di Tola M, Marino M, et al. Usefulness of the organ culture system when villous height/crypt depth ratio, intraepithelial lymphocyte count, or serum antibody tests are not diagnostic for celiac disease. Transl Res. 2013; 161(3):172-80.

FOOD ALLERGIES AND INTOLERANCES

Alfredo Di Leo, Tiziana Larussa*
*In memoriam

LEARNING OBJECTIVES

- To define food allergies and intolerances and their differences.
- To know the diagnostic and treatment management of food allergies.
- To define the key concepts of lactose intolerance.
- To understand the less common forms of pharmacologic intolerance.

CLASSIFICATION

Adverse food reactions represent a remarkably interesting area, mainly for the media attention to the population involved. These reactions can be classified as toxic and non-toxic (**Figure 20.1**).

Toxic reactions are secondary to the ingestion of substances contained in the food causing gastrointestinal symptoms. Among these are: mushroom intoxication, the scombroid syndrome (diarrhoea, hypotension, dyspnea, and bronchospasm secondary to the ingestion of fish inadequately preserved and containing high quantities of his-

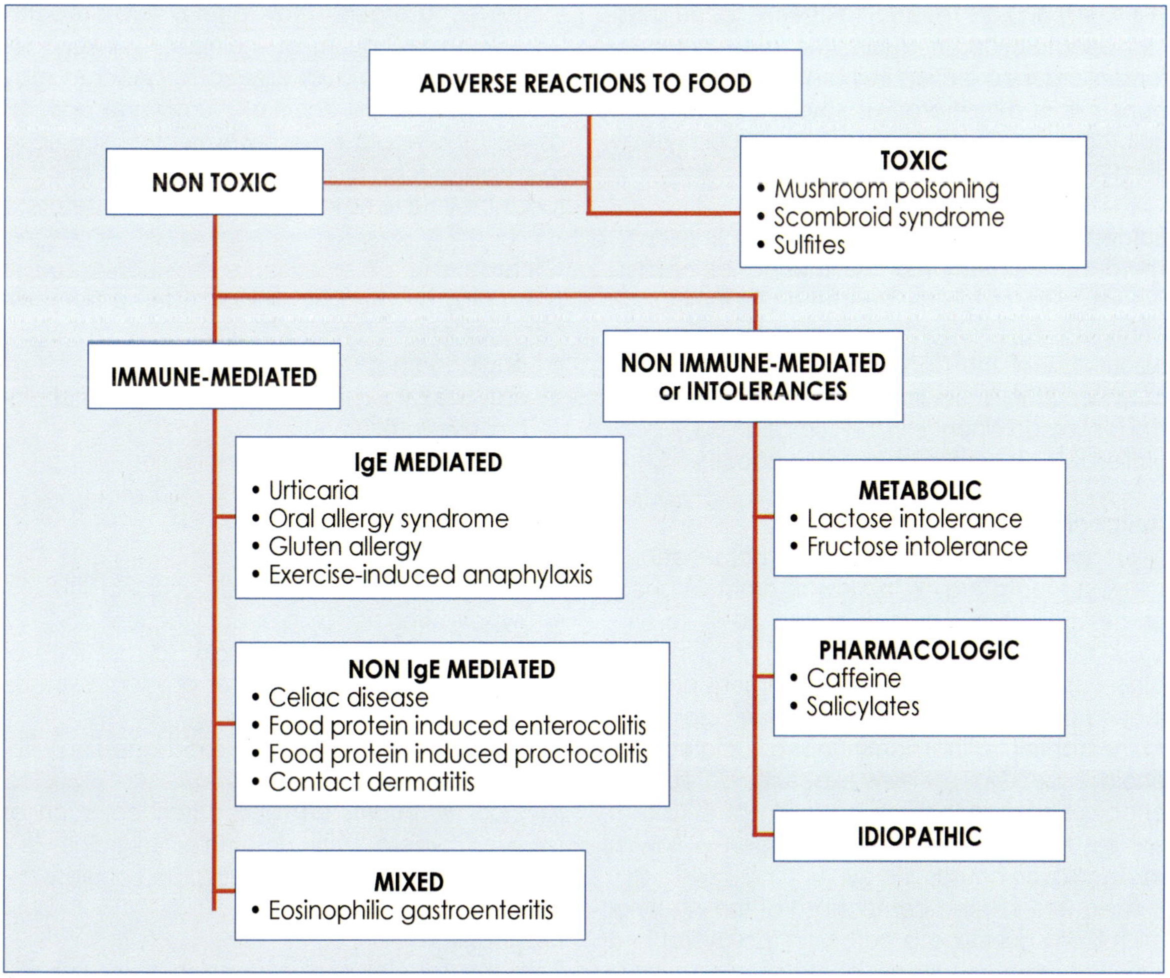

Figure 20.1 Classification of food allergies and intolerances.

tamine) and the sulfite syndrome (contained in wines and causing anaphylaxis).
Non-toxic reactions differ by (depend on the) individual susceptibility and can be divided into immune-mediated (more properly called food allergies) and non-immune mediated (food intolerances).

IGE-MEDIATED FOOD ALLERGIES

Definition and Subclassification

On the basis of the immunologic mechanism, food allergies can be divided into IgE-mediated and non-IgE mediated (Figure 20.1).
IgE-mediated food allergies are caused by an inappropriate production of immunoglobulins belonging to the E class (IgE) directed towards particular food antigens that are recognised as "strangers" by the immune system. Most of these food antigens have a glicoproteic and hydrosoluble nature, they have a high molecular weight (10-70 kD) and are resistant to chemical and physical denaturation. In adults, the most common food allergens are dried fruit (especially peanuts), eggs, milk and its derivatives, soy, fish, shellfish, and fruit (cherries, peaches, apricots), although every food is potentially allergenic.

Epidemiology

The public perception of the importance of allergic reactions to food exceed the predominance of these reactions identified in clinical studies.
About 25% of the population (adults/children) is convinced they suffer from a food allergy, although the real predominance in the European adult population is 1-2%. Among children it is about 5-8%.

Aetiopathogenesis

A fundamental pathogenetic phenomenon underlying food allergy is the loss of oral tolerance, or the loss of the immune system's ability to suppress an immunological response to antigens that otherwise would be innocuous. Allergens are normally processed in the lymphoid tissue associated to the gastrointestinal system (gut-associated lymphoid tissue, GALT), where exposure to Treg lymphocytes stimulates the production of IL-10 that ensures tolerance towards the antigen. A flaw in this regulation causes allergy.
Furthermore, altered composition of the intestinal microbiota could be a cofactor. The microbiota is an important modulator of the immune system because it regulates the balance between lymphocytes Th1 and Th2 and immunotolerance. Clear scientific evidence demonstrates that it has an aetiopathogenetic role in the development of food allergies. It has actually been proved that in a person with food allergies there is a high concentration of Stafilococcus aureus and Clostridia, as well as a low percentage of Bacteroides e Bifidobacteria as compared to a non-allergic individual.
Additionally, a genetic background is also responsible for susceptibility to develop food allergies: mutations in the gene of filaggrin have been linked to peanut allergy.
When a predisposed individual is first exposed to a food antigen, he/she will produce an abnormal amount of specific IgEs for that antigen that will be bound to the mastocytes and basophils membrane. As soon as contact further occurs, antigens will bind the specific IgEs and cause the degranulation of immune cells with secretion of large amount of histamine that causes clinical manifestations of different grade of severity.
Moreover, allergens may display cross-reactivity: via a mechanism of molecular mimicry, for instance, an individual allergic to peaches may be allergic also to cherries, plums, and apricots as well. This would explain why persons sensitized to a kind of food may result reactive also to other foods they have never been exposed to before.

Clinic

There may be multiple clinical pictures. The most common are:

- angioedema;
- oral allergy syndrome (oropharyngeal itch, labial swelling);
- diarrhoea and/or abdominal pain;
- nausea and vomiting;
- itch;
- hives;
- asthma, rhinitis, cough, otitis, conjunctivitis;
- hypotension similar to anaphylactic shock;
- exercise-induced anaphylaxis (a rare form of anaphylaxis occurring after physical exercise due to cereal ingestion).

The onset of symptoms follows food ingestion within a few minutes or hours.
Atypical symptoms are also described, such as fatigue, hyperactivity, insomnia, migraine, osteo-muscular pains, night sweats, and enuresis.

Diagnosis

Both the familial and personal histories are important. If a patient does not have parents with known allergies he/she has a risk to develop allergies of 1-15%; having one affected parent carries a risk of 40%, having two up to 80%. Accurate history can reveal the food that elicits a reaction within a short period of time (from a few minutes to 2 hours after ingestion). Moreover, clinical manifestations are often stereotyped and can be elicited by the ingestion of the food in question.

The oral provocation test, or more precisely the double blind placebo controlled challenge, is considered the diagnostic gold standard. It is performed in two days and consists in the administration of the dry or lyophilized allergen in a carrier food on one day, and of the placebo in the carrier food or vice versa on the following day. The allergen dose is progressively increased for monitoring the patient's clinical picture and the eventual onset of typical symptoms. The provocation test should be carried out in a protected environment, and immediately interrupted if severe reactions occur (anaphylaxis); it should never be performed as a diagnostic test in children with a history of anaphylactic reactions. In this clinical context, cutaneous provocation tests and laboratory tests have an important role. To recognise the IgE-mediated reactions, cutaneous tests performed with the prick test method, using standardised food extracts, are very useful. Vegetal extracts and fruit can be tested with the prick by prick method (applying small amounts of fresh food directly to the skin). The negative predictive value and the prick test specificity are very high (95%), but their positive predictive value and sensitivity are about 50%. Sensitivity is lower in the elderly and in patients treated with corticosteroids and antihistamines that may produce false negatives. Another useful test to identify IgE-mediated reactions is the search for in vitro specific food antibodies (radioallergosorbent test, RAST) in peripheral blood. For RAST a low positive predictive value and a high predictive negative value are described as well. Finally, all laboratory tests imply false positives: patients may result hyper-sensitive to antigens despite having never shown symptoms after ingestion of that food. Positivity should be discussed as far as its potential connections with the clinic and the patient's history.

Therapy and Prevention

The total elimination of the food in the diet that causes allergy is the fundamental therapeutic principle. However, this strategy may result difficult for several reasons. First, the so-called occult allergens may be present in unsuspected foods (for instance, fish jelly in cakes or casein in wine). Another problem is the scarce clarity on product labels. This may happen because an allergen can be defined in non-comprehensible terms for a non physician (whey, lactalbumins, caseinates identify milk proteins), or simply because texts are small or in a foreign language. Also, the caption "spices and flavors" may hide tricks. Finally, cross-reactivity may make the list of foods to be eliminated longer.

Immunotherapy consists in administering increasing doses of the antigen so as to induce a response of tolerance to it. It can be administered in sublingual, subcutaneous or epicutaneous route. It works by inducing an allergen specific-Th2 lymphocyte shift toward a Treg phenotype which secretes IL-10 and TGF-beta. Unfortunately, the clinical studies that have investigated this technique are heterogeneous with a very small sample size, making further controlled trials necessary to confirm the efficacy of these therapies and define their safety profile. Omalizumab, a monoclonal antibody directed against IgE, has already been approved and demonstrated good effectiveness, by reducing the IgE titer. Other monoclonal antibodies, such as reslizumab and mepolizumab (anti-IL-5) and Etokimab (anti-IL-33) are under investigation.

As for prevention, during pregnancy and breastfeeding a balanced diet is recommended without any restrictions, with exclusive breastfeeding for at least 4-6 months, while if breastfeeding is not possible, formulations of hypoallergenic milk should be used for 4 months. After the fourth month avoiding or increasing the consumption of allergenic foods is not necessary.

NON IGE-MEDIATED FOOD ALLERGIES

Food protein enterocolitis is a typically pediatric syndrome that occurs within the third month of life with vomiting, diarrhoea, and malabsorption. The more frequent causative antigens are cow milk proteins or soy. In some cases positivity may be found in the occult fecal blood test. Treatment is based on elementary or oligoantigenic diets or on the use of hydrolysed milk. Allergic eosinophilic proctocolitis also appears during the first months of life and is caused by allergy to milk proteins. The symptoms (diarrhoea and haematochezia) appear immediately after the exposure to the antigen (within a few hours) and rapidly disappear after the elimination of the food from the diet.

Its distinctive histopathological feature is mucosal oedema with eosinophil infiltration. Coeliac disease is treated in a separate chapter, although its classification under food allergies proposed by the American Society of Allergy is incorrect, since it is an autoimmune disorder.

FOOD INTOLERANCES

Definition, Pathogenesis, Clinic, and Diagnosis

These non-immunomediated adverse reactions to foods can be divided into enzymatic and pharmacological according to their pathogenic mechanism. The enzymatic ones are due to enzymatic deficiencies that do not allow proper metabolization or digestion of the food in question, including lactose, fructose, trehalose, and saccharose/isomaltose intolerance. The pharmacological ones are due to chemical substances (caffeine, salicylates, benzoate, histamine) that, not degraded because of genetic predisposition, cause typical symptoms.

Lactose Intolerance

In the small intestine two genes regulate the metabolism of lactose. One is lactase-phlorizin hydrolase (LPH) that encodes lactase, an enzyme on the microvilli of enterocytes that is responsible for the degradation of lactose into glucose and galactose. The other one, the MCM6, regulates the activity of LPH. Primary lactose intolerance is due to a genetic mutation of LPH, and it is extremely rare. Secondary intolerance is much more common: after a damage of the small intestinal mucosa (infections, inflammatory diseases, chemotherapy, or radiotherapy), lactase expression is reduced. Moreover, with age and in particular after weaning, a physiological reduction of lactase expression occurs, which can explain the onset of intolerance. However, in some persons lactase expression does not decline with age and this event may be related to the presence of the variants 13910C >T and 22018G >A of the MCM6 gene. These variants are more common among peoples traditionally devoted to pastoralism in the North Europe, which explains why lactose intolerance is less common in those areas (10%) than in Afro-American populations (80-90%). From a pathogenetic point of view (**Figure 20.2**), the missing degradation of lactose leads to its transiting in the large intestine where microbial flora metabolizes it, producing gas (hydrogen, methane, carbon dioxide) that causes bloating, abdominal pain, abdominal distension, abnormal bowel sounds, flatulence, and production of short chain fatty acids (SCFA) that recall water by osmosis and cause diarrhoea. For diagnosis, a very important role is the clinic and history coupled with the diary of the patient's diet to trace the association between symptoms and the food causing them. Moreover, fundamental for confirmation of diagnosis is the lactose breath test, which entails the administration of a solution

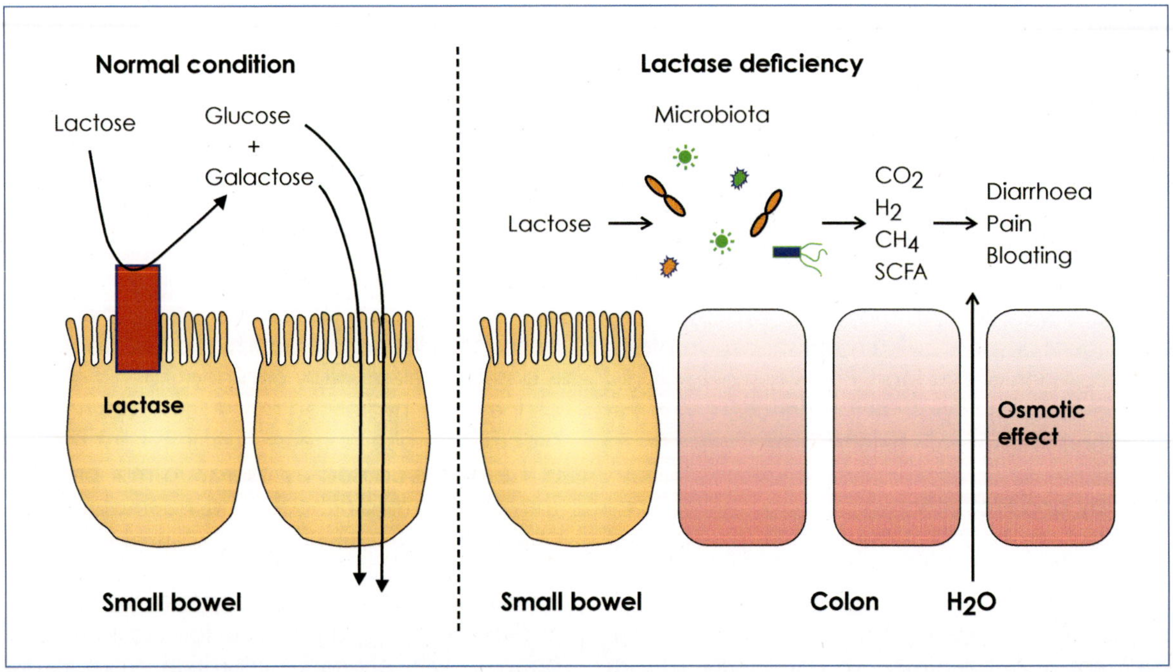

Figure 20.2 Pathophysiology of lactose intolerance. SCFA: Short-Chain Fatty Acids.

of 25 or 50 g of lactose, and measurement of the exhaled hydrogen: when a value >10 ppm over the baseline is found, the diagnosis is confirmed.
Therapy consists of the exclusion of foods containing lactose. Initially, a rigorous (or strict) 4 weeks' exclusion diet is suggested to achieve a complete regression of symptoms. Later, a gradual reintroduction of small amounts of lactose can be attempted to identify the personal limit of tolerance to lactose that varies significantly among individuals (the majority can eat <12 g of lactose). Yogurt is allowed because it contains lactic ferments that produce beta-galactosidase. Also, prehydrolysed milk can be introduced as well. Moreover, enzymes like tilactase or beta-galactosidase can be prescribed before a meal when the total absence of lactose in the food is uncertain.

Pharmacologic Intolerances

Pharmacologic intolerances are basically due to pharmacologically active substances, naturally present in foods or added (additives or colorings). The most common are intolerance to histamine and salicylates.
Susceptible individuals have primary defect of the enzymes needed for the metabolism of the substance in question. For example, in persons with a histamine intolerance there is a deficiency in the diamine-oxydase enzyme (DAO), necessary for the catabolism of exogenous histamine. Ingesting food with a high level of histamine (red wine, seasoned cheese) may block the already reduced activity of DAO (black tea, some food colorings, alcohol) or trigger endogenous histamine release (wheat germs, walnuts, acetaldehyde), resulting in clinical reactions that resemble food allergy:

- cardiogenic shock;
- respiratory symptoms (rhinorrhoea, nasal obstruction, asthma);
- hypotension or hypertension, arrhythmias;
- cutaneous signs (rash, itch, flush, hives);
- gastrointestinal symptoms (meteorism, abdominal cramping, diarrhoea);
- migraine.

Another example of pharmacological food intolerance is the reaction to salicylates present in foods and spices such as curry, paprika, cinnamon, peppers. Diagnosis relies on identifying the triggers containing salicylate and then testing whole blood (heparinised) incubated with 5-acetilsalicylic acid and arachidonic acid.
Finally, the Chinese restaurant syndrome has been described for monosodium glutamate intolerance, a flavour enhancer. It usually appears 15-20 minutes after exposure with flushing, migraine, muscular stiffness, sweating, paraesthaesia, nausea, and diarrhoea. For histamine intolerance a diet excluding the foods that induce endogenous histamine release or contain histamine is mandatory. For salicylate intolerance, foods and drugs containing salicylates and/or colourings and/or benzoic acid should be avoided. Pharmacologically, a therapy with anti-leukotrienes such as montelukast can be prescribed.

KEY CONCEPTS

- Food allergies can be IgE-or non IgE-mediated.
- The gastroenterological clinic (abdominal pain, diarrhoea) often accompanies extra-intestinal symptoms (rhinitis, dermatitis, hives, asthma, anaphylactic shock).
- The triggering antigen is frequently a proteic one, and the most commonly involved foods are peanuts, dried fruit, eggs, soy, fish, crustaceans, and fruit.
- The gold standard for diagnosis is the oral provocation test, but prick test and RAST can be used despite a low sensitivity and a high specificity.
- The treatment of food allergy is based on the exclusion of allergens from the diet. Lactose intolerance is a secondary phenomenon in most cases.
- The lactose breath test is the diagnostic gold standard.

REFERENCES

- Misselwitz B, Butter M, Verbeke K, Fox MR. Update on lactose malabsorption and intolerance: pathogenesis, diagnosis and clinical management. Gut. 2019;68(11):2080-91.
- Sicherer SH, Sampson HA. Food allergy: A review and update on epidemiology, pathogenesis, diagnosis, prevention, and management. J Allergy Clin Immunol. 2018;141(1):41-58.
- Prince BT, Mandel MJ, Nadeau K, Singh AM. Gut Microbiome and the Development of Food Allergy and Allergic Disease. Pediatr Clin North Am. 2015;62(6):1479-92.
- De Martinis M, Sirufo MM, Suppa M, Ginaldi L. New Perspectives in Food Allergy. Int J Mol Sci. 2020;21(4):1474.

CHAPTER 21

DIVERTICULAR DISEASE

Rosario Cuomo, Giovanna Del Vecchio Blanco

LEARNING OBJECTIVES

- To define the diagnostic criteria of diverticular disease.
- To identify the different clinical profiles of diverticular disease.
- To provide adequate diagnostic data.
- To provide the criteria for proper indications for medical or surgical therapy.

DEFINITION

"Diverticulosis" consists of the formation diverticula in the colon. The most common type of diverticula are "pseudo-diverticula", i.e., herniations affecting only the mucosa and submucosa. Herniation occurs in the muscular colonic wall where the perforating arteries cross the circular muscle layer, generally between the mesenteric and lateral teniae coli (**Figure 21.1**). True diverticula are, instead, congenital and are characterized by the herniation of all the layers of the visceral wall. Diverticula occur more frequently among the elderly, and often as multiple lesions. In 65% of cases, they affect the sigmoid colon (**Figure 21.2**).

The mere presence of diverticula in the colon, without symptoms, is defined diverticulosis. Symptomatic uncomplicated diverticular disease is a syndrome characterized by recurrent abdominal symptoms (pain and swelling), closely resembling the irritable bowel syndrome. Acute diverticulitis is a condition secondary to diverticular inflammation and is characterized by an acute episode of severe abdominal pain, protracted in time and localized in the lower left quadrant; it is often associated with altered bowel habit, leukocytosis and fever. Acute diverticulitis may become complicated by the onset of concomitant access, intestinal perforation and/or peritonitis.

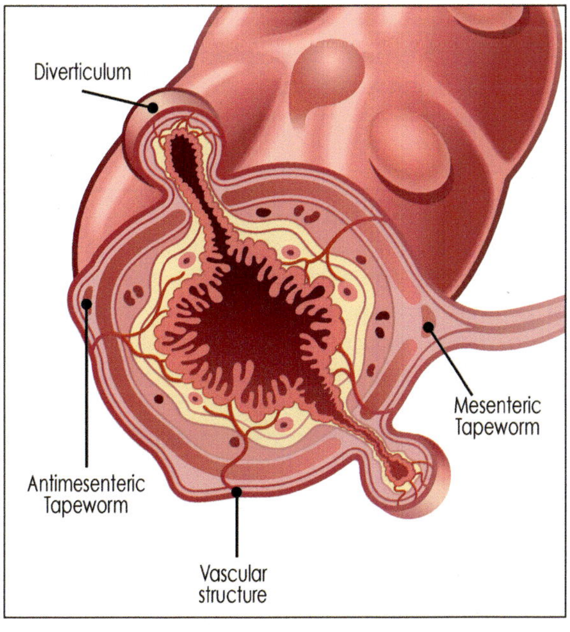

Figure 21.1 Drawing shows colonic diverticula.

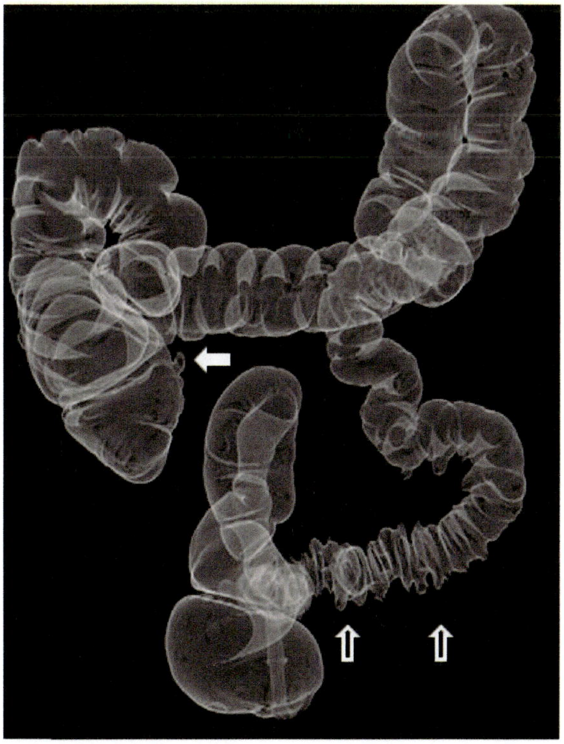

Figure 21.2 Virtual colonoscopy shows right colon diverticulum and multiple diverticula of the left colon (Courtesy of Dr Roberto Fiori).

EPIDEMIOLOGY

Diverticula disease is rather common in industrialized countries, with high prevalence rates in the United States and increasing prevalence in Europe, given the longer life expectancy. Prevalence rates in the English population are calculated to be about 35% among individuals aged above 60 years; the global incidence is about 1.55 cases every 1000 inhabitants and 5.75 cases in those over 75 years of age, with slightly higher rates for females. In most cases, diverticular disease has a favorable diagnosis and a low complications rate. Only 2.5-6.2% of affected individuals develop diverticulitis; mortality rates in the US for this condition are equal to 1.0%, with a 4.3% surgical mortality. Recently, hospitalization rates have increased due to acute episodes, and data from general medicine units in the UK reported a two-fold increase in perforations due to diverticular disease from 1990 to 2005. According to recent data, recurrence rates for diverticulitis show a 9% prevalence at 1 year and a 13% prevalence at 2 years; higher rates have been recorded both for complicated diverticulitis and among women. The presence of one or more comorbidity—quite common in the elderly—increases mortality rates by six-fold.

PATHOPHYSIOLOGY

There are 3 main agents involved in the formation of colon diverticula:

- low dietary fiber intake;
- altered structure of the colonic wall;
- altered motility, with consequent increase in endoluminal pressure.

A low fiber diet has a pathogenic role in the development of diverticulosis. The evidence in support of this theory is that diverticular disease is common in western countries where the intake of dietary fiber is generally low, and less frequent in countries characterized by a higher intake of dietary fiber (i.e., Asia and Africa). The occurrence of diverticulosis in populations who migrate from areas with a low prevalence of this condition to areas with higher prevalence, as well as the lower incidence rate among vegetarians, confirms the pivotal role of dietary fiber.
Changes affecting the connective tissue of the intestinal wall also seem to have a key role in the genesis of diverticula. Indeed, there is a high prevalence of diverticulosis among patients with connective tissue diseases, such as Enlher-Danlos' and Marfan's syndromes. Elastin and collagen—two of the main components of the extracellular matrix—seem to be especially involved in the pathogenic mechanism of diverticular disease. Electronic microscopy studies on affected subjects have detected a 200% increase in elastin deposits between teniae muscle cells, with consequent thickening of the colonic wall. An increased type III collagen synthesis has been described, correlated to age, and increased tissue expression of the metalloproteinase inhibitors that regulate tissue deposition of collagen in the colonic wall. The progressive elastosis of colonic teniae seems to be ascribable to the increased proline content, used as additive by the food industry. Therefore, the formation of colonic diverticula may be favored by the progressive hardening/stiffening of the intestinal wall, due to the increased collagen content.
Altered intestinal motility has also been detected in the pathogenesis of diverticular disease. Increased intraluminal colonic pressure has been observed in several studies, both in resting conditions and following different stimuli (food, cholinergic drugs), supporting its role in the genesis of diverticula, especially involving the left colon. As intraluminal pressure in the right colon is lower, other factors – including genetics and structural wall alterations – may be involved in the pathogenesis of diverticula in this region, a condition typical of Asian populations. Altered motility and intestinal sensitivity also seem to play a role in the genesis of pain in symptomatic uncomplicated diverticular disease.
Additionally, altered intestinal bacterial flora (dysbiosis) as well as intestinal mucosal inflammatory response have been postulated as having a role in the development of this condition—particularly in the pathogenesis of diverticulosis.

CLINICAL PROFILE

In most cases (an estimated 80%), the presence of diverticula is asymptomatic; their diagnosis is often an occasional finding during instrumental diagnostic tests performed for other medical indications. Clinically, we may identify three conditions:

- asymptomatic diverticular disease, or simply "diverticulosis";
- symptomatic uncomplicated diverticular disease;
- diverticulitis.

Diverticulosis does not require any specific follow-up. Symptomatic uncomplicated diverticular disease is characterized by abdominal pain of variable intensity—even at night, generally localized in the lower left quadrant, but sometimes irradiating to the whole abdomen. Patients often complain of abdominal distension and irregular bowel movements (constipation and/or diarrhoea), with passage of mucus with the feces; pain is often partly or totally relieved after a bowel movement and/or passing gas. This stage does not present with fever, leukocytosis or evidence of peritoneal irritation, and the clinical profile may resemble the irritable bowel syndrome.

Diverticulitis mainly presents with pain involving the lower left quadrant; pain intensity and the extent of the general clinical profile are associated with the extension of the inflammatory process, which may be localized or diffuse. Pain may irradiate posteriorly, to the left side, to the inguinal region or the lower abdominal quadrant. Nausea and vomiting are generally absent, except in case of intestinal occlusion; conversely, changes in bowel habit are quite common. Patients with acute diverticular disease often refer of urinary symptoms, indicating that the inflammation has extended to the bladder wall. This would account for symptoms such as dysuria, vesical tenesmus, and frequent micturition, whereas the onset of urinary infection may suggest a colo-vesical fistula. Mild fever is a typical symptom of diverticulitis; leukocytosis, increased erythrocyte sedimentation rate (ESR) and C-reactive protein (C-rp) indicate intestinal wall inflammation.

In about 5% of patients, symptomatic diverticular disease leads to complications—namely abscess, perforation, fistula, intestinal occlusion, and diverticular bleeding.

Abscess formation is the most frequent complication of acute diverticular disease. It is the consequence of a covered perforation/micro perforation of a diverticulum (**Figure 21.3**). The abscess may be distinctly delimited within the peri-diverticular space or extend to the adjacent recess, reaching the ischioanal fossae. Symptoms are pain, fever, sometimes with nausea and vomiting. For the definition of abscess extension, see the four stages of the disease described in Hinchey's clinical classification (**Table 21.1**).

Intestinal perforation is a condition occurring when there is rupture of a diverticulum, or an abscess formed within the abdominal cavity. The perforation of a diverticulum leads to the severe clinical condition of acute abdomen, with sudden abdominal pain involving the lower quadrants and irradiating to the whole abdomen and requiring timely diagnosis and surgical treatment. A clinical

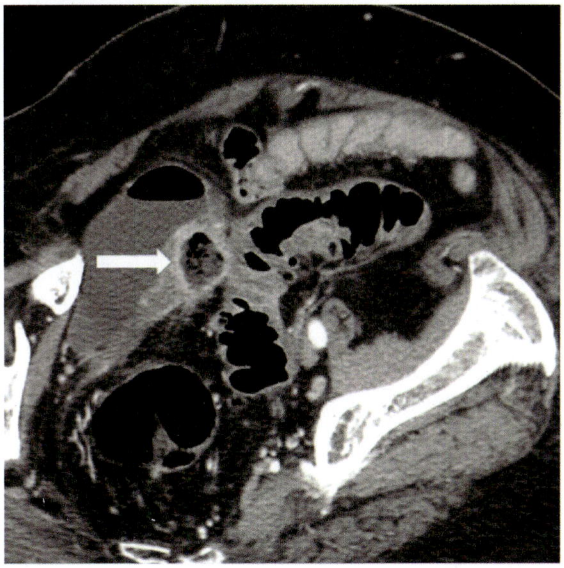

Figure 21.3 Virtual colonoscopy shows diverticulitis complicated by the presence of an abscess (arrow) in the middle third of the sigmoid adjacent to the bladder. The thickening of the sigma wall is well evident. (Courtesy of Dr Roberto Fiori.)

sign is the presence of free gas in the peritoneal cavity, detectable by both percussion and abdominal X-rays.

The occurrence of fistulisation derives from a diverticulitis associated to an abscess which, by erosion, penetrates the wall and opens into the intestinal lumen and the adjacent structure. This may lead to colovesical, colocutaneous, colovaginal and coloenteral fistulas. In rarer cases, the fistula may penetrate the ureter or the peritoneum. Characterising symptoms of a fistula are pneumaturia, fecaluria, and recurrent vaginal infections.

Intestinal occlusion may be due to acute stenosis during an intercurrent episode of acute diverticulitis and is correlated to pericolic flogosis and/or compression of the abscess, or even to a stenosis consequent to fibrosis following recurrent acute diverticulitis.

Table 21.1 Modified Hinchey classification of acute diverticulitis

- 0 Mild clinical diverticulitis
- Ia Confined pericolic inflammation or phlegmon
- Ib Pericolic or mesocolic abscess
- II Pelvic, distant intra-abdominal, or retroperitoneal abscess
- III Generalized purulent peritonitis
- IV Generalized fecal peritonitis

Adapted from (Wasvary H et al. 1999).

Intestinal bleeding is a quite common complication, occurring in about 3-5% of patients with diverticulitis. About 30-40% of intestinal bleeding episodes are due to diverticular bleeding. Diverticular bleeding is caused by the erosion of diverticular wall vessels and may even be independent of the underlying acute inflammation. Non-steroid anti-inflammatory drugs (NSAID) favor the onset of diverticular bleeding. In most cases, bleeding stems from an arteriole – and is therefore of moderate intensity. In about 70-80% of cases, spontaneous healing occurs; should this not be the case, treatment consists of surgical treatment, with intestinal resection of the affected segment.

INSTRUMENTAL DIAGNOSIS

Symptomatic diverticular disease is a distinct disease from other conditions with similar symptoms, i.e., irritable bowel syndrome, appendicitis, chronic inflammatory intestinal diseases, ischaemic colitis, colorectal cancer, gynecological diseases (ovarian cyst rupture, ovarian torsion). As the clinical diagnosis is inaccurate in 34 to 67% of cases, the diagnosis needs to be confirmed by instrumental examination, especially before scheduling the patient for surgery.

A colonoscopy provides information on the extent of the diverticular disease (**Figure 21.4**) and on the presence of the mucosal alterations (inflammation) of the peridiverticular region; The examination should not be carried out in the acute stage of the disease, given the high risk of perforation by the accidental insertion of the probe in a diverticulum and/or by the insufflation of air into the colon. An indication for a colonoscopy is the presence of intestinal bleeding possibly due to a diverticulum, to diagnose the origin of the bleeding and for treatment purposes. An arteriography may be necessary in case of massive bleeding.

The histological assessment performed during the colonoscopy shows mucosal changes surrounding the diverticulum only in case of diverticulitis and its complications. Whereas the diagnosis on surgical samples is rather clear-cut – i.e., differentiate between chronic inflammatory diseases and diverticular inflammation – there is controversy over the diagnosis of bioptic material collected during a colonoscopy. A small percentage of patients may develop a condition defined as segmental colitis associated with diverticulosis (SCAD), which is characterized by chronic inflammation involving the interdiverticular mucosa of the colon segment involved. The rectum and the right colon are spared by this inflammatory state.

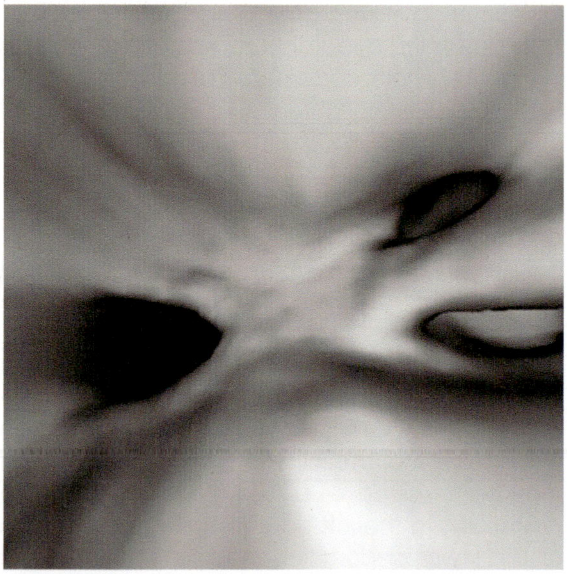

Figure 21.4 Colonoscopy shows colonic diverticula.

A computerized tomography (CT) scan with contrast media provides important information especially in the presence of diverticulitis with or without extraintestinal complications. In the last few years, standard CT and opaque enema have been replaced by multilayer CT and virtual colonoscopy (VC) or colonography (**Figure 21.5**). The latter test is used mainly for the diagnosis of diverticular disease and enables an uneventful examination of

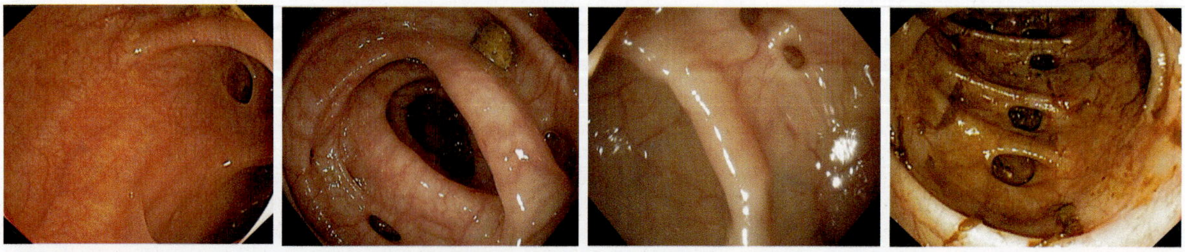

Figure 21.5 Diverticular orifices at virtual colonoscopy. (Courtesy of Dr Roberto Fiori.)

the colonic lumen, the intestinal wall, the pericolic space and the perivesical area, also to identify air within the bladder— suggesting the presence of a colovesical fistula.
The magnetic resonance is a possible alternative to CT and is especially interesting because it is devoid of ionizing radiations. Nevertheless, compared to tomography, it is longer and may be altered by the presence of artifacts due to movement—particularly common in the elderly.
The ultrasound scan is a useful, highly specific, and highly sensitive diagnostic tool, provided it is performed by an expert operator. It is useful to diagnose septic complications such as abscesses or fistulas.

THERAPEUTIC OPTIONS

Asymptomatic diverticulosis does not require any pharmacological treatment; there is limited evidence suggesting an increase in dietary fiber.
Rifaximine, a non absorbable oral antibiotic, if associated with higher fiber intake, may improve symptoms in patients with diverticular disease. The use of mesalazine (a local anti-inflammatory agent) to relieve symptoms is controversial; it is nevertheless ineffective in preventing diverticulitis. Patients with diverticular disease who take aspirin and NSAIDs on a regular basis are at greater risk of developing diverticulitis and diverticular bleeding, whereas diverticular perforation is an untoward effect of opioids and corticosteroids.
Management of patients with acute diverticulitis depends on the severity (complicated/uncomplicated) and complexity (presence of abscess, fistula, etc.) of the condition. Systemic antibiotics may improve the clinical profile and need to be prescribed considering the specific case of each patient. Severe and complicated forms of acute diverticulitis require hospitalization, intestinal rest and wide-spectrum antibiotics. Treatment of an abscess may require drainage.
Elective surgery may be considered in patients with symptomatic diverticular disease, complicated by fistulas or stenosis, and should be performed during quiescence of symptoms. There is controversy over the role of the patient's age when considering the surgical option. Indeed, some studies have shown that patients aged less than 50 years have greater likelihood of recurrence, given the longer life expectancy, and would therefore benefit from surgical treatment.
Immunocompromised patients or those on immunosuppressive treatment, with chronic renal failure or collagen diseases, are at greater risk of perforation during episodes of acute diverticulitis; a suitable therapeutic option in these cases is conservative treatment of the acute episode, followed by elective surgical resection. Surgery consists of resection of the sigma or in a left haemicolectomy with a colo-colic anastomosis, without need for a temporary protective stoma. Emergency intestinal resection (in the presence of bleeding or in case of perforation) is generally achieved as a two-step approach, according to Hartmann's technique. The first step consists of a resection of the affected segment and a cutaneous protective stoma; the second step is performed a few months later to reinstate intestinal continuity. In case of diffuse peritonitis due to perforation, a recent approach is the laparoscopic lavage of the peritoneal cavity as emergency treatment, with elective surgery of the affected segment scheduled subsequently. Surgical treatment, especially elective surgery, is increasingly more often performed laparoscopically, with results comparable to laparotomy in terms of functional results, but with the advantage of lower levels of post-surgical pain, post-surgical infections, and faster recovery time.

KEY CONCEPTS

- There is an increasing prevalence of diverticulosis, although in most cases, the outcome of the disease is favorable and the complications rate low.
- A high fiber intake in patients with diverticular disease decreases the risk of symptoms onset and complications.
- Mortality is higher in the presence of comorbidities.
- Symptomatic diverticular disease may have symptoms like irritable bowel syndrome.
- A virtual colonoscopy should be considered in the diagnostic workup in case of symptomatic diverticular disease.
- Colonoscopy is indicated in case of gastrointestinal bleeding to exclude other pathologies other than diverticulitis and for the treatment of bleeding
- The management of patients with acute diverticulitis depends on the severity and complexity of the condition.

REFERENCES

- Collins D, Winter DC. Modern concepts in diverticular disease. J Clin Gastroenterol. 2015; 49:358-69.
- Cuomo R, Cargiolli M, Cassarano S, et al. Treatment of diverticular disease, targeting symptoms or underlying mechanisms. Curr Opin Pharmacol. 2018; 43:124-31.
- Lips LM, Cremers PT, Pickhardt PJ, et al. Sigmoid cancer versus chronic diverticular disease: differentiating features at CT colonography. Radiology 2015; 275:127-35.
- National Institute for Health and Care Excellence. Diverticular Disease: Diagnosis and Management. NICE guideline NG147. 2019.
- Peery AF, Shaukat A, Strate LL. AGA Clinical Practice Update on Medical Management of Colonic Diverticulitis: Expert Review. Gastroenterology. 2021;160:906-11.
- Pfützer RH, Kruis W. Management of diverticular disease. Nat Rev Gastroenterol Hepatol. 2015;12:629-38.
- Strate LL, Morris AM. Epidemiology, pathophysiology, and treatment of diverticulitis. Gastroenterology 2019;156:1282-98.
- Vaidya KK, Floch MH. Diverticular disease: paradigm shifts in pathogenesis and treatment. Curr Treat Options Gastroenterol. 2015;13:143-55.

CHAPTER 22

PROCTOLOGY

Giovanni Egidio Maconi, Alfredo Papa

LEARNING OBJECTIVES

- To know the main anorectal pathologies and their epidemiological relevance.
- To know the pathophysiological bases and the various modalities of clinical presentation of anorectal pathologies.·
- To be able to formulate a correct diagnosis of anorectal diseases.
- To know the main therapeutic approaches to anorectal diseases.

INTRODUCTION

Pathology of the lower rectum, anal canal, and perineum is common and a cause of considerable distress. The prevalence of anorectal disorders in the general population is probably much higher than would appear if based solely on clinical encounters, because many patients are embarrassed by anorectal symptoms, and tend to avoid seeking medical help. Self-diagnosis and treatment are common. When a physician is consulted, it is usually for what the patient regards as "haemorrhoids". This is a common disorder; along with anal fissures and pruritus ani, they account for approximately 70% of complaints involving the anorectum. Nonetheless, various other disorders present with similar "haemorrhoidal" symptoms.

The rectum is the lower tract of the large intestine, extending for 10 to 15 cm above the anal canal. It is is roughly 4 cm long, begins at the anorectal junction and ends at the anal verge (anal orifice). The dentate or pectinate line marks the midpoint of the anal canal, where the mucosal columnar epithelium of the proximal portion of anus ends, and the dermal squamous epithelium of the distal portion begins (**Figure 22.1**). The mucosa above the dentate line is not supplied by sensory nerve fibers. As a result, many diagnostic (e.g., biopsies) and surgical procedures (e.g., haemorrhoid band ligation) can be performed in this area of the anal canal without anesthesia. In contrast, the area below the dentate line is abundantly supplied with sensory nerve fibers. Indeed, the perianal dermal area is one of the most sensitive areas of the body. Anal glands drain into the crypts of Morgagni at the dentate line, and most rectal abscesses and fistulae originate in these glands.

The anal canal receives its blood supply from the superior, middle, and inferior haemorrhoidal arteries, which are branches of the inferior mesenteric, hypogastric, and internal pudendal arteries, respectively. Arterial blood flow is somewhat less abundant posteriorly, which may be an important factor in the postulated role of ischaemia as a determinant of anal fissure chronicity: the posterior wall of the anus is the site of 90% of all anal fissures. The anal canal is drained by veins of the systemic and portal systems. The internal haemorrhoidal plexus drains into the superior rectal vein and then through the inferior mesenteric vein into the portal vein. This explains why rectal varices develop during portal hypertension in cirrhosis. The distal part of the anal canal is drained by the external haemorrhoidal plexus and then through the middle rectal and pudendal veins into the internal iliac vein (systemic circulation).

The muscles surrounding the anorectum are important for maintaining fecal continence and allow-

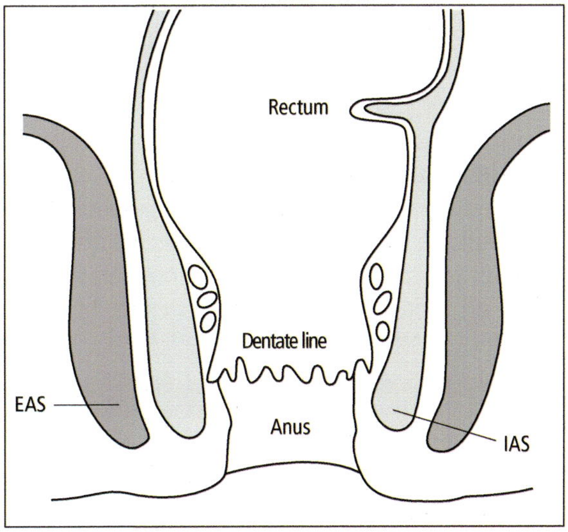

Figure 22.1 Schematic depiction of the anatomy of the anorectal region. IAS = internal anal sphincter; EAS = external anal sphincter.

ing evacuation. The internal anal sphincter (IAS) is the thickened continuation of the circular smooth muscle of the rectum. Maintenance of normal anal pressure depends largely (80%) on the IAS, which is therefore important for continence. Nevertheless, partial surgical resection of this sphincter (lateral internal sphincterotomy), which is currently used to treat anal fissures, can be carried out without causing fecal incontinence. The external anal sphincter (EAS) contributes to the remaining 20% of anal pressure. It is composed of a layer of voluntary skeletal muscle arranged as a tube, surrounding the IAS. Proximally, the EAS fuses with the puborectalis muscle, the tonic contraction of which is responsible for maintaining the recto-anal angle in resting state.

The tone of the sphincters of the anus determines its physiological and persistent closure.

Only when the combined action of the "mass movements" of the colon brings its contents into the rectum and induce its distension, this determines the involuntary relaxation of the IAS (rectal-anal inhibitory reflex) and the initial passage of material into the anal canal. Here, the rectal content comes in contact with the mucosa of the anal canal, richly innervated and equipped with specific receptors that distinguish intraluminal content characteristics, in particular, its solid, liquid or gaseous consistency. This generates contraction of the EAS or, as conditions allow complete relaxation of the pelvic floor muscles and the anal sphincters to allow the passage of gas or defecation. Closely related to the mechanism of defecation is fecal continence, ensured not only by tonic contraction of the anal sphincters but also by maintenance of the anorectal angle by the puborectal muscle. Under normal conditions, 80% of pressure in the anal canal is sustained by contraction of the IAS and 20% by the EAS.

The most common symptoms of ano-perianal disease include anal pain, ano-rectal bleeding, prolapse (haemorrhoids, mucosa or the entire rectal wall), anal pruritus, purulent discharge from the the anus or fistulas around the anus, swellings or lumps in or around the anus, constipation or fecal obstruction, difficulty in passing stool, and incontinence to flatus or feces (**Table 22.1**).

Ano-rectal and perianal diseases usually do not require extensive diagnostic workup. Key to diagnostic workup is accurate collection of the patient's history, followed by confirmation of lesions by visual inspection, digital examination, and anoscopy or proctoscopy. The latter still play a key role in the detection of anal diseases. Depending on the presence of specific symptoms and potential differential diagnosis, however, additional studies may be necessary. When a more proximal lesion is suspected, sigmoidoscopy or colonoscopy with biopsy should be done. An essential part of the workup of colorectal diseases, involves assessment of anorectal physiology with procedures like endoanal ultrasonography, anal manometry, and/or defecography. Fistulography is no longer used and now is replaced by magnetic resonance imaging (MRI), while computerized tomographic (CT) scan is used in selected cases, mainly in acute conditions. Successful interaction with the patient can greatly facilitate diagnosis, and definition of treatment, with optimal compliance of the patient.

Proctological disorders can be grouped into five broad categories: prolapse, inflammatory, suppurative, functional, and neoplastic diseases. Anorectal disease characterised by prolapse may include haemorrhoidal disease, as well as the various forms of rectal prolapse.

The inflammatory lesions consist mainly of anal fissures, solitary rectal ulcer, and proctitis (infectious and non-infectious forms). Almost all suppurative anorectal diseases stem from infections of the anal glands, which lead to the formation of abscesses and fistulas.

Functional disorders are mainly related to altered motility of the pelvic floor muscles. The increased and/or uncoordinated activity of these muscles can lead to non-relaxing pelvic floor dysfunctions. These disorders may be associated with pain and/or impairment of defecation (primary anorectal constipation - obstructed defecation), urination, and/or sexual intercourse. All these functions require relaxation and coordination of pelvic floor muscles and the urinary and anal sphincters. Decreased motility, by contrast, can lead to fecal incontinence, urinary incontinence or both.

Functional anorectal disorders can have severe negative effects on quality of life; they are discussed extensively elsewhere in this book. Functional disorders can also be the cause of idiopathic pruritus ani and unexplained anal pain. Anal cancers include adenocarcinomas (which develop from the columnar epithelium of the mucosa), lymphomas (which arise from mucosal lymphoid tissue), and keratinizing squamous cell carcinomas (which develop in the anodermal squamous epithelium).

Table 22.1 Symptoms of anorectal and perianal lesions.

Symptoms	Most Frequent Causes
Anal pain	• Thrombosed haemorrhoids • Anal fissure • Perianal abscesses & fistulas. • Anal malignancy
Anorectal bleeding	• Haemorrhoids • Anal fissures • Inflammatory bowel disease (IBD) • Non-IBD proctitis • Neoplasia (polyps, malignancy) • Anal fistula • Solitary rectal ulcer
Prolapse	• Haemorrhoids • Rectal prolapse (mucosal or complete) • Polyps (anal or rectal) • Hypertrophied anal papillae
Anal pruritus	• Mucus leak from haemorrhoids or prolapse • Discharge and soiling from anal fissure or fistula • Anal skin tags, papilloma, condyloma • Skin lesions (dermatitis, psoriasis,) • Worm infestation (*Enterobius vermicularis*) • Following surgical anorectal procedures • Anal incontinence • Inadequate or overzealous hygiene
Pus discharge from and around the anus	• Anal fistula, anal fissure with suppuration • Proctitis (IBD and non-IBD) • Anal malignancy • Solitary rectal ulcer • Suppuration in thrombosed haemorrhoids
Lump or mass in or around the anus	Painful masses • Abscess/haematoma/fistula • Thrombosed haemorrhoids • Inflamed sentinel pile of anal fissure • Malignancy Painless masses • External anal tags • Fibrous polyp, hypertrophied anal papillae • Papilloma, condyloma
Constipation or fecal obstruction	• Fecal impaction • Pelvic and anorectal neuromuscular disorders
Incontinence to flatus or feces	• Debilitating conditions (advanced age, mental illness) • Neurological disorders • Post-operative • Obstetrical injury • Rectal prolapse • Severe diarrhoea • Overflow incontinence with fecal impaction

HAEMORRHOIDAL DISEASE

The exact incidence of haemorrhoidal disease is unknown, but 10 to 25% of the adult population are thought to be affected. Symptoms like prolapse, bleeding, pain, and itching are more common in older individuals, with peak prevalence between 45 and 65 years. Emorrhoidal disease (HD) has been attributed to diverse factors, including constipation and prolonged straining. Familial history of HD, postural habits, low-fiber diet, and increased resting anal pressure due to hypertone of the internal anal sphincter are considered risk factors for HD.

Pregnancy favors congestion of the anal cushions and the development of symptomatic haemorrhoidal disease, which resolves spontaneously shortly after delivery. Alcohol and spicy foods, as well as severe diarrhoea, may trigger recurrence of HD symptoms. The incidence of haemorrhoids in patients with chronic liver disease is no higher than that in the general population. Anorectal varices develop in up to 80% of patients with portal hypertension, but they can be easily distinguished from haemorrhoids.

Internal haemorrhoids originate from the inferior haemorrhoidal venous plexus, above the dentate line, and are covered by mucosa. External haemorrhoids develop from the more distal portion of the same venous plexus, located below the dentate line, and are covered with squamous epithelium. Mixed diseases characterized by both forms are not uncommon. Internal haemorrhoids are generally classified into four grades based on their appearance and degree of prolapse (**Figure 22.2**): Grade I, haemorrhoids bleed but do not prolapse. Grade II, haemorrhoids prolapse through the anus when the patient strains, especially during defecation, but they reduce spontaneously. Grade III, haemorrhoids prolapse through the anus on straining and require manual reduction. Grade IV, haemorrhoid prolapse cannot be reduced.

Acutely thrombosed, incarcerated internal haemorrhoids and thrombosed haemorrhoids involving the circumferential prolapse of the rectal mucosal prolapse are also classified as grade IV.

External haemorrhoids are visible at the anal verge. They may form residual redundant skin tags from previous episodes of external haemorrhoidal inflammation and edema or thrombosis. They can interfere with perianal hygiene and cause irritation and itching.

A definitive diagnosis of haemorrhoidal disease relies on a detailed patient history and clinical ex-

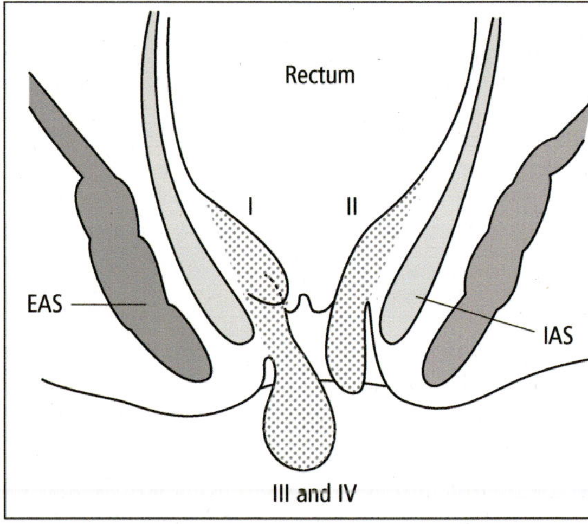

Figure 22.2 Schematic depiction of internal haemorrhoids, which are commonly classified in four degrees: grade I, bleed but do not prolapse; grade II, prolapse through the anus on straining but reduce spontaneously; grade III, prolapse through the anus on straining and require manual reduction; and grade IV, the prolapse is irreducible. IAS= internal anal sphincter; EAS = external anal sphincter.

amination, including digital exploration and anoscopy performed with the patient lying on his/her left side. Size and location of the haemorrhoids, as well as severity of inflammation and bleeding, should always be established. Flexible sigmoidoscopy should be performed in patients with haemorrhoidal disease or other anorectal symptoms. Patients with rectal bleeding who are at increased risk for colorectal cancer (e.g., over the age of 50, with a positive family history) should undergo colonoscopy to exclude cancer as the cause of bleeding. The perianal area should be inspected for anal skin tags, external haemorrhoids, perianal dermatitis caused by anal discharge or fecal soiling, fistula-in-ano, and anal fissure. The haemorrhoid classification system is useful for identifying the most appropriate and effective treatment.

The first-line therapy for haemorrhoid symptoms is conservative and consists of increasing fluid and fiber intake, appropriate modification of toilet behavior, and phlebotonic drugs consisting of plant extracts (i.e., flavonoids) and synthetic compounds (i.e., calcium dobesilate). The bleeding and pain of grade I haemorrhoids and the prolapse associated with grade II haemorrhoids that do not respond to this approach can generally be safely and satisfactorily resolved with office-based procedures, such as sclerotherapy, infrared photocoagulation, thermocoagulation (heater probe), multipolar electrocoagulation (BICAP) or radiofrequency ablation, and rubber-band ligation (**Figure 22.3**).

The last method may also be effective for grade III haemorrhoids although positive results will likely require a larger number of treatment sessions. Surgical therapy is the best choice for the management of persistently symptomatic grade III or IV haemorrhoids. It includes excisional haemorrhoidectomy, stapled haemorrhoidopexy, and Doppler-guided ligation of the haemorrhoidal artery. For acutely thrombosed external haemorrhoids, the best solution is excision and clot evacuation, which should ideally be performed within 72 hours of symptom onset. Residual haemorrhoids are banded or excised later.

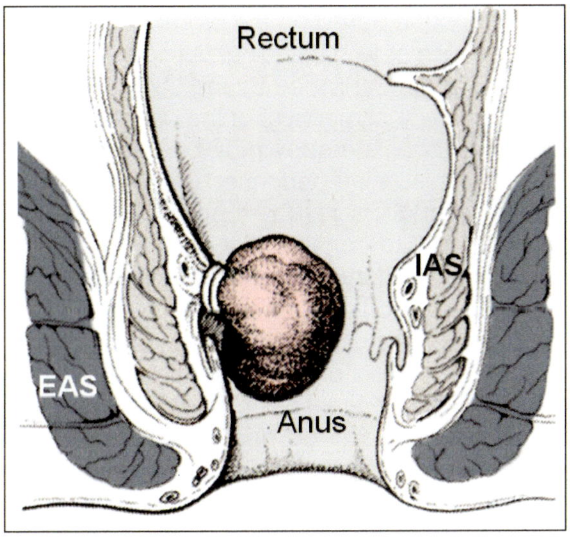

Figure 22.3 Schematic depiction of rubber-band ligation, currently the most common office procedure for the treatment of grade II or III haemorrhoids. IAS= internal anal sphincter; EAS= external anal sphincter.

RECTAL PROLAPSE

Rectal prolapse involves the protrusion of one or more layers of the rectal wall through the anal canal. Partial prolapse is limited to the mucosal layer. It may be occult or manifest and associated with haemorrhoidal disease (**Figure 22.4**). Mucosal prolapse is classified as first degree when the prolapsed tissue is visible below the anorectal ring on straining, second-degree when it reaches the dentate line, and third-degree when it arrives at the anal verge. Complete (full-thickness) rectal prolapse is classified in four types: grade 1 with prolapse up to the anal verge; grade 2 with prolapse outside the anus that reduces spontaneously; grade 3 with prolapse outside the anus that can be manually reduced; and grade 4 with prolapse that cannot be reduced manually. Accurate identification of the type and degree of prolapse is important for choosing the appropriate treatment.

Rectal prolapse is most common among older women, but it can occur at any age, even during childhood. The primary mechanism is excessive straining, which over many years gradually weakens the pelvic floor and its supporting structures. Most patients present with anal protrusion or symptoms of obstructed defecation or fecal incontinence. Predisposing factors include pre-existing dysmotility, dyssynergic defecation, and intussusception (also known as internal rectal prolapse).

Intussusception is characterized by full-thickness prolapse of the rectal wall that does not protrude through the anus. Rectal prolapse and intussusception may coexist with rectocele. The latter is an abnormal sac-like protrusions of the rectal wall — towards the vagina (anterior wall prolapse) or less commonly towards the sacrum (posterior wall prolapse) — that often becomes visible during defecation. Rectocele is common in adult women (20%) and frequently is small (<2 cm) and asymptomatic, and does not require treatment. Rectocele is believed to be the result of weakness of the rectovaginal septum and/or pelvic floor, but the exact cause is not known. Obstetric injuries and multiple vaginal deliveries have been proposed as precipitating factors, although rectocele is also seen in nulliparous women. Sixty percent of patients with rectocele have various patterns of dyssynergic defecation.

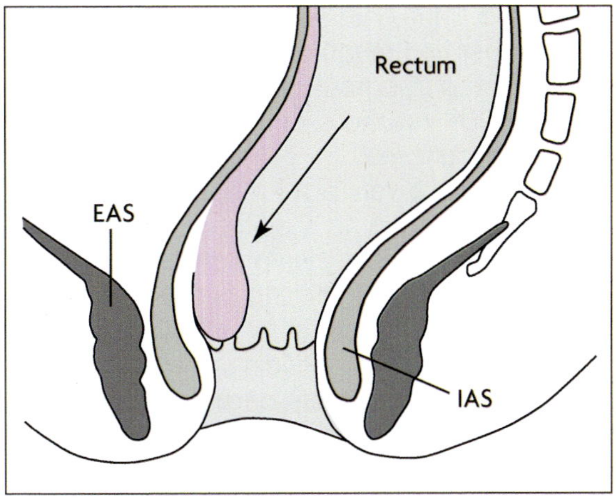

Figure 22.4 Schematic depiction of occult prolapse of the rectal mucosa. During defecation, straining is increased to overcome the mechanical obstacle of the anterior mucosal prolapse, thereby aggravating the prolapse. IAS= internal anal sphincter; EAS= external anal sphincter.

The diagnosis of rectal prolapse is predominantly clinical. Visualization of the prolapse may be possible only when the patient is straining. If doubts arise, imaging studies, including fluoroscopic or dynamic magnetic resonance defecography, can confirm the diagnosis, and endoscopy may be useful for identifying associated colonic disorders.

Nonsurgical management (e.g., increased fiber and water intake, fiber supplements, biofeedback) is often sufficient for first- or second-degree mucosal prolapse.

These therapeutic measures can also help alleviate constipation and incontinence before and after surgery for full-thickness prolapse. Transanal procedures, such as rubber-band ligation or mucosal excision, can be used in patients with second- and third-degree mucosal prolapse. Several surgical procedures have been advocated for the treatment of full-thickness rectal prolapse, including laparotomy and laparoscopic trans-abdominal approaches, stapled transanal rectal resection, and robotic rectal resections. However, in the absence of data from well-controlled randomized studies, the relative efficacies of these procedures remain to be established.

ANAL FISSURE

An anal fissure is a linear ulcer (a longitudinal "cut") of the anoderm, distal to the dentate line. Approximately 90% of anal fissures are located in the mid-posterior portion of the anus and 10% occur in the anterior wall. Fissures that develop in any other area of the anus and those that do not heal (with proper treatment) should raise the suspicion of associated diseases, such as perianal Crohn's disease (CD), infectious lesions (HIV-related ulcer, syphilis), or cancers.

An anal fissure is very painful, because it involves the multilayer squamous epithelium of the anoderm, which is richly innervated with pain fibers. During defecation, stretching of the lesion causes pain, which may persist for a few hours, and is often associated with bleeding. The pain can be so severe that the patient begins to avoid defecating, which results in hardening of the feces and exacerbation of symptoms.

An anal fissure is considered to be acute when lasting fewer than 6 weeks, is superficial, and has well-demarcated borders. Chronic fissure lasts for more than 6 weeks, has keratinous borders, is associated with a sentinel skin tag and hypertrophied anal papillae, and is usually so deep that the fibers of the IAS may be visible (**Figure 22.5**).

The aetiology of anal fissures is unknown. Vascular mechanisms, increased tone of the IAS, trauma, and stress have been hypothesized as potential causes. The posterior area of the anoderm has been shown to be less richly perfused than other anodermal areas, and the blood flow to this area is diminished even further by the increased tone in the IAS. These observations suggest that the fissure could be a form of ischaemic ulceration. Contributing roles have also been attributed to anodermal trauma caused by the passage of hard stools or explosive diarrhoea.

The diagnosis is based on the presence of intense pain, sometimes with bleeding, during or after defecation, and is confirmed by thorough inspection of the posterior commissure of the anus. Digital examination and anoscopy may be very painful if not impossible, unless performed under anesthesia. An acute anal fissure is a superficial lesion that responds well to conservative measures, such as dietary interventions (increased fiber and water intake, fiber supplements, stool softeners), warm water sitz baths, and analgesics. Proper anal hygiene and regularization of bowel habits can reduce the risk of recurrence. For longer-standing fissures, the measures described above will provide only transient relief. The goal of treatment for chronic anal fissures is to reduce the pressure within the

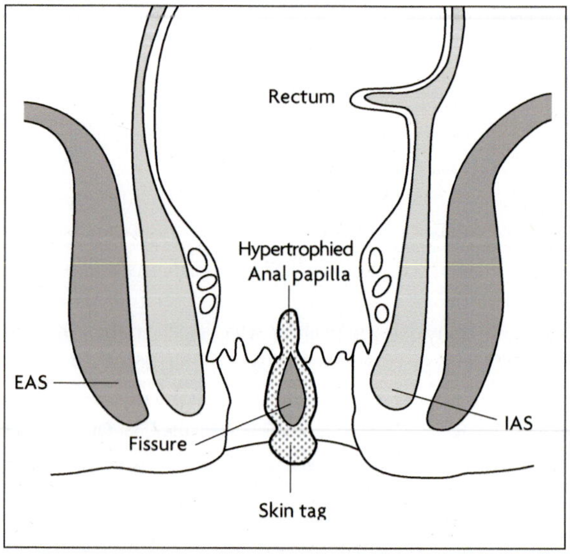

Figure 22.5 Schematic diagram of an anal fissure at the anal verge, which may extend to the dentate line. Chronic fissures may be associated with a hypertrophied anal papilla and skin tags. IAS= internal anal sphincter; EAS= external anal sphincter.

anal canal by decreasing the tone of the anal muscle, thereby promoting healing of the fissure (4). A number of medical and surgical approaches have been proposed for this purpose. Topical application of nitrates (glyceryl trinitrate) and calcium channel blockers (nifepidine, diltiazem) are successful in 50% to 80% of cases. Injections of botulinum toxin into the IAS or anal dilatations by means of specific devices are also used, but the benefits of these approaches have not been well documented. The major drawbacks of these non-surgical therapies are their adverse effects and decreasing efficacy over time.

Surgery is still the most reliable solution for chronic relapsing anal fissure and patients refractory to drug therapy. Controlled lateral internal sphincterotomy is widely regarded as the "standard treatment" for chronic anal fissure.

SOLITARY RECTAL ULCER SYNDROME

The solitary rectal ulcer syndrome (SRUS) is an uncommon benign disorder, affecting usually young adults and often related to abnormal defecation. It is underdiagnosed, with an estimated annual prevalence of one in 100,000 persons. Clinical features include rectal bleeding, copious mucus discharge, prolonged excessive straining, perineal and abdominal pain, feeling of incomplete evacuation, constipation, and - rarely - rectal prolapse. The cause and pathogenesis are still unknown, but multiple mechanisms are likely involved. Ischaemic mucosal injury, resulting from the pressure of impacted stools in the rectum, and local trauma due to internal intussusceptions, rectal prolapse or repeated self-digitation, may be contributing factors. Descent of the perineum and abnormal contraction of the puborectalis muscle during straining on defecation may induce trauma and compression of the anterior rectal wall.

Dyssynergia with paradox anal contraction is present in a variable percentage (25-82%) of patients with SRUS.

Diagnosis is based on clinical, endoscopic, and histological findings, as well as on the results of imaging studies (e.g., defecography, dynamic MRI). Colonoscopy should also be performed, with biopsy of both normal- and abnormal-appearing rectal mucosa. Ulcers range in size from 0.5 to 4.0 cm, are usually located on the anterior wall of the rectum and are covered by a layer of white, grey, or yellowish slough. A solitary rectal ulcer is a misnomer because multiple ulcers are found in 40% of patients, while 20% of patients have a solitary ulcer, and the remaining lesions differ in shape and size, and include hyperemia and polypoid lesions of the mucosa. Differential diagnosis includes rectal CD, proctitis, and malignant lesions. Histological hallmarks of SRUS include diffuse collagen deposition in the lamina propria, hypertrophy of the muscularis mucosa with upward extension of muscle fibers into the space between the crypts, and glandular crypt abnormalities.

Treatment options include dietary measures (increased fiber and water intake, bulking agents like bran or psyllium), topical drugs (sucralfate, mesalazine, steroids, and/or fibrin sealants), biofeedback, and surgery. Responses improvement in symptoms and endoscopic findings–vary widely. The choice of treatment should be based on the severity of symptoms and whether there is a rectal prolapse.

PROCTITIS AND PERIANAL INFECTIONS

Proctitis is an acute or chronic inflammation that is limited to the lower 15 cm of the rectum. Presenting symptoms include anorectal discharge (mucoid, mucopurulent, or bloody), anal pain, burning, and/or itching, and tenesmus. On flexible sigmoidoscopy, the rectal mucosa appears friable and diffusely erythaematous, with red spots and erosions.

The most common and best-known form is idiopathic ulcerative proctitis, but there are several sexually transmitted infectious forms frequently seen in individuals who are immunodeficient and in men who have sex with men. The most common are gonorrheal and syphilitic proctitis (caused by *Neisseria gonorrhoeae* and *Treponema pallidum*, respectively) and forms caused by *Chlamydia trachomatis* (lymphogranuloma venereum), herpes simplex virus (HSV) type II, human papillomavirus (HPV), or cytomegalovirus (CMV) (7). Multimicrobial infections are by no means rare. The pathogens listed above preferentially infect the rectal mucosa, but HSV, HPV, and *Treponema pallidum* can also infect the squamous epithelium of the anal canal. The proctitis may also be associated with perianal lesions, such as the vesicles, pustules, and ulcers caused by HSV or warts (condyloma acuminate) caused by HPV. The latter is usually confined to the anal and perianal areas, but involvement of the proximal rectal mucosa is not uncommon.

Treponema pallidum infection can also cause masses in the anal canal and ulcers, which are typically painless with well-defined, indurated margins, and clean bases, sometimes associated with tender inguinal lymph nodes.

Non-infectious forms of proctitis can be caused by drugs - non-steroidal anti-inflammatory drugs (NSAIDs) in particular -, radiation therapy, trauma, foreign bodies, and allergic processes.

The diagnostic workup of proctitis and perianal lesions should include endoscopic evaluation (flexible sigmoidoscopy or, if CD is supected, ileo-colonscopy), histological assessment of anorectal biopsies, serologic tests for specific infectious agents, smears and cultures of perianal material and a rectal swab. Infectious proctitis should be treated with specific antibiotics and antivirals; non-infectious forms can be managed with topical formulations containing mesalazine or steroids.

Perianal skin lesions are common and vary widely in form and severity (erythema, pustules, nodules and suppurating nodules, subcutaneous microabscesses, pseudokeloids, etc.). They are mainly caused by bacterial infections (hidradenitis suppurativa) or fungal infections (candidiasis) or scratching.

The most common bacteria involved in hidradenitis suppurativa include *Streptococcus milleri, Staphylococcus aureus,* anaerobic streptococci, *Bacteroisdes* species, *Escherichia coli, Klebsiella,* and *Proteus*. These infections are often associated with diabetes, poor nutrition, impaired immunity, and/or fecal incontinence. Erythaema can also be caused by skin irritants like soaps or proctologic creams or underwear made of synthetic materials. The infectious lesions should be treated with specific antimicrobial agents; those caused by sensitization can be managed with antihistamines or topical steroids.

ABSCESSES AND FISTULAS

Anorectal abscesses and fistulas are common and highly debilitating suppurative disorders caused in up to 80% of cases by infection of the anal glands. Symptoms vary from anal pain and purulent discharge to bleeding and incontinence. They are the cause of significant morbidity and have a strong negative impact on quality of life.

Nearly all anal glands extend into the intersphincteric space. As a result, this is the area where abscesses generally form. From here, tracts or tunnels may extend in various directions: upward, downward, around the anus itself. When the tract reaches the skin surface or another epithelialized surface like that of the vagina, the result is a fistula.

Anal abscesses and fistulae can be the result of Crohn's disease, trauma, hidradenitis suppurativa, tuberculosis, perianal actinomycosis, or sexually transmitted infections (especially HIV and *Chlamydia trachomatis*). Local infection related to an anal fissure, carcinoma, or a foreign body may also cause a fistula.

Abscesses are classified according to their extension as perianal (the most common), ischiorectal, intersphincteric, or supralevator (**Figure 22.6**). The last type is the rarest, accounting for <10% of all abscesses.

Fistulas are classified on the basis of their relation to the internal anal sphincter, the external anal sphincter, and the puborectalis. The number of fistulae, the internal and external openings of each tract, the presence of blind tracts or extensions, and the presence of active sepsis within the site of the cavity should also be noted. Fistulae-in-ano can be broadly classified as high or low, depending on whether or not they transverse the levator-ani muscle (see Figure 22.6).

The diagnosis of anorectal abscesses and fistulas is based on the presence of typical symptoms, the most common of which are swelling, throbbing, continuous pain, discharge, and fever. In the presence of an anal abscess, digital examination may be impossible because of pain. Examination

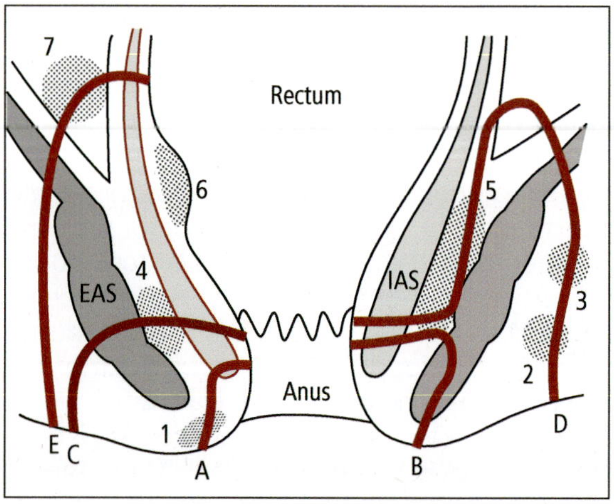

Figure 22.6 Schematic diagram of the topographic classification of anorectal abscesses and fistulas.
Topography of abscesses: 1. perianal abscess; 2. low intersphincteric abscess; 3. high intersphincteric abscess; 4. low ischiorectal abscess; 5. high ischiorectal abscess; 6. submucosal abscess; 7. suprasphincteric abscess.
Topography of fistulas: A. superficial fistula; B. intersphinceteric fistula; C. transphincteric fistula; D. suprasphincteric fistula; E. extrasphincteric fistula. Superficial and intersphincteric are also referred to as low and simple fistulas, while transphincteric, suprasphincteric, and extrasphincteric forms are also referred to as high and complex fistulas.

under anesthesia (EUA) is associated with a diagnostic accuracy of 90%. Magnetic resonance imaging also offers high accuracy (76-100%), with findings that can change surgical management in 15-21% of cases. Endoscopic ultrasound offers similar accuracy (56-100%) and modifies surgical management in 10–15% of cases.
Computed tomography (CT) is less helpful and generally used only in acute conditions and when MRI is contraindicated.
Fistulography is no longer used in practice. Among the emerging diagnostic techniques, transperineal ultrasound has been suggested as an inexpensive, painless, prompt, and widely available technique. Since the presence of concomitant rectal inflammation has therapeutic relevance, flexible proctosigmoidoscopy should be used routinely in the initial evaluation.
Treatment of abscesses requires incision and drainage: antibiotic therapy alone is not sufficient. An abscess that is not drained can spread to adjacent tissues, producing potentially life-threatening necrotizing infections.
Treatment of anal fistulae is a challenge that requires specialist skills. Surgical intervention varies according to the type of fistula, therefore precise characterization and classification of the lesion are essential to optimize outcomes. The goals of therapy are to alleviate symptoms, achieve persistent closure of the fistula, and minimize the risk of recurrent lesions and infections. Combined medical (systemic antibiotics) and surgical therapies offer the best outcomes. The course of the fistulous tract influences the choice of surgical procedures.
Options include fistulotomy, fistulectomy, seton placement, transanal advancement flaps, diverting ostomy, and proctectomy. A seton is a fine rubber sling or heavy nylon suture that is passed through the fistula (from the anal canal to the opening on the perianal skin surface) and tied loosely.
This is usually a temporary preoperative measure that allows the fistulous tract to drain before surgical repair, thereby preventing the internal accumulation of pus. However, setons can also be used therapeutically as cut seton with gradual division of the anal muscle, thereby minimizing the risk of fecal incontinence.

PRURITUS ANI

Pruritus ani affects 1–5% of the population and is more common in men. It is a chronic itching localized to the anus and perianal skin. Pruritus ani is classified as idiopathic when no cause is found. In approximately 75% of cases, it is the result of an underlying anorectal or dermatological disorder (secondary pruritus ani), and specific treatment of the primary disorder leads to resolution of symptoms. Leakage of stool or mucus (secondary to fecal incontinence or prolapse of haemorrhoids or rectal mucosa) can cause irritation and itching. Other causes include contact dermatitis, psoriasis, infections (candidiasis), parasites (*Enterobius vermicularis*), systemic diseases (diabetes mellitus, lymphoproliferative disease), anal or colorectal cancer, certain medications, and diet (common offenders include caffeinated drinks, alcohol, milk products, peanuts, spices, citrus, grapes, tomato, and chocolate).
Any underlying disorder should be treated. Patients with idiopathic pruritus ani should be helped to eliminate potential dietary causative factors and modify their personal hygiene habits. They often attribute the itching to poor hygiene and may become overzealous in keeping the perianal area clean. Excessive cleaning, particularly with the use of brushes and/or caustic soaps, irritates the sensitive anal and perianal region and exacerbates the pruritus instead of relieving it.

IDIOPATHIC ANAL PAIN

Pain in the anorectal region in the absence of underlying diseases or anatomic abnormalities is not uncommon. Diagnosis is based on clinical presentation, which is categorized in three different clinical entities: coccygodynia, levator ani syndrome, and proctalgia fugax.
Coccygodynia manifests as pain or aching discomfort in or around the coccyx and is typically caused by trauma or arthritis. The pain can be reproduced by digital rectal examination. Treatment of the acute phase includes warm sitz baths, NSAIDs, and stool softeners.
The levator ani syndrome mainly affects women under the age of 45. The discomfort is described as tenderness or an aching sensation high in the rectum. In general, it does not disturb the patient's sleep. It is usually exacerbated by defecation and sitting, while walking or lying down may bring some relief. At the rectal examination, the levator muscle may feel like a tight band that is tender on palpation.
Proctalgia fugax mainly occurs in young men. The pain is described as a sharp cramp lasting a few seconds or minutes which may awaken the pa-

tient from sleep. The digital rectal examination is normal.
The pathogenesis of levator ani syndrome and proctalgia fugax is unknown, but both disorders appear to be related to anorectal and pelvic muscle dysfunctions. Treatment involves reassurance, warm sitz baths, regulation of bowel habits, perineal strengthening exercises, biofeedback, drug therapies (muscle-relaxing agents), acupuncture, and psychotherapy.

ANAL CANCER

Anal cancers are infrequent, accounting for only 2% of gastrointestinal tract malignancies. The vast majority are squamous cell cancers (80%) or adenocarcinomas (15%). The presenting symptoms are often identical to those of more common benign lesions of the anal canal (e.g., haemorrhoids). Some cancers are discovered incidentally during digital rectal examination. Pain in the early stages is usually absent.
There may be a palpable mass (external or internal), or cancer can present as an ulcer, polyp, or verrucous growth. The development of anal cancer has been associated with HPV and HIV infections, history of sexually transmitted diseases, history of cervical cancer, and the use of immunosuppressive drugs. Most tumours respond well to combined treatment with chemotherapy and pelvic radiation.
Anal squamous cell carcinoma in situ (also called Bowen's disease, squamous intraepithelial lesions, or intraepithelial neoplasia) is considered a premalignant lesion. Progression from low-grade to high-grade lesions has been described, similar to that observed in the uterine cervix.
The rare intraepithelial mucinous adenocarcinoma, also referred to as Paget's disease, arises from the dermal apocrine sweat glands and appears as an erythaematous, eczematoid plaque. It is more common in women and manifests with intractable itching.
Primary colorectal lymphomas are very rare and most are B-cell non-Hodgkin lymphomas. Anal malignant melanoma is also rare and carries a poor prognosis.

KEY CONCEPTS

- Anorectal diseases are divided five main categories: prolapse (haemorrhoidal, rectal), inflammatory pathologies (fissure, solitary ulcer, proctitis), suppurative (abscess and fistulae), functional, and neoplastic.
- The most common symptoms of anorectal diseases are pain, anorectal bleeding, anal pruritus, anal prolapse, excretion of pus from the anus or perianal fistulas, nodules or anal or perianal masses, constipation from difficult evacuation, and fecal incontinence.
- Haemorrhoidal disease is classified in 4 grades based on the severity of haemorrhoidal prolapse. Less than 10% of patients need surgery.
- An anal fissure is a longitudinal ulceration of the anal canal which causes acute anal pain during and after defecation. Therapy includes topical muscle relaxants and, in resistant forms, the partial sphincterotomy of the internal anal sphincter.
- Proctitis is an acute or chronic inflammation of the anorectal mucosa. It can be of infectious, non-infectious or idiopathic origin.

REFERENCES

- Abramowitz L, Weyandt GH, Havlickova B, et al. The diagnosis and management of haemorrhoidal disease from a global perspective. Aliment Pharmacol Ther. 2010;31 Suppl 1:1-58.
- Cone MM1, Whitlow CB. Sexually transmitted and anorectal infectious diseases. Gastroenterol Clin North Am 2013;42:877-92.
- Jacobs D. Clinical practice. Hemorrhoids. N Engl J Med 2014;371:944-51
- Qing-Chao Zhu, Rong-Rong Shen, Huan-Long Qin, Yu Wang. Solitary rectal ulcer syndrome: Clinical features, pathophysiology, diagnosis and treatment strategies. World J Gastroenterol 2014; 20: 738-744
- Sahnan K, Adegbola SO, Tozer PJ, Watfah J, Phillips RK. Perianal abscess. BMJ 2017 Feb 21;356-475.

CHAPTER 23

COLORECTAL NEOPLASIA

Luigi Ricciardiello, Mariabeatrice Principi

LEARNING OBJECTIVES
- To know the benign and malignant neoplasms of the colon and rectum.
- To know the risk factors that predispose to benign and malignant neoplasms of the colon and rectum.
- To know the inherited syndromes that predispose to colorectal cancer.
- To know the therapeutic approach and prevention of colorectal tumours.

Colorectal neoplasms include benign forms, including adenomas, and malignant tumours, in particular colorectal adenocarcinoma (CRC). CRC is one of the major causes of cancer incidence and death worldwide. Despite the reduction in incidence rates due to the implementation of screening program in industrialized countries, the rapid change towards a more westernized lifestyle in developing countries has increased the prevalence of CRC in populations that were historically less susceptible to the disease. Premalignant lesions, whose removal reduces the risk of malignant progression, usually precede CRC. Risk factors for CRC are age, obesity, and positive family history for CRC, and hereditary syndromes with high susceptibility to cancer.

ADENOMATOUS POLYPS, NON POLYPOID LESIONS, AND SERRATED POLYPS

Polyps are macroscopically visible protrusions on the mucosal surface of the intestine, ranging from a few millimeters to centimeters. Macroscopically, they can be classified as sessile (with a broad base) or pedunculated (with a stalk), and can be single or multiple. A polyp may consist of inflammatory tissue or it can be a congenital lesion, a benign neoplasm (a potential cancer precursor) or made of malignant cells (cancer).
Histologically, benign colorectal tumours can be classified as:

- Neoplastic mucosal polyps. This group comprises adenomatous polyps and serrated adenomas; in most cases they are benign neoplastic lesions, with potential malignant transformation.
- Non-neoplastic mucous polyps. This group includes inflammatory, hyperplastic, and hamartomatous polyps. Inflammatory polyps are found more frequently in inflammatory bowel diseases (IBD), in ulcerative colitis (UC) and Crohn's colitis, and they can differ size. Hyperplastic polyps are very common in the elderly and are often small. Both inflammatory and hyperplastic polyps have no potential for malignant transformation. Juvenile polyps and Peutz-Jeghers polyps are hamartomas, which characterize specific forms of polyposis.
- Submucosal lesions. The most frequent are lipomas, leiomyomas, fibroids, lymphoid nodules, and benign carcinoids (generally non-secretory type).

Polyposis is characterized by the presence of at least 20 polyps.

Adenomatous Polyps

Adenomatous polyps are benign neoplastic lesions that, based on their histological characteristics, are divided into: tubular, tubulo-villous, and villous. Adenomas show cellular and structural atypia that characterize the degree of dysplasia divided into a low and high grade.
The presence of high-grade dysplasia (with no invasion of the base or stalk) is actually intraepithelial or in situ carcinoma whose removal is curative. Tubular adenomas are the most frequent, while the tubulo-villous may be of variable size between 1 and 10 cm in diameter. Villous adenomas grow more frequently in the rectum and are usually larger than tubular and tubulo-villous and occur as non-pedunculated lesions with a velvety cauliflower-like surface.
The malignant potential of adenomas depends on the degree of epithelial dysplasia, the size, the presence of the villous component, and the number. Most CRCs derive from pre-existing adenomas. Overall, the whole sequence takes about 10-12 years.

Non-Polypoid Neoplastic Lesions

In addition to its typical presentation as polypoid lesions, CRC can develop from non-polypoid neoplasms. Non-polypoid lesions include slightly elevated, completely flat and depressed forms, plus two flat-depressed variants. The overall incidence of cancer in non-polypoid neoplasms is 10-40%, and 1-35% in polypoid lesions.

Serrated Polyps

Serrated shape reflects the jagged/saw-toothed aspect of the crypt due to inappropriate growth of epithelial cells organized into intraluminal formations. Sessile serrated adenomas, mostly reaching >1 cm in size, are prevalent in the proximal colon (from the cecum to the splenic flexure), and are characterized by crypts that, focally or in more or less extended areas of the polyp, show minimal architectural dysplastic changes.
In serrated adenomas (including serrated polypoid adenoma) a recognizable serrated pathway persists together with nuclear and cytological alterations attributable to dysplasia. Both lesions, together with mixed serrated polyps (consisting of areas of serrated dysplasia and of traditional adenomatous dysplasia) are potentially premalignant neoplasms (serrated adenoma-carcinoma sequence).

Clinical Features

Most adenomas are asymptomatic and are usually found during colonoscopy for CRC screening, but also as an incidental finding during other procedures performed for unrelated symptoms. Symptoms and signs associated with adenomas, particularly those larger than 1 cm in size, are anemia, chronic occult blood loss in stool or rectal bleeding, sudden changes in bowel habits (e.g., constipation followed by diarrhoea), abdominal pain, rectal prolapse, intestinal obstruction due to of a voluminous adenoma.
Villous adenomas may lead to a hypersecretory syndrome characterized by hypokalemia and deep mucus secretion.

FAMILIAL POLYPOSIS

Polyposes are commonly distinguished in hereditary and non-hereditary polyposis syndromes (**Table 23.1**). Familial polyposis are rare, inherited conditions with an exceedingly high risk of developing malignant tumours.

Table 23.1 Familial polyposis.

Hereditary Polyposis

- Adenomatous polyposis
  Familial adenomatous polyposis (FAP, familial adenomatous polyposis)
  Variants of familial adenomatous polyposis
  Gardner's syndrome
  Turcot syndrome
  Mitigated form of familial adenomatous polyposis
  MUTYH polyposis
- Hamartomatous polyposis
  Poutz Joghers syndrome
  Juvenile polyposis

Non-Hereditary Polyposis

- Cronkhite-Canada syndrome
- Hyperplastic polyposis
- Nodular lymphoid hyperplasia

Familial Adenomatous Polyposis

Familial adenomatous polyposis (FAP) is an autosomal-dominant inherited disease (frequency 1/10.000 newborns) characterized by hundreds to thousands of adenomatous polyps in the gastrointestinal tract (**Figure 23.1**); polyps appear early (usually around the age of 16) and are found in adults over the age of 40. Polyps can develop in the colon, but also in the stomach (where they are usually glandular polyps without dysplasia) and in the duodenum.
There are rare variants of FAP associated with extraintestinal features: Gardner's syndrome, where FAP is associated with osteomas and benign soft tissue tumours (desmoid tumours, epidermal cysts, fibroids, lipomas, etc.); and Turcot syndrome, asso-

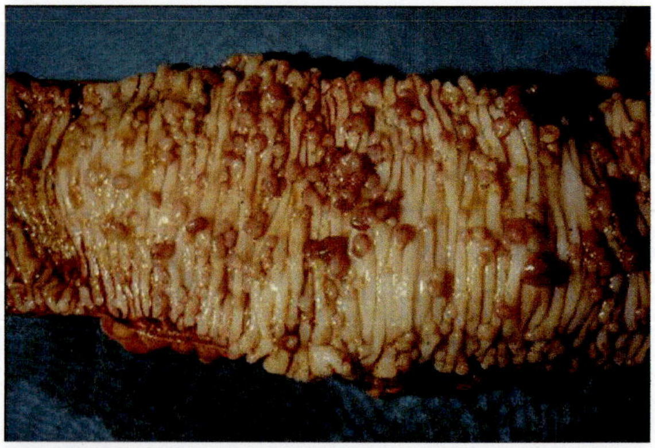

Figure 23.1 Macroscopic appearance of familial adenomatous polyposis.

ciated with brain tumours such as medulloblastoma. Accidental detection of congenital hypertrophy of the retinal-pigment epithelium is frequent in patients with FAP. The attenuated form of familial polyposis (AFAP) is characterized by the presence of <100 adenomas mainly located in the right colon (proximal to the splenic flexure).
In AFAP the average age of cancer onset is 49 years.
The genetic basis of FAP, demonstrable in about 70-90% of patients, is the germline mutation of the adenomatous polyposis coli (APC) gene located on the long arm of chromosome 5. Thus, the disease can be diagnosed through genetic testing. Mutations in the central portion of the gene are associated with a classical phenotype of the disease, while those occurring in the proximal or distal regions are associated with the attenuated forms.
A form of recessive adenomatous polyposis is due to the biallelic inactivation of the MUTYH gene. Affected persons have clinical features phenotypically similar to those in patients with AFAP.
In a patient carrying an APC gene mutation, the risk of developing adenocarcinoma is almost 100% and can develop in young-adulthood, a few years after the appearance of adenomas.
Genetic diagnosis should be performed in pre-adolescence to start endoscopic surveillance by the age of 10-12 with a yearly colonoscopy.
When the disease is no longer manageable endoscopically due to the number and size of polyps, patients are referred to elective prophylactic surgical treatment.

Hereditary Hamartomatous Polyposis

Peutz-Jeghers syndrome and juvenile polyposis are familial polyposes characterized by the development of hamartomatous polyps. Polyps can develop throughout the gastrointestinal tract, especially in the small intestine in Peutz-Jeghers syndrome and in the colon in juvenile polyposis. In patients with Peutz-Jeghers syndrome, mucocutaneous pigmented spots are often observed on the lips, mouth, and skin. Hamartomas can cause bleeding, intussusception or obstruction. The lifetime risk for colorectal cancer is 39% for juvenile polyposis. Patients with Peutz-Jeghers syndrome have an exceedingly high risk of developing cancer, in particular those involving the pancreas, breast, and colorectum.
Treatment consists of endoscopic removal of the polyps, or surgical resection of affected intestinal segments. The genetic basis of Peutz-Jeghers syndrome is the germline mutation of the STK11 gene. Juvenile polyposis can be caused by either mutations BMPR1A or SMAD4, both involved in TGF-B signaling.

COLORECTAL MALIGNANT NEOPLASMS

Malignant tumours are mostly adenocarcinomas, called CRC. Malignant non-epithelial tumours include lymphomas and sarcomas. Although it is rare, there is also the possibility of metastatic tumours to the colon (from melanomas, breast and lung cancers).

Colorectal Cancer (CRC)

CRC accounts for 95% of all malignant tumours involving the colorectum; in terms of incidence, it is the third in men and second in women, and the fourth and the third cause of cancer death in men and women, respectively.
When diagnosed, CRC are often in an advanced stage, with a 5-year overall survival rate of approximately 50%. In Italy, estimated new CRC cases are approximately 30 35,000 each year, with 15-18,000 deaths. In most cases, colorectal cancers develop from adenomatous polyps.
Identification of adenomatous polyps and their endoscopic removal significantly reduces the risk of malignant evolution (by interrupting the adenoma-carcinoma sequence), thus justifying CRC prevention programs.
The main risk factors for CRC are age, family history/hereditary syndromes, obesity, dietary, and lifestyle factors (**Table 23.2**). Most CRCs are diagnosed in adults aged >50 years. About 20% of CRCs develops in younger persons or in those with a positive family history for the disease, suggesting a hereditary susceptibility (familial CRC). In familial CRC the risk of developing the disease is 2 to 6 times greater than in the general population.
Approximately 4% of patients with CRC have one of the two inherited syndromes: FAP (1%), and Lynch syndrome (LS) or HNPCC (hereditary non-polyposis colorectal cancer) (3%) (**Figure 23.2**).
There is an increased risk of developing CRC in persons with inflammatory bowel diseases (ulcerative colitis and Crohn's colitis), especially long-term pancolitis (more than 7 years). In these conditions, CRC develops from adenomatous dysplasia found on flat mucosa or raised lesions with dysplasia-RLD (adenoma-like or not adenoma-like). In these patients, if high-grade dysplasia or multifocal low-grade dysplasia is found, total colectomy is recommended.

Table 23.2 Risk factors for colorectal carcinoma onset.

- Age: >50 years
- Familiarity/hereditary
  Family history of adenomatous polyps or CCR
  Family polyposis in the colon (adenomatous and hamartomatous)
  Hereditary non-polyposis colorectal cancer (HNPCC)

- Other risk factors
  Chronic inflammatory diseases of the colon (ulcerative colitis, Crohn's colitis)
  Acromegaly
  Immunodeficiency disorders (AIDS)
  Overweight/obesity
  Carcinogens and environmental/dietary mutagens
  High-calorie, hyperlipidic, and low-fibre diet
  Overweight, sedentary life style
  Alcohol, smoking

- Associated conditions
  Internal urinary differences
  Streptococcus bovis

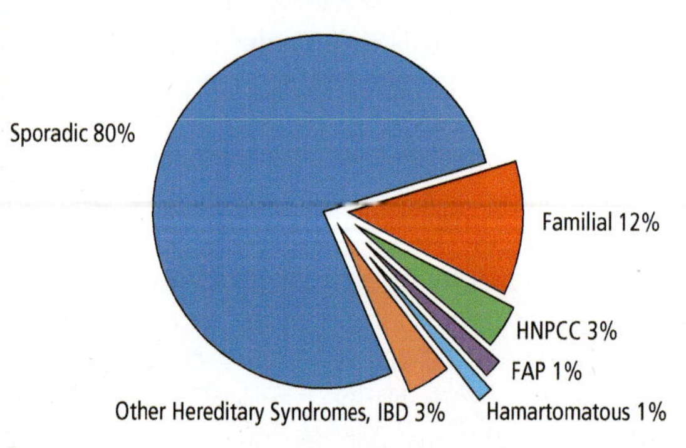

Figure 23.2 Prevalence of colorectal cancer.

There are several dietary and lifestyle factors predisposing to CRC: obesity, overweight and sedentary lifestyle, hypercaloric, hyperlipidic and low-fiber diet, alcohol and smoking. Many prospective studies have shown a significant increase in colon cancer risk in individuals with a body-mass index (BMI) >30. Studies carried out on animals indicate a strong association between a high-fat diet and the risk of developing colorectal cancer. Furthermore, an inconsistent association between red meat intake and colorectal cancer risk has been shown.

Contrary to the effects of a high-fiber low-fat diet, a low-fiber diet leads to a high concentration of secondary bile acids and their metabolites, mutagens and fecal carcinogens; their prolonged contact with the intestinal mucosa due to slow transit might lead to molecular changes. Recently, a protective role of aspirin against the development of sporadic colorectal cancer has been demonstrated. This has also been found in patients affected by LS.

Pathogenesis of CRC

The exact cause of CRC development is not fully known. However, much of the knowledge about its pathogenesis derives from studies addressing the adenoma-carcinoma sequence, and focused on the molecular pathways.

Adenoma-Carcinoma Sequence

There are two critical steps involved in CRC development: one called "initiation" that marks the transition from normal epithelium to adenoma; and the second called "promotion" that involves the transition from adenoma to carcinoma. It is hypothesized that different carcinogens might be responsible for specific genetic alterations in these two phases.
Almost all CRCs are believed to develop from pre-existing adenomas (80% from adenomatous polyps, 20% from serrated adenomas). The likelihood of the adenoma-carcinoma sequence is supported by:

- Epidemiological data: same prevalence of adenomas and cancer by age, population and geographical areas; age distribution curves indicating that adenomas precede cancer; same risk factors for adenomas and cancer.
- Clinicopathological evidence: endoscopic removal of adenomas reduces CRC incidence; screening reduces CRC incidence and mortality; adenomas and cancer distribution in the colon and rectum have the same distribution; coexistence of cancer foci on adenomas or residual adenomatous tissue in cancers.
- Genetic evidence: progression from normal mucosa to adenoma and cancer is determined by a succession of genetic alterations involving oncogenes, tumour suppressor genes, and genes encoding DNA repair proteins.

Genetic Alterations

To date, there are three known alternative molecular pathways that can lead to the development of colorectal cancer. The early event linking the three pathways is the derangement of the WNT system (involving APC-β-catenin) due to either mutations or epigenetic changes (**Figure 23.3**):

- CIN or chromosomal instability pathway. This is characterized by widespread chromosomal alterations and aneuploidy. This pathway is the most frequent in sporadic cancer and characterizes cancers developing in the setting of FAP. While germline mutations of the APC gene are the cause of FAP, its somatic mutations are considered the key initial step in the normal mucosa-adenoma-carcinoma sequence.
  The APC gene encodes a tumour suppressor protein. Its mutation causes a failure of the β-catenin destruction complex, β-catenin cytoplasmic accumulation, followed by nuclear translocation. This leads to increased transcription of oncogenes, with altered cell cycle and increased proliferation, and failure in controlling intercellular contacts. The pathway is characterized by the following consecutive molecular alterations: K-RAS gene mutations (characterizing the transition from small to large adenomas), p53, SMAD4 and DCC losses (deleted in colon cancer) (in an advanced stage of carcinoma). CIN+ tumours arise more frequently in the left colon.
- MSI or microsatellite instability. This is due to a failure in one of the DNA mismatch repair (MMR) proteins (due to mutations or epigenetic silencing due to promoter hypermethylation). While the germline mutations of some of the MMR genes (hMLH1, hMSH2, hMSH6, hPMS2, EPCAM) cause LS or HNPCC, hMLH1 gene promoter hypermethylation causes spo-

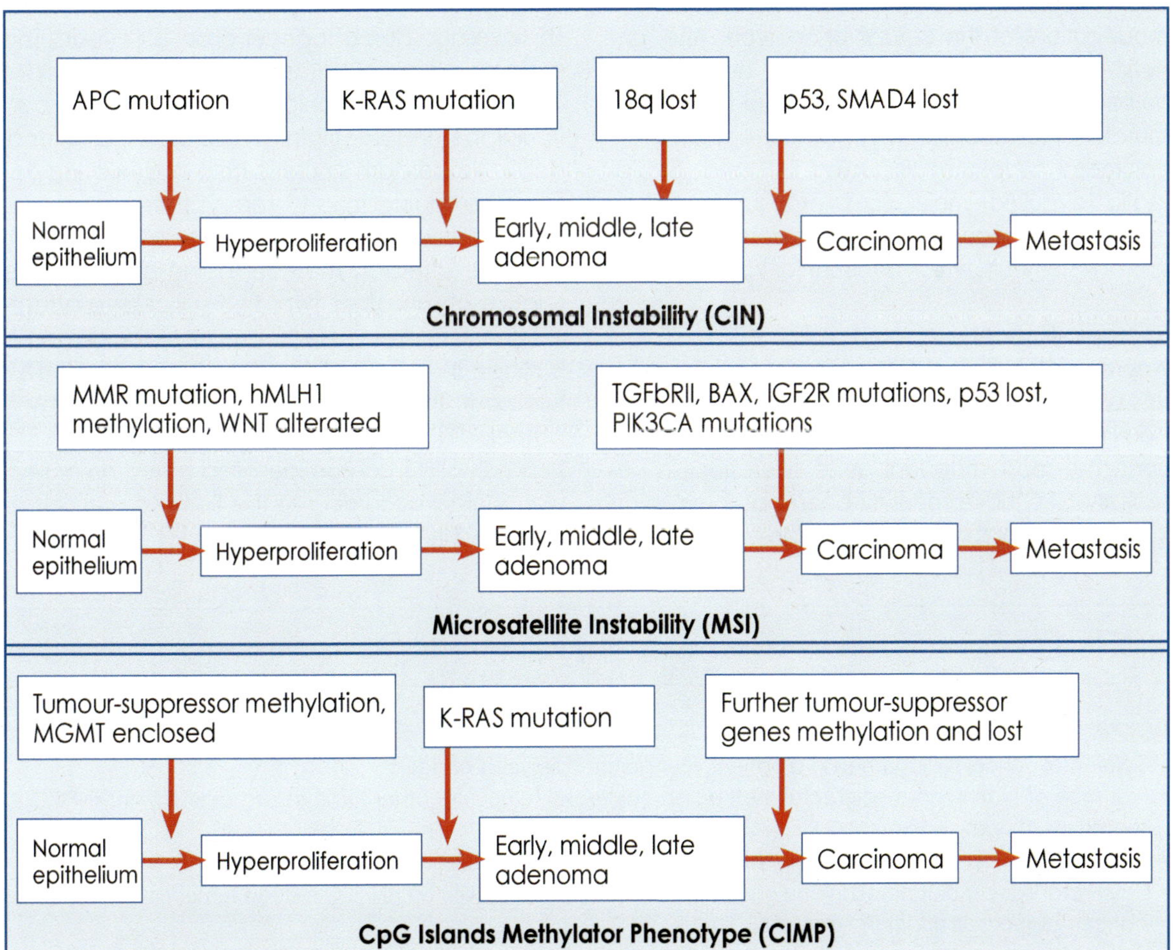

Figure 23.3 Genetic alterations involved in colorectal carcinogenesis. Three dominant genetic pathways are distinguished in the different clinical-pathological forms of CRC: the WNT pathway responsible for chromosomal instability (CIN) and dominant in sporadic and familial CRC prevalent in the left colon; the DNA pathway mismatch repair (MMR) responsible for the instability of microsatellites (microsatellite instability-MSI) and dominant in the hereditary CRC typically arising in the right colon; and the pathway of the CIMP (CpG islands methylator phenotype) dominant in CRC that develops from serrated adenoma (blocked pathway)

radic cancers with MSI. Microsatellites are highly repetitive sequences that populate the coding regions of tumour suppressor genes: failure in one of the MMR proteins leads to progressive accumulation of alterations in microsatellite sequences of tumour suppressor genes. MSI+ cancers arise more frequently in the proximal colon.

- CIMP or CpG islands methylator phenotype. This is characterized by widespread gene promoter hypermethylation (and subsequent silencing), particularly in tumour-suppressors. The pathway is more frequently associated with CRCs that develop from serrated adenoma. CIMP + CRCs have a high frequency of B-RAF gene mutations (in particular V600E), a kinase of the Ras family. BRAF mutation leads to reduced apoptosis.

Genetic alterations lead to changes in cell proliferation, differentiation, apoptosis, polarization, and modifications of the cellular phenotype. Also, genetic alterations can be inherited or acquired. Inherited genetic alterations (usually due to germline mutations) lead to the development of hereditary colorectal neoplasms (including FAP and LS). Somatic (acquired) molecular alterations (mutations or epigenetic changes) lead to the development of sporadic tumours, which account for 95% of CRCs.

Sporadic Cancer

Approximately 80% of CRCs are defined "sporadic", although all CRCs have an acquired genetic component in the form of multiple somatic mutations. The most important gene alterations in hereditary CRC have recently been observed even in familial or sporadic CRC in variable percentages. Approximately 85% of colorectal tumours follow the chromosomal instability pathway described above, while 15% of sporadic CRCs follow the microsatellite instability pathway, as in the case of LS.

Lynch Syndrome or Hereditary Non Polyposis Colorectal Cancer (HNPCC)

Lynch syndrome (LS), also known as hereditary non polyposis colorectal cancer (HNPCC) is an autosomal dominant form of CRC, with high penetrance (80-85%) of colorectal cancer and accounts for 3-5% of all cases.

The genetic basis is the germline mutation of one of the DNA MMR genes. LS cancers are frequently located proximally to the splenic flexure, feature a quasi-diploid karyotype and, while histologically aggressive, they tend to have more indolent clinical evolution.

The average age at cancer onset is 44 years. The syndrome is also characterized by a high risk of developing extracolonic tumours involving in particular the endometrium, ovary, ureter, and renal pelvis. Amsterdam II criteria help in identifying patients belonging to a LS family: the presence of three relatives with HNPCC-associated tumours, with one affected member being a first degree relative of the other two; two successive affected generations; in at least one case the diagnosis is made in a patient younger than age 50; FAP ruled out; the diagnosis must be confirmed by a pathologist.

Persons with LS can be identified based on molecular analysis according to the Bethesda guidelines presented in **Table 23.3**.

Table 23.3 Bethesda criteria for the molecular diagnosis of HNPCC (Lynch syndrome).

Tumours must be genetically tested for HNPCC if:

- Colorectal cancer is diagnosed in a patient younger than 50 years of age
- Presence of synchronous colorectal methacron colorectal tumour, or other tumours associated with HNPCC #, regardless of age
- Colorectal cancer with MSI * histology diagnosed in a patient younger than 60 years of age
- Colorectal cancer diagnosed in one or more first-degree relatives with an HNPCC-related tumour, with one of the cancers diagnosed under the age of 50
- Colorectal cancer diagnosed in two or more first- or second- degree relatives with HNPCC-related tumours, regardless of age

Tumours of the colon, endometrium, stomach, ovary, pancreas, ureter and renal pelvis, biliary tract, and brain (usually glioblastoma - as in Turcot syndrome), adenomas of the sebaceous glands and keratoacanthomas (Muir-Torre syndrome), carcinoma of the small intestine

* Presence of infiltrating tumour lymphocytes, Crohn-like lymphocyte reaction, mucinous differentiation, signet ring cells, medullary growth model

In persons with a genetic mutation in one of the DNA MMR genes, screening with yearly colonoscopy should start at the age of 20-22 years.

Clinical Aspects

Symptoms are related to the cancer stage and location. In the cecum and the right colon the symptoms tend to appear late and the first sign may be microcytic anemia from chronic blood loss, fatigue or dyspnea, and unexplained weight loss. For cancers arising in the sigmoid colon or rectum, symptoms may be acute rectal bleeding, abdominal discomfort or tenesmus.

Later symptoms may include a palpable mass or obstructive symptoms such as abdominal cramp-like pain, changes in bowel habits and urogenital disorders. The main symptoms and their frequency in CRC are: occult bleeding (75%), rectal bleeding (58%), anemia (57%), abdominal pain (52%), weight loss (39%), constipation and anorexia (27 %), diarrhoea (22%), nausea and vomiting (22%), tenesmus (10%).

The main complications are: acute and chronic intestinal bleeding, occlusion, perforation, invasion and compression of adjacent organs (bladder, ureters, vagina, local nerves), local (peritoneum, lymph nodes), and distant metastases (liver, lung, brain and bones).

Rectal exploration is the first approach in recent rectal bleeding or tenesmus. However, diagnostic confirmation of neoplasia is made by colonoscopy (**Figure 23.4**) demonstrate a polyp, typically larger than 1-2 cm with an uneven surface, or an easily bleeding ulcerated mass or a stricturing lesion. Biopsies of lesions performed during colonoscopy can confirm the diagnosis: 95% of cases are adenocarcinomas, the remaining 5% are lymphomas, carcinoids or other lesions.

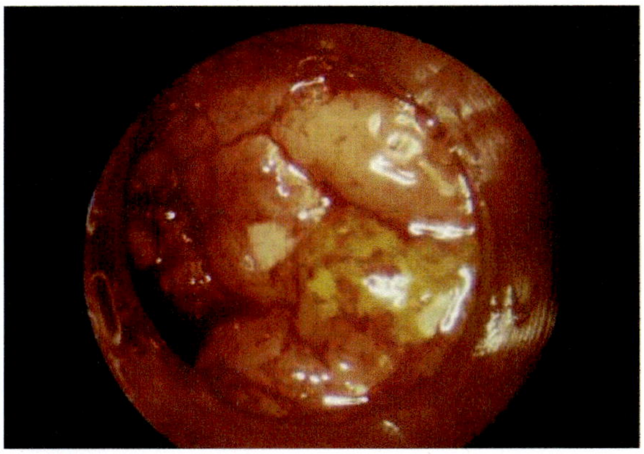

Figure 23.4 Endoscopic aspects of colonic adenocarcinomas.

Laboratory tests, including serum dosage of tumour antigens such as carcinoembryonic antigen (CEA), CA19-9 and others, are of little diagnostic use. CEA can be increased in various conditions including smoking and liver disorders; high levels of CEA can appear late or not occur; nonetheless, its presence or reappearance in the post-surgical period carries an unfavorable prognosis.

Concerning treatment, sometimes CRC is completely removable by endoscopy (polypectomy, mucosectomy or endoscopic submucosal dissection) and curative in intramucosal cancer. However, surgical removal is required in most cases.

Differential Diagnosis

Symptomatic CRC may initially be confused with various benign conditions with similar clinical features. Intestinal bleeding can simulate: haemorrhoids, anal fissures, colonic diverticulosis, angiodysplasias, and intestinal idiopathic inflammatory diseases.

Changes in bowel habits may raise the suspicion of irritable bowel syndrome, diverticular disease or inflammatory bowel disease. Abdominal pain raises the suspicion of diverticulitis, functional, ischaemic or inflammatory bowel disease.

The cause of these symptoms needs to be carefully sought, especially it of recent onset and in people over 50 years of age.

Staging

It is essential for the prognosis and for the choice of treatment. The most widely used test is abdominal-pelvic CT; further investigations are decided according to symptoms and tumour characteristics. The most commonly used staging classification systems are the TNM and Dukes.

Table 23.4 presents the stages according to TNM and Dukes and their correlation with prognosis.

Surgical Treatment

Surgical treatment is based on the removal of tumour mass, satellite lymph nodes, resectable metastases, and possibly the removal of contiguous organs if involved by neoplastic infiltration. The extent and types of colonic resection are related to tumour location. Removal of neoplastic lesions is performed according to the principles of oncological radicality.

In recent years, colon surgery has undergone considerable changes with the introduction of laparoscopic techniques. Colonic tumours can be treated by laparoscopic resection.

When applicable, the laparoscopic approach has considerable advantages over open surgery: cos-

Table 23.4 Colorectal carcinoma: correlation between stage according to TNM and Dukes and prognosis at 5 years after surgery.

Stage I - Dukes A	T1-2, N0, M0	Mucosa, submucosa, muscolaris	• 5-year survival in 80-100% • No adjuvant chemotherapy
Stage II - Dukes B	T3-4, N0, M0	Peritoneum Pericolic tissue	• 5-year survival in 50-75% • Chemotherapy?
Stage III - Dukes C	T1-4, N1-3, M0	Stage I or II + lymphnodes	• 5-year survival in 30-50%
Stage IV - Dukes D	T1-4, N1-3, M1	Stage III + distant metastases	• 5-year survival in 5%

metic advantages of a laparotomy, post-operative pain, less use of analgesics, rapid recovery of intestinal functions earlier re-feeding, with shorter hospital stay, and faster return to work.

Oncological Treatment
Complementary treatment to non-curative surgery (II, III and IV) comprises chemotherapy, immunotherapy and adjuvant radiotherapy. Adjuvant chemotherapy has proven efficacy (prolonged survival) in patients with lymph node involvement or other unfavorable prognostic factors (stage III). Radiotherapy, in combination with chemotherapy, has a therapeutic role for locally advanced rectal carcinoma, in the preoperative phase to reduce the neoplastic mass (debulking), and in the post-operative phase to reduce local recurrences.

PREVENTION OF COLON CANCER

Epidemiological (high incidence and mortality) and evolutionary characteristics (slow adenoma-carcinoma sequence) of CRC, besides the availability of appropriate diagnostic and therapeutic tools, make this tumour an ideal target for effective prevention. Prevention is addressed to asymptomatic patients and aims at eliminating risk factors associated with cancer development (primary prevention), or early diagnosis and removal of the disease (secondary prevention).
Primary prevention in the general population aims at reducing the risk of developing adenomas.
The increased incidence of cancer among immigrants from low-incidence to high-incidence areas highlights the role of environmental factors in the development of CRC, markedly related to Western lifestyles and to economically developed areas. However, the specific role of nutritional and dietary factor on carcinogenesis, as protective (a diet rich in fiber, fruit, and vegetables, calcium, vitamins D and B6), or promoting factors (consumption of red meat and cooking at high temperatures with carbonization), is still controversial. A protective effect is recognized for physical activity. Conclusive evidence is provided by the protective effects of aspirin on sporadic CRC. Secondary prevention follows well-defined guidelines.
In the general population (>45-50 years), screening with a fecal occult blood test can be performed at home and repeated every two years. Today's screening programs rely on fecal immunochemical test (FIT) or fecal occult blood test (FOBT), which use specific antibodies recognizing human haemoglobin. Screening allows selection of persons for colonoscopy. The World Health Organization in 1968 defined criteria for effective screening guidelines:

- high incidence of disease;
- high mortality/morbidity ratio;
- latent stage of disease;
- efficacy of early treatment in reducing mortality;
- availability of easy-to-apply, acceptable-to-the-population, inexpensive and accurate screening tools; adequate distribution of facilities within the territory;
- favorable cost/effectiveness ratio;
- acceptable follow-up resulting from diagnosis and treatment.

Colorectal cancer has all these characteristics.
In high-risk populations (personal or family history of adenomas or cancer, or for IBD or hereditary syndrome surveillance) colonoscopy should be performed directly with the frequency depending on the underlying conditions. Colonoscopy can identify cancer precursors (adenomas) or to diagnose

cancer at an early stage, thus providing a favorable prognosis. In Italy, recent data indicate that CRC mortality rates have declined with the wider implementation, thus confirming the effectiveness of preventive initiatives. Fecal DNA tests can detect mutations associated with neoplasia with a sensitivity of up to 87% for cancer and up to 40% for advanced adenomas but they are not applicable for population screening initiatives.

Cost and accessibility of virtual colonoscopy (VC) do not make this test available as a population-based screening test. Furthermore, the diagnostic accuracy in detecting small polyps is unsatisfactory. International guidelines do not specifically agree on the use of VC in screening. Sigmoidoscopy is used in some European countries as a first-level screening test, followed by total colonoscopy if positive for adenomas or cancer.

KEY CONCEPTS

- Colorectal carcinoma (CRC) is third in incidence among cancers in men and second in women.
- The risk of malignant progression of adenomatous polyps depends on histological type, size and number of polyps.
- The greatest risks of developing colorectal carcinoma are: age over 50 years, presence of adenomatous polyps, positive family history, obesity, familial polyposis, and Lynch syndrome.
- Familial adenomatous polyposis (FAP) inevitably leads to the development of carcinoma even at a young age.
- CRC has ideal characteristics for primary and secondary prevention.
- Primary prevention can prevent adenoma onset by targeting lifestyles or through chemoprevention. Current evidence does not provide specific recommendations for the general population, but only generic indications for adopting a healthy lifestyle.
- Secondary prevention can reduce CRC incidence and mortality by interrupting the adenoma-carcinoma sequence. The best test for this purpose is colonoscopy.
- Prevention of colon cancer in populations at average-risk, can detect advanced adenomas (and their removal) or early CRC through the administration of a first-level test (fecal occult blood or sigmoidoscopy) followed, if positive, by colonoscopy.
- Surveillance can prevent cancer in persons with increased risk (personal history of adenomas or CRC; family history of CRC) or high risk (hereditary syndromes and IBD); and it is performed with colonoscopy.

REFERENCES

- Annese V, Beaugerie L, Egan L, et al. European evidence-based consensus: inflammatory bowel disease and malignancies. JCC 2015; 945-65.
- Atkin WS, Edwards R, Kralj-Hans I, et al. Once-only flexible sigmoidoscopy screening in prevention of colorectal cancer: a multicentre randomised controlled trial. Lancet. 2010; 375:1624-33.
- Benson AB 3rd, Arnoletti JP, Bekaii-Saab T, et al.; National Comprehensive Cancer Network. Colon cancer. J Natl Compr Canc Netw. 2011 Nov; 9(11):1238-90.
- Chan AT, Giovannucci EL. Primary prevention of colo-rectal cancer. Gastroenterology. 2010; 138:2029-43.
- Colorectal cancer: diagnosis and management. Clinical guideline CG131. NICE November 2011 (https// www.nice.org.uk/guidance/cg131).
- Lieberman D. Progress and challenges in colorectal cancer screening and surveillance. Gastroenterology. 2010; 138:2115-26.
- Segnan N, Armaroli P, Bonelli L, et al. Once-only sigmoidoscopy in colorectal cancer screening: follow-up findings of the Italian Randomized Controlled Trial-SCORE. J Natl Cancer Inst. 2011; 103:1310-22.

CROHN'S DISEASE

Livia Biancone, Alessandro Armuzzi

LEARNING OBJECTIVES

- To provide the epidemiology, anatomiclinical characteristics, clinical outcome, course, and complications of Crohn's disease.
- To understand difficulties in diagnosis and indications for diagnostic techniques in Crohn's disease.
- To learn the indications for medical and surgical treatments for Crohn's disease.

INTRODUCTION

Crohn's disease (CD) is a chronic inflammatory bowel disease (IBD) of unknown ethology. Intestinal lesions may involve any section of the gastrointestinal tract, from the mouth to the anus. The disease was first described by Burril Crohn, Leon Ginzburg, and Gordon Oppenheimer. In 1960, Henry Lockhart-Mummery and Basil Morson, first described the possible involvement of the colon in CD.

CD is characterized by a chronic relapsing course with recurrent relapse and remission of symptoms. In subgroups of patients, CD may also be associated with extraintestinal manifestations. As the aetiology of CD is currently unknown, no curative treatments are currently available for the disease, However, growing knowledge about its pathogenesis has led to the development of highly effective treatment for the disease.

Due to its chronic course, patients with CD require continuous medical treatment, clinical assessments and, often, surgical treatment for the post-surgical recurrence of lesions.

In CD the lesions more frequently involve the distal ileum and the colon, with a segmental distribution, and damaged areas interspersed with areas free of alterations. The inflammation involves all the layers of the intestinal wall, unlike ulcerative rectocolitis. The predominant type of intestinal lesions may be fibrosing (associated with frequent obstruction), penetrating (associated with the more frequent development of abscesses) or non-penetrating (or inflammatory) non-stenosing. However, these three characteristics can coexist in the same patient or evolve during the course of the disease. CD is also characterized by a high tendency to recurrence of intestinal lesions after surgical resection, generally starting from areas close to anastomosis.

EPIDEMIOLOGY

CD is more frequent in industrialized countries (North America, Northern Europe). This finding suggests the role of environmental factors in the pathogenesis of the disease.

Incidence and Prevalence

The incidence of Crohn's disease has nearly quadrupled during the last 25 years, especially in Northern Europe (11.4/100,000/year; prevalence 262/100.000) and in North America (23.8/100.000/year; prevalence 318.5/100.000). In Italy, the estimated incidence is 6.9/100.000 inhabitants/year and the prevalence 86/100.000 inhabitants, with no significant differences between genders, as recently reported in an epidemiologic study performed in Central Italy.

Crohn's disease is the main organic cause of recurrent abdominal pain in persons15-25 years old.

CD is diagnosed in more than 2/3 of cases before the age of 35 and, in 25% of cases before the age of 20 years.

The peak incidence occurs at the age between 15 and 40 years, although the second peak incidence is observed between the age of 50 and 60 years.

During the last decades, diagnosis of CD has progressively declined.

Risk Factors

The aetiology of CD is still unknown. However, the following main risk factors for the disease have been identified.

*The Authors wish to thank Dr. Benedetto Neri for his assistance.

Familial History of IBD

The role of genetic and family history is supported by several observations. Approximately 12% of patients have a sibling with a diagnosis of Crohn's Disease or ulcerative colitis (UC). The relative risk for a CD patient to have a child carrying the same disease is about 10 times higher than the general population and there is a high concordance for CD in homozygotic twins.

Cigarette Smoking

Cigarette smoking is the only environmental risk factor associated with the disease. Smoking is associated with a higher risk of developing the disease [odds ratio (OR) 1.76; 95% confidence interval (CI) 1.4-2.2], a more severe course and earlier recurrence after surgery.

Appendectomy

Appendectomy is associated with a higher risk of developing CD [relative risk (RR) 1.6] particularly within the first year after surgery (RR 6.5), showing a progressive reduction of risk over time. This observation indicate one of the diagnostic difficulties in CD, as acute appendicitis may be the initial manifestation of the disease.

Other Factors

Among other risk factors, the use of oral contraceptives, antibiotics at a young age (OR 1.74; 95% CI 1.3-2.2), NSAIDs use and diet (rich in fat and poor in fibers) have been suggested. However, no defined aetiological association has been demonstrated for any of these factors.

PATHOLOGICAL ANATOMY

Macroscopic Appearance

Intestinal lesions in CD are characterized by three main features:

- possible involvement of any area of the gastrointestinal (GI) tract
- patchy distribution
- involvement of all the layers of the bowel wall (**Table 24.1**).

Although any area of the GI tract may be involved in CD, lesions more frequently involve the terminal ileum (30-40%), the terminal ileum and colon (40-55%) or the colon only (5-10%). Lesions show a typical patchy distribution with focal areas affected and unaffected by chronic inflammation.

The main macroscopic alterations of the affected areas are mainly by bowel wall thickening (**Figure 24.1**), due to edema, inflammatory infiltration

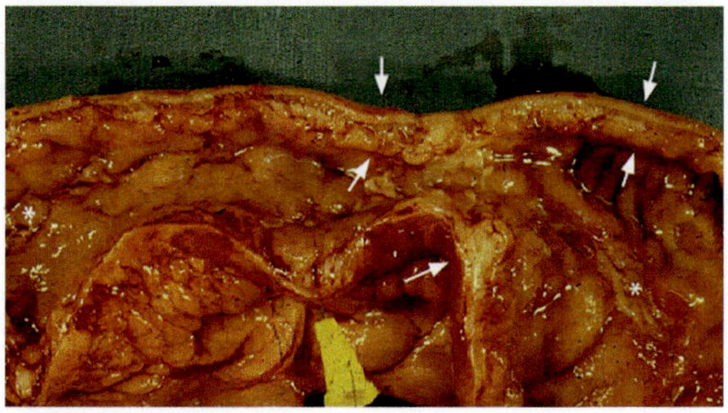

Figure 24.1 Macroscopic appearance of an ileal surgical specimen from a Crohn's Disease patient. The figure shows a marked tickening of the bowel wall (arrows) due to fibrosis, with lumen narrowing, diffuse ulcerations (*) surrounded by oedema of the mucosa, giving rise to a "cobblestone" appearance of the tract.

Table 24.1 Main lesions in Crohn's Disease.

Macroscopic Lesions	Microscopic Lesions
Focal distribution	Focal aggregates of lymphocytes-macrophages, granulomas
Increased bowel wall thickness	Edema, muscular thickness,fibrosis
Intestinal fissures	Deep and not wide ulcers
Transmural distribution	Inflammation of all layers of the bowel wall
Serositis	Perivascular inflammatory infiltrate
Stenosis	Fibrosis after mucosal healing of ulcers, edema
"Cobblestone" appearance	Focal aggregates of lymphocytes-macrophages, granulomas, oedema of mucosa and submucosa
Fistulae	Deep fissures arising from ulcers passing through bowel wall layers, with loop adhesion
Aphthous ulcers	Superficial ulcers with focal aggregates of lymphocytes-macrophages in mucosa

and fibrosis. The inner bowel wall layer shows serpiginous ulcers, often evolving into deep ulcers. Inflammatory involvement of the sierosa and the development of fissures may cause adhesions giving rise to fistulization.

Bowel wall thickening and fibrotic tissue may determine the development of strictures that differ in relation to the site, extent, severity, and number of lesions (Table 24.1). The lesions of CD and its complications affect its course.

Anatomopathological Features and Phenotypic of the Disease

The pattern of CD lesions may be categorized in three main subgroups that may co-exist in the same patient or evolve the one into the other:

- Fibrostricturing disease. Characterised by lumen narrowing (**Figure 24.2 A**) and stenosis. These are caused by wall thickening due to local inflammation and/or, more often, by fibrotic tissue developing after healing of ulcers. The stenotic tract may be single or multiple, variable in length, often localized in the distal ileum and associated with dilation of the GI tract above the stenosis.
- Penetrating disease. Characterised by fistulas, tracts covered by epithelium and communicating between the intestinal areas and adjacent intestinal loops or other organs. Fistulae originate from fissures and adhesions due to inflammation of serosa. Fistulae in CD may form communication between intestinal loops (enteroenteric fistulas) (**Figure 24.2 B**), with the skin (enterocutaneous fistulas), the bladder (enterovescical fistulas), the ureter (enteroureteral fistulas) or the vagina (enterovaginal fistulas). One of the orifices of the fistulae may also end in the retroperitoneum and, more often, in the mesentery, thus causing abscesses.
- Non stricturing-non penetrating disease. Characterized by bowel wall thickening due to inflammation of the GI tract, without the development of fistulae or stenosis (**Figure 24.2 C**). The tract shows small and superficial ulcers (aphthous ulcers), as an expression of recent lesions (**Figure 24.2 D**) and/or deeper ulcers and fissures often in communication often surrounded by swollen mucosa due to edema, thus assuming the typical macroscopic cobblestone aspect (**Figure 24.2 E**).

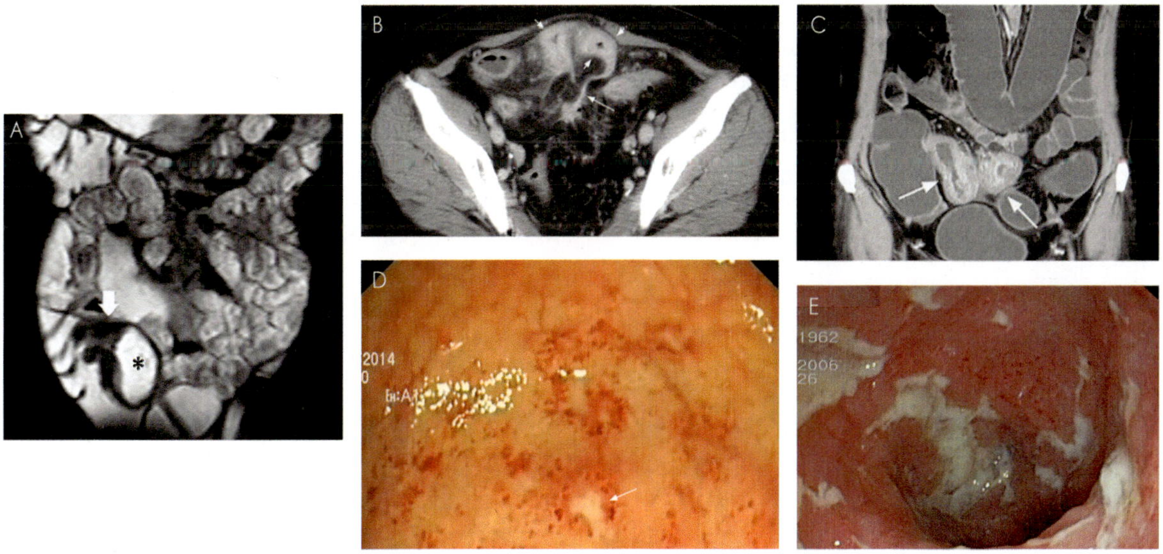

Figure 24.2 Crohn's Disease: Anatomoclinical characteristics.

A) Fibrostricturing CD. Entero-MRI image showing stenosis of the terminal ileum at the ileo-cecal valve, with marked thickening of the bowel wall (arrows) associated with dilation of the ileal loop above the stenosis (*).

B) Fistulizing/penetrating CD. Entero-CT scan showing thickening of the bowel wall (short arrows) associated with entero-enteric fistulae (long arrows).

C) Entero-CT images from a Crohn's Disease patient with ileal disease showing increased bowel wall thickness associated with contrast enhancement after intravenous contrast and dilation of the ileum and colon after contrast given by mouth and as an enema.

D) Endoscopic images of aphthoid ulcers of the intestinal mucosa (arrows).

E) CD of the ileum showing a prevalent inflammatory (or non-stricturing non-penetrating) pattern, with deep ulcers surrounded by areas of mucosa swollen due to oedema ("cobblestone" appearance).

Microscopic Appearance

CD is histologically characterized by a chronic granulomatous inflammation (Table 24.1).

The main lesions are non-caseating granulomas, patchy and transmural inflammation with focal infiltration of lymphocytes and fissures. Granulomas may be detected in approximately 60% of patients, constituted by epithelioid cells, Langhans-like giant cells, without necrosis. Although the presence of granulomas is specific for CD, their absence does not rule out diagnosis of the disease, as granulomas are detected only in a small percentage of patients. Inflammation of the bowel wall is characterized by aggregates of inflammatory cells (mainly T-lymphocytes and macrophages) with patchy and multifocal distribution localized in multiple bowel wall layers, particularly in the submucosa. In some patients, fibrosis may develop due to fibrotic healing of the lesions leading to stenosis.

The extent and severity of lesions, as assessed macroscopically and histologically, are independent of clinical activity of the disease.

Aetiology

The aetiology of CD remains unknown. Current evidences suggest that, in genetically predisposed individuals, a dysregulation of the host immune response towards luminal antigens (mainly the resident bacterial flora) is able to determine or at least to maintain and perpetuate local inflammatory processes. Several agents have been proposed, though none of them has been shown to play a role in the aetiology of CD.

Microbiota

Disbiosys has been suggested in CD, as supported by a reduced number of *Bacterioides* and *Firmicutes*, associated with an increase Gammaproteobacteria and Actinobacteria.

Approximately 1/3 of patients show an increase in entero-invasive *Escherichia coli* able to cross the mucosal barrier, adhere and invade intestinal epithelial cells, and survive and replicate within macrophages, thus inducing the release of high levels of TNF-α. Preliminary evidence also shows lower concentrations of *Faecalibacterium prausnitzii*, a commensal bacterium with anti-inflammatory properties. Recently, the microbiota of patients with CD has also been associated with an increase in viral species (e.g., caudovirales) and fungi.

This hypothesis is partially supported by two observations:

- treatments that modulate intestinal bacterial flora, e.g., probiotics and antibiotics, may modify CD;
- surgical diversion of the luminal content by temporary ileostomy with fecal diversion, improves the clinical course of the disease and also prevents post-operative recurrence.

Furthermore, surgical recanalization with the passage of luminal content through the anastomosis is followed by the post-operative recurrence of the disease

However, no aetiologic agents have been identified in CD.

Immune Response

CD is characterized by T-lymphocytes and macrophages activation with a prevalent 'cell-mediated immune response.

Prevalent T-helper lymphocytes type 1 activation leading to higher levels of Interferon gamma (IFN-gamma), interleukin 12 (IL-12), IL-18, IL21 and tumour necrosis factor-α (TNF-α) has been demonstrated in tissue biopsy from CD patients.

Genetic Susceptibility

Genome-wide association studies have identified more than 200 alleles associated with IBD, 37 currently appear to be more specifically associated with CD. Genes associated with bacterial components, innate immunity and related to the Th17 immune response (NOD2, ATG16L1, LRRK2, IRGM, Il23R, HLA, STAT3, JAK2) or to inadequate function of the mucosal epithelial layer (MUC2) have been described.

An inappropriate host immune response towards intestinal bacterial components has been postulated as a keyfactor in the pathogenesis of the disease.

Genetic variations have been reported in a minority of patients with CD (about 12%), thus supporting the role of epigenetics and environmental factors in the pathogenesis of the disease.

CLINICAL PRESENTATION

CD can have extremely variable onset, symptoms, and clinical course.

Crohn's Disease

In about 10% of CD patients, symptom onset can be acute, with severe abdominal pain, fever, leukocytosis, thus miming acute appendicitis. In subgroups of patients, several years before the onset

of typical intestinal symptoms, perianal disease, extraintestinal manifestations (involving the joints, skin, eyes or liver) or growth delay may develop before the diagnosis of CD.
In the majority of patients, however, typical but non-specific symptoms are observed at disease onset, including recurrent abdominal pain, diarrhoea with or without blood, weight loss, low-grade fever, fatigue. The time interval between symptoms onset and diagnosis of CD may vary between 0 and 4 years (mean, 8-9 months). During this period, an erroneous diagnosis of appendicitis, adnexitis or irritable bowel syndrome (IBS) may be often made.

Anatomo-Clinical Features

CD shows a wide spectrum of clinical and anatomopathological features mainly related to the characteristics of the lesions (site, extent, type, duration, complications, previous intestinal resections) and of the host (age, gender, lifestyle, smoking habits, psychosocial conditions, familial history of IBD). The main variable is the site of the lesions, which can involve the jejunum, ileum, ileum-colon, colon, or rectum, and anal canal. The presence of lesions related to the disease in the upper GI tract (oral mucosa, oesophagus, stomach, duodenum) is generally associated with more typical localizations of the disease. Perianal disease is characterized by anal and/or perianal lesions, like skintags, fistulae, and abscesses. The extension of lesions, from a few centimeters to over 1 meter, can influence the course of the disease, while the type or behavior of the disease, fibrostenosing, fistulizing or predominantly inflammatory forms, is often associated with subocclusive symptoms, fever, diarrhoea, and nutritional deficits, respectively.

Signs and Symptoms

The type and severity of symptoms are related to the characteristics of the host and the lesions. Adominal pain, together and chronic diarrhoea, is the most frequent symptom.
Chronic diarrhoea may be the direct expression of lesions or related to malabsorption of biliary acids with steatorrhea, more frequent in patients with previous ileal resection.
Rectal bleeding and tenesmus may develop in patients with lesions involving the sigmoid colon and the rectum. Abdominal pain is mostly located in the mesogastrium c and the right iliac fossa; it may vary in severity and frequency, with a possible occurrence at night with no resolution after diarrhoea. In the presence of stenosis, the pain is recurrent and mostly related to bowel tenderness, dilation of small bowel loops, while in the inflammatory and penetrating patterns of the disease the pain is more frequently continuous as an expression of severe inflammation. Fever may range from less than 38°C to high fever, may be related to disease activity or to development of abscesses. Abdominal masses, usually painful on palpation and localized in the right iliac fossa, are characteristic and may be due to wall thickening, perivisceral inflammation, and eventually to such complications as stenosis, fistulization or abscesses. Weight loss may be due to reduced caloric intake, malabsorption or increased catabolism related to inflammation. In children growth deficit is a classic symptom of the disease.
Perianal fistulas may appear years before the onset of intestinal symptoms, with a chronic recurrent course, no tendency towards spontaneous healing but rather a marked tendency to develop complications including abscesses. Anal lesions, include perianal cutaneous hyperemia and edema, skin tags, ulcers and fissures. Extraintestinal manifestations include articular (peripheral arthritis, ankylosing spondylitis, sacroileitis), cutaneous (erythema nodosum, pyoderma gangrenosum), ocular (uveitis, iridocyclitis, episcleritis) manifestations. These are more frequently observed in young patients with colonic or perianal involvement of lesions. Hepatobiliary (primary sclerosing cholangitis) and thromboembolic complications are also reported. Biliary and renal stones are common in ileal disease, consequent to of bile acid malabsorption due to extensive ileal lesions or resections. Renal amyloidosis is rare, potentially evolving into chronic renal failure.

NATURAL HISTORY

Clinical Course

CD is typically chronic, with recurrent phases of remission and relapse of the disease. The probability of remission after a period of activity is very high (>90%), as is the rate of relapse at one year (>60%). In the course of disease, abdominal complications like stenosis, fistulae, and abscesses may develop and require surgical resection. Severity of the disease is related to young age at diagnosis, proximal bowel bowel lesions, fistulizing pattern, perianal disease, need for steroids at disease onset.
However, after a variable time interval, surgical resection is followed by recurrence of lesions. Recurrent lesions initially include aphthous ulcers, followed by more severe deep lesions (endoscopic recurrence), which is not necessarily associated

with intestinal symptoms (asymptomatic recurrence). Postoperative recurrence may lead to the development of new complications requiring further resection. The clinical course of CD is more aggressive in patients with symptom onset at a young age, familial IBD, smokers, and with penetrating behavior at disease onset.

Complications

Local and systemic complications may develop in CD (**Table 24.2**). Local complications may co-exist and their frequency increase according to duration of the disease. These include: internal fistulae (entero-enteric, enterovesical, rectovaginal) or external (entero-cutaneous) (**Figure 24.2 B**), obstructions, perforations, haemorrhage, abscesses. Fistulae are often associated with stenoses and subsequent development of abscesses, with a poor tendency towards spontaneous healing. Stenosis is more common in patients with ileal disease (complicated by obstructions in 50% of cases), giving rise to subobstruction or overt obstruction. The development of small bowel or colonic adenocarcinoma in lesions is a rare but possible complication. Anal lesions are more frequently associated with colonic localization of disease.

DIAGNOSIS

Criteria

The diagnosis of CD is often difficult due to the lack of specific symptoms and/or of a gold standard diagnostic work up.

Diagnosis

Diagnosis is based on clinical history, clinical assessment, physical examination, biochemical alterations, and radiological, endoscopic, and histologic finding. Among possible objective finding, fistulas and extraintestinal manifestations may suggest CD.

Physical examination may reveal pain in the right iliac fossa or the mesogastrium or an of abdominal mass. Diagnostic examinations do not provide specific alterations pathognomonic for CD but they are often useful to rule out other diseases with similar clinical manifestations.

Differential Diagnosis

Differential diagnosis comprises: ulcerative colitis; infectious colitis or enterocolitis including tuberculosis, *Yersinia* ileitis, *Clostridium difficile* pseudomembranous colitis, enterocolitis related to *Salmonella*, *Shighella* and *Campylobacter*, viral colitis, including colitis related to cytomegalovirus (CMV), and parasitic colitis including colitis due to *Entamoeba*; irritable bowel syndrome; lymphomas; ischaemic colitis, radiation colitis; colorectal cancer (CRC); segmental colitis associated with diverticula (SCAD); appendicitis; intestinal or pelvic endometriosis; coelicac disease, chronic ulcerative non granulomatous jejuno-ileitis; other rare diseases, including eosinophil gastroenteritis, microscopic colitis or amyloidosis.

Unclassified IBD (IBD-U) and Indeterminate Colitis

CD and UC share common clinical and ethiopathogenetic characteristics, although often with different pathological features, clinical course and differential diagnosis. However, in 5% to 10% of patients, differential diagnosis between CD limited to the colon and UC is not feasible, at least at symptom onset. Such cases fall under the definition of "Indeterminate colitis" or of "Unclassified IBD (IBD-U)" in patients with or, respectively, without colectomy and histological assessment of the entire colon (vs. endoscopic biopsies for IBD-U).

Table 24.2 Main clinical features of Crohn's Disease.

Local	Systemic
Fistulae	Cuteneous: erythaema nodosum, pyoderma gangrenosus
Abscesses	Ocular: uveitis, iridocyclitis, episcleritis
Obstruction, sub-obstruction	Articular: arthritis, ankylosing spondylitis, sacroileitis
Perforation	Hepatobiliary: primary sclerosing cholangitis, cholangiocarcinoma, gallbladder stones
Haemorrhage	Kidney: renal oxalate lithiasis; amyloidosis
Adenocarcinoma of the small bowel or of the colon-rectum	Thromboembolic disease

As medical treatment is substantially comparable between patients with CD limited to the colon and UC, this differentiation assumes relative therapeutic relevance.
Differently, in patients eligible for surgery, discrimination between the two diseases is clinically relevant. This is because after removal of the colon and rectum (proctocolectomy) and ileal pocket packaging ("pouch"), about 40% of patients with unclassified colitis will develop characteristics typical of CD, associated with the frequent development of complications, including the need to convert the pouch into a final ileostomy.
In patients with undetermined and unclassified colitis, the study can be performed using an endoscopic videocapsule that visualizes of aphthous ulcers compatible with CD and not detectable by conventional radiology, as well as the histological review of the surgical specimen.

Scores for Assessing CD

CD is clinically characterized by recurrent phases of activity and remission. Clinical assessment, physical examination, biochemical examinations, and diagnostic procedures concur not only to establish diagnosis, but also to determine the extent of the disease. Clinical activity may be defined by specific scores for standardized and quantitative of clinical evaluation. The CD activity index (CDAI) is the most widely used clinical score for assessing the clinical activity of CD. The final CDAI score results from the sum of the following 8 variables multiplied by a coefficient: number of liquid/semiliquid stools, abdominal pain, and general well being during the last seven days, presence of extraintestinal manifestations, use of antidiarrhoics, abdominal mass, haematocrit and body weight. The resulting CDAI score identifies patients in clinical remission (<150) or in clinical activity (>150). Besides the CDAI score, other indexes have been proposed for assessing CD, including clinical scores (Harvey-Bradshaw, HBI), endoscopic score (Simple Endoscopic Score for CD – SES-CD), and radiologic scores (Magnetic Resonance imaging index of Activity – MaRIA). These additional scores have been proposed for assessing the grade of activity of CD and responsiveness to drug treatments.

Diagnostic Tests

Biochemical Examinations

Blood chemistry can disclose sideropenic hypochromic microcytic anemia (due to bleeding, increased catabolism related to chronic inflammation, lower intake) or macrocytic anemia (due to reduced absorption of vitamin B12 and/or folic acid). During clinical activity of the disease frequent findings include leukocytosis, higher ESR, C reactive protein, and alpha-1-acid glycoprotein. Additional findings include hypoalbuminemia (due to intestinal loss or lower intake), hypocholesterolemia, hypotriglyceridemia, deficiency of vitamin D3 and B12, folic acid, (due to malabsorption), and electrolyte imbalance (due to chronic diarrhoea). Stool tests for bacteria and parasites are mandatory to rule out the infectious diseases in differential diagnoses. Diagnosis of IBD may also be supported by the finding of elevated fecal calprotectin, a protein present within granulocytes in the stools, which can be also used to monitor the efficacy of treatments.

Endoscopic Examinations

Colonoscopy with visualization of the ileum (ileocolonoscopy) is the gold standard as it allows visualization of the mucosal surface and bioptic sampling of lesions. Ileocolonoscopy visualizes mucosal lesions surrounded by uninvolved tissue. CD lesions more frequently observed include aphthous ulcers or confluent ulcers of various morphology, surrounded by edematous mucosa, giving rise to the typical "cobblestone" appearance, and stenosis often not allowing passage of the endoscope (see Figure 24.2).

Oesophagogastroduodenoscopy (EGDS)

It is recommended in upper GI symptoms (nausea, vomiting, epigastric pain) to detect the possible presence, in 1-3% of patients, of oesophageal, gastric or duodenal lesions associated with the typical ileal and/or colonic localizations.

Radiological Techniques

Radiological imaging is crucial to support or confirm clinical suspicion of CD, to define localization, extent, presence of intra-abdominal complications, and disease activity. Among the currently available techniques, the higher accuracy is obtained with entero-CT, entero-MRI, and intestinal ultrasound. These techniques have recently replaced traditional radiological studies including radiological examination of small bowel using barium, small bowel follow-through and double-contrast examination of the colon.
Intestinal ultrasound, entero-CT and entero-MRI reveal bowel wall thickening due to inflammation. Complications such as stenosis, fistulas, and abscesses may be accurately detected after di-

lation of the small bowel loops using contrast (non absorbable electrolytic solutions like polyethylene glycol or PEG), given by mouth or by naso-gastric-tube for entero-CT or entero-MRI. The three examinations have comparable diagnostic accuracy, differ by indication in relation to their characteristics: for example, entero-CT and entero-MRI are mainly used for detecting complications and in patients with acute symptoms; entero-MRI and ultrasonography are also used as preliminary examinations in the diagnosis of disease and for assessing its course, as they both are non-invasive and do not expose patients to ionizing radiations (**Figure 24.3**).

The plain film of the abdomen is still useful for the diagnosis of obstruction (i.e., allows detection of air-fluid levels and dilation of bowel loops) and intestinal perforation.

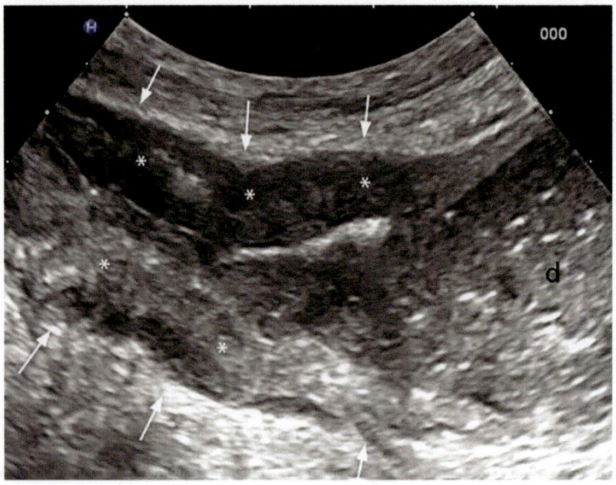

Figure 24.3 Image from an ultrasound examination of the ileum in a CD patient, showing a markedly increased bowel wall thickness (*), with dilation of the proximal ileal loop (d), thus suggesting the presence of stenosis.

TREATMENT

Medical Treatment

As the aetiology of CD is still unknown, no curative therapies are currently available. Targets of medical treatment include: a) induction of remission; b) maintenance of steroid-free remission; c) mucosal healing; d) prevention of post-operative recurrence.

In general, patients with mild-to-moderate CD can may be managed in outpatient while those with severe disease often require hospitalization.

In patients with active CD, corticosteroids still represent the most effective conventional treatments. Methylprednisolone (iv o im) or prednisone (by mouth) (0.75-1 mg/kg) can induce remission in 65-85% of patients. Abuse or inappropriate use of corticosteroids may raise the risk of infections and complications.

Bowel rest (parenteral or enteral nutrition) or antibiotics (ciprofloxacin and metronidazole) may increase the efficacy of corticosteroids. About 30 to 40% of patients responsive to corticosteroids develop steroid-dependence or, more rarely, become steroid-refractory.

In such case, recent drugs (first clinical trial in 1995), in biological therapies, including monoclonal anti-TNF-α antibodies (infliximab or adalimumab), anti-alpha 4/beta 7 may be indicated, in addition to integrin (vedolizumab) or p40 interleukin 12/23 anti-subunit (ustekinumab). The first of these drugs to be developed and more widely used today are the anti-TNFα monoclonal antibodies (infliximab or biosimilars and adalimumab).

Biological therapies, administered by intravenous infusion (infliximab or biosimilars, vedolizumab, or first administration of ustekinumab) or subcutaneous (adalimumab or subsequent administration of ustekinumab) may induce clinical remission and endoscopic resolution in patients refractory to conventional therapies and the closure, at least temporarily, of refractory perianal fistulae in 70 and 50% of patients, respectively. Since these drugs modulate the immune system, they are not devoid of possible side effects.

Among these, the most important are bacterial or viral infections and the slatentization of tuberculosis infection (especially with anti TNFα), which must be excluded before treatment. In moderately active ileal CD, a systemic low bioavailability steroid, such as budesonide (9 mg/day), which is associated with fewer side effects, may be indicated. The use of conventional immunosuppressants long used for CD, such as thiopurines (azathioprine, and its metabolite 6-mercaptopurine), as well as methotrexate, are predominantly indicated for the maintenance of remission. These slow-acting drugs are indicated in patients with chronically active or steroid-dependent disease. Thiopurines are efficacious in the treatment of perianal fistulas and extraintestinal manifestations, albeit less so than anti-TNFα. Some antibiotics are also temporarily effective in reducing intestinal inflammation and treatment of extraintestinal and clinical manifestations due to bacterial overgrowth. Metronidazole and ciprofloxacin are particularly effective in ileococcal and colic disease and in human disease. In the maintenance of remission, immunosuppressive agents and biological therapies may delay clinical exacerbation of disease. However, in relation to the greater risk of side effects, the latter are reserved for patients with a cortico-dependent profile or in more severe disease. Prevention of post-surgical recurrence is predominantly treated with mesalazine and azathioprine.

Surgical Treatment

Surgical indications for CD include acute and chronic complications and treatment failure. Chronic complications include fibrostricturing stenoses, cancerization of colinic or small bowel lesions. Drug intolerance and the development of fistulae, particularly involving other organs (e.g., bladder, ureters, and gynecological tract) may also be observed. Acute complications include intestinal obstruction, perforation or the development of abscesses, haemorrhage, and systemic toxic colitis.

Persistently active disease despite second-line treatments or also the need for corticosteroids to maintain remission, termed steroid-dependence, are considered a failure of medical treatment. The surgical indication may also become an emergency, due to peritonitis because of perforation, toxic colitis, haemorrhage or septic shock. Urgent surgery is rare in CD, and has progressively declined in recent years. Resolution of septic complications by percutaneous drainage of the abscess is the preferred approach, when compared to surgical treatment which, possibly, should be delayed after drainage of the abscess.

Intestinal obstruction is a relatively common event in CD. As obstruction most often involves the small bowel, a non-surgical approach of the obstruction should be initially preferred, as positioning a naso-gastric-tube and administration of systemic corticosteroids (iv) is effective in most patients. This modality of treatment allows to plan adequate evaluation of the GI tract and, if necessary, elective surgical treatment using mini-invasive techniques.

Surgical treatment is performed in about 70-80% of CD patients within 20 years from the diagnosis. As multiple resections are often required (from 30 to 70% of cases according to different studies), due to disease recurrence, surgery must be finalized for maximum intestinal sparing.

In CD, intestinal resection is the most common surgical approach, accounting for 70-80% of surgical procedures performed for ileo-colitis, more frequent in stenosis or fistulae. It constitutes the first choice for patients with fistulizing complications and in Crohn's colitis (total colectomy with ileo-rectal anastomosis or total proctocolectomy with teminal ileostomy when the rectum also is severely involved).

Non-resective surgery. Strictureplasty is a technique for treating stenosis without resecting the involved intestinal tract.

The major benefit of strictureplasty is its ability to preserve the small bowel and reduce the risk of short bowel syndrome, a feared complication following extensive or multiple intestinal resections, characterized by malabsorption. It is the preferred treatment in patients with short stenosis, particularly if multiple, in patients with previous intestinal resections and in limited stenosis of the duodenum. The main non-resective surgical techniques include: strictureplasty according to Heineke–Mikulicz (**Figure 24.4 A**), strictureplasty according to Finney (**Figure 24.4 B**), and the Michelassi's tech-

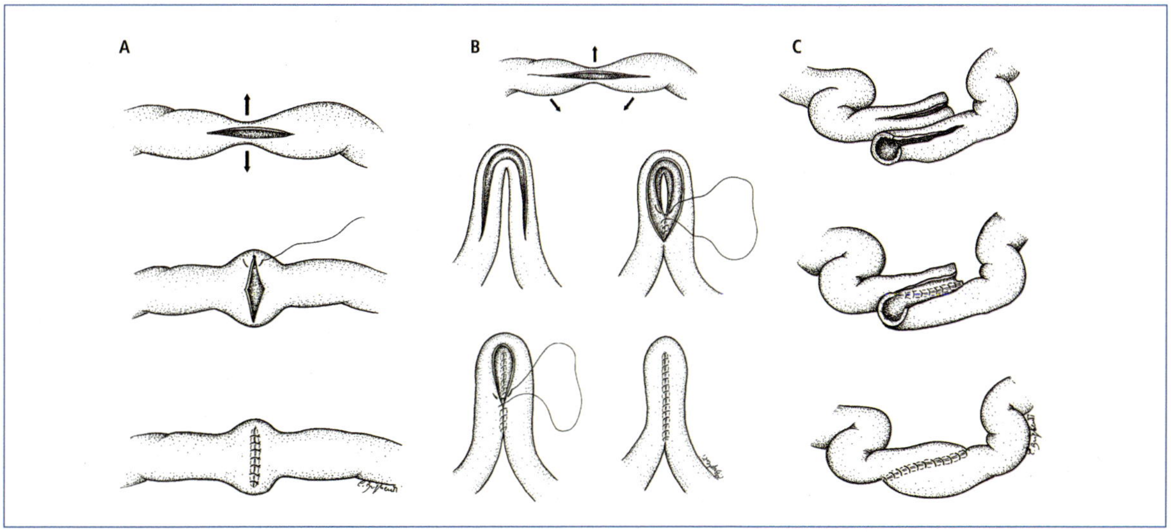

Figure 24.4 Schematic illustrations of strictureplasty according to Heineke-Mikulicz (A), to Finney (B) and to Michelassi (C)

nique (side-to-side isoperistaltic strictureplasty), which is used for treating extensive stenotic tracts (>20 cm) or numerous and close short stenoses (**Figure 24.4 C**).

Surgery of perianal disease. Perianal CD is relatively common, associated with the development of abscesses, fistulae, and anal stenosis.

Therapeutic approach includes, as a first step, surgical exploration under anesthesia (EUA), a procedure useful for defining the characteristics and the severity of perianal disease, for treating abscesses and sepsis, and for preventing recurrence of the abscess by positioning loose setons to drain the fistulae, thus optimizing medical treatment.

Pelvic MRI with contrast is the most useful pre-operatory diagnostic technique to characterize perianal disease.

Proctectomy with permanent stomy may be required for more severe perianal disease resistant to medical treatment, with multiple fistulae not responsive to combined medical and mini-invasive surgical therapy.

KEY CONCEPTS

- Crohn's Disease is a chronic inflammatory disease of unknown aetiology, characterized by recurrent phases of remission and relapse of symptoms, mainly diarrhoea, abdominal pain, weight loss, fever.
- Intestinal lesions in Crohn's Disease may Involve any area of the gastrointestinal tract, although more frequently the terminal Ileum and the colon. Typical features include transmural Inflammation, focal and patchy lesions, and fibrostricturing, fistulizing or non-penetrating non-fistulizing behavior.
- The diagnosis may be difficult, as there is no a gold standard diagnostic approach. Endoscopic and radiological findings may help to support diagnosis, to define disease activity and complications, and for assessing its course.

REFERENCES

- Di Domenicantonio R, Cappai G, Arcà M, Agabiti N, et al. Occurrence of inflammatory bowel disease in central Italy: a study based on health information systems. Dig Liver Dis. 2014;46(9):777-82.
- Gionchetti P, Dignass A, Danese S, Magro Dias FJ, et al. European Crohn's Colitis Organization. 3rd European Evidence-based Consensus on the Diagnosis and Management of Crohn's Disease 2016: Part 2: Surgical Management and Special Situations. ECCO.J Crohns Colitis. 2017;11(2):135-49.
- Gomollón F, Dignass A, Annese V, Tilg H, et al. ECCO. 3rd European Evidence-based Consensus on the Diagnosis and Management of Crohn's Disease 2016: Part 1: Diagnosis and Medical Management.J Crohns Colitis. 2017;11(1):3-25.
- Ng SC, Shi HY, Hamidi N, Underwood FE, et al. Worldwide incidence and prevalence of inflammatory bowel disease in the 21st century: a systematic review of population-based studies. Lancet. 2018;390 (10114):2769-78.
- Torres J, Mehandru S, Colombel JF, Peyrin-Biroulet L. Crohn's disease.Lancet. 2017;389(10080):1741-55.

ULCERATIVE COLITIS

Fabiana Castiglione, Maurizio Vecchi

LEARNING OBJECTIVES

- To know the definition, epidemiological characteristics, and aetiological hypotheses of ulcerative rectocolitis.
- To know its main anatomopathological characteristics and clinical picture.
- To understand the most effective diagnostic modalities and other diseases in differential diagnosis.
- To learn the natural history of the disease and its complications.
- To know the main medical and surgical therapeutic guidelines.

INTRODUCTION

Ulcerative colitis (UC) is a chronic inflammatory bowel disease (IBD) affecting the large intestine, whose lesions always affect the rectum and may extend proximally in a continuous manner to include partially or the entire colon. Inflammation only affects the most superficial layer of the intestinal wall, i.e., the mucosa. UC may affect the rectum (proctitis) or the sigmoid and rectum (proctosigmoiditis), or may involve the colon up to the left flexure (left-sided colitis), to the transverse colon (subtotal colitis) or to the cecum (pancolitis). However, its extension can vary between patients and in the individual patient during evolution of the disease.

Disease severity at clinical presentation is determined by the extent and intensity of the inflamed lesions. Rectal bleeding is the characteristic symptom, and it is often associated with tenesmus (urgency to defecate, even when the rectum is empty). In the most extensive forms, diarrhoea, abdominal pain, fever, weight loss, extra-intestinal manifestations, and intestinal complications may be associated with symptoms and signs. Long-term UC is also a risk factor for the development of colorectal cancer.

EPIDEMIOLOGY

UC is widespread throughout the world, however, its incidence is much higher in the Western industrialised countries. This specific geographic distribution likely reflects a combination of genetic and environmental factors (eating habits, intestinal bacterial flora, cigarette smoking), which influence the disease's further development. In Italy, the incidence is to 5-10/100,000/year, with an estimated prevalence of 80-100 patients/100,000 inhabitants and without significant differences between North and South regionas of the country. Based on the exemptions for pathology, it can be assumed that in Italy there are between 80 and 100,000 patients with UC. The disease can manifest at any age, but it usually begins between 20 and 40 years, and it affects men and women equally. Risk factors influencing disease development are a family history of chronic inflammatory bowel disease (the highest risk factor), abstinence from tobacco smoking, and lack of appendectomy. About 3-5% of patients have a family member who also suffers from Crohn's disease (CD) or UC. Tobacco smoking plays a protective role in UC, as the disease is more common in non-smokers and especially in ex-smokers. The positive effect of smoking on UC is also confirmed by the finding that the disease course is more favorable in tobacco smokers. Appendectomy seems to be another protective factor for the development of UC.

ANATOMICAL PATHOLOGY

Macroscopic Features

At the time of diagnosis, lesions usually only affect the rectum in 10-15% of cases, the sigmoid-rectum in 30-40%, the segment of the colon up to the splenic flexure in 20%, up to the transverse colon in 15%, and the entire colon in about 15%.

The rectum is inflamed in all patients, and the le-

*The Authors wish to thank Dr Anna Testa for her assistance.

sions can extend from the rectum to the rest of the colon in a uniform and continuous manner. The continuity of the lesions is a characteristic of the disease. During the course of UC, the colonic mucosa appears edematous, hyperemic, and granular and may present erosions and ulcerations. The extent, number, and severity of lesions are related to the severity of the disease course. Over time, polypoid lesions (so-called "pseudopolyps" characteristic of UC) of variable shape, size, and number may develop; they result from regeneration of the epithelium, following the healing of inflamed mucosa. Changes in the extent of lesions can be observed in the same patient during the course of the disease.

Microscopic Features

The inflammation caused by UC is typically limited to the most superficial layers (mucosa and submucosa). Also, at the microscopic level, an important feature is the uniform and continuous distribution of inflammation. Edema of the lamina propria is observed, with dilated and congested vessels and extravasated red blood cells and leukocytes, with inflammatory cells infiltrating the lamina propria; the lamina propria is composed of neutrophils, lymphocytes, plasma cells (basal plasmocytosis), macrophages, eosinophils and mast cells.

Neutrophils tend to invade the epithelium of the crypts, giving rise to crypt abscesses which are characteristic, but not specific, of the disease. Epithelial damage is a characteristic of UC and, in addition to erosive lesions and ulcers, there is a reduction in goblet cell secretion (mucin depletion) and derangement of glandular architecture caused by crypt reduction and distortion (**Figure 25.1**).

Ulcers can extend to the muscular layer of the colon only in the most severe forms of UC and in the presence of toxic megacolon; in such cases, the colon can undergo ischaemic necrosis.

The histological picture shows no signs of active inflammation only on complete remission; nonetheless an abnormal glandular architecture remains, with the continued presence of atrophic and distorted crypts, which are easily recognizable as evidence of a history of UC.

Dysplasia can be observed in patients suffering from long-term illness. It can be classified as "low grade", "high grade" or "indefinite", and it is associated with an increased risk of developing adenocarcinoma. Dysplastic lesions may be present in isolated polypoid lesions or on flat or atrophic mucosa. These lesions predispose to colorectal cancer. For this reason, patients with long-term UC are advised to undergo periodic endoscopic examination.

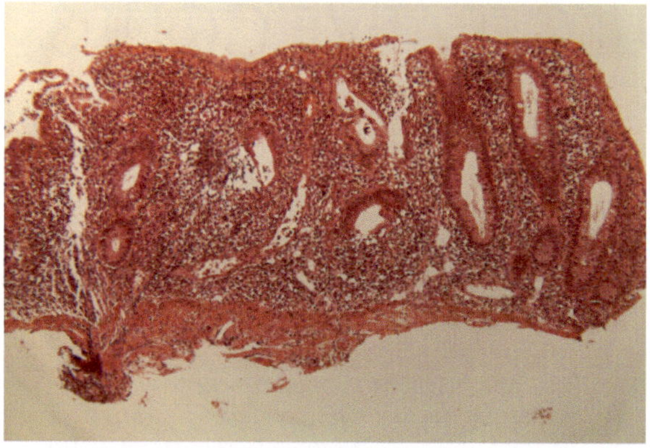

Figure 25.1 Histological features of active UC: typical findings include loss of surface epithelium, reduction/disappearance of goblet cells, dense acute and chronic inflammatory infiltrate in the lamina propria, presence of crypt abscesses (Courtesy of Dr. G. Ronchi).

AETIOLOGY AND PATHOGENESIS

The exact cause of UC remains unknown. Currently, the best supported theory is that it is caused by an abnormal immune response to intestinal lumen antigens (from food or, most probably, bacteria) in genetically predisposed persons. Epidemiological and experimental study findings have suggested a genetic predisposition to the disease, even if, still today, it has not been possible to identify a single gene or multiple genes that characterize its transmission and heterogeneous phenotypes. This seems to suggest that UC is a polygenic disease and that genetic screening is useless in clinical settings. A variety of experimental data have suggested the role played by intestinal bacterial flora, though no reproducible variations in intestinal bacterial populations have ever been identified in humans and the use of antibiotics has never had a significant therapeutic effect. Conversely, numerous experimental data and the excellent response to drugs affecting the immune system have underscored the important involvement of immune mechanisms in the pathogenesis of mucosal damage.

CLINICAL PRESENTATION

The disease is characterized by alternating phases of acute inflammation, or flares, in which symptoms and characteristic signs of the clinical manifestations are clearly evident, with periods of disease inactivity or remission, in which symptoms are absent and clinical well-being is normal. Rectal bleeding is the most characteristic sign of acute phases. The absence of blood in the stool for the entire duration of the disease can be considered a diagnostic exclusion criterion. Sometimes, especially when inflammation is limited to the rectum, bleeding may be the only symptom, in some cases associated to the passage of air and mucus (without diarrhoea or sometimes, even with constipation). In such cases, diagnosis may be very late because the clinical manifestation indicates the presence of haemorrhoids: this delay should be avoided due to the proven tendency of proctitis and distal forms to extend up to or beyond the splenic flexure. In other cases, especially if the extent of inflammation is greater, diarrhoea may also accompany rectal bleeding – even at night and it may contain visible amounts of blood – abdominal pain and rectal tenesmus. The latter is an expression of inflammation of the rectum and is a typical symptom. Abdominal pain is generally not very intense; it is often widespread in all quadrants but mainly in the left, and only partially relieves with bowel emptying. At onset, in most cases, symptoms are relatively mild and worsen progressively if left untreated. In some cases, however, the disease can begin very acutely; this occurs particularly in cases of extensive colitis. In such cases, clinical manifestations can mimic those of acute infectious colitis, where systemic symptoms such as fever, dehydration, electrolyte imbalance, and tachycardia may also present. Indeed, infection involving intestinal pathogens may contribute to the onset or exacerbation of symptoms of UC, making differential diagnosis even more difficult. Significant objective findings are the observed in cases of particularly serious flare-ups, with abdominal distension and reduced intestinal peristalsis. Regarding blood tests, iron-deficiency anemia is observed in more than half of cases during acute phases and it is generally secondary to blood loss. Hypoalbuminemia, also severe degree, is frequently observed during flare-ups and is caused by a reduction in caloric intake but mostly by intestinal protido-dispersion.

An increase in inflammatory markers, particularly ESR and PCR, is observed in moderate-to-severe forms of UC, where it may represent both an index of disease activity and a predictor of disease course. During severe flares, leukocytosis, hypokalemia, and metabolic alkalosis are also observed. An increase in platelets, fibrinogen, and mucoproteins is also frequent.

Evaluation of Severity

Accurate assessment of symptoms intensity is essential for initiating therapeutic treatment. For clinical purposes, the classification of Truelove and Witts (Truelove and Witts' severity index) is still widely used (**Table 25.1**); on the basis of a few detectable parameters and with a few modifications, this classification allows to distinguish active disease phases in four forms (mild, moderate, severe, and fulminant) and thus provides important evaluations for prognostic and therapeutic purposes.

The extent of lesions reflects both the intensity of disease and the presence of systemic symptoms (the greater the extension, the more severe are diarrhoea and bleeding, possible dehydration and possible hydroelectrolytic disorders, including serious ones).

Table 25.1 Severity Index of UC (Truelove & Witts criteria, partially modified).

Mild Colitis	Moderate Colitis	Severe Colitis	Fulminant Colitis
<4 bowel movements/day	4-6 bowel movements/day	>6 bowel movements/day	>10 bowel movements/day
Infrequent bleeding	Moderate bleeding	Frequent bleeding	Abundant bleeding
Normal Hb	Normal Hb	<75% of normal Hb	The need of blood transfusion
Normal ESR	≤30	>30	>30
Normal Temperature		Normale/Elevated Temperature	Elevated Temperature
Normal Heart Rate		Normal/Elevated Heart Rate	Elevated Heart Rate

DIAGNOSIS

When UC manifests with highly characteristic features, it is easy to consider a specific set of diagnostic tests. However, diagnostic delay is possible and can be partially justified by the more elusive types of presentation that can be confused with other conditions (haemorrhoidal bleeding).

Laboratory Exams

Traditionally, the most commonly used laboratory tests include complete blood count, which can disclose anemia (usually hypochromic and microcytic), which is attributable to the lack of iron due to chronic iron-loss or linked to chronic inflammation. Anemia can be so severe as to require blood transfusions.

Elevation of inflammation markers (ESR, C-reactive protein, and α-1 acid glycoprotein), thrombocytosis and leukocytosis are infrequent and, if present, are often associated with more severe and /or more extensive phases of illness. In order to exclude clinical manifestations caused by an infection or a parasitic infestation of the intestine, it is necessary to perform coproculture and parasitological examination of feces; for the latter, at least 3 samples are needed to increase sensitivity. Recently, a high prevalence of fecal positivity for *Clostridium difficile* and/or mucosal cytomegalovirus infection (CMV) has been reported in acute phases of the disease; however, the precise role of these infections, whether precipitating or aggravating factors, has not been clarified yet.Nevertheless, their specific search (associated with CMV in the blood) is necessary because findings may eventually result in important changes in treatment. In recent years, laboratory tests have been developed to measure the fecal excretion of specific proteins that are markers of local inflammation (calprotectin*, lactoferrin). These tests have high predictivity in differentiating organic disease from a functional disorder and a good predictive value of recurrence in patients with UC in remission.

Endoscopic Imaging

Ileocolonoscopy is the cornerstone examination in the diagnosis of UC. Even if no pathognomonic endoscopic lesions are found, some are considered highly indicative in differential diagnosis and other clinical forms with similar presentation (**Table 25.2**), with sensitivity and specificity higher than 90% (**Figure 25.2**).

Colonoscopy also allows evaluation of the extent and activity of disease, thus providing useful parameters for instituting appropriate therapy. It also provides biopsy samples for histological evaluation to confirm the diagnosis (see Table 25.2, Figure 25.1). Evaluation of the terminal ileum (retrograde ileoscopy) should be performed in all patients to exclude CD.

Furthermore, in severe colitis, careful endoscopic examination, limited to the distal segments and with low air insufflation, is also useful for prognostic purposes, since some findings, such as denudation of the colonic mucosa and the presence of deep ulcerations, are associated with an increased risk of surgical intervention.

Radiological Imaging

Contrast-free radiological examination of the abdomen is useful in patients with severe disease to evaluate signs of perforation (free air in the peritoneum), gaseous distension of the colon (toxic megacolon) or other warning signs of a negative evolution (for example, gaseous distension of loops of the small bowel). The double-contrast barium enema examination, once a cornerstone in the diagnosis of UC, is no longer used, while the diagnostic effectiveness of other radiological examinations (colon-MRI, colon-CT) is still under study, although none of these can, at the moment, replace colonoscopy with biopsies.

NATURAL HISTORY, DISEASE COURSE, AND COMPLICATIONS

After resolution of the onset episode of UC, the natural evolution of the disease is characterized by recurring episodes of acute inflammation, or flare-ups, with reappearance of symptoms may be absent, in which there may be a total disappearance of signs and symptoms. Today's therapies generally allow control of acute flare-ups and maintenance of clinical remission.

In a smaller percentage of patients (10 to 20%) the disease has, a chronically active course in which periods of remission are absent or may be achieved with pharmacotherapy but not maintained

* Fecal calprotectin, a protein derived from neutrophils degranulation, currently appears to be the most sensitive marker of intestinal inflammation. It correlates well with endoscopic indexes of disease activity and, therefore, is useful for facilitating initial diagnosis and for monitoring disease activity and response to treatment.

Table 25.2 Endoscopic and histological features in the differential diagnosis of UC (see also Figure 25.2)

	Endoscopy	Histology
Ulcerative colitis	Proximal extent from the rectum; diffusely edematous colonic mucosa; hyperaemia; friability; erosions, superficial ulcerations; sometimes spontaneous bleeding	Widespread architectural alterations in colonic mucosa, acute and chronic inflammation of colonic mucosa; mucin depletion; frequent crypt abscesses;architectural distortion and atrophy of crypts
Crohn's disease	Segmental inflammation; ulcerations (often deep); stenosis; ileus usually involved	Focal architectural alterations; transmural inflammation, with possible granulomas; possible presence of crypt abscesses
Ischaemic colitis	Often involving the splenic flexure and descendant colon; rarely present in the rectum	Mucosal necrosis; capillary swelling; fibrosis (if chronic)
Collagenous colitis	Normal	Subepithelial collagen band with thickness >10 μ; Chronic inflammation of the lamina propria
Lymphocytic colitis	Normal	Chronic inflammation of the lamina propria, with increased intraepithelial lymphocytes >20%
Infectious colitis	Variable	Predominantly neutrophil infiltrate; crypt abscesses present, though without crypt distortion
Pseudomembranous colitis	Edema; yellow-whitish plaques attached to the mucosa	Similar to ischaemic colitis; fibrinous and purulent exudates
Amoebic colitis	Focal ulcers; stenosis	Similar to ulcerative colitis; amoebe noticeable with Schiff colouring
Radiation colitis	Multiple telangiectatic lesions, especially in the rectum and sigma	Vasculitis, widespread collagen, fibrosis deposition
Gonococcal proctitis	Granularity and nodularity of the rectal mucosa	Intense neutrophil infiltrate; Gram + bacteria

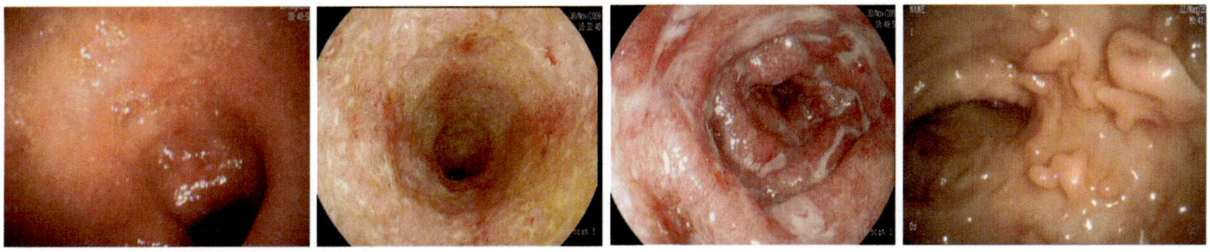

Figure 25.2 Endoscopic appearance of UC with mild (a), moderate (b), severe (c) activity, or in remission with pseudopolyps (d)*.
a) diffuse mucosal edema with loss of vascular pattern, granularity, mild erythaema, minor erosions.
b) More intense edema and erythaema, granularity, diffuse erosions
c) Ulcers, erythaema, nodularity, spontaneous bleeding
d) Mucosal atrophy with reduction of vascular pattern, no signs of active inflammation, pseudopolyps

* Mayo endoscopic score: 1) Mild activity: mild erythaema, reduced vascular pattern, mild mucosal friability 2) Moderate activity: marked erythaema, absence of vascular design, moderate mucosal friability, erosions 3) Severe activity: spontaneous bleeding,

for long periods (e.g., steroids). In a very small percentage of patients, however, after the initial phase of acute inflammation, further relapses are no longer observed and signs of disease seem to disappear: it is possible that, in these patients, there may be other forms of colitis– most probably acute self-limited colitis. In patients with a typical disease pattern, subsequent flare-ups, which may be similar to those observed during the onset episode, have the same degree of severity generally proportional to the extent and severity of organ involvement.
Rectal bleeding is the hallmark symptom of the disease. In some cases, bleeding can be so intense as to become a true emergency in patient management, requiring repeated blood transfusions - or even - emergency surgery.
Relapses can usually be prevented and controlled with medical therapy, however, in about 15% of cases the disease becomes severe and requires intensive or semi-intensive medical management. In such cases, it is important to exclude the presence of a concurrent *Clostridium difficile* or cytomegalovirus infection.
Fulminant colitis is a particularly severe flare-up of the disease and manifests with bloody diarrhoea, abdominal pain, and fever (Table 25.1); this type of colitis is present in 1-2% of patients with UC. Signs of systemic sepsis with tachycardia, hypotension, and leukocytosis are common. Standard first-line medical treatment includes administration of fluids and intravenous steroids, if there are no signs of peritonitis.
A contrast-free radiograph of the abdomen is necessary to rule out perforation or toxic megacolon. Toxic megacolon manifests as an acute gaseous dilatation of a part of the colon, usually the transverse colon (diameter >6cm), evaluated by computed tomography of the abdomen. It is associated with signs of systemic toxicity and its incidence varies between 2% and 7%. Hypokalemia, anti-diarrhoeal therapy, colonoscopy or barium enema are risk factors for toxic megacolon.
Patients require close clinical and radiological monitoring, as well as aggressive medical therapy, due to the high risk of perforation. If improvement in 24-48 hours is not achieved or if there is clinical deterioration or if signs of perforation appear, emergency surgery is necessary. Perforation, which can occur even in the absence of toxic megacolon, increases the risk of mortality from 4 to 40%. About a third of patients with UC have extra-intestinal manifestations (**Table 25.3**). Many, in particular cutaneous and ocular manifestations are often related to disease activity and tend to improve during periods of remission.
Conversely, there is no change in the natural history of ankylosing spondylitis or sclerosing cholangitis in relation to intestinal inflammation or following colectomy. Both conditions are, however, extremely demanding for the patient because the first can cause serious functional limitations to the spinal column, while the latter can evolve into cirrhosis of the liver, and further into cholangiocarcinoma.
UC is a risk factor for the development of colorectal cancer. The risk depends on the duration and extent of disease, but also on other factors including family history of colorectal neoplasia, co-existence of primary sclerosing cholangitis, and persistence of disease activity.
In specialist centers treating more severe patients, the risk at 20 years after onset of disease varies from 10 to 20% and increases by 1-2% each year that follows. However, population studies indicate far less relevant data. Colonoscopy surveillance in cancer

Table 25.3 Extra-intestinal manifestations commonly associated with UC.

Organ	Complication	Related to Disease Activity
Liver	Steatosis	Yes
	Sclerosing cholangitis	No
Skin	Erythema nodosum	Yes
	Pyoderma gangrenosum	Yes
Joints	Peripheral arthritis	+
	Axial Spondiloarthropathy	No
Eye	Episcleritis, uveitis	Yes

prevention identifies mucosal dysplasia or a neoplasm at an early stage. Since dysplasia usually occurs 7 to 10 years after disease onset, endoscopic surveillance should be initiated from that time and continued at intervals from 1 to 3 years, in relation to the patient's cancer risk. In this context, multiple and random biopsies should be taken (4 radial biopsies from every 10 cm of the colon), in addition to biopsy of evident mucosal lesions.

Enhanced endoscopy techniques for targeted biopsy sampling such as chromoendoscopy, autofluorescence, and confocal laser endomicroscopy are becoming widespread. The histological diagnosis of dysplasia is not always easy, especially in the presence of acute inflammation, because of the difficulty in differentiating dysplasia from mucosal variations due to inflammation. Biopsy samples should be classified as: negative, undefined for dysplasia, low-grade dysplasia, and high-grade dysplasia. When high-grade dysplasia is confirmed, colon resection is indicated. The presence of low-grade dysplasia or an undefined specimen for dysplasia necessitates surveillance at short intervals.

MEDICAL THERAPY

Medical therapy of UC is mainly aimed at:

- control and regression of inflammation during flare-ups (acute phase therapy);
- maintainence of remission (maintenance therapy).

In recent decades, there has been much progress in therapeutic options for the medical treatment of UC.

From a practical point of view, it can be very useful to identify the stage of severity of UC (mild, moderate, and severe) according to the Truelove and Witts severity index, which was later modified to include the most severe form, fulminant (Table 25.1). In addition to clinical activity of the disease, the therapeutic approach to UC is also guided by the extent of disease, which is an important factor to consider when deciding which drug and/or which drug formulation may be the most appropriate for the individual patient.

Mild-to-Moderate Flares

Mild-to-moderate forms of UC do not require hospitalisation; aminosalicylates are the first choice of drugs for their documented efficacy and low probability of side effects. Among aminosalicylates, mesalazine is the most widely used.

The various formulations of oral mesalazine are able, albeit in different ways, to transport the active drug to the colon, where it exerts its therapeutic activity in contact with the colonic mucosa. These preparations, when used >3 g/day, induce clinical remission in 40-60% of patients in 4-8 weeks. In addition to oral controlled release formulations, a variety of other preparations of mesalazine for rectal use (suppositories, enemas, gels and foams) have been developed. Mesalazine in the form of suppositories is particularly effective in proctitis, while enemas, gels, and foams induce remission after 6-8 weeks of treatment in 70-80% of patients with mild-to-moderate flares of UC that do not extend beyond the sigmoid colon. When the extent of the disease exceeds the sigmoid colon, oral therapy is recommended. Oral and local combination therapy is the most successful treatment.

In patients who do not respond to salicylic therapy, either traditional corticosteroids or the more recently introduced low-bioavailability corticosteroids should be prescribed, both of which can be used in oral and rectal treatments. Initially, topical corticosteroid beclometasone dipropionate (3 mg/day) should be taken in the evening. The combination of topical beclometasone dipropionate and topical aminosalicylates may be more effective than single administration. If topical therapy does not induce remission, physicians should opt for oral treatment with the more recent low-bioavailability corticosteroids (beclometasone dipropionate 5-10 mg/day or MMX-budesonide, 9 mg/day). Alternatively, a full dosage of prednisone (50 mg/day) or methylprednisolone (40 mg/day) for 2-4 weeks should be prescribed, with subsequent gradual tapering. In general, corticosteroid therapy will induce clinical remission in 70-80% of patients. In mild or moderate UC, in which dependence on steroid therapy (steroid-dependent forms) is observed, immunomodulator drugs may be used, particularly azathioprine or 6-mercaptopurine Azathioprine (at a dosage of 2-2.5 mg/kg/day) and 6-mercaptopurine (1-1.5 mg/kg/day) may allow for progressive reduction of steroid doses, up to complete withdrawal, and may extend the remission phase in a high percentage of patients. The potentially long latency of these drugs prevents their use in the steroid-resistant forms. Such patients, but also the steroid-dependent, may respond to monoclonal antibodies that work against TN-

F-α. This therapy consists of induction treatment and subsequent administration for maintenance therapy. The most commonly used drugs are infliximab (intravenous administration) and adalimumab/golimumab (subcutaneous administration).
More recently, a new therapy for steroid dependent or steroid refractory patients with a different target compared to TNF, such as anti-integrin therapy, has been developed. These drugs are needed for the migration of immune cells into inflamed tissues.
Vedolizumab is the new drug with such a mechanism of action*.

Severe Colitis

Incidence of severe episodes of UC is not high and its prevalence is in steady decline due to quicker and more effective therapeutic approaches. In these forms, there is extremely elevated risk of toxic megacolon and worsening of clinical conditions into systemic inflammatory response syndrome (SIRS) and/or multiple organ failure syndrome (MOFS). The specific therapeutic measures to be taken in the severe forms of UC are known as the "Oxford regimen" (**Table 25.4**).
According to the most widely acknowledged criteria, these therapeudic measures should be continued for at least 5 days and, in case of non-response, the patient should be referred for surgery or salvage therapy with monoclonal anti-TNFα or with intravenous cyclosporine.

Table 25.4 Treatment scheme for acute severe colitis (modified version of "Oxford Regimen").

Hospitalisation
Rest
Intensive clinical-instrumental and medical-surgical monitoring
Corticosteroids (intravenous)
Administration of liquids/electrolytes/blood transfusions
Low-residue diet/non-oral nutrition
Low-molecular-weight heparins (LMWH)
Topical therapy (mesalamine/steroids)
Antibiotics (?)

Maintenance Therapy

In general, maintenance therapy is indicated in all UC patients in remission after an acute phase, regardless of the extent of disease. Indeed, it has been shown that continuous oral administration of aminosalicylates, at dosages >1.6 g/day, is able to significantly reduce the risk of relapse as compared with placebo. Topical treatment is very effective in the acute phases of the most distal forms of UC and it has also been proposed as maintenance therapy in such cases, even considering its limits regarding patient compliance.
In patients with proctitis, maintenance therapy with mesalazine suppositories is effective and well tolerated. Maintenance therapy with corticosteroids, even at low bioavailability, should not be considered due to their low efficacy and numerous side effects. In patients with frequent relapses despite amynosalycilates treatment, it is possible to use azathioprine or 6-mercaptopurine. Maintenance therapy with azathioprine or 6-mercaptopurine is also indicated in patients with steroid-dependent forms of UC.
In these patients, maintenance treatment with anti-TNF or Vedolizumab is possible option for maintenance therapy.
In patients with remission induced by anti-TNF therapy or who have been treated for a severe or fulminant attack, it is possible to use azathioprine or an anti-TNF drug as maintenance management therapy.

SURGICAL THERAPY

Approximately 15-20% of patients with UC require surgery due to complications or failure to respond to medical therapy.
The rationale behind surgical treatment of UC is the fact that the disease affects only the colon and the rectum and, therefore, a proctocolectomy is substantially curative.
In summary, the reasons for opting for surgery include: no response to medical treatment; dependence on the use of steroids; need to suspend therapy due to side effects or dysplasia or cancer. In order to optimize surgery outcomes, patients should not undergo surgery if severely malnurished, excessively immunocompromised or weakened by the effects of immunomodulatory therapy.

* At present, a further therapeutic option is Tofacitinib, an inhibitor of Janus Kinases (JAK), proteins that are involved in regulating intracellular transduction of several pro-inflammatory cytokines.

In fact, timely surgical treatment is a predictor of a favorable prognosis. In other circumstances, surgery may urgently be needed due to complications such as toxic megacolon, intestinal bleeding or perforation.

Types of Surgical Procedures

There are various types of procedures to treat UC. The choice of the type of intervention for each individual patient depends on an appropriate balance between the patient's history, intestinal function, and residual disease.

Proctocolectomyileal-Anal Pouch

This is the most widely used surgical procedure today and involves resection of the colon and rectum, with the creation of a pouch made out of the last piece of the ileum (small intestine) that is attached to the anal canal (ileal pouch-anal anastomosis - IPAA).

The operation can be performed in two stages: the first is the proctocolectomy, the preparation of the pouch and the ileo-anal anastomosis, with the creation of an exclusionary ileostomy. The second stage takes place a few months later and involves closing of the ileostomy. In the most acute cases, it should be performed in three stages (colectomy, proctectomy, recanalization). The procedure can be performed in laparoscopy, which has been used with increasing frequency because associated with less post-operative pain, shorter hospitalisation time, faster patient recovery, and better aesthetic results. The most common complication is pelvic sepsis, which occurs in 5-8% of patients. Risk factors include poor nutritional status and immunosuppressive treatment. Anastomotic dehiscence is the most frequent cause of failure, while patient mortality is less than 1%.

After the operation, the frequency of evacuations is 4-6 in the following 24 hours; daytime incontinence is exceptional, while night incontinence, which is generally modest, is relatively frequent. Some patients need to use a protective diaper while sleeping.

The use of antidiarrhoeal drugs is frequent and ranges from 50-75%, however, their use is reduced to 25-30% of cases after one year. During the first year, bowel adaptation occurs with an increase in the capacity of the pouch, which ensures a better functional result. Surgery reduces female fertility but does not compromise the possibility of pregnancy.

Quality of life is better than in patients undergoing terminal ileostomy and also compared to those with active colitis. Ten years after surgery, removal of the pouch is necessary in 2-9% of cases. The most significant long-term complication is pouchitis. Clinically, it is characterized by increased bowel frequency associated with haematochezia, abdominal cramps, and fever.

The aetiology of pouchitis is unknown; it is believed to be the result of an immune response to an alteration in bacterial flora. The diagnosis is made by endoscopy, which indicates an ulcerative inflammation of the ileal mucosa, with varying degrees of severity. It is estimated that the incidence of pouchitis is 15% at one year, 36% at 5 years, and 46% at 10 years after the operation. Pouchitis usually responds to treatment with antibiotics, and the need to remove the pouch entirely occurs only in a few cases.

Colectomy with Ileorectal Anastomosis

Colectomy with ileum-rectal anastomosis consists in removing the colon, while preserving the rectum and intestinal transit with colorectal anastomosis.

It is indicated in cases in which the rectum presents a disease in a phase of mild activity or if differential diagnosis with Crohn's colitis is doubtful, or if the patient is of childbearing age to avoid any complications that prevent pregnancy, or, if anatomical features make the preparation of the pouch impractical.

The operation is performed in a single procedure and without the need for a protective stoma, and it guarantees good intestinal functioning if the disease in the rectum is in remission. It is not recommended in the presence of active proctitis or rectal dysplasia. Long-term complications include recurrence of disease activity in the residual rectum and rectal cancer, for which endoscopic surveillance is necessary.

Proctocolectomy with Ileostomy

This procedure involves surgical removal of the colon, rectum, and anus, with the creation of a permanent ileostomy.

It is recommended in patients who are not eligible for reconstructive treatment (neither of the two types of surgery described above) or in reoperation due to failure of restorative proctocolectomy (see above).

Emergency Surgery

Fulminant/UC and toxic megacolon may require urgent surgical intervention. In this case, a three-stage procedure is recommended.

KEY CONCEPTS

- Ulcerative Colitis (UC) is a chronic inflammatory disease of the colon of unknown aetiology.
- The lesions in ulcerative rectocolitis are limited to the rectum-colon, involving the rectum in all patients, but potentially extending proximally to the cecum. Inflammation limited to the mucosa, continuity of lesions, and involvement of the rectum are typical of the disease.
- The course of ulcerative rectocolitis is generally intermittent chronic, with acute phases interspersed with periods of clinical quiescence.
- The constant sign of acute phases is the loss of bright red blood alone or mixed with feces, often accompanied by rectal tenesmus; in more limited cases (proctitis) these may be the only signs of disease. When inflammation is more extensive, abdominal pain, fever, tachycardia, anemia, and dehydration may also occur.
- Medical therapy is generally able to reverse symptoms in active phases and to maintain the remission phases for a long time.
- Nevertheless, 20% of patients undergo surgical therapy, usually due to non-response to medical therapy for acute complications or the onset of colorectal neoplasia. Surgery entails removing the colon and, in most cases, the rectum.

REFERENCES

- Choi CH, Rutter MD, Askari A, et al. Forty-year analysis of colonoscopic surveillance program for neoplasia in ulcerative colitis: an updated overview. Am J Gastroenterol. 2015 Jul;110(7):1022-34.
- Harbord M, Eliakim R, Bettenworth D, et al. Third European evidence-based consensus on the diagnosis and management of ulcerative colitis. Part 2: Current management. J Crohn Colitis. 2017:1-24.
- Maaser C, Sturm A, Vavricka SR, et al.; European Crohn's and Colitis Organisation [ECCO] and the European Society of Gastrointestinal and Abdominal Radiology [ESGAR]. ECCO-ESGAR Guideline for Diagnostic Assessment in IBD Part 1: Initial diagnosis, monitoring of known IBD, detection of complications. J Crohns Colitis. 2019;13(2):144-64.
- Magro F, Gionchetti P, Eliakim R, et al. Third European evidence-based consensus on the diagnosis and management of ulcerative colitis. Part 1: Diagnosis, Extra-intestinal Manifestations, Pregnancy, Cancer Surveillance, Surgery, and Ileo-anal Pouch Disorders. J Crohn Colitis. 2017:1-39.
- Sturm A, Maaser C, Calabrese E, et al.; European Crohn's and Colitis Organisation [ECCO] and the European Society of Gastrointestinal and Abdominal Radiology [ESGAR]. ECCO-ESGAR Guideline for Diagnostic Assessment in IBD Part 2: IBD scores and general principles and technical aspects. J Crohns Colitis. 2019;13(3):273-84.
- Ungaro R, Mehandru S, Allen PB, Peyrin-Biroulet L, Colombel JF. Ulcerative colitis. Lancet. 2017;389(10080):1756-70.

OTHER INFLAMMATORY COLITIS

Walter Fries, Angelo Viscido

LEARNING OBJECTIVE

- To know other forms of inflammatory colitis, their epidemiology, clinical presentation, principle diagnostic criteria, and basics of therapy.

The 'other inflammatory colitis' include all pathologies that cause diarrhoea due to an inflammatory process of the colon, but distinct from that of the classical entities like ulcerative colitis or Crohn's disease including the inflammatory bowel disease undefined (IBDU). Due to their aetiology, they may be classified as idiopathic and secondary.
Among the idiopathic diseases, there are the acute self-limiting colitis (ASLC) and the (primary) microscopic colitis. The ASLC may be considered an infectious colitis if the identification of an infectious agent remains unsuccessful.
Secondary colitis comprise the colitis associated to diverticula (SCAD), diversion colitis, actinic or radiation-induced colitis, and ischaemic colitis.
Among all these other inflammatory colitis, the most frequent in the general population are the microscopic colitis. Recent epidemiologic studies have revealed that their incidence is close to that of classical inflammatory bowel diseases. They represent the most frequent finding in patients aged over 50 years that undergo colonoscopic evaluation for chronic unbloody diarrhoea.

MICROSCOPIC COLITIS

The microscopic colitis is characterized by the presence of chronic or recurrent watery diarrhoea (without blood) with normal appearing colonic mucosa at colonoscopy. Histologic examination reveals an inflammatory process limited to the mucosa. The absence of macroscopic lesions has conferred the denomination of this pathology. Other investigations, like radiology, do not reveal any alteration. Diagnosis is based on the clinical picture and on histologic examination. There are two main forms of microscopic colitis: the lymphocytic colitis and the collagenous colitis. Their description is quite recent and diagnostic criteria have been established and validated in 1989.

Histopathology

The diagnosis of microscopic colitis is based on microscopic examination.
Typical histologic lesions of the microscopic colitis, especially that of collagenous colitis, are present in the ascending colon and may be absent in the descending and sigmoid colon, and rectum. For this reason, biopsies should be performed also on the right colon.
Lymphocytic colitis is characterised by (**Figures 26.1, 26.2**):

1. an increase of intraepithelial lymphocytes within the colonic epithelium (≥20 lymphocytes per 100 epithelial cells);
2. a chronic inflammatory infiltration of the lamina propria;
3. a basement membrane with normal thickness (around 3 μm);
4. a conserved glandular architecture (there may be a mild damage of the epithelium that may present with areas of degeneration or detachment).

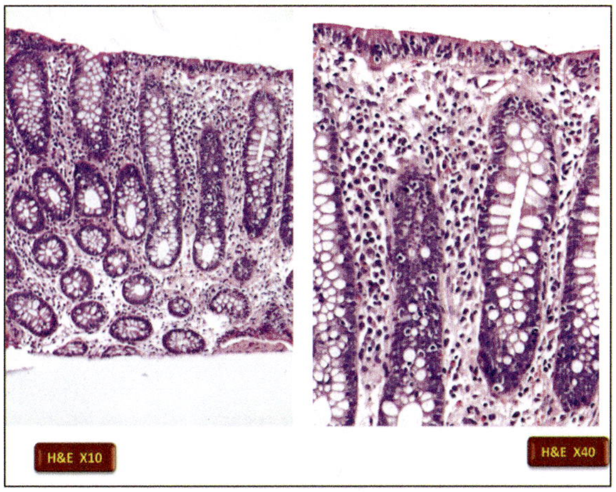

Figure 26.1 Lymphocytic colitis. Haematoxylin-Eosin stain (H&E). Two different magnifications (x10 on the left, and x40 on the right) demonstrate the increase of intraepithelial lymphocytes within the colonic epithelium, a chronic inflammatory infiltration of the lamina propria, a conserved glandular architecture, a basement membrane with normal thickness (around 3 μm).

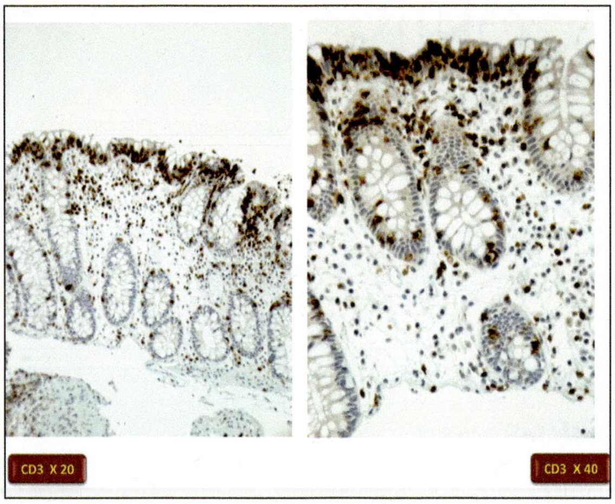

Figure 26.2 Lymphocytic colitis. Immunohistochemistry by anti-CD3 antibodies (T-cells co-receptor). Staining indicates T lymphocytes.

Collagenous colitis is characterised by (**Figure 26.3**):

1. thickening of subepithelial collagenous layer ≥10 μm;
2. chronic inflammatory infiltrate of the lamina propria;
3. conserved glandular architecture (there may be a mild damage of the epithelium that may present with areas of degeneration or detachment).

The increased thickness of collagenous fibres may be continuous or patchy.

In normal conditions, the basement membrane is constituted by type IV collagenous fibres, laminin and fibronectin. In case of collagenous colitis, the basement membrane is composed by type VI collagen and tenascin, variants produced during tissue repair mechanisms. The increased thickness of the basement membrane may thus be a reactive process due to inflammation.

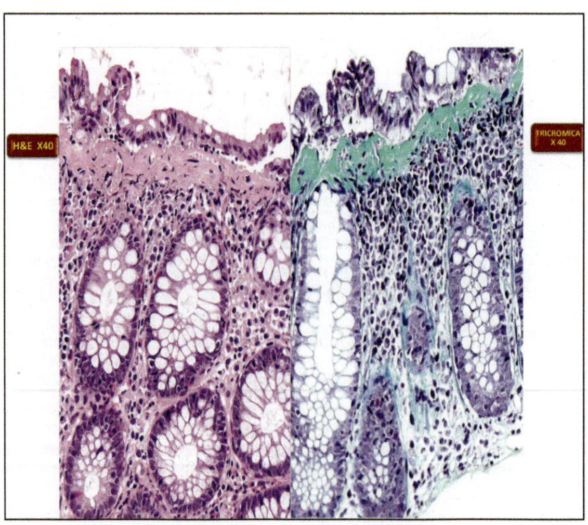

Figure 26.3 Collagenous colitis. Haematoxylin-Eosin stain (H&E) on the left. Trichrome staining on the right. Both demonstrate thickening of subepithelial collagenous layer ≥10μm (more evident by trichrome staining), chronic inflammatory infiltrate of the lamina propria, conserved glandular architecture.

Epidemiology

Microscopic colitis is rather frequent, in fact, it is diagnosed in 10-20% of patients who undergo colonoscopy for chronic or recurrent unbloody diarrhoea. Population studies report a variable incidence rate of 1 to 12 new cases per 100,000 persons/year with the mildly higher prevalence of lymphocytic colitis. Frequency is similar between Europe and North America. Prevalence ranges from 123/100,000 (Sweden, 2008) up to 219/100,000 (USA, 2010) for both forms.

The incidence rates of microscopic colitis are constantly and rapidly increasing over the past years, maybe due to the more frequent use of routine biopsies also on apparently normal colon mucosa. Mean age at diagnosis is over 50 years of age (between 53 and 69 years) and a Canadian study has revealed that people of over 65 years of age have a fivefold risk compared to younger people. However, every age may be affected by these pathologies. The frequency of microscopic colitis is higher in females with a 3:1 ratio with respect to males.

Aetiology and Pathogenesis

The diagnosis of microscopic colitis relies on microscopic morphology and thus, it is likely the same term may be used in forms with different aetiology. For this reason, it has been proposed to distinguish primary and secondary microscopic colitis. The idiopathic form is considered by some researchers a subtype of inflammatory bowel disease. The aetiology of primary microscopic colitis is unknown and most likely multifactorial. The most studied factors are:

Genetic susceptibility. Familiarity with microscopic colitis has rarely been described. Relatives affected by inflammatory bowel disease have been reported in 12% of patients with microscopic colitis. An association with HLA-DQ and with single nucleotide polymorphisms (SNP) of genes encoding tumour necrosis factor-α (TNF-α) and metalloproteinase-9 (MMP-9) have been reported.

Hormonal factors. The higher prevalence in females has led to suggest a role for hormonal factors. Oestrogens and progesterone do have a protective effect on the intestinal barrier in experimental models. The reduction of these hormonal levels with ageing may, therefore, favour the occurrence of this form of colitis.

Immune factors. The association of microscopic colitis with many autoimmune diseases such as coeliac disease, thyroiditis, rheumatoid arthritis, and diabetes has led to the hypothesis that lymphocytic and collagenous colitis may belong to the autoimmune diseases. Their prevalence in middle-aged women has strengthened this hypothesis.

Luminal factors. It has been observed that the exclusion of intestinal transit by means of an ostomy induces the regression of the histologic alterations of microscopic colitis.

Drugs. Some drugs, such as non-steroidal anti-inflammatory drugs, proton pump inhibitors, antidepressants and antipsychotic, have been implicated in the development of microscopic colitis.

Clinical Presentation

Symptom onset may occur at every age, although it is observed more often in women over 50 years of age. The predominant symptom is watery diarrhoea. Frequently, abdominal pain and weight loss are associated. In the majority of cases, diagnosis is made various years after symptom onset. The natural course of the disease is chronic and frequently characterized by an alternation of clinical flares and remission. The inflammatory-type diarrhoea depends in its severity on the intensity of the inflammatory infiltrate in the colon mucosa. Although microscopic colitis negatively impacts on the quality of life, the natural history seems to be benign. An anti-diarrhoeal based therapy together with anti-inflammatory (mesalazine) drugs are generally efficacious. Intestinal or general complications are rare and the risk of colorectal cancer seems not to be increased in these diseases.

Therapy

Therapy is not different between the two histologic entities. Therapy of secondary forms due to some categories of drugs is based on treatment interruption of the drug suspected to be the cause of colitis.

Aims of the therapies are to (1) induce and to (2) maintain clinical remission. The symptom diarrhoea is the main cause of complaint and therefore first-line treatments target this symptom using anti-diarrhoeal drugs like loperamide. The only drug tested in a randomized clinical trial is represented by budesonide, a new generation steroid with a rapid first-pass metabolism in the liver. Withdrawal of this drug, however, is followed by recurrence of symptoms in many patients (60-80%). Prolonged administration of low-dose budesonide may maintain prolonged remission.

Diversion Colitis

Diversion colitis is an inflammatory process that develops in a segment of the colon surgically excluded from intestinal transit by means of ileostomy or colostomy. Endoscopic evaluation of the excluded colon may reveal any grade of inflammation up to ulcerations. Histologic examination shows the presence of an inflammatory infiltrates with conservation of crypt architecture. Topical administration of short-chain fatty acids (SCFA) is efficacious because these fatty acid represent the main fuel for colonocytes. Definitive therapy is based on surgical recanalization.

Segmental Colitis Associated with Diverticulosis (SCAD)

No epidemiologic data are available on this entity. It represents a non-specific form of colitis that remains confined to the area involved by diverticula. By endoscopy, SCAD may present with areas with erythaema and friability of the mucosa around the diverticular orifices. Sometimes a more diffuse pattern may be present but always limited to intestinal segments bearing diverticula. Typically the rectum and proximal segments to diverticula are spared. The clinical picture is characterized by diarrhoea with mucus and blood with or without abdominal pain. This entity is more frequent in males over 50 years of age. Histology is non-specific (**Figure 26.4**). Normally, inflammation is self-limiting but may require therapy with mesalazine or steroids. Only in refractory cases, a surgical option may be required.

Ischaemic Colitis (IC)

It represents an entity with very scant epidemiologic data. Generally, it involves subjects over 60 years of age with a higher frequency in females. Risk factors are represented by vascular surgery

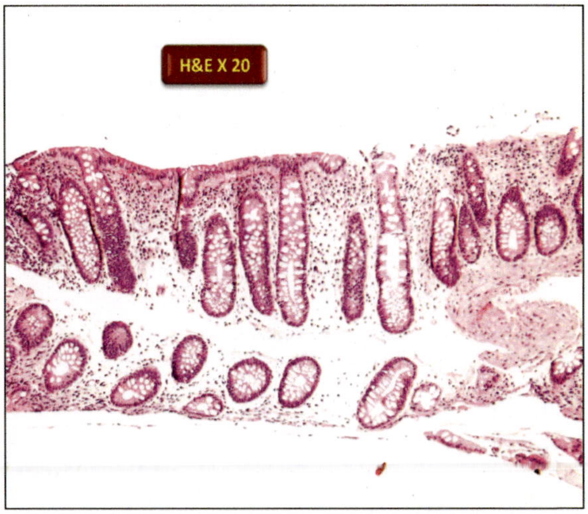

Figure 26.4 Segmental Colitis Associated with Diverticulosis (SCAD). Haematoxylin-Eosin stain (H&E). It is evident an inflammatory infiltrate of both epithelium and lamina propria, with conserved glandular architecture. Epithelial damage is also present.

(e.g., surgery for abdominal aortic aneurysms) or by cardiac failure con sudden reduction of the cardiac output.

In younger subjects, IC is associated with vasculitis, thrombophilia, or the use of drugs (agonists or antagonists of serotonin and its receptors, oestrogens) or drug abuse (cocaine, methamphetamines).

A classification distinguishes the non-gangrenous forms (reversible, transitory, ulcerative ischaemic colitis, ischaemic stenosis) that represent 80-85% of cases from the gangrenous form and the fulminating ischaemic colitis.

A segmental pattern is frequent with the left colon being the most frequently involved part of the colon in 75% of patients (descending and sigmoid colon). Less frequent is an isolated location at the right colon (10-25%) or the splenic flexure. The rectum is always spared.

Diagnosis is based on plain abdominal X-Ray film (in order to exclude perforations), CT-scan evaluation in order to exclude thromboembolism, and proctosigmoidoscopy. The endoscopic findings depend on severity and timing. Initially, there may be present submucosal bleeding spots that may re-absorb within 48 h or evolve in ulcerations. Typical diagnostic features are the segmental location with a longitudinal ulcerated stripe. Examination with Doppler-ultrasonography may be helpful to put in evidence a reduced or absent blood flow in the colon wall. Laboratory investigations include the white blood cell count, inflammatory parameters, lactate-dehydrogenase, lactate, and creatine phosphokinase.

The clinical picture is variable comprising a transitory colitis, forms resembling ulcerative colitis, up to fulminating colitis. Symptoms consequently may vary from crampy abdominal pain with or without faecal urgency to bloody diarrhoea or frank rectal bleeding, or acute abdomen.

Actinic Colitis/Proctitis

Actinic proctitis develops in subjects that underwent radiotherapy for gynecologic, urologic, or rectal tumours. Around 75% of patients will develop rectal symptoms during radiotherapy and in 20% of those patients, the situation will evolve into chronic proctitis. In most severe cases, perianal fistulas, stenosis or faecal incontinence may occur. The clinical picture is represented by urgency, pelvic pain, and poorly formed stools mixed with mucus and blood. On histology, the acute phase is characterized by colonocytes with giant nuclei, fibroblastic proliferation, and absence of mitotic activity, whereas in the chronic phase vascular alterations and platelet thrombi are present always accompanied by fibrosis of the lamina propria end crypt distortion. Therapy is based on the topical administration of mesalazine and/or steroids.

Drug-Induced Colitis

Diagnosis of drug-induced colitis or entero-colitis is based on an accurate investigation of patients' drug history. Among the most common pharmacological agents leading to colon inflammation are non-steroidal anti-inflammatory drugs (NSAIDs), bisacodyl, carbamazepine, statins, isotretinoin, and some chemical drugs etc. Histologic examination is non-specific showing frequently an abundant eosinophilic infiltrate while therapy is based on individuation and withdrawal of the responsible agent.

More severe clinical scenarios may be provoked by some new anti-tumour agents, the checkpoint inhibitors, monoclonal agents stimulating the anti-tumour immune response. Among these are the anti-cytotoxic T-lymphocyte–associated antigen-4 (CTLA-4), programmed cell death 1 (PD1), and anti–programmed death-ligand 1 (PD-L1). Gastrointestinal adverse reactions range from simple diarrhoea (10-20%) to severe colitis (around 1%).

Histologic examination reveals acute colitis with crypt abscesses and glandular aggression. Besides a rich neutrophil infiltrate there are CD-8 positive lymphocytes. Based on clinical and endoscopic features, several grades of severity determine treatments ranging from anti-diarrhoeal drugs (grade 1), high dose systemic steroids (grade 2), or biotechnologic agents, e.g., anti-TNFs (grade 3); in some extremely severe cases colectomy may be indicated.

KEY CONCEPTS

- Besides the classic forms of inflammatory bowel diseases, there are other diseases that cause diarrhoea characterized by an inflammatory process of the colon. These conditions are referred to as "other inflammatory colitis".
- Microscopic colitis is characterized by the chronic or recurrent presence of watery diarrhoea (without blood) and normal colon mucosa at endoscopy; on histological examination there is an inflammatory process located at the mucosa level.
- Microscopic colitis has an incidence similar to that of classical intestinal inflammatory diseases. It is the most frequent diagnosis in people over 50 undergoing colonoscopy for chronic diarrhoea without blood.
- Diversion colitis consists of an inflammatory process that develops in the mucosa of a tract of the colon that has been excluded from intestinal transit following an ileostomy or colostomy. It regresses after surgical recanalization surgery.
- Segmental colitis associated with diverticulosis (SCAD) is a non-specific form of colitis that involves the colon mucosa involved in diverticula.
- Ischaemic colitis is caused by reduction of blood flow to the intestine due to vascular surgery, heart failure with sudden reduction of cardiac output, vasculitis, thrombophilic diathesis, or drugs.
- Actinic colitis occurs in patients undergoing radiation therapy for gynecological, urological or rectal neoplasms.

REFERENCES

- Boland K, Nguyen GC. Microscopic Colitis: A review of collagenous and lymphocytic colitis. Gastroenterol Hepatol. 2017;13:671-77.
- Pardi DS. Diagnosis and management of microscopic colitis. Am J Gastroenterol 2017; 112:78-85.
- Miehlke S, Guagnozzi D, Zabana Y, et al. European guidelines on microscopic colitis: United European Gastroenterology and European Microscopic Colitis Group statements and recommendations. United European Gastroenterol J. 2021;9:13-37.
- Tong J, Zheng Q, Zhang C, Lo R, Shen J, Ran Z. Incidence, prevalence, and temporal trends of microscopic colitis: a systematic review and meta-analysis. Am J Gastroenterol 2015;110:265-76.
- Verhaegh BPM, Münch A, Guagnozzi D, et al. Course of Disease in Patients with Microscopic Colitis: A European Prospective Incident Cohort Study. J Crohns Colitis. 2021;15:1174-83.
- Olsen LM, Engel PJH, Goudkade D, et al. Histological disease activity in patients with microscopic colitis is not related to clinical disease activity or long-term prognosis. Aliment Pharmacol Ther 2021;54:43-52.
- Chande N, Al Yatama N, Bhanji T, Nguyen TM, McDonald JW, MacDonald JK. Interventions for treating lymphocytic colitis. Cochrane Database Syst Rev 2017;7: CD006096.
- Kafil TS, Nguyen TM, Patton PH, MacDonald JK, Chande N, McDonald JW. Interventions for treating collagenous colitis. Cochrane Database Syst Rev. 2017;11: CD003575.
- Sebastian S, Wilhelm A, Jessica L, Myers S, Veysey M. Budesonide treatment for microscopic colitis: systematic review and meta-analysis. Eur J Gastroenterol Hepatol. 2019;31:919-27.
- Collins M, Soularue E, Marthey L, Carbonnel F. Management of Patients With Immune Checkpoint Inhibitor-Induced Enterocolitis: A Systematic Review. Clin Gastroenterol Hepatol. 2020;18:1393-1403.

LIVER FUNCTION AND MECHANISMS OF ACUTE AND CHRONIC HEPATIC INJURY

Ludovico Abenavoli Montebianco, Leonardo Baiocchi

LEARNING OBJECTIVES

- To know the anatomy of the liver.
- To know the physiology of liver function.
- To know the mechanisms of acute and chronic hepatic injury.
- To know the pathophysiology of non-cholestatic hepatic injury.

ANATOMY OF THE LIVER

The liver is the largest gland in the human body. Its weight range is 1.2-1.5 kg. It has two surfaces, an anterior-posterior or diaphragmatic surface and a postero-inferior or visceral surface. Hepatic blood inflow is via the hepatic artery and the portal vein, while outflow is sustained by the hepatic veins, which converge in the inferior vena cava.
The hepatic parenchyma is organized in lobules, in the form of a polygonal pyramid with a tapered apex 1 mm in diameter and a height of about 1.5-2 mm, delimited by connective tissue (**Figure 27.1**). Each lobule consists of laminae formed by a single layer of hepatocytes. The laminae are perforated and anastomosed to each other, thus delimiting the hepatic sinusoids. The center of the lobule is occupied by the central vein, a tributary of the hepatic vein, in which the sinusoids converge. The area where three or more adjacent lobules come into contact with a stellate aspect is the portal tract. The inter-lobular branches of the portal vein, the hepatic artery, and the bile duct (together forming the portal triad) are located in the portal tract. The functional unit of the liver is the Rappaport acinus. The acinus is an area of parenchyma located between two central veins. At the periphery the acinus incorporates part of the portal tract. In the acinus three zones are recognized according to the distance from the nutritive vessels. Zone 1 contains the maximum blood supply, while zone 3, the most peripheral one, is more affected by ischaemic damage.

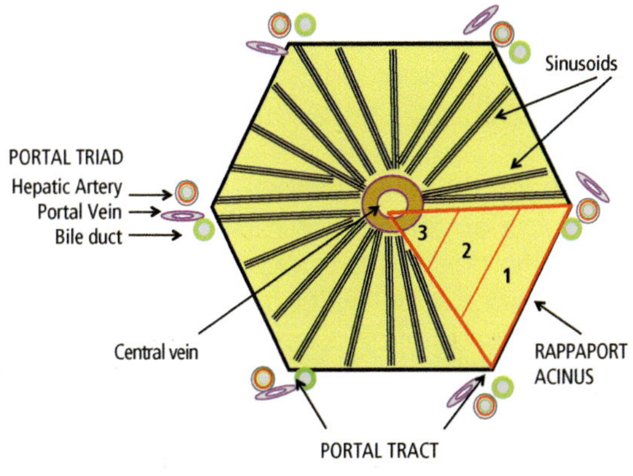

Figure 27.1 Diagram of a hepatic lobule.

LIVER CELLS

Hepatocytes

Hepatocytes are the most numerous cells in the liver. Their structure and metabolism vary according to their distance from the inflow of portal blood. Hepatocytes closer to the portal tract have a higher metabolism and a greater number of mitochondria because they receive more arterial blood than the hepatocytes of the intermediate zones and the areas surrounding the central vein (**Figure 27.2**).

Hepatic Stellate Cells (Ito Cells)

Ito cells are of mesenchymal origin and much less numerous than hepatocytes. They are located between the laminae, at the base of the hepatocytes and have a star-like, irregular shape.
Their cytoplasm is rich in lipid vesicles containing

*The Authors wish to thank Dr. Francesco Santopaolo for his assistance.

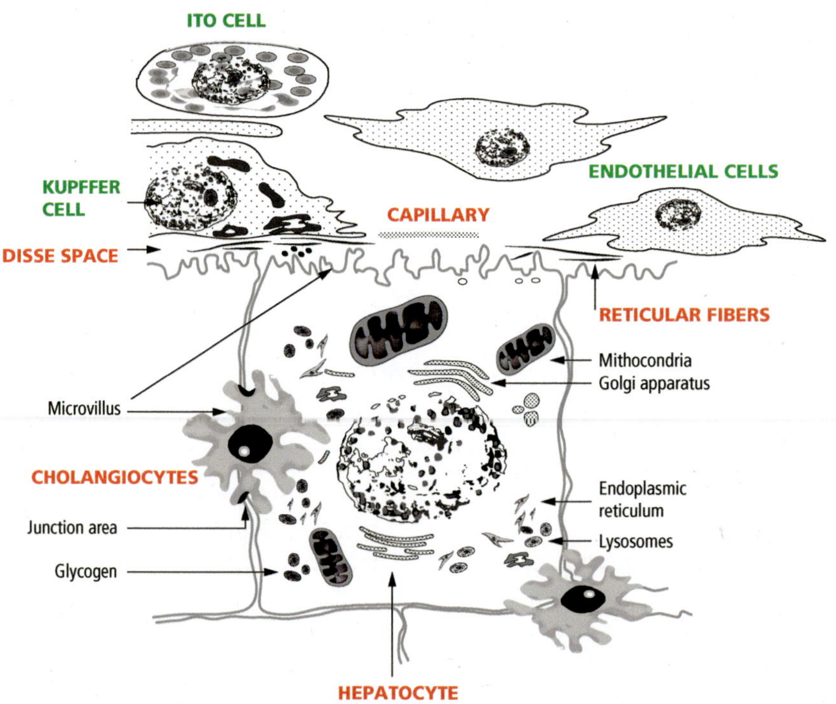

Figure 27.2 Diagram of liver histology.

vitamin A. They produce matrix constituents, including collagen. They are essential in the regeneration of the liver after injury by producing growth factors and contributing to the restoration of liver homeostasis (Figure 27.2).

Endothelial Cells

They constitute the endothelium of the sinusoids. They are flattened and protrude into the lumen of the sinusoids with the nucleus-containing portion. They have often overlapping margins, especially where the largest sinusoidal fenestrations are located. They have no particular features, except for low mitochondrial content. The luminal surface has small pinocytotic vesicles and short and poor microvilli (Figure 27.2).

Kupffer Cells

They are the macrophages of the liver, derived from monocytes and located in the lumen of the sinusoids. They have subtle amoeboid cytoplasmic extensions that come into contact with endothelial cells. They are located in the sub-endothelial space or inserted in the endothelial wall. Kupffer cells are recognizable by their large and clear nucleus. Unlike endothelial cells, there are numerous microvilli, invaginations, and pseudopodia on their surface. They exert intense phagocytic activity and are part of to the mononuclear phagocyte system (Figure 27.2).

Cholangiocytes

For the features of these cells in normal and pathological conditions, refer to specific chapters (Figure 27.2).

LIVER FUNCTION

The liver is the metabolic factory of our body. It carries out numerous functions:

1. Production and secretion of bile to emulsify fats.
2. Carbohydrate metabolism:
   - gluconeogenesis (synthesis of glucose from amino acids, lactic acid or glycerol);
   - glycogen synthesis (complex molecule, polysaccharide of glucose);
   - glycogenolysis (degradation of glycogen by the enzyme phosphorylase to provide energy by secreting glucose into blood circulation).
3. Metabolism of hormones (insulin and sex hormones)
4. Synthesis and degradation of various plasma proteins with specific functions:

- Albumin (oncotic function. It is also a carrier protein and inhibits some proteases);
- Transferrin, ceruloplasmin, haptoglobin, lipoprotein (carrier function);
- α1-antitrypsin, α- and β-globulins (inhibition of proteases);
- hormones (intra- and inter-cellular messengers);
- coagulation factors I (fibrinogen), II (thrombin), V, VII, IX, X and XI, as well as protein C, protein S, hepcidin and antithrombin.

Furthermore, hepatocytes are involved in the deamination and transamination of amino acid through enzymes called transaminases, which convert the non-nitrogenous component of amino acids into glucose and lipids. Hepatocytes synthesize non-essential amino acids.

5. Lipid metabolism (synthesis of cholesterol and triglycerides). Most of the fatty acids are captured by the liver and esterified to triglycerides, they can be esterified with cholesterol, incorporated into phospholipids or oxidized to CO2 or ketone bodies.
6. Haemoglobin catabolism and formation of bile pigments.
7. Metabolism of exogenous toxins and drugs through the recruitment of numerous enzymatic systems, largely cytochrome P450.
8. Conversion of ammonia into urea through the Krebs-Henseleit cycle.
9. Deposit of substrates and coenzymes such as glycogen, vitamin B12, iron, copper.
10. Haematopoiesis in fetal life. In the fetus until the third month, the liver is the main site of production of red blood cells. It is replaced by the bone marrow at 32 weeks of gestation.

MECHANISMS OF ACUTE AND CHRONIC HEPATIC INJURY

The mechanisms underlying acute and chronic hepatic injury are extremely complex and at present not fully clarified. For learning purposes we can refer to a chain of events involving the cellular biochemical system of hepatocyte (**Table 27.1**). Except for the few cases in which a direct cytopathic mechanism may be recognized (e.g., ischaemic damage, hepatitis A, some toxins), as a general rule exogenous or endogenous injury to hepatocytes, invariably elicits an inflammatory reaction by the immune system. Moderate inflammatory reaction, as observed in self-limiting injury, plays an important role in repairing the damage and restoring normal physiological functions. However, if the inflammatory response is excessive or persistent, massive cell loss due to necrosis or apoptosis and the establishment of fibrotic processes may ensue (**Figure 27.3**). The main factors in hepatic injury are:

- inflammation;
- necrosis and/or cell apoptosis;
- fibrosis in chronic inflammation.

Liver Inflammation

Liver inflammation invariably occurs following insults accompanied by cellular stress. It is due to resident hepatic cells (Kupffer cells, stellate cells, endothelial cells) and cells that are recruited in response to damage (monocytes, macrophages, dendritic cells, and natural killer cells).

Necrosis of hepatic cells does not appear to be an indispensable element in the initial development of inflammatory response.

The initiation of inflammation is characterized by activation of resident macrophages and release of chemokines.

The pro-inflammatory cytokines are interleukin-1 β, interferon-γ, followed by tumour necrosis factor-α (TNF-α), and interleukin-6, resulting in the recruitment and translocation of inflammatory cells and inducing the production of cell adhesion molecules such as ICAM-1 and VCAM-1. The inflammatory cell infiltrate can consist of granulocytes, macrophages and plasma cells and T and B lymphocytes.

Table 27.1 Factors involved in liver injury.

Type of Liver Damage	Inflammation	Necrosis/Apoptosis	Fibrosis
• Ischaemic	+/-	+++	-
• Acute (viral or toxic*)	+++	+++	-
• Chronic	++	++	+/-
• Chronic with cirrhosis	++/-	++/-	+++

* Grade of inflammation is usually high but may vary according to poisoning.

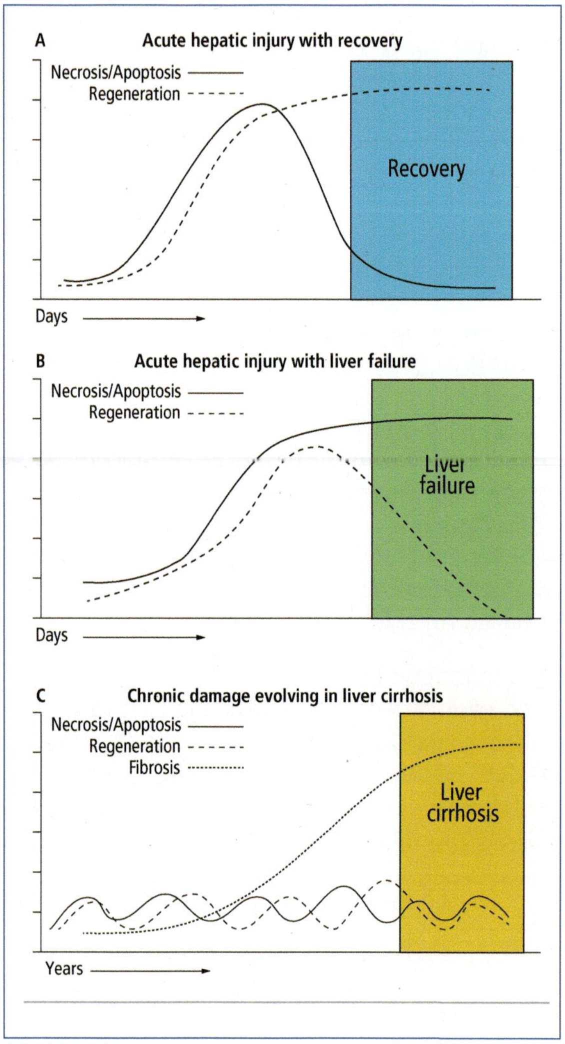

Figure 27.3 Liver injury.

Apoptosis and/or Cellular Necrosis

Following an inflammatory stimulus, especially a response to the production of TNF-α and interleukin-6, numerous biological factors are activated that can result in apoptosis and/or cellular necrosis.

Apoptosis is a process of programmed cell death characterized by cell volume reduction, chromatin condensation, DNA fragmentation with preserved cell integrity. Councilman's bodies visible under light microscopy are the morphological equivalent of hepatocytes in apoptosis. Instead, necrosis is characterized by cell swelling and rupture of the cell membrane, with consequent release of the intracellular content in the surrounding spaces.

During acute or chronic injury, hepatocytes show aspects compatible with necrosis and apoptosis, for which the term "necro-apoptosis" has been coined. In support of this definition, in vitro data demonstrate that TNF-α can cause hepatocyte death by both modalities. Cell death of a single hepatocyte due to either apoptosis or necrosis caused by the cellular ATP content, as only adequate cellular concentrations of ATP allow apoptosis.

When hepatic damage results in necro-apoptosis, the same inflammatory mediators stimulate the production of other factors that induce cell proliferation and hepatic regeneration.

Therefore, a mechanism is established that can regulate the simultaneous removal of excessively damaged cells and their replacement through the proliferation of healthy cells. In this way, minor injury is usually repaired without significant consequences.

However, a large acute injury, usually of toxic or viral origin, can cause significant hepatic necrosis, unaccompanied by adequate reparative processes and resulting in severe hepatic failure.

Liver Fibrosis

A variable degree of liver fibrosis is present in chronic liver disease. When subversion of the liver architecture is complete, the clinical picture that results is that of cirrhosis. The most reliable hypothesis for the onset of liver fibrosis is that it is stimulated by signals deriving from hepatocyte necrosis or apoptosis.

Necro-apoptosis stimulates hepatic stellate cells during chronic hepatic injury. Hepatic stellate cells shift from a quiescent phenotype to myofibroblast with chemotactic, contractile and matrix remodeling. Following activation of stellate cells, there is an increase in protein deposition in the extracellular matrix consisting of type I and III collagen, fibronectin, and laminin. The imbalance between fibrogenesis and fibrolysis results in an increased deposition of these proteins in the extracellular matrix, with invasion of the spaces by hepatocytes in necro-apoptosis.

Collagen deposition results in the formation of bridges between the portal tract and the central vein to generate hepatocyte nodules surrounded by collagen, with consequent architectural alteration of the liver.

The process of liver fibrosis was long considered irreversible. However, based on experimental and clinical data, it was observed that regression of fibrosis, even if partial, is possible. In particular, regression may be observed when chronic injury is repaired. Moreover, other therapeutic strategies are being evaluated to limit activation of stellate cells, determine their apoptosis, reduce deposition of extracellular collagen, and facilitate its degradation.

KEY CONCEPTS

- The liver is the metabolic factory of our body ; it its major functions are the synthesis and degradation of organic substances.
- It is a possible target of acute or chronic injury, with persistence of damage.
- The main factors in hepatic injury are inflammation, necrosis/cell apoptosis and, in case of chronic injury, fibrosis.
- When liver fibrosis is complete, the result is altered architecture with the clinical and anatomopathological picture of cirrhosis.

REFERENCES

- Brenner C, Galluzzi L, Kepp O, Kroemer G. Decoding cell death signals in liver inflammation. J Hepatol. 2013;59:583-94.
- Mehal W, Imaeda A. Cell death and fibrogenesis. Semin Liver Dis. 2010;30:226-31.
- Novo E, Cannito S, Paternostro C, et al. Cellular and molecular mechanisms in liver fibrogenesis. Arch Biochem Biophys. 2014;548:20-37.

CHAPTER 28

NATURAL HISTORY OF LIVER DISEASE

Vincenza Calvaruso, Pietro Lampertico

LEARNING OBJECTIVES

- To summarise the natural history of liver disease, especially viral chronic hepatitis and non-alcoholic steatohepatitis.
- To focus on diagnostics in the course of chronic hepatitis.

INTRODUCTION

Liver disease may have an acute or chronic course. The acute course is due to the rapid elimination of the pathogen, the chronic one is due to its persistence.

ACUTE HEPATITIS

Acute hepatitis is defined as a necroinflammatory process of the liver parenchyma that resolves within 6 months of the onset. The main and common feature of all types of acute hepatitis is the significant elevations in transaminases (>10 times the upper limit of normal). The other clinical manifestations depend on the extent of cellular necrosis. It is possible to distinguish different scenarios:

- the "transaminitis", i.e. the isolated elevations in aminotransferases without clinical signs;
- anicteric hepatitis, accompanied by vomiting, nausea, fever, anorexia, asthenia, abdominal pain but without jaundice;
- icteric hepatitis (with jaundice, without encephalopathy);
- acute liver failure (ALF) (characterized by reduction of coagulation factors and/or encephalopathy). ALF is associated with high mortality and often requires liver transplantation. Even the most severe forms of acute hepatitis do not evolve to chronicity. The causes of hepatitis are summarized in **Table 28.1**.

CHRONIC HEPATITIS – GENERAL CONSIDERATIONS

Chronic hepatitis (CH) is defined as a clinical-pathological entity characterized by persistence over time (≥6 months) of hepato-biliary necrosis, due to widespread inflammation of the liver, associated with a variable degree of fibrosis (as a repair phenomenon). The major causes of CH are shown in **Table 28.2**:

- most of CH are viral (high prevalence of HCV in Italy);
- chronic alcoholic hepatitis is second in frequency, predominates in some social contexts and is more frequent in the North than in Southern Italy;
- non-alcoholic steatosis (NAFLD = Non-Alcoholic Fatty Liver Disease) is increasing with a prevalence of 25% in Italian population;
- autoimmune hepatitis predominates in women;
- haemochromatosis and Wilson's disease are relatively rare causes of CH; they have genetic origin and often occur in relatives.

The natural history of chronic hepatitis of any aetiology is similar. The disease mostly begins asymptomatically. In fact, most patients have no episodes of acute hepatitis;
the aetiologies that most frequently begin with acute icteric hepatitis in severe forms
are the chronic hepatitis D virus and the autoimmune hepatitis.

Table 28.1 Major causes of acute hepatitis.

- Hepatitis A, B, C, D, and E virus; Epstein-Barr virus, Cytomegalovirus
- Drugs/Toxic
- Alcohol

Note: Elevated transaminases, sometimes very high, may be due to hepatic ischaemia or the passage of a gallstone through the ductus choledochus

Table 28.2 Major causes of chronic hepatitis.

- Hepatitis B, C and D virus
- Alcohol
- Non-alcoholic steatohepatitis
- Type 1 and type 2 autoimmune hepatitis
- Primary biliary cholangitis (PBC), primary sclerosing cholangitis (PSC)
- Drugs
- Haemochromatosis
- Wilson disease

Note: Chronic hepatitis from hepatitis E virus in transplant recipients.

Episodes of jaundice reported in childhood/adolescence from elderly patients with CH
are often due to a hepatitis A virus and are irrelevant. In the case of a chronic viral hepatitis, whether subclinical or in the form of acute hepatitis, the disease occurs usually asymptomatically; the only indicator is the alteration in transaminases, but sometimes the patients maintain the transaminases within the limits of normal; liver function remains intact. The patient with CH may feel asthenic; the symptom is difficult to evaluate, due to both the depression caused by the knowledge of the disease and to the disease itself. However, the presence of systemic symptoms such as fever, weight loss, intense asthenia in a non-cirrhotic patient with altered liver enzymes should elicit the suspect of systemic causes (lymphoma, other haemopathy, amyloidosis) that may compromise liver biochemistry. Liver damage may remain stable or evolve slowly without clinical problems; transaminases remain altered, sometimes fluctuating over time, but function and other liver parameters remain stable; patients with chronic HCV infection and normal transaminases are more likely to have a slow progressing mild hepatitis, however it is not uncommon to observe cases of cirrhosis even in patients without alteration of liver transaminases; This mild variant of the liver disease is less probable in active HBV infection and rare in HDV and autoimmune hepatitis. With the persistence of the inflammatory process, a progressive increase of fibrotic lesions in liver parenchyma is observed. Then the fibrous septa expand to the portal tract, with formation of porto-portal bridging and veno-portal bridging, until completely alteration the normal liver architecture achieving the histological picture of cirrhosis. Any CH may potentially evolve to cirrhosis. The process evolves subclinically for many years; also the initial cirrhosis is an anatomical fact, it does not affect the liver function that remains compensated (**Figure 28.1**).

The evolution to cirrhosis is associated with the development of portal hypertension, initially asymptomatic, then clinically manifested with splenomegaly.

By abdominal ultrasound is possible observe the increased diameter of portal vein. Another ultrasound finding is the inversion of the portal flow and a reduced splenic and superior mesenteric veins respiratory excursions.

Endoscopy can show congestive gastropathy and oesophageal varices. Symptoms of liver failure may appear, the earliest of which is usually the ascites. The time interval from the beginning of the CH and liver failure is widely variable; it may be very rapid (within one year) in autoimmune hepatitis, short (5 years) in chronic HBV hepatitis and long (20 to 30 years if there are no comorbidities) in HCV hepatitis and NASH.

In the long period of asymptomatic CH, the only sign of disease, when present, is represented by the persistence of altered liver enzymes. The other laboratory tests reflecting the liver function change only in advanced disease.

In nodular evolution of CH a progressive decline in the number of platelets is observed. This is an early sign of disease evolution even before the deterioration of liver synthesis activities. The decrease in pseudo-cholinesterase occurs relatively early but is poorly specific.

Albuminemia, INR and cholinesterase (CHE) decrease only late; elevations in bilirubin are a poor prognostic sign. The Child-Pugh score is able to classify the severity stage of cirrhosis (**Figure 28.2**). The evolution of liver fibrosis can be evaluated with the liver biopsy or, in recent years, with non-invasive tools. Although liver biopsy remains the most accurate resource for determining the degree of fibrosis evolution, it is not well accepted by the patient and leads to possible complications. Non-invasive methods have been developed in the last decade; the most used is the hepatic ela-

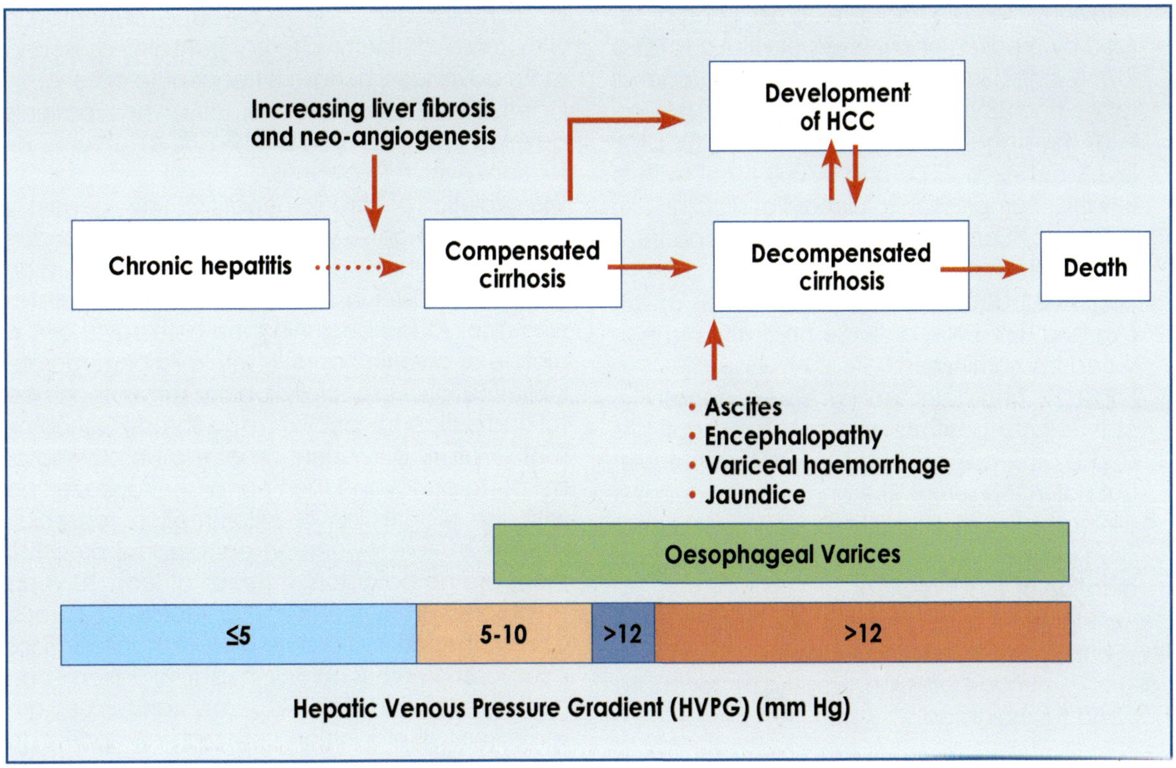

Figure 28.1 The natural history of chronic liver disease

stography (Fibroscan), which has been considered reliable for the exclusion or diagnosis of cirrhosis mostly in viral hepatitis. Serum fibrosis markers such as Fibrotest, Biopredictive, Fib-4, APRI (AST/Platelets) are less used in clinical practice.

CHRONIC HEPATITIS B (HBV)

Most patients remain asymptomatic for many years although some may complain of non-specific disorders such as asthenia. Symptoms of liver failure appear only late when the disease progresses to cirrhosis and to hepatic decompensation. The progression of chronic hepatitis to liver cirrhosis and hepatocellular carcinoma (HCC) depends on numerous factors such as viral replication levels (HBV-DNA), advanced age, male gender, family history of HCC and/or cirrhosis, African race, obesity, diabetes mellitus, C >B viral genotype, precore or core promoter mutants, co-infection (with HCV/HDV or HIV), alcohol and aflatoxins.
The cumulative incidence of cirrhosis in patients with untreated chronic hepatitis is 8-20% at 5 years and in patients with cirrhosis the cumulative risk of decompensation is 20% at 5 years. The annual risk of developing HCC in patients with chronic hepatitis is 0.3-0.6% and 2-5% in patients with cirrhosis. HBV-DNA suppression, after antiviral therapy with nucleoside or nucleotide analogues, reduces the risk of progression to cirrhosis and to HCC. Furthermore, it significantly reduced the risk of hepatic decompensation in cirrhotic patients.
The combination of serological (HBsAg, HBeAg and anti-HBe), virological (HBV-DNA), biochemical (ALT) and fibrosis (invasive and non-invasive) markers allows to define five phases in the natural history of HBV, characterized by different prognosis, therapeutic indications and monitoring strategies. The new nomenclature proposed in the latest European Guidelines for the Study of the Liver is based on the description of the two main characteristics of chronicity: infection vs hepatitis.

- *Phase 1*, HBeAg-positive chronic HBV infection (previously termed "immune-tolerant") characterized by high levels of HBsAg and viremia, but ALT within the normal range and HBeAg positivity;
- *Phase 2*, HBeAg-positive chronic hepatitis B (previously termed "immuno-reactive HBeAg positive") defined by HBsAg and HBeAg positivity, high levels of ALT and HBV-DNA, histological evidence of chronic hepatitis or cirrhosis;
- *Phase 3*, HBeAg-negative chronic HBV infection

(previously termed "inactive carrier") characterized by medium or low levels of HBsAg (<1,000 IU/ml), anti-HBe positivity, ALT within the normal range and HBV-DNA <2.000 IU/ml; some patients at this stage, however, may have HBV-DNA levels between 2,000 and 20,000 IU/ml, with a low risk of progression to cirrhosis or HCC;

- *Phase 4*, HBeAg-negative chronic hepatitis B (previously termed 'immuno-reactive HBeAg negative') defined by moderate levels of HBsAg and HBV-DNA, anti-HBe positivity and elevated transaminases;
- *Phase 5*, characterised by HBsAg negativity, anti-HB-core positivity with or without anti-HBs and by the presence of HBV-DNA in the liver but not in the serum. This phase represents the clinical cure of hepatitis B, spontaneous or drug-induced, but does not represent the eradication of viral infection.

Generally, antiviral treatment is reserved for phases 2 and 4, the monitoring for phases 1 and 3. In case of immunosuppression, prophylaxis for phase 1, 3, and 5 is indicated.

CHRONIC HEPATITIS C (HCV)

In Europe, HCV primary infection is responsible for about 10% of cases of hepatitis, asymptomatic in most cases. Against the benign nature of primary infection, exposure to HCV is complicated by a high risk of chronicity in about 80% of cases. Evolution is more frequent after asymptomatic primary infection (90%) rather than after primary infection with jaundice (50-80%). Majority of patients has a completely asymptomatic infection that is detected by the elevation of the transaminases; in about a quarter of the cases, signs of cirrhosis are present at presentation. Young patients (<35 years old) usually have a mild disease.

15-35% of subjects with an HCV infection exhibit normal transaminases at the first evaluation. Transaminases can remain persistently normal; they can fluctuate within the limits of the normal range and transiently rise above the threshold values; in some cases they can reactivate permanently after years.

Sudden transaminase peaks in subjects that had normal enzymes for years are typical of HCV genotype 2 infection; these peaks recede in intensity within a few months but often do not fall within the threshold values. This is a sign of florid disease onset. Although transaminases remain normal, liver fibrosis may develop despite biochemical silence.

In asymptomatic older subjects a presentation with more distinctly altered transaminases and more advanced disease is frequent to observe.

Often the ALT increase abruptly when patients develop cirrhosis. At least 10-20% of chronic infections evolve to cirrhosis.

The evolution of chronic hepatitis is slow, generally lasts no less than 20 years (if there are no concurrent causes that accelerate it). The progression of fibrosis is faster in old patients and accelerates with age. At the beginning the histology shows a picture of chronic hepatitis with mild or moderate inflammation - especially lobular rather than portal and periportal- and with mild fibrosis; Concomitant steatosis is frequent reported. Fibrous septa, first porto-portal and then porto-central develope with the progression of inflammation (especially if this is more evident in porto-portal areas). If there are no cofactors, it needs at least 10 years to progress from Metavir 1 to Metavir 2 fibrosis. Chronic hepatitis C has no typical manifestations compared to other chronic hepatitis; patients can complain of asthenia, γ-glutamyltransferases are sometimes disproportionately high compared to the ALT. Elevations in gammaglobulins is late and generally follows the development of cirrhosis. An early and progressive decline in platelets is often observed in the course of chronic hepatitis C, unrelated to clinical signs of portal hypertension such as splenomegaly and oesophageal varices; this provides a reliable indicator of disease progression even in the absence of any other clinical or biochemical signs of evolution. Once cirrhosis is established, the time interval leading to the development of portal hypertension or liver failure is 5-10 years. HCV cirrhosis is a major risk factor for the development of HCC, with an annual risk of 1-5%.

It is relevant to remember that HCV infection has been also associated with a lot of different extrahepatic manifestations. HCV infected patients are at higher risk of mixed cryoglobulinemia, lymphoma, lichen planus, Sjögren's syndrome, porphyria cutanea tarda, rheumatoid-like arthritis, depression, chronic kidney end-stage renal disease, type 2 diabetes and cardiovascular disorders/ mortality.

Also in the case of hepatitis C, viral eradication is associated with a significant reduction in progression to cirrhosis, decompensation of disease and HCC.

In the last years, with the availability of direct antiviral drugs (DAAs) it is possible to achieve a sustained virological response in almost all cases, regardless of viral load and genotype, as well as the stage of the disease.

Cofactors for Fibrosis Progression in Patients with Chronic Hepatitis C

Various factors accelerate the progression of chronic hepatitis C to fibrosis/cirrhosis (**Table 28.3**). In subjects >50 years the evolution is faster than in the younger patients; males are more susceptible than women, perhaps due to the inhibitory effect of estrogens on fibrosis. Alcohol use above 20 g/day is a factor of progression, such as cigarette or cannabis smoking. Various metabolic alterations accelerate the evolution, especially liver steatosis, diabetes mellitus, obesity, insulin resistance. The risk of insulin resistance and type 2 diabetes mellitus is increased in subjects with HCV genotype 1 or 4; in this context the fibrosis formation and progression are more rapid. Liver steatosis is also common in patients with HCV genotype 3; it is directly induced by the virus, is not associated with the progression of HCV and regresses with the therapy. A direct role of iron accumulation on the activation of HCV is uncertain.

Co-infection with HBV, including an occult infection with this virus, accelerates the progression. About 30% of patients with HIV are co-infected with HCV; therefore, it is indicated to search for anti-HCV in all HIV-positive subjects. It remains uncertain whether the evolution of HCV hepatitis is accelerated in patients with high CD4 + levels and in those who start therapy against HIV (HAART), when they are not yet immunocompromised; However, since survival of HIV subjects has increased with the efficacy of HAART, there is more time for the development of complications HCV-related; Furthermore, cirrhosis from HCV has become a major cause of mortality in coinfected HIV-HCV patients. There is insufficient evidence that HCV accelerates the evolution of HIV infection. Patients with HIV often will develop drug-related liver disease.

Table 28.3 Factors that accelerate the progression of liver fibrosis in patients with chronic hepatitis C

- Alcohol
- Age >50 years
- HBV coinfection
- HIV coinfection
- Immunosuppression
- Obesity
- Steatosis
- Smoking
- Menopause

CHRONIC HEPATITIS D (HDV)

It shows no different histological and clinical features compared to other chronic liver disease, in particular hepatitis B. It is characterized by greater histological aggressiveness and faster progression to cirrhosis and to HCC; the prototype is the still young HBsAg-positive patient with frank liver cytolysis and low HBV-DNA levels.

CHRONIC HEPATITIS E (HEV)

It can rarely develop in immunocompromised and transplanted patients, those receiving chemotherapy and HIV-infected.

NON-ALCOHOLIC FATTY LIVER DISEASE (NAFLD)

Non-alcoholic fatty liver disease (NAFLD) is now the most frequent cause of chronic hepatopathy in outpatients, with a prevalence in abdominal ultrasound of 25% in the Italian population. It includes a wide spectrum of disorders characterized by lipid accumulation in the liver (>5%) in the absence of significant alcohol consumption: the majority of patients (70-80%) have a simple steatosis (NAFL), while the more progressive form of the disease, the non-alcoholic steatohepatitis (NASH), is characterized by the presence of micro and macrovesicular steatosis induced by hepatocellular damage and/or inflammation, with or without fibrosis. It is thought that a percentage ranging from 10 to 20% of NAFLD evolves to NASH, which will therefore have a prevalence of 2-3% in the general population. NASH may develop advanced fibrosis (30-40% of patients) or even cirrhosis (10-15% of patients).

The clinical importance of NAFLD is also linked to the independent effect of promoting cardiovascular damage, to the progression to other chronic liver diseases and to the associated risk of neoplasia (hepatic and extrahepatic). The development of NASH recognizes a multifactorial pathogenesis. Factors involved are represented by:

- severity of insulin resistance and steatosis with induction of lipid pathways, development of oxidative stress and mitochondrial damage;
- alterations of the microbiota and intestinal permeability;
- any systemic pro-inflammatory status secondary to release of cytokines and/or adipokines (visceral adipose tissue dysfunction);

- hereditary variants that can influence hepatic lipid metabolism, the inflammatory response and the fibrosis process.

Factors associated with increased disease severity are: age, type 2 diabetes mellitus, elevated insulin levels, high body mass index (BMI >30 kg/m2), chronic elevations in transaminases, presence of genetic risk factors (homozygous for I148M variant of PNPLA3).

In the United States and European countries, NASH is now becoming the leading cause of hepatocellular carcinoma in patients with chronic liver disease and one of the growing indications of liver transplantation.

KEY CONCEPTS

- Acute liver disease is often symptomatic and easily diagnosed. However, can be asymptomatic and without jaundice, and therefore the diagnosis is possible only by detection of high levels of transaminases.
- Chronic liver disease remains totally asymptomatic for years; its assessment requires the determination of the transaminases. The detection of liver biochemistry remains the only diagnostic tool of chronic hepatitis; it is therefore used as a screening tool particularly in patients at risk (addicts, poly-transfusions, sexually promiscuous subjects, hepatotoxic drugs, etc.).

REFERENCES

- EASL recommendations on treatment of hepatitis C: Final update of the series. Journal of Hepatology 2020 vol. 73 j 1170–1218.
- EASL 2017 Clinical Practice Guidelines on the management of hepatitis B virus infection. Journal of Hepatology 2017; 67:370–398.
- EASL Clinical Practice Guidelines on hepatitis E virus infection. Journal of Hepatology 2018 vol. 68 j 1256–1271
- Di Marco V, Calvaruso V, Ferraro D et al. Effects of Eradicating Hepatitis C Virus Infection in Patients With Cirrhosis Differ With Stage of Portal Hypertension. Gastroenterology 2016;151:130–139.
- de Franchis R; Baveno VI Faculty. Expanding consensus in portal hypertension: Report of the Baveno VI Consensus Workshop: Stratifying risk and individualizing care for portal hypertension. Journal of Hepatology. 2015 Sep;63(3):743-52.
- Non-alcoholic fatty liver disease in adults 2021: A clinical practice guideline of the Italian Association for the Study of the Liver (AISF), the Italian Society of Diabetology (SID) and the Italian Society of Obesity (SIO). Dig Liver Dis. 2022 Feb;54(2):170-182.
- Francque SM, Marchesini G, Kautz A et al. Non-alcoholic fatty liver disease: A patient guideline. JHEP Rep. 2021 Sep 17;3(5):100322.

CHAPTER 29

DIAGNOSTICS

Alessandro Federico, Saveria Lory Crocè

LEARNING OBJECTIVES

- To give knowledge for a correct interpretation of laboratory analysis.
- To know the main exams to be used for a correct diagnostic approach.
- To know the main features of invasive and non-invasive instrumental exams used for the definition of liver diseases stage.

ROUTINARY LIVER TESTS

The use of biochemical tests plays an important role in diagnosis and management of liver diseases. They are often defined incorrectly "tests of liver functionality" including liver enzymes, expression of hepatocyte damage, cholestasis and tests that show the synthetic liver function. Liver tests, commonly used in clinical practice, are listed in **Table 29.1**.

Hepatocellular Damage: AST and ALT

Transaminases or aminotransferases (aspartate aminotransferase, AST or GOT; alanine aminotransferase, ALT or GPT) are localized in hepatocytes and they are sensitive markers of their damage. They participate in gluconeogenesis by catalysing the transfer of amine groups from aspartate or alanine to ketoglutaric acid forming respectively oxaloacetic acid and pyruvic acid. ALT is in highest concentration in hepatocytes compared to other tissues and it is considered a more specific marker of liver damage. On the contrary, AST is in a lot of tissue including the muscle (myocardium and skeletal muscles), kidney and brain. AST/ALT ratio more than five with normal or mild elevated ALT is appealing of compromission of skeletal muscle (i.e., rhabdomyolysis) or of significative muscle activity. AST are localized in cytoplasm and mitochondria, whereas ALT are only localized in cytoplasm (**Figure 29.1**).

About 80% of AST activity into the liver is derived from mitochondrial isoenzyme, whereas in the serum it is due to cytosolic isoenzyme. Hepatocyte necrosis or their membrane damage with increase permeability induces AST and ALT release in the blood. Levels up to 300 UI/L are not usually specific and they can highlight in each hepatopathy. Levels more than 1000 UI/L are exclusively associated to an extended hepatocellular necrosis, more commonly caused by:

- pharmacological damage;
- acute ischaemia;

Tabella 29.1 The most common liver tests and their meaning.

Hepatocellular Damage Aspartate aminotransferase (AST, GOT) Alanine aminotransferase (ALT, GPT)
Cholestasis Alkaline Phosphatase (AP) γ-glutamyltransferase (γ-GT)
Protein Synthesis Albumin Prothrombin Activity (PA/INR)
Captation Capacity, Conjugation A and Escretion of Hepatocyte Fractionated and total bilirubin

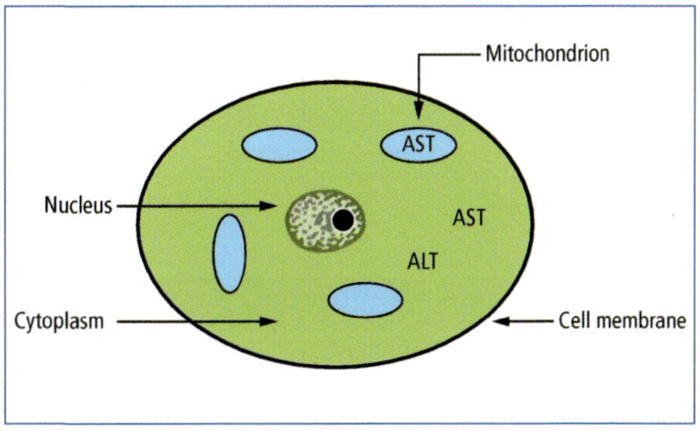

Figure 29.1 AST and ALT localization into hepatocyte.

*We thank Dr. Marcello Dallio, Resident Physician in Gastroenterology, University of Campania "Luigi Vanvitelli", Naples, Italy for the English translation.

- acute viral hepatitis;
- Aautoimmune hepatitis;
- Wilson's disease.

Biliary obstruction (i.e., lithiasis of choledochus), which can cause a fast increase of biliary system pressure and can determine an acute and transitory increase in AST and ALT levels

ALT are present in high concentration in periportal hepatocytes (region 1 of Rappaport) and in low concentration in pericentral lobular hepatocytes (region 3 of Rappaport) (**Figure 29.2**).

Hepatocytes situated around central-lobular vein receive a lower oxygen amount and so they are more sensitive to necrotic damage in case of acute liver ischaemia (acute hypotension or sever cardiopathy). Pericentral lobular necrosis causes a fast transaminase increase with higher AST levels compared to ALT in the first few days after the acute event. Transaminases are catabolised from liver and their level reduces slowly, since ALT biological half-life is longer than AST one.

Transaminases alterations are observed on all chronic liver diseases. Among non hepatic pathologies, a hypertransaminasemia can be observed in tyreopathy, celiac disease, muscle diseases and anorexia.

In alcoholic hepatopathies AST/ALT ratio is generally >1. When it is >3 it is highly suggestive of alcoholic hepatopathy. It depends on mitochondrial damage induced by alcohol with consequent AST release in the blood. A ratio >1 is also correlated to the development and progression of fibrosis to cirrhosis in all chronic hepatopathies forms, also non-alcoholic ones.

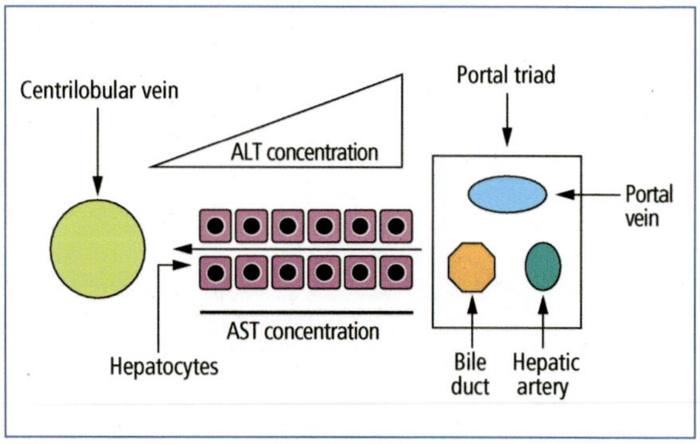

Figure 29.2 Different concentrations of AST and ALT in relation to hepatocyte localisation.

Cholestasis: Alkaline Phosphatase and γ-Glutamyltransferase

Alkaline phosphatase (FA) includes a group of enzymes that catalyse hydrolysis of some organic phosphate esters. They are in canalicular membrane of hepatocyte and epithelium of biliary system, in osteoblast membrane, in the brush border of small intestine cells, in proximal tubules of the kidney, in the placenta and in white blood cell. Most of serum FA is of bone and liver origin. The distinction among the different isoenzymes is performed by electrophoresis. An isolated increase of FA, with normal levels of γ-glutamiltransferase (γGT), occurs in youth age (increase of bone isoenzyme), in bone diseases (rickets, osteomalacia, Paget's disease) and in third trimester of pregnancy (increase of placenta isoenzyme). There are rare liver disorders characterized by the isolated increased of FA, among which benign recurring intrahepatic cholestasis and progressive familiar intrahepatic cholestasis. FA increase, higher than 2-3 times compared to the standard, is peculiar of intra or extrahepatic cholestasis, even if this observation isn't useful to differentiate between intra and extrahepatic ones. The concomitant association with γGT increase can confirm liver and cholestatic origin of hyper FA.

γGT is an enzyme that catalyse the transfer of peptides of gamma-glutamic group, such as glutathione, to other peptides or amino acids. It is present in liver, kidney, pancreas, intestine, and spleen. In the liver γGT is localized in hepatocyte membrane, particularly in peri-central lobular region and biliary epithelium. γGT is a sensitive marker of liver damage and biliary system, but it is characterized by a lack of specificity. The increase can express cholestasis, but also alcoholic abuse, drug-induced liver damage, diabetes, hyperthyroidism, chronic obstructive pulmonary disease, and kidney failure.

Protein Biosynthesis: AP/INR and Albumin

In the liver, albumin synthesis and most of coagulation factors occur. Therefore albumin and prothrombinic activity (AP)/International Normalized Ratio (INR) are the real test that express synthetic liver function. Albumin has a biological half-life of about 21 days, for this reason its level could not be compromised in acute hepatitis. In chronic hepatitis and cirrhosis low levels of albumin are markers of advanced disease. Hypoalbuminemia is not a specific sign of hepatopathy, since it is also observed in malnutrition, in infections, in nephrotic syndrome or protein losing enteropathy.

AP/INR measure the activity of coagulation factors synthesized in the liver and dependent K vitamin. Coagulation factors have a shorter biological half-life compared to albumin. Therefore AP/INR is a good test to measure liver function in case of acute liver failure.

Captation Capacity, Conjugation, and Excretion of Hepatocyte: Total and Fractioned Bilirubin

Bilirubin is the terminal product of eme (eme + globin) metabolism. In physiological conditions, a man everyday produces 250-350 mg of unconjugated bilirubin composed by:

- *emocatheresis percentage* that derives from red blood cell destruction;
- *erythropoietic percentage* that derives from inefficient erythropoiesis;
- *hepatic percentage* that derives by catabolism of emeproteic molecules contained in hepatocytes (i.e., cytochrome P450, etc.).

These three percentages represent unconjugated bilirubin, commonly knows as "indirect". In the blood, unconjugated bilirubin is mainly bound to albumin. Albumin can bind bilirubin up to a ratio of 8,2 mg of bilirubin per one albumin gram (i.e., in a patient of albuminemia of 4 g/dL, bilirubin can bind up to a concentration of about 32 mg/dL). The stability of albumin-bilirubin complex is very important, since it prevents that bilirubin can be damaging for the brain (nuclear jaundice) and kidney (it alters Na^+/H^+ exchange). In the vascular antipode of hepatocyte, bilirubin separates itself from albumin. The transport through the membrane occurs via passive diffusion and for the activity of a transportation protein. The passage of bilirubin is bidirectional. Conjugated bilirubin, commonly known as "direct", is more fastly picked up. Inside the hepatocyte, unconjugated bilirubin is transported through endoplasmatic reticulum by two carrier proteins (protein z and ligandin). Glucuronation occur in endoplasmatic reticulum due to diphosphate glucuronyltransferase. This process produces monoglucuronide and diglucuronide bilirubin (highly represented). Conjugated bilirubin reaches biliary pole of hepatocytes (probably by diffusion in cytoplasm), therefore it passes in the bile through a transportation system (MRP2). In Figure 29.3, diagnostic iter in case of serum evidence of hyperbilirubinemia is exemplified.

DIAGNOSTIC EXAMS

Diagnostic exams aim at confirming or excluding hypotheses done on the basis of clinical history and physical exam. It is important to take into consideration that the diagnosis is rarely based on a single exam and that a lot of tests contribute to the diagnosis, but they are not conclusive. In order to diagnose correctly, it is necessary to take into consideration patient's features (gender, age, race, geographical area), clinical history and epidemiological knowledge.

Viral Markers

Hepatitis C Virus Infection (HCV)

Diagnosis of HCV infection is based on two serological tests: anti-HCV antibodies research, that are indirect marker of infection, and HCV-RNA research, that is a direct marker of infection. Immunoenzymatic test (EIA III) for the detection of anti-HCV antibodies has a sensibility higher to 99% and a negative result therefore sufficient to exclude an HCV chronic infection. High sensibility and economicity make it suitable for screening and diagnostic test in patients with signs of chronic liver disease. The research of viral genome (HCV-RNA) in plasma or in patient's serum is performed by very sensitive molecular technologies, such as Reverse Transcriptase-Polymerase Chain Reaction (RT-PCR) and Transcription-Mediated-Amplification (TMA) and they are available qualitative and quantitative tests. In diagnosis of chronic infection, qualitative HCV-RNA determination must be required only in case of positivity for anti-HCV antibodies. However if a recent infection is suspected (1-4 months), HCV-RNA research should be performed independently form the result of anti-HCV test, because it allows to diagnose the infection also during the period of "non immunological reactivity", when anti-HCV antibodies are not yet developed. Qualitative HCV-RNA is necessarily performed in transfusional centres, in order to increase the safety of blood transfusion. HCV-RNA quantitative tests, performed with PCR real-time technology, are able to give information about circulating virus quantity and they have the same sensitivity, guaranteed by qualitative tests. These tests do not have to be used for clinical monitoring of patients because HCV-RNA quantity does not correlate with prognosis and it does not give information about progression on liver damage, but they are very useful to monitor the response to antiviral treatment, since they can detect difference in the concentrations of HCV-RNA in the order of 1 Log.

Virus C hepatitis has got a genomic variability that has led to the distinction of six different genotypes and into the genotypes it is possible to identify different subtypes with a homology higher than 90%

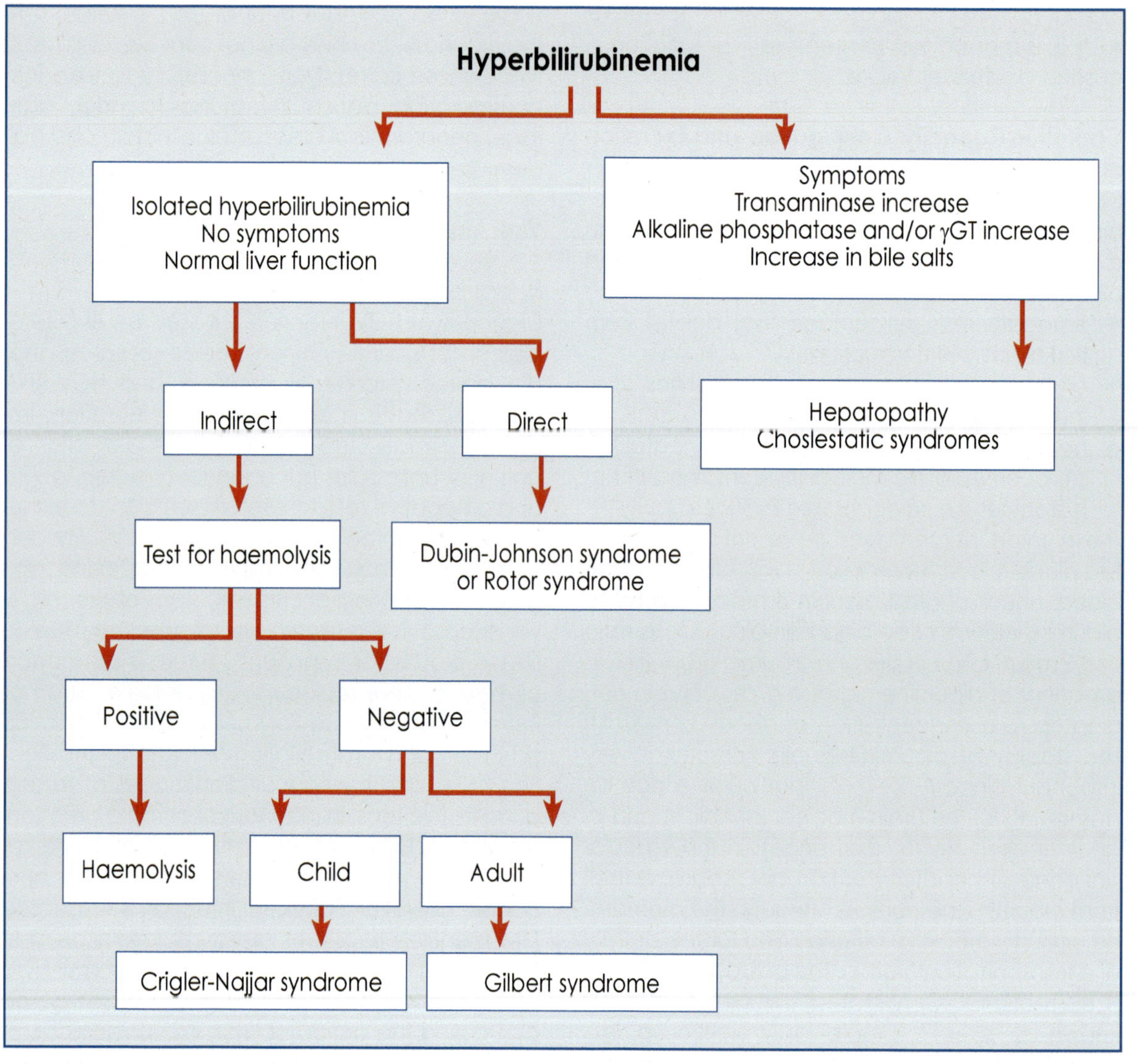

Figure 29.3 Diagnostic iter of hyperbilirubinemia.

In Italy, the infection with genotypes 1, 2 and 3 covers more than 90% of cases of infection due to genotype 4, spread in groups of immigrants from Middle East and North Africa. The determination of viral genotype performed by biomolecular technology has a practical relevance, because the different genotypes have a different sensitivity to antiviral drugs and their characterization represents an important element in therapeutic decision.

Virus B Infection (HBV)

In order to diagnose and check clinical and therapeutic monitoring of acute and chronic HBV infection, serological markers and HBV-DNA quantification in serum are used (Figures 29.4 and 29.5). Serum markers, performed by immunoenzymatic techniques, include the research in serum of HBsAg (surface antigen of hepatitis B virus, which indicates an active HBV infection; the research of HBeAg antigen and anti-HBe antibody that allows to diagnose the type of chronic B virus hepatitis (positive HBeAg or negative HBeAg) and to determine the state of chronic carrier without HBV symptoms; the research of anti-HBc antibody, which, if isolated, indicate a previous one HBV infection; the research of anti-HBs antibody that indicate the protection against HBV infection after acute hepatitis, resolved spontaneously or after the vaccination. In patients with chronic HBV hepatitis it is necessary to perform the research of antibodies against hepatitis D virus (HDV) because the co-infection HBV-HDV in Italy and in immigrants from Easter Europe is relatively frequent (7-12%). Serum levels of HBV-DNA are useful to define and differentiate the patients who are chronic carriers without symptoms from those with active chronic disease. The quantitative dosage of HBV-DNA with real-time PCR is considered the most suitable method because is very sensitive and has got a wide dynamic range of quantification (1 to 7-8 logarithms).

Hepatitis A Virus (HAV)

The diagnosis of hepatitis A virus is more simple. The presence in serum of anti-HAV IgG antibody (IgG anti-HAV) indicates a previous and healed HAV infection, whereas the presence of anti-HAV IgM antibodies IgM (IgM anti-HAV) allows doing diagnosis of acute HAV hepatitis.

Test for Diagnosis of Autoimmune Hepatitis

The diagnosis of autoimmune hepatitis is based on composite scores, including non-organ specific autoantibodies direct against antigens present in all tissues (elements of cytoskeleton, mitochondrial antigens, nuclear components, ribosomial antigens)

In the diagnostic iter of autoimmune type 1 and 2 hepatitis *Anti Nuclear Antibodies* (ANA), *Anti Smooth Muscle Antibodies* (SMA) and *Anti Liver/Kidney Microsome* (LKM) are commonly researched; in the hypothesis of a primitive bile cholangitis *Anti Mitochondrial Antibodies* (AMA) researched; if sclerosing cholangitis is suspected *Anti-Neutrophil Cytoplasmic Antibodies* (ANCA) are researched.

To research auto antibodies in serum, indirect immunofluorescence method (IFI) is used. It is based on the capacity of antibodies against human immunoglobulins, conjugated with fluorescent substances, to detect the presence of antibodies fixed to specific antigens, expressed in substrates that consist of cells in culture or sections of murine or monkey tissue fixed on slide.

For the correct evaluation of tests it is necessary to define antibody pattern that, even if not specific, is associated more frequently to a type of autoimmune disease, and intensity of fluorescence that is expressed with a quantitative evaluation obtained by performing sequential dilutions of serum until to the disappearance of fluorescence.

Exams for the Diagnosis of HereditaryStorage Disease

Wilson's Disease

The dosage of ceruloplasmin is used if Wilson's disease is suspected. Ceruloplasmin is a glycoprotein produced by the liver, which binds to copper molecules to allow the transportation in the bile and kidney for their elimination through urine. The levels of ceruplasmin in serum are usually measured with immunoenzymatic method and normal values are included between 20 and 60 mg/dL. In Wilson's disease, the values can be lower than 10 mg/dL, but about the half of patients affected by active Wilson's disease can have values of ceruplasmin lower than the standard levels.

Haemochromatosis

In patients with a possible iron accumulation in the liver, the percentage of saturation of transferrin and serum levels of ferritin should be measured.

The value of saturation of transferrin is the percentage given by the ratio between plasmatic iron level (quantity of iron transported in the blood) and TIBC (capacity of proteins in haematic circle to bind the iron). The percentage of saturation of transferrin is calculable by the following formula:

$$\text{saturation of transferrin} = (\text{plasma iron level/TIBC}) \times 100.$$

Normal values of saturation are lower than 45%. In patients with saturation of transferrin higher than 45% it is necessary to perform the research of genetic mutation that are associated to haemochromatosis. Elevated serum levels of ferritin help to confirm the diagnosis of haemochromatosis and they can be useful as predictors of liver fibrosis. Ferritin values lower than 1000 ng/dL indicate that is very improbable the presence of liver cirrhosis in patients with haemochromatosis, whereas values higher than 1000 ng/dL, if associated to other bioumoral tests, physical signs and indicative instrumental data of chronic liver damage, can help to do diagnosis of liver cirrhosis.

Deficit of α1-Antitripsine

Deficit of α 1-antitripsine (AAT) is a genetic disease that is a genetic disease that is occurred with a pulmonary emphysema and other clinical manifestations. It is characterized by low levels of AAT, glycoprotein produced by the liver with inhibitory function of proteasis. The lack of this protein is mainly due to hereditary deficiency and numerous genetic variants that cause the production of reduced levels of antitripsin (50-80% of the normal). α1-antitripsine is dosed on the blood with an immunofelometric method and normal values are 90 205 mg/dL.

Evaluation of Liver Fibrosis

Liver Biopsy

The main aim of liver biopsy is to obtain useful information to define the prognosis and for therapeutic decisions. Particularly, biopsy is indicated to know the severity of the disease, both in terms of extension of necro-inflammatory injuries (grading) and quantity of fibrosis (*staging*). In the clinical practice, the pathologists use systems of "semiquantitative evaluation" that express with a number (usually from 1 to 4) or with an adjective (mild, moderate, grave) the severity of the degree of inflammation and the stage of fibrosis. Moreover, through the biopsy it is possible to evaluate the histological specific characteristics that are associated to clinical picture such as alcoholic and non-alcoholic steatosis, the inflammatory infiltrate on viral hepatitis, plasmacellular infiltrate of autoimmune hepatitis, alterations of cholangiocyte and small bile ducts in primitive bile cholangitis or sclerosing cholangitis, iron accumulation in haemochromatosis or copper accumulation in Wilson's disease. Through the current techniques, the complication of a bioptic exam of the liver is represented by pain (easily controllable) and unusually by bleeding.

Non Invasive Methods for Evaluation of Liver Fibrosis

Fibroscan

In the last few years new instrumental and lab approaches are developed for non invasive evaluation of liver fibrosis. The most promising method is based on the liver elastography (Fibroscan). Fibroscan is an instrument based on the principle of elastometry, which evaluates the elasticity of the liver. The system consists of a low frequency probe that include an ultrasound transductor built on the axis of a vibrator. A low frequency vibration is transmitted by the vibrator to the liver tissue through the transductor. The vibration induces the wave that spreads through the liver. At the same time, the ultrasounds pulse-echo follows the wave and measures the velocity that is directly correlated to elasticity of liver tissue. The results registered in real time by the same transductor and expressed in kilopascal (kPa). The increase of consistence of liver tissue determines the velocity of propagation of the wave, therefore in patients with mild fibrosis and liver characterized by normal elasticity low values in kPa are registered, whereas in patients with advanced fibrosis or cirrhosis the registered values are more elevated.
New elastography techniques, based on Acoustic Radiation Force Impulse (ARFI), both point-shear wave elastograpy (pSWE) and two-dimensional shear wave elastography (2D-SWE), are becoming widely used, especially in the last few years. Cut-off values to stage liver fibrosis were recently published and are summarized in the **Table 29.2**.
Liver stiffness was found to be directly related to fibrosis severity and CSPH, defined as an increased pressure gradient in hepatic veins >10 mmHg. In terms of portal hypertension, liver stiffness is a reliable indicator of increased intrahepatic resistances and does not account for the hyperdyna-

Table 29.2 Current recommendations for interpretation of liver stiffness values.

Current Recommendations for Interpretation of Liver Stiffness Values Evaluated by pSWE in Patients with Viral Hepatitis and NAFLD

<5 kPa (1.3 m/sec)	High probability for ruling-**out compensated advanced chronic liver disease** (cACLD)
<9 kPa (1.7 m/sec)	In absence of suggestive clinical signs, this cut-off can exclude **compensated advanced chronic liver disease** (cACLD)
9-13 kPa (1.7-2.1 m/sec)	High probability for **compensated advanced chronic liver disease** (cACLD), but need to be correlated with clinical, laboratory and ultrasound findings
>13 kPa (2.1 m/sec)	Diagnostic for **compensated advanced chronic liver disease** (cACLD)
>17 kPa (2.4 m/sec)	Suggestive for clinically significant portal hypertension (CSPH)

mic splanchnic circulation, this is the main reason behind the development of stiffness studies on the spleen. Portal hypertension leads to spleen congestion, thus increasing its stiffness.
However, actual guidelines do not specify cut-off values for this new method, given the fact that up until the last two-three years the evidence was not so abundant.

Abdominal Ultrasonography

Even liver ultrasonography has an important role in diagnostics of liver diseases. Through the observation of specific signs such as nodularity of liver surface, hypertrophy of caudate lobe and blood-flow velocity recording characteristics of sovrahepatic veins, the ultrasonography can give useful information about fibrosis progression.
To evaluate portal hypertension, ultrasonography exam has to evaluate the patency of portal vein and the presence of collateral or ascites circles, and to measure the size of portal vein, the dimension of the spleen and the velocity of portal flow. It is necessary to evaluate the content ot bladder and the possible dilation if bile ducts in case of benign or malign obstruction. Finally, ultrasonography is crucial in the surveillance of patients affected by liver cirrhosis, since they can develop hepatocellular carcinoma.

Haematochemical Tests of Fibrosis

They are good markers of presence or absence of fibrosis or cirrhosis. It is not yet clear their role in the distinction of different stages of fibrosis, its progression and regression. Indirect markers reflect the liver function that reduced with the progression of fibrosis; whereas direct marker reflect the extracellular matrix considering molecules involved in liber fibrogenesis.
Among the indirect markers, there is APRI (AST/*Platelet Ratio Index*), validated in chronic C virus hepatitis, and Fibrotest that used five biochemical parameters and two clinical one. Among direct marker there are hyaluronic acid and PIIINP (terminal ammine and serum peptide of procollagen III). Enhanced Liver Fibrosis (ELF) score was developed combining clinical and biochemicals parameters of fibrogenesis.

Invasive Method for the Evaluation of Portal Hypertension

Hypertension evaluation is a key point in diagnostic iter in patients with liver advanced fibrosis or cirrhosis. Digestive endoscopy is the first level method for the evaluation of patient with portal hypertension. The presence of oesophageal or gastric varices is sufficient to do a diagnosis of cirrhosis with portal hypertension, whereas the evaluation of the dimension of oesophageal varices (small, medium and big, on the basis of the percentage of occupation of oesophagus ray) and the presence of some pathognomonic signs (red signs) allow identifying subjects who can show digestive haemorrhage.
Hepatic Venous Pressure Gradient (HVPG) is the direct marker and was validated as indicator of portal pressure in liver cirrhosis. This technique, eco-guided, is performed by the introduction of a radiopaque balloon catheter under fluoroscopic control through jugular vein, up to one of the liver veins, where the measurement of free hepatic venous pressure (FHVP = *Free Hepatic Venous Pressure*) and the pressure obtained by occluding the vein (WHVP = *Wedged Hepatic Venous Pressure*) are carried out. The hepatic venous pressure gradient (HVPG) is the result of WHVP-FHVP. This method is able to distinguish the liver cirrhosis in clinical stage defined as: absence of non clinically significative portal hypertension HVPG between 6 and 10 mmHg); significative clinically portal hypertension (HVPG >10 mmHg). The value of HVPG >10 mmHg was identified as predictive of the development of complication of cirrhosis (appearance of oesophagus/gastric varices, haemorrhage caused by varices and ascites) and death.

KEY CONCEPTS

- Liver test performance represents the first main step for hepatopathy diagnosis and management.
- Routinary liver test (AST, ALT, γGT, alkaline phosphatase, total and fractionated bilirubin, Quick time, total proteins and electrophoresis express the cytolitic and cholestatic damage and liver protidosynthetic capacity.
- In hepatological evaluation of patients must be performed and taken into consideration all liver tests.

REFERENCES

- Barr RG, Wilson SR, Rubens D, Garcia-Tsao G, Ferraioli G. Update to the Society of Radiologists in Ultrasound Liver Elastography Consensus Statement. Radiology 2020; 296:263-274
- de Franchis R. Baveno VI Faculty. Expanding consensus in portal hypertension: report of the Baveno VI Consensus Workshop: stratifying risk and individualizing care for portal hypertension. J Hepatol. 2015;63:743-52.
- European Association for Study of Liver. EASL 2017 Clinical Practice Guidelines on the management of hepatitis B virus infection. J Hepatol. 2017;67:370-98.
- European Association for Study of Liver. EASL Recommendations on treatment of hepatitis C 2018. J Hepatol. 2018 Aug;69(2):461-511.
- European Association for the Study of the Liver; Asociacion Latinoamericana para el Estudio del Higado. EASL-ALEH clinical practice guidelines: non-invasive tests for evaluation of liver disease severity and prognosis. J Hepatol. 2015;63:237-64.
- Kwo PY, Cohen SM, Lim JK. ACG Clinical Guideline: Evaluation of Abnormal Liver Chemistries. Am J Gastroenterol. 2017;112:18-35.

CHAPTER 30

VIRAL HEPATITIS

Alessia Ciancio, Vito Di Marco

LEARNING OBJECTIVES

- To know the epidemiology, pathogenesis and clinic of hepatitis A, B, C, D, and E.
- To know how to distinguish acute from chronic hepatitis.
- To know how to assess the patient with viral hepatitis based on medical history, physical examination, and which II and I level tests to order.
- To know how to identify patients eligible for antiviral treatment.
- To know the available drugs, their mechanisms of action, their efficacy, and side effects.

Hepatitis is commonly the result of a viral infection; the most common are the hepatotropic viruses (Hepatitis A virus (HAV), Hepatitis B virus (HBV), Hepatitis C virus (HCV), Hepatitis D virus (HDV) and Hepatitis E virus (HEV)) that affect mainly, though not only, the liver. Viral hepatitis can also be observed in systemic virosis caused by cytomegalovirus, Epstein-Barr virus, adenovirus, Herpes virus and Coxsachie virus and Coronavirs-19. A particularly severe acute hepatitis occurs during yellow fever.

Viral hepatitis can be acute, with a more or less symptomatic clinical course and healing with elimination of the virus, or chronic, with persistence of long-term viral infection, associated with progressive liver disease. In general, hepatitis is classified as acute or chronic based on the duration of the inflammation and insult to the hepatic parenchyma. Chronic viral hepatitis of any aetiology can progress to cirrhosis; progression is partly linked to the aetiology of the disease (generally is faster in chronic hepatitis D than in chronic hepatitis C) or in presence of co-factors, such as alcohol abuse, that accelerate its evolution, or other viruses (HIV, HBV/HCV). In the acute forms, insufficient liver function can occur, depending on the extent of liver injury, which in severe cases may result in acute hepatic failure (AHF) with hepatic coma and death unless urgent liver transplant is performed.

ACUTE HEPATITIS

Acute viral hepatitis refers to necroinflammatory liver damage caused by hepatotropic virus infection that persists for less than six months. Hepatocyte necrosis and inflammation of liver tissue underlie the most common symptoms and clinical signs such as anorexia and jaundice and the appearance of abnormal serum liver test values. The objectives of the physician are to evaluate the severity of acute disease, define the aetiology of acute hepatitis, identify patients at high risk to develop fulminant hepatitis, evaluate the probability of chronic evolution, the opportunity of antiviral therapy, and establish prophylactic actions to reduce the risk of virus transmission to sexual partners and cohabiting family members.

There are two clinical patterns of acute viral hepatitis:

- symptomatic form characterised by jaundice preceded by or associated with anorexia, nausea and vomiting, abdominal pain, flu-like syndrome;
- asymptomatic form diagnosed based on the finding of elevated serum level (often 10-20 times the upper normal limit) of alanine aminotransferase (ALT) and aspartate aminotransferase (AST) without symptoms or signs of acute liver damage.

The symptomatic clinical pattern is more common in adult patients with epidemic HBV or HAV infection, while the asymptomatic presentation is characteristic of HBV infection in children and HAV or HEV infection in developing countries where transmission is endemic. Acute HCV infection is more often asymptomatic and the elevated serum AST/ALT levels is often less severe. Patients with immunodeficiency disorders or under immunosuppressive therapies are more likely to have the asymptomatic form if they have an acute viral infection.

Pathophysiologic Features

Typical acute viral hepatitis causes diffuse necroinflammatory damage of the lobular parenchyma with increased cellularity, pleomorphism of hepatocytes and spotty necrosis. Two mechanisms of parenchymal necrosis can be observed during viral acute hepatitis: eosinophilic degeneration with the formation of eosinophilic or acidophilic bodies that induce apoptosis and lytic necrosis and ballooning degeneration leading to lytic necrosis. The mechanisms of liver regeneration are characterized by mitosis and nucleation of hepatocytes; inflammation reactions include proliferation of Kupffer cells and infiltration of sinusoids and the portal tract by inflammatory mononuclear cells. Cholestasis is mild and appears late in the course of acute hepatitis, and steatosis is mild or absent. Inflammatory mononuclear cells expand the portal tracts, but piecemeal necrosis is rare and very mild. Bridging necrosis and multilobular necrosis or massive necrosis develops in more severe cases. Fibrosis of the portal tract and proliferation of bile ducts are absent. In acute hepatitis associated with systemic viral infection (cytomegalovirus, Epstein-Barr virus, adenovirus and herpes virus), liver damage may be focal or massive, depending on the severity of infection. In fulminant hepatitis, the liver undergoes massive multilobular or bridging necrosis.

Diagnostic Criteria

When a patient presents the clinic pattern of acute hepatitis, the physician must seek additional information to confirm diagnosis, identify the virus infection, and evaluate the risk of liver failure. A rational approach to diagnosis must start from careful clinical history taking and search for the potential source of virus infection.
The main elements to verify are:

- recent travel to areas endemic for viral hepatitis (HAV and HEV);
- infection occurring during a well-defined family or community outbreak of viral hepatitis (HAV, HBV, HEV);
- parenteral drug abuse including intranasal cocaine use (HBV, HCV);
- tattoos, acupuncture, or ear piercing (HBV, HCV);
- unprotected sexual intercourse (HBV, HAV, HCV), particularly in men who have sex with men (MSM).

The physician should ask the patient to list currently used medications and herbal products to rule out the drugs known to cause hepatotoxic injury; and alcoholic hepatitis should be considered in patients with a history of alcohol abuse. A complete physical examination is appropriate, but there are no specific physical signs of acute hepatitis. In addition to jaundice, hepatomegaly can be found.

Blood Tests

To establish the severity of acute hepatitis it is advisable to perform laboratory tests, and to establish the aetiology it is necessary to search for specific serological markers. Serum levels of AST and ALT are elevated in acute hepatitis: ALT levels over five times the upper normal limit, and over ten times the upper normal limit in most cases of symptomatic hepatitis. Typically, ALT levels are higher than those of AST. In asymptomatic patients, elevated enzymes levels may be the only sign of disease, while in symptomatic patients, the serum levels of bilirubin are elevated. Bilirubin peak, generally, follows ALT peak. The serological diagnosis of acute hepatitis is presented in **Table 30.1**.

Therapy

There are no specific treatments for acute hepatitis and major emphasis is placed on prevention of transmission.
Persons with uncomplicated acute hepatitis do not require hospitalization and are managed at home with outpatient follow-up. Intensive care management is pivotal in patients with fulminant hepatitis. Age, encephalopathy, serum bilirubin and INR, and creatinine serum levels are important predictors of outcome and suggest the urgency of OLT.

Hepatitis A Virus (HAV)

HAV is a small RNA virus, a member of the genus *Hepatovirus*, spread by the fecaloral route, either via person-to-person contact or via consumption of contaminated food or water. Causes acute hepatitis only. Fulminant hepatic failure develops in less than 1 percent of patients with hepatitis A. HAV is ubiquitous and the incidence of HAV has declined substantially since implementation of vaccination. In high endemic areas, HAV infection is usually acquired in infancy and the majority of people less than 20 years of age are immune to the virus. In developed countries, HAV usually occurs sporadi-

Table 30.1 Serological diagnosis of acute hepatitis.

Hepatitis	Serological Markers
Hepatitis A	anti-HAV IgM
Hepatitis B	HBsAg, anti-HBc IgM
Hepatitis D	HDV Ag, anti-HDV IgM
Hepatitis C	Anti-HCV, HCV-RNA
Hepatitis E	anti-HEV IgM

cally or in outbreaks in at-risk persons, particularly travelers or tourists who have visited developing countries and men who have sex with men (SMS). Symptoms develop 15 to 45 days after infection and often with abrupt onset with fever, fatigue, anorexia, nausea, vomiting, abdominal distress, and myalgia, with dark urine and pale stools.

In children, HAV infection is often asymptomatic or causes mild symptoms, whereas in more than 70% of adults, infection often presents with symptoms and jaundice. Symptoms end in 2-4 weeks and serum AST/ALT levels return to normal within 3 to 4 months.

The standard for diagnosis of acute HAV infection is the detection of IgM anti-HAV antibodies in serum. IgM anti-HAV is detectable from the onset of symptoms and usually remains positive approximately 3-24 weeks, although low levels of IgM anti-HAV remain detectable for more than 12 months. Total anti-HAV, which is a mixture of IgG and IgM, is also positive at onset of infection. High serum levels of IgG anti-HAV remain detectable for life and are interpreted as a marker of previous infection. HAV infection can have a protracted course (over 3-4 months) and a biphasic pattern with a second AST/ALT peak, but never causes chronic hepatitis. The prognosis of HAV hepatitis is invariably favorable even in rare cases presenting a protracted course. Acute HAV infection does not require specific therapy.

Hepatitis B Virus (HBV)

The hepatitis B virus has a partially double stranded circular DNA genome of about 3.2 kilobase pairs. The envelope gene of HBV produces the surface antigen (HBsAg), hepatitis B core antigen (HBcAg) is the major product of the nucleocapsid gene, while hepatitis B antigen (HBeAg) is a secreted product of the same gene. The transmission routes are parenteral (drug abuse, tattoo, body piercing, acupuncture, aesthetic or otherwise called cosmetic treatments), unprotected sexual intercourse with at risk partners, men who have sex with men, heterosexual persons who have multiple sex partners or contact with sex workers or perinatal by an HBsAg-positive mother. HBV infection has a long incubation period, ranging between 40 and 180 days, during which the person is infectious. In adults, the onset of disease is insidious with malaise, anorexia, and nausea. These symptoms precede the onset of jaundice. The duration of jaundice ranges from a few days to several weeks.

Serum HBsAg positivity in patients with acute hepatitis suggests that HBV is the causative agent, but the standard for diagnosis of acute HBV hepatitis is the detection of serum IgM anti-HBc. IgM anti-HBc is detected at the onset of acute hepatitis and persists for 3-12 months. At the onset of symptoms both HBeAg and HBV-DNA can be detected in the serum and usually disappear after the AST/ALT peak. Anti-HBe antibodies appear in serum shortly after the disappearance of HBeAg, although both may be positive for a short time.

Total anti-HBc, including both IgM and IgG antibodies, is present at onset of acute hepatitis B. When the acute hepatitis subsides, IgM anti-HBc disappears, but IgG anti-HBc persists for life. HBsAg remains detectable during the course of acute hepatitis and disappears during convalescence. Anti-HBs arise after HBsAg is no longer detectable and remain present for life in most people. The prognosis of typical HBV hepatitis is good and more than 95% of adults recover without sequelae. The persistence of abnormal ALT values for more than 6 months after the onset of acute hepatitis suggests progression to chronicity.

Treatment for acute HBV is mainly supportive, because in adults the progression in the chronic form is observed in only about 5% of patients. Patients with a severe (such as those who develop a coagulopathy [INR >1.5]) or a protracted course (such as persistent symptoms or marked jaundice [bilirubin >10 mg/dL] for more than four weeks after presentation) should be treated with nucleos(t)ide therapy.

Hepatitis D

HDV is a small defective RNA virus that causes hepatitis only in patients with concurrent HBV infection; the simultaneous presence of HBsAg is required for complete virion assembly and secretion.

Acute HDV infection may present as coinfection with HBV or superinfection in a chronic HBsAg carrier. The two forms have different serological patterns. The standard diagnosis of acute HDV hepatitis relies on the detection of HDV antigen (HDV Ag) in serum during the early stage of infection and of anti-HDV antibodies (anti-HDV Ab). IgM anti-HDV is detected early during the course of acute HDV hepatitis. Acute HDV hepatitis can be referred to as coinfection if IgM anti-HBc is present, since this marker suggests a concomitant acute B infection.

There is no specific treatment for acute HDV infection.

Hepatitis C

HCV is a single stranded RNA virus. The routes of transmission are similar to those of hepatitis B, but the efficiency of sexual, household, and perinatal transmission is much lower. Onset of symptoms occurs usually 2 to 26 weeks after infection, but most cases are asymptomatic and only 25% of patients develop jaundice. Anti-HCV antibodies can be detected in about 90% of patients with HCV acute hepatitis during 3-4 weeks of illness. However, the diagnostic window between the acute onset and anti-HCV seroconversion can be as long as 6-9 months. Moreover, in the absence of well-documented anti-HCV seroconversion, anti-HCV cannot differentiate between acute, chronic or past infection. The standard diagnosis relies on the detection of HCV-RNA in serum by polymerase chain reaction (PCR) that can be detectable as early as one to two weeks after exposure. A common aspect of acute HCV infection is its high probability to induce chronic liver disease. In fact, 50-85% of patients with acute infection develop chronic liver disease and 20% will progress to cirrhosis. There is not any recommendation for an immediate treatment: patients could undergo antiviral therapy during acute infection rather than waiting six months to determine whether chronic infection has been established

Hepatitis E

HEV is a single stranded RNA virus and, like HAV, causes acute epidemic hepatitis. Virus transmission occurs by the fecaloral route and transmission is associated with contamination of food or water source in developing countries. In developed countries, hepatitis E is mostly locally acquired zoonotic infection. An important route of infection is consumption of infected pork products that have been undercooked or consumed without cooking. A few HEV infections have demonstrated a possible transmission by blood transfusions or by vertical transmission. The incubation period is approximately 15-60 days. Around three weeks post-infection, HEV RNA is detected in blood and stool, with viremia lasting approximately 3-6 weeks. The anti-HEV IgM can be measured early in the serum of infected persons and is then replaced by anti-HEV IgG. Immunosuppressed patients can fail to clear HEV infection, and chronic HEV infection has been defined as persistent HEV replication for 6 months. The vast majority of patients with acute HEV are asymptomatic; in symptomatic patients, jaundice is usually accompanied by malaise, anorexia, nausea, vomiting, abdominal pain, but also diarrhoea, arthralgia and pruritus. Acute HEV infection does not require antiviral therapy. Very few case reports are available on ribavirin treatment for severe acute HEV infection, except in pregnant women as its teratogen activity

CHRONIC HEPATITIS

The chronic types of viral hepatitis are characterized by a course that exceeds 6-12 months of persistent infection. Generally follow an acute, symp tomatic or asymptomatic phase, which does not recover but persists with subsequent chronicity; they frequently have a subtle, asymptomatic outset, and are incidentally discovered during examination or visits for other reasons, or late with symptoms and signs of complications (ascites, digestive bleeding, encephalopathy or hepatic cancer), when already in the cirrhotic phase. Viruses that, in addition to acute hepatitis, cause chronic hepatitis are:

- Hepatitis B Virus (HBV);
- Hepatitis C Virus (HCV);
- Hepatitis D Virus, (HDV);
- Chronic hepatitis caused by hepatitis E virus (HEV) has been reported in the immunocompromised.

Chronic HBV Hepatitis

In Italy, the prevalence in the general population of HBV chronic infection, higher in the past, is now estimated to be <1%, with prevalence clearly higher in immigrants, with great variability in relation to the country of origin.

Epidemiology

After primary infection, less than 10% of healthy adults and up to 90% of children become chronic carriers of the virus. According to the 2016 Polaris Observatory Study, around 364 million people live in the world with a chronic HBV infection. The prevalence of hepatitis B varies between countries; in industrialized countries, it is generally less than 2%. In Italy, the number of HBsAg carriers is less than 1%, the majority of which is over 50 years old, but the prevalence of HBV infection in immigrants is much higher than in Italians, exceeding 8% in some groups. The epidemiology of HBV in Italy has undergone a radical decrease in recent decades, because of improvement in public hygienic and socioeconomic conditions, campaigns for the prevention of HIV infection, which shares the same transmission routes with HBV, vaccination against HBV. In Italy, vaccination, which became mandatory in 1991 for all newborns and children up to age 12 years in 2003 remained mandatory only for newborns, thus boosting the protection of the entire population up to 40 years of age. Another measure that contributed to the epidemiological trend was the introduction, in 1991, of mandatory screening for women in the third trimester of pregnancy, which allowed prophylaxis in births by HBsAg-positive mothers.

Natural History and Clinical Manifestations

The virological evolution of chronic infection B is conventionally divided into five successive phases:

1. HBeAg-positive chronic HBV infection (without clinical evidence of disease, previously termed 'immune tolerant' phase);
2. HBeAg-positive chronic HBV hepatitis (with clinical evidence of disease, previously termed immune reactive phase);
3. HBeAg-negative chronic HBV infection (without clinical evidence of disease, previously termed 'inactive carrier');
4. HBeAg-negative chronic HBV hepatitis (with clinical evidence of disease, previously termed HBeAg negative chronic hepatitis);
5. occult infection.

The different stages of chronic HBV infection may occur over time, according to the virological stages of chronic HBV infection as presented in **Table 30.2**. The first four phases are characterized by the presence of HBsAg and are defined based on the HBeAg/anti-HBe serological status and serum HBV-DNA titer; while occult infection is defined by the absence of HBsAg in the blood and by the presence of HBV-DNA in the liver. Patients in immunotolerance may remain so for a long time or may demonstrate a progressive transition in the phase of immunoclearance, which corresponds to the phase of chronic HBeAg positive hepatitis.

From clinical point of view, we can distinguish:

-HBeAg positive chronic hepatitis, with persistently altered transaminase levels with moderate fluctu-

Table 30.2 Virological phases of HBV infection.

	HBeAg Positive		**HBeAg Negative**		
	Chronic Infection	**Chronic Hepatitis**	**Chronic Infection**	**Chronic Hepatitis**	**Occult Infection**
Old terminology	Immune tolerant	Immune reactive HBeAg positive	Inactive carrier	HBeAg negative chronic hepatitis	Occult infection
HBsAg	High	High/intermediate	Low	Intermediate	Negative
HBeAg	Positive	Positive	Negative	Negative	Negative
antiHBe	Negative	Negative	Positive	Positive	Positive/ Negative
HBV DNA	>107 IU/mL	104-107 IU/mL	<2,000 IU/mL	>2,000 IU/mL	<200 IU/mL
HBV-DNA in the liver	Positive (++)	Positive (+)	+	Positive/+	Positive (+)
ALT	Normal	Elevated	Normal	Elevated	Normal
Liver disease	None/minimal	Moderate/severe	None	Moderate/severe	None
Disease progression	Low	Moderate to high	Very low	Moderate to high	no
Treatment	**Not indicated**	**Indicated**	**Not indicated**	**Indicated**	**Not indicated**

ations, and high HBV-DNA levels; the key histologic finding is hepatic necroinflammation of variable entity. The patient with HBe-Ag positive chronic hepatitis may remain in this phase over time, often with disease progression to cirrhosis and possibly hepatocarcinoma, or transition in the anti-HBe positive phase (anti-HBe seroconversion) with remission of disease and asymptomatic carrier status, or progression to chronic anti-HBe positive hepatitis.

- Chronic anti-HBe positive hepatitis, in which a continuous necroinflammatory process characterizes the disease in about 30-40% of cases and in the remaining from the fluctuating trend of HBV-DNA and hepatic cytolysis (and related transaminases) is interspersed with periods of biochemical remission and absence or minimal viral replication determinable in the blood. It is the most represented form of chronic hepatitis B (> 85% of cases) in Italy and is supported by HBV variants unable to express HBeAg (HBeAg-minus). The infection remains long asymptomatic; the disease is diagnosed at an age between 35-40 years and reaches the cirrhotic stage at an average age of 45 years. The difference between chronic HBV-infected HBV-positive HBV and HBeAg-negative HBV is presented in **Table 30.3**.
- 'Asymptomatic' carriers of HBV, with non-progressive chronic infection - generally with positivity for HBsAg and anti-HBe, normal transaminases, undetectable or low-dose HBV-DNA, absence of signs or symptoms of liver disease. The inactive asymptomatic carrier may remain so over time or demonstrate viral reactivation with recovery of activity and disease development. These individuals should be monitored over time without antiviral therapy and should avoid as far as possible exposure to other hepatotoxic factors (alcohol, other hepatitis viruses, drugs, etc.) and, as far as possible, drugs that may influence immune control (cortisone, immunosuppressants, cytostatic, immunomodifying biological drugs), which are potentially capable of reactivating the virus and liver disease.

In chronic infection, the patient often comes to the doctor's attention for increased transaminase levels or the occasional finding of HBsAg, in the absence of a history of previous active infection and in complete absence of symptoms. In other cases, chronic HBV hepatitis occurs with non-specific digestive symptoms or with chronic asthenia and, more rarely, with rheumatological systemic signs or with vasculitis and panarteritis. If the chronic infection is long lasting and has not been identified or has been neglected, the diagnosis of related HBV chronic liver disease may be delayed in the presence of complications such as decompensated cirrhosis or a hepatocarcinoma.

HBV and Pregnancy

HBV infection does not influence the course or outcome of pregnancy and pregnancy does not influence the course of HBV liver disease; however, a study involving women with chronic HBV-related hepatitis, reported an increased risk of gestational diabetes, antepartum haemorrhage, and preterm delivery, while in decompensated cirrhosis, the likelihood of carrying out a pregnancy it is 50%. In cirrhotic women, there is an increased risk of worsening of portal hypertension during pregnancy, with a consequent increase in decompensation or oesophageal varices bleeding, for which a gastroscopy starting from the second trimester is appropriate. In finding varicose veins at risk, there is indication of treatment; beta-blockers can be used. During pregnancy, the immune response to HBV decreases with increased HBV-DNA and decreased transaminases, but after delivery returns with reduction in HBV-DNA and increased transaminases. All women with chronic HBV-related hepatitis should receive

Table 30.3 Clinical differences between chronic wild-type HBV infection and chronic HBeAg minus infection.

	HbsAg+ Wild Type	HBeAg - Type
Age (years)	<40	>40
ALT	Stable	Variable
Viremia	Stable	Variable
Parenteral risk factors	Presents	Absent
Progression	50%	>80%
Response to interferon	Pretty good	Poor

a quantify HBV-DNA quantification test at the end of the second trimester before considering eventual antiviral prophylaxis in the third trimester (**Table 30.4**), if the HBV-DNA titer is high (>200.000 IU/mL) o l'HBsAg >4 log10). Antiviral prophylaxis with TDF should start at week 24–28 of gestation and continue for up to 12 weeks after delivery

There is no evidence that caesarean delivery decreases the risk of maternal foetal transmission of HBV. Breastfeeding is not contraindicated unless the mother is on antiviral therapy.

Treatment Options

In recent years, new antiviral drugs for chronic hepatitis B have boosted the efficacy and safety rates, prolonging patient life expectancy and enhancing the control of the evolution of liver injury. The aim of treatment is to promote the loss of HBsAg and the appearance of HBsAg antibodies (anti-HBs seroconversion). However, this result is achieved only in a small number of patients; in most cases, the persistent suppression of viral replication (HBV-DNA negative) is obtained, leading to a reduction in necroinflammatory hepatic activity, arrest or delay of progression of fibrosis and/or the appearance of cirrhosis and its complications, but without the permanent elimination of the virus. In practice, the treatment aims to transform a viremic patient with chronic hepatitis (active infection), both HBeAg + and HBeAg-, into an inactive anti-HBe positive carrier without disease, with undetectable serum HBV-DNA.

Treatment Indications

The indication for treatment depends on the degree of fibrosis, the level of HBV-DNA (>2000 IU/mL) and of transaminases, regardless of the HBe- Ag disease. The study of fibrosis usually requires a liver biopsy, because Fibroscan is not considered reliable in recognizing intermediate fibrosis in chronic hepatitis B. If the patient is HBeAg positive, the transaminase levels are normal (in some controls over six months), and the HBV-DNA titer is high; in the immunotolerant phase, there is no indication to treat, unless there is a positive family history of liver cancer or cirrhosis or evidence of significant fibrosis on liver biopsy. The patient should be monitored every six months. Patients with normal transaminases but HBeAg negative and HBV-DNA not determinable or present at low titer, classified as inactive carrier, should not be treated but rather monitored once a year.

Treatment should be considered in HBeAg positive and negative patients, with a bioptic evidence of moderate to severe hepatic fibrosis or in patients with mild fibrosis based on age, favorable prognostic factors (HBV-DNA with a low titer, genotype A, B, and C), and based on patient's motivation. Treatment is always "mandatory" in patients with cirrhosis even if ALT levels are normal and HBV-DNA levels are <2000 IU/mL but still detectable and should be "immediate" in patients with decompensated disease.

Table 30.4 Recommendations during pregnancy in women with HBV chronic infection.

Condition	Recommendations
WOMAN OF CHILDBEARING AGE without advanced fibrosis	Delay therapy until the child is born
FIRST TRIMESTER	Screening for HBsAg is strongly recommended
PREGNANT WOMEN with moderate or severe liver fibrosis	Therapy with Tenofovir is recommended
PREGNANT WOMEN already on NA therapy	Tenofovir should be continued while Entecavir or other NA should be switched to Tenofovir
THIRD TRIMESTER	In pregnant women with high HBV DNA levels (>200,000 IU/mL) or HBsAg levels >4 log10 IU/mL, antiviral prophylaxis with Tenofovir should start at week 24–28 of gestation and continue for up to 12 weeks after delivery
BREAST FEEDING	It is not contraindicated in HBsAg positive untreated or treated women

Therapeutic Strategies

Italian guidelines have proposed an algorithm, the "Stresa paradigm", that recommends indications for treatment and type of drug to be used in relation to stage of disease. The scheme attributes to interferon a priority role in initial or mild forms of disease, a role that decreases with progression of fibrosis, and recommends a rational choice based on favorable criteria of response. The Stresa paradigm allows therapy with oral antiviral agents, so called nucleoside/nucleotide analogs (NUC), from the forms with substantial fibrosis to liver biopsy (Ishak >S3 or Metavir >F2) in increasing indication with the increase in fibrosis and particularly in decompensated cirrhosis or in conditions at risk of decompensation. (**Table 30.5**)
Two therapeutic modalities are recognized, depending on the drug used.

Interferon therapy

Interferons (IFN) are a family of cytokines produced by cells in response to various stimuli; the control of viral replication and disease occurs through immune modulation. IFN therapy is limited over time, usually no longer than 12 months, depending on the stage of disease. In the treatment of chronic HBV hepatitis, alpha-interferons are used, available in Italy in a pegylated form, i.e., slow release and weekly administration, at a dosage of 180μg.
The main indication is in the early stages of disease, in young and in HBeAg- positive person; a reduction (or loss) of HBsAg in association with a decrease in viremia and normalization of transaminases is predictive of response. Response to therapy is achieved not only when serum HBV-DNA is no longer determinable, but also in low residual viremia such as in spontaneous inactive carriers

Table 30.5 Indications for treatment in patients with HV infection.

Condition	Recommendations	Treatment
HBeAg +ve chronic infection (normal ALT and high HBV-DNA levels)	Treatment not indicated but patients should be followed with periodical assessments	
HBeAg +ve chronic infection older than 30 years	Patients may be treated	Interferon (or NA)
HBeAg +ve chronic infection with family history of HCC or cirrhosis	Patients can be treated	Interferon (or NA)
HBeAg -ve chronic infection	Treatment not indicated but patients should be followed with periodical assessments	
HBeAg -ve chronic infection with family history of HCC or cirrhosis	Patients can be treated	Interferon (or NA)
HBeAg +ve chronic hepatitis with HBV-DNA >2000 U, increased ALT and fibrosis >F2	Patients should be treated	Interferon or NA
HBeAg -ve chronic hepatitis with HBV-DNA >2000 U, increased ALT and fibrosis >F2	Patients should be treated	Interferon or NA
Patients with compensated or decompensated cirrhosis (regardless of HBV-DNA or ALT levels)	Treatment is mandatory	NA
PREGNANT WOMEN with HBV-DNA >200.000 IU/mL or HBsAg >4 log10 IU/mL	Antiviral prophylaxis should start at week 24–28 of gestation and continue for up to 12 weeks after delivery	Tenofovir

(HBV-DNA <2000 IU/mL). IFN therapy is successful in about 20-30% of patients with positive HBeAg chronic hepatitis and in 10-25% of patients with chronic anti-HBe positive hepatitis, with differences depending on the stage of disease and viral genotype. Treatment with IFN can be burdened by side effects, including asthenia, hyporexia/anorexia, flu-like syndrome, headache, myalgia, local reactions at the injection site; adverse events such as neutropenia and thrombocytopenia require a dose reduction or suspension in 10 to 40% of patients. Usually, the use of IFN is contraindicated in patients with decompensated liver disease, leukopenia and/or severe thrombocytopenia, severe and uncontrolled depression, current pregnancy, active autoimmune diseases, epilepsy, active drug addiction, and heart failure.

Therapy with oral antiviral drugs

Oral antiviral agents (NUC) are divided into nucleosides, such as lamivudine (LMV) and entecavir (ETV), and nucleotides such as tenofovir disoproxil fumarate (TDF) and tenofovir alafenamid (TAF, tenofovir prodrug but with greater safety for bone metabolism and renal function). This therapy achieves and then maintains inactive carrier status through prolonged control of viral replication with these drugs; NUCs cannot eradicate HBV, but only inhibit replication, so that HBV-DNA remains undetectable in serum. Benefits of NUC are oral administration, high rate of control of viremia (>90%), and minimal side effects. NUC therapy is indicated especially in patients with advanced liver disease or contraindications or intolerance to peg-IFN or in patients who have not responded to a previous peg-IFN cycle. The current indication is to use third generation NUCs, i.e., entecavir and tenofovir, because of their greater antiviral efficacy, with minimal risk of viral resistance, even when used for decades. They are administered orally in a single daily dose. Both decrease HBV-DNA levels and normalize transaminases within a few months. After five years of maintenance therapy with the two drugs, the response is maintained in more than 95% of treated patients, but the elimination of HBsAg remains un- common, especially in HBeAg-negative patients. For these reasons, oral therapy with NUC is indefinitely maintained in the majority of patients and is suspended only if HBsAg is definitively eliminated and no signs of cirrhosis. Response to ETV and TDF therapy in cirrhotic patients is very efficient (>90%), similar to non-cirrhotic forms, and free of side effects. Therapy clearly improves liver function immediately, and in the long term induces regression of fibrosis. Treatment with antivirals in decompensated cirrhosis should be started immediately. The disadvantage, real with first-generation NUC (like lamivudine), potential with second-generation NUCs, is the risk of emergency of viral variants, due to the appearance under pharmacological pressure of mutations in the reverse transcriptase gene that make the virus resistant to therapy, with loss of response, increased HBV-DNA, rise in transaminase levels, and delay recovery from hepatitis. The treatment of pregnant women with TDF in the third trimester of pregnancy is recommended to reduce the risk of HBV transmission to the unborn child; the drug has proven effective in reducing vertical transmission and without risk of teratogenicity.

Chronic HDV Hepatitis

The prevalence of HDV in HBsAg-positive chronic liver disease decreased from 25% in the 1970s to 8% at the end of the last century thanks to the aggressive vaccination campaigns against HBV. In recent years, the prevalence rate increased, due to the influx of immigrants from areas where HDV remains endemic (i.e., Moldavia, Mongolia and some areas in Africa). The current prevalence of infection in HBsAg carriers with chronic hepatitis is around 11%. As with HBV infection, chronic hepatitis D patient characteristics have also changed. Having decreased the reservoir of HDV infection and new infections, the current type of chronic hepatitis D is represented by patients who acquired the infection many years before, when the virus was endemic in Italy, and have often developed cirrhosis in the meantime. Clinical-histological progression of hepatitis D towards cirrhosis is frequent and observed in 85% of cases after superinfection and is usually more rapid than in chronic hepatitis B (in about 5-10 years). Once the cirrhotic state is reached, a clinically stable situation is often established, compatible with prolonged survival. In immigrants with more recent infections, the clinic resembles a florid chronic hepatitis, characterized by inflammation and conspicuous cytolysis.

Therapy

Interferon (IFN) remains the only treatment for chronic hepatitis D, but the results are limited. With Peg-IFN α-2a, at a dose of 180 µg/week for 12-18 months, virological response is obtained in about 25% of patients, but the response in cirrhotic patients is lower. Viral relapses are frequent after the therapy has been discontinued. This is explained by the fact that HDV is highly infectious in HBsAg, therefore the only valid goal of therapy is elimination of HBsAg. No response was observed with antivirals treatment based on directed drugs against HBV, neither with LMV, ETV and TDF, nor with the combination of these antivirals and Peg-IFN with or without ribavirin. Newer agents, having novel mechanisms of action, with or without Peg-IFN show more promise. As examples, Lonafarnib, a specific inhibitor of HDV prenylation, or Bulevirtide (Myrcludex B), which blocks entry of HBV and HDV. Both drugs show decline in HDV RNA levels during treatment. There is no HDV vaccine to prevent superinfection in HBsAg carriers, but HBV vaccination is effective prophylaxis against hepatitis D.

Chronic HCV Hepatitis

Hepatitis C virus infection can be initially asymptomatic, so that the acute phase of infection often goes unnoticed and is diagnosed in the chronic phase, usually following the occasional finding of a transaminase elevation or appearance of signs or symptoms of liver disease that lead patients to seek the causes. Symptoms are generally not very specific and include fatigue or digestive symptoms. Some patients with chronic HCV infection may have extra-hepatic disorders secondary to the C virus's ability to cause clinical manifestations outside the liver, such as mixed cryoglobulinemia, lymphomas or alterations in glucose and/or lipid metabolism. Mixed cryoglobulinemia, a circulating immune complex disease whose production is secondary to a B-cell lymphoproliferative process, is the extrahepatic disease most closely related to HCV infection. Only a minor proportion of persons with chronic HCV infection have symptoms such as asthenia, arthralgia, and cutaneous purpura. In severe cases, impairment of the function of the kidneys and peripheral and/or central nerves may also occur. Persons with chronic HCV infection also have a relatively higher risk of developing lymphoproliferative diseases than the general population, and a risk of developing lymphomas derived from peripheral B-lymphocytes (centrofollicular lymphoma, chronic lymphatic leukemia, immunocytoma, lymphoma of the marginal area).
Clinical and experimental studies have shown a correlation between HCV infection and metabolic abnormalities, such as insulin resistance, hepatic steatosis, and type 2 diabetes mellitus. These clinical manifestations are secondary to the ability of the C virus to interfere directly with insulin signal transduction pathways (HCV genotype 1) and with lipid metabolism (HCV genotype 3). Finally, recent clinical studies have reported an increase in atherosclerotic disease, cardiovascular changes, and mortality from cardiovascular events and a chronic deficit of serum vitamin D levels in subjects with chronic HCV infection.
Clinically, chronic HCV infection is characterized by alterations in transaminase level, with large fluctuations, but in a large percentage of patients with chronic HCV infection (20-30% of cases) transaminases remain persistently within normal values, which does not necessarily rule out significant hepatic injury. The course of chronic hepatitis is clinically silent; nevertheless, about 25% of chronic infections evolve towards cirrhosis. Once cirrhosis is established, the time interval leading to the development of portal hypertension or hepatic failure is 5-10 years. HCV cirrhosis is the major risk factor for the development of hepatocellular carcinoma, although cases of HCC have also been reported in persons with chronic HCV infection without cirrhosis. The natural history of chronic hepatitis is slow, generally taking about 20 years if there are no concurrent causes to speed up the process (alcohol, coinfections with other viruses, iron, drugs, age, and sex).
There are non-modifiable factors and modifiable factors, on which it is possible to intervene. Non-modifiable risk factors include age at the time of infection and gender. Studies have documented that advanced age at the time of infection and a longer time of infection are independently associated with faster progression of liver fibrosis. Males generally have a more rapid progression of liver disease than females. The lower rate of progression of liver fibrosis in women is lost after menopause, suggesting an antifibrogenic protective role of oestrogen. The modifiable risks factors of progression of hepatic fibrosis are: lifestyle habits; viral coinfections; and metabolic factors. Consumption of alcohol can accelerate the progression of liver disease in individuals with hepatitis C. Alcohol by itself, if consumed in high concentrations is a risk factor for chronic liver disease and even in small amounts, is significantly greater in hepatitis C. The consumption of alcohol of any kind, even in moderate quantities, should be avoided. Cannabis consumption is associated with a higher frequency of advanced liver fibrosis in individuals with HCV hepatitis. In contrast, coffee consumption seems to play a protective role in the progression of chronic HCV hepatitis. Other cofactors are viral coinfections, mainly in substance abusers or in transfused subjects before 1992. Coinfection with the hepatitis B virus leads to significant acceleration of progression, which has been greatly reduced with the introduction of universal vaccination for hepatitis B. An emerging problem is coinfection with HIV. In patients with HIV infection, thanks to retroviral therapies, life expectancy has increased

significantly, but increased survival is characterized by accelerated progression of chronic HCV hepatitis in cirrhosis, so that today the complications of HCV-induced liver cirrhosis are the most frequent cause of death in HIV-positive persons. Some metabolic alterations can interfere with the progression of liver fibrosis. For example, obesity, and in particular visceral obesity, insulin resistance, diabetes, and steatosis, are associated with a faster progression of hepatitis C infection. This evidence has led to the identification of targets to delay the evolution of liver disease. In patients with hepatitis C infection, diet, regular physical activity and, ultimately, body weight reduction improve insulin sensitivity and are associated with a slower evolution of liver injury. Patients should be educated about the benefits of regular to physical activity and a balanced diet for the maintenance of adequate body weight. The efficacy of drugs with insulin-sensitizing activity, albeit conceptually useful, has yet to be evaluated in patients with hepatitis C. Finally, low serum vita- min D levels and, less frequently, hepatic iron accumulation or genetic mutations in the HFE gene may contribute to faster progression of liver disease.

HCV and Pregnancy

The risk of HCV transmission from mother to newborn is less than 5%. In about a third of cases, the transmission of the virus has occurred already in utero. Although a spontaneous elimination rate of 25-30% of HCV has been reported, in other studies, including Italian ones, the percentage of chronic infection has been high. In HCV-positive women without cirrhosis of the liver, pregnancy does not usually give rise to complications. However, some studies have shown that HCV-positive pregnant women have an increased risk of gestational cholestasis compared to HCV-negative women. In HCV-positive women, transaminases often drop and normalize during pregnancy, while plasma HCV-RNA rises during the second or third trimester. In contrast, viremic titers decrease after pregnancy; spontaneous HCV elimination after delivery is attributed to the loss of pregnancy-induced immunosuppression, with consequent vigorous postpartum reconstitution of the immune response against HCV by T lymphocytes. There is no evidence that caesarean delivery decreases the risk of maternal-foetal transmission of HCV. Breast-feeding is not contraindicated.

Therapy

The treatment of HCV infection has undergone a profound innovative revolution in recent years, thanks to the development of drugs with direct antiviral action, which can be used orally, with an excellent safety profile and very high therapeutic efficacy. These drugs, called direct acting antivirals (DAA - Direct Antiviral Agents) ensure complete and definitive elimination of the virus in over 95% of treated patients. The new therapeutic schedule based on the combination of different DAAs has completely replaced traditional interferon-α and ribavirin therapies, which were the standard for hepatitis C, but with important limits for safety and clinical use, given the numerous contraindications, with even reduced efficacy in various patient subgroups. The new antiviral drugs (DAA) became available in Italy in the first half of 2015.

The new DAA became available in Italy in 2015; all patients who present with a chronic HCV infection, regardless of the degree of fibrosis, are eligible for reimbursement of DAA drugs. In this way, the national plan foresees for the control of virus hepatitis possible definitive elimination of HCV infection from the population over the next 10 years.

The New HCV Oral Antiviral Drugs

In 2015, new direct antiviral drugs (DAA) for the treatment of chronic C virus hepatitis became available in Italy.

They include various classes of drugs:

- viral polymerase inhibitors, directed against the NS5B protein of HCV, with the denomination ending in -buvir. The first member of this drug class is sofosbuvir, directed against the catalytic site of the viral polymerase (nucleoside inhibitor, NI). It is active against all HCV genotypes and has a high genetic barrier (i.e., it is very difficult for the virus to become resistant to the drug). It is therefore the reference drug for therapy, in combination with other DAAs in oral combination regimens (without interferon);
- inhibitors of HCV (PI) protease with the denomination ending in -previr. Currently, grazoprevir, glecaprevir and voxilaprevir, the latter coformulated with sofosbuvir and velpatasvir in a single molecule, are available;
- inhibitors of NS5A, a viral protein essential for replication and assembly of HCV, with the denomination ending in -asvir. In Italky, currently are Velpatasvir, coformulated in a single tablet with sofosbuvir, pibrentasvir, and elbasvir are available.

These DAAs are used in different oral combinations based on viral genotype and liver disease stage. With these treatment schemes it is possible to obtain a complete and definitive eradication of the virus (SVR-supported virological response, which is documented by the absence of HCV-RNA in the blood 12 weeks after the end of the therapeutic cycle) in about 95-98 % of patients treated. Therapy schedules are generally very well tolerated and can also be used in very advanced or decompensated liver disease (cirrhosis Child-Pugh B or C). These drugs have also revolutionized the management of liver transplantation in patients with related HCV disease, allowing patients to be transplanted without replicating virus and thus avoiding the recurrence of post-transplantation hepatitis C, previously unavoidable in 100% of cases.

Chronic HEV Hepatitis

Hepatitis E has long been considered a self-limiting disease. However, recently, some organ transplant patients and subsequent immunosuppressive therapy have developed chronic HEV infection, defined by the detection of persistent HEV-RNA in serum and feces for 6 months or more. In all studies, a frequency of chronicity was reported in about 1% of observed cases, and in patients undergoing liver transplantation a high rate of evolution in cirrhosis and graft failure was observed. Chronic HEV hepatitis has also been reported in HIV-positive patients and in immunosuppressed patients (HIV, chemotherapy or haematological or rheumatological diseases). So far, chronic hepatitis has involved persons with HEV genotype 3 infection. In organ transplant receiving immunosuppressive treatment, and affected by chronic HEV hepatitis, viral clearance is required to avoid the risk of progressive and rapid liver injury.

Before considering antiviral treatment, suspension, or reduction of the dose of immunosuppressive therapy (in particular of drugs acting on T cells) should be evaluated, if possible; viral clearance in 30% of patients results in reduction of immunosuppression. Antiviral therapy is necessary in patients in which it is impossible to reduce immunosuppressive treatment and those in which HEV-RNA clearance is not achieved after reduction of immunosuppression. Treatment options are not yet well defined: ribavirin has been used successfully in monotherapy only in a series of cases and controlled clinical trials. The dose of ribavirin is 600 to 1000 mg daily for 12 weeks with SVR rate around 80%. Anaemia was the most common side effect and required a reduction in ribavirin dose. Patients who fail to achieve an SVR, pegylated interferon-alfa could be considered. However, interferon has an immunostimulatory effect that can increase the risk of acute rejection in all organ transplant settings. For this reason, interferon cannot be used in kidney transplant recipients due to the increased risk of acute rejection.

KEY CONCEPTS

- Infection with hepatitis viruses is the most frequent cause of acute hepatitis.
- Acute HAV and HEV infections heal spontaneously whereas infection with HBV, HDV, and HCV often progress to chronic hepatitis.
- Assessment of the severity of disease in chronic hepatitis B is essential for therapy planning liver infection without disease does not require specific therapies, whereas chronic active hepatitis B is treated with specific and effective therapies.
- Chronic hepatitis D is a severe form of chronic hepatitis that evolves into cirrhosis in the short to medium term. The therapy for active chronic hepatitis D is peg-IFN for 12-18months.
- The evolution of chronic HCV-related hepatitis is influenced by different cofactors that influence with the progression of liver fibrosis.
- The treatment of HCV infection has recently undergone a profound innovative revolution, thanks to the development of drugs with direct antiviral action, which can be used orally, with an excellent safety profile - also in advanced or decompensated liver disease - and very high therapeutic efficacy (over 95% of success).

REFERENCES

- European Association for the Study of the Liver. EASL Clinical Practice Guidelines: management of chronic hepatitis B infection. J Hepatol. 2017;67:370-98.
- European Association for the Study of the Liver. EASL Recommendations on treatment of hepatitis C 2018. J Hepatol. 2018;69(2):461-511.
- The World Health Organization. Hepatitis B. https://www.who.int/news-room/fact-sheets/detail/hepatitis-b (Accessed on August 23, 2020).
- World Health Organization. Global progress report on HIV, viral hepatitis and sexually transmitted infections, 2021. Available at: https://www.who.int/publications/i/item/9789240027077.

ALCOHOL-RELATED LIVER DISEASE

Manuela Merli, Vincenzo Cardinale

LEARNING OBJECTIVES

- To recognise the presence of and know how to define the extent and duration of an incongruous use of alcohol over time.
- To know the main pathogenetic mechanisms of alcohol-induced liver injury.
- To recognise alcohol-related liver disease and its cofactors, know how to define the stage, the possible evolution, and therapeutic management.

INTRODUCTION

Alcohol-related organ disorders are extremely common conditions in the population and their onset depends not only on the amount of ethanol, but also and above all on the type of drinking (even occasional excessive drinking is a risk factor). Many of these organ diseases, such as chronic pancreatitis, dilated heart disease, peripheral neuropathy or Wernicke's encephalopathy can begin early in the youth or young adult age group. The estimate of daily alcohol consumption can be made using an arbitrary unit, called alcohol unit (AU) or drink. The AU corresponds to 12-13 g of ethanol; this amount is contained in a 125 mL wine glass, or in 330 mL of beer or in 40 mL of spirit. Alcohol-related liver disease (ALD) is defined as acute or chronic liver damage caused by the incongruous consumption of alcohol-related beverages. There is no dose of alcohol consumption defined as harmless since the organ damage from alcohol is influenced by several cofactors. However, the acceptable daily intake limit is a maximum of 20 g/day for females and 30 g/day for males. Alcohol addiction is instead described as the set of physiological, behavioural, and cognitive alterations in which the consumption of alcohol plays a high priority role.

EPIDEMIOLOGY

Scope of the Problem

In Europe, the population over 15 years of age consumes an average of 11.3 liters of pure alcohol per year (Status report on alcohol consumption, harm, and policy responses in 30 European countries 2019). This figure has not undergone significant changes in the last 10 years despite attempts in European countries to implement campaigns to contain the consumption of alcohol-related beverages. In 2016, the consumption of alcohol-related beverages was responsible for 5.5% of the deaths observed in 30 European countries. In the younger sections of the population, alcohol plays a proportionately more important role in mortality than it does between adults and the elderly. In the 15-19 age group this percentage rises to 19% and in the 20-24 age group to 23.3% of causes of death, depending on the mortality from road accidents caused by the use of alcohol. Around 1 in 5 deaths between 15-19 years and around 1 in 4 deaths in the 20-24 age group in Europe have been caused by alcohol, bringing the ratio of alcohol-related deaths in adolescents/young adults to in the adult population at a worrying proportion of about 4:1. In Italy, (data 2017-2020 Istituto Superiore di Sanità) less than half of adults (18 and 69 years) declare that they do not consume alcohol-related beverages, but almost 1 in 6 people use it at a "greater risk" for health , by quantity or method of recruitment. These are more frequently young people (between 18-24-year-olds the share is close to 33%), men and people socially more advantaged, without economic difficulties or with a high level of education. The consumption of "higher risk" alcohol remains a prerogative of residents in Northern Italy (with an increasing trend). Binge drinking, which has been slowly and steadily increasing since 2008, is also a prerogative of Northern Italy and in particular of the Northeast. Binge drinking is defined as the consumption of at least 5 alcohol-related units between meals over a period of approximately 2 hours. During 2020, the closures of the premises imposed by the containment measures of the Covid pandemic partially reduced the share of binge drinking while the habitual high consumption of alcohol, which involves a smaller share of the population, slowed the reduction that was observed before the 2018. Still in the 2017-2020 four-year period, 61% of the over-65 population declared that they do not habitually consume alcohol-related beverages, while 20% reported moderate consumption and consumption at risk for health, equal to more than one unit on average. alcohol content (AU) per day, the remaining 19%. Worrying is the number of people over 65 who take alcohol despite having an absolute contraindication, such as 28% of people with liver disease (14% also consume more than 1 AU per day). In 2018 in Italy, 8.7% of the accidents detected by the Carabineers and the Traffic Police were alcohol-related (this percentage was 7.8% in 2017). Also in 2018, the data obtained from the Hospital Discharge Forms (SDO) revealed a total of 55,032 hospital discharges, characterized by having indicated at least one pathology attributable to alcohol with a clear prevalence of chronic liver diseases, such as steatosis, hepatitis, and cirrhosis (56.2% of cases). The attention of health professionals to the problem of inadequate use of alcohol still appears too low: just 10% of consumers at "greatest risk" report having received advice to drink less from a doctor or other health professional.

Natural History

Incongruous use of alcohol can cause a spectrum of hepatic damage ranging from mild steatosis to established cirrhosis to hepatocellular carcinoma. Fat accumulation in hepatocytes is present in about 90% of those with incongruous use of alcohol. Although steatosis can be resolved rapidly with abstinence, fibrosis progression occurs in 10-20% of subjects, and cirrhosis may occur in 10% of cases within 5 years in subjects who continue to take more than 50 g of alcohol per day. A particularly evolving picture is that of steatohepatitis (ASH), which occurs in about 10-35% of subjects who take more than 50 g of alcohol per day. ASH is an important clinical entity for the following reasons: (1) this entity is a documented precursor of cirrhosis, with a long-term risk 9 times higher than patients with simple steatosis, (2) patients may develop portal hypertension even in the absence of cirrhosis and, (3) patients with severe illness have consequently very high short-term mortality rates. With the continued incongruous use of alcohol (more than 50 g per day), micronodular cirrhosis develops in 8-20% of cases. Over time, this lesion may evolve to the deposition of broad bands of fibrosis that separate nodules of hepatic tissue (macronodular cirrhosis). Hepatocellular carcinoma typically develops in this context.

PATHOPHYSIOLOGY/PATHOGENESIS

Metabolism of Ethanol and Pathogenesis of Alcohol-Related Liver Disease (ALD)

The pathogenesis of alcohol-related liver injury is complex and involves several interrelated mechanisms that participate in the onset and progression of the injury itself. Ingested ethanol is more than 80% absorbed by the duodenum and jejunum. The lower amount of body water in women results in a higher blood concentration at the same quantity ingested. The amount of ethanol that reaches the liver is also influenced by the activity of the gastric alcohol/dehydrogenase (ADH) (first pass metabolism), in turn influenced by the concentration of ethanol in beverages (works more if the drink contains more ethanol), from the habit of drinking (it works less for a continuous use of alcohol), from sex and age (it works less in young women, after 50 years its activity is equal between the two sexes), and from the assumption of some drugs. Through the portal vein, ethanol reaches the liver where it is mainly metabolized in the hepatocytes of the pericentral zone, the area with the lower tension of O_2, which explains the predominantly centro-lobular localization of damage. The alcohol metabolism systems are different and come into operation in relation to the amount of ethanol taken and the duration of consumption (**Figure 31.1**). The main detoxification system is the enzyme NAD-dependent Alcohol Dehydrogenase (ADH), present in the cytosol of hepatocytes, which oxidizes ethanol to acetaldehyde and NADH + H^+. Acetaldehyde in turn is oxidized by Aldehyde Dehydrogenase (ALDH) in acetate and NADH + H^+. The acetate is converted into Acetyl-CoA which can be used in the Krebs cycle or as a substrate for the synthesis of fatty acids. For higher or continuous alcohol concentrations another metabolic pathway is activated: the Microsomal Ethanol Oxidizing System (MEOS); its activation results in accelerated metabolism of ethanol, drugs and toxic substances (with possible interferences between them and influence on the bioavailability of the drugs themselves). Acetaldehyde is a highly reactive toxic compound that is responsible for many of the systemic effects of alcohol, such as nausea, headaches, and flushing. In addition, acetaldehyde is particularly toxic to hepatocytes,

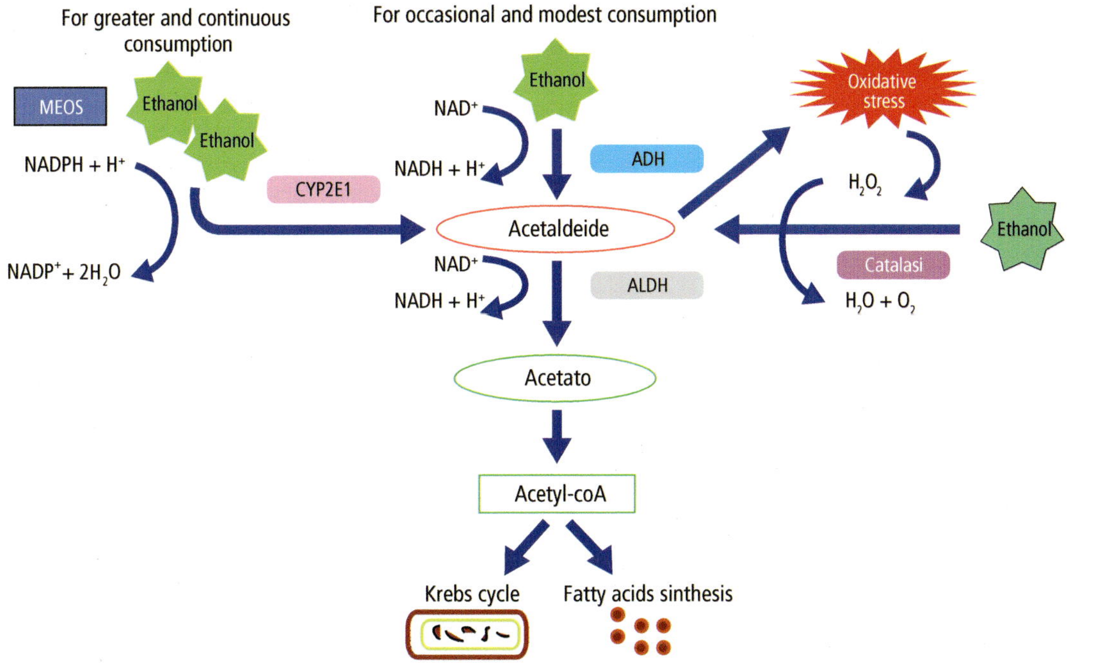

Figure 31.1 Metabolic pathways of ethanol oxidation. Legend: Nicotinamide adenine dinucleotide phosphate (NADP); Alcohol Dehydrogenase (ADH) NAD-dependent; Aldehyde Dehydrogenase (ALDH); Microsomal Ethanol Oxidizing System (MEOS); Cytochrome P 450 2E1 (CYP2E1), H_2O_2, hydrogen peroxide; H_2O, water; Acetyl coA: Acetyl coenzyme A.

as it binds to the microtubule and microsomal system proteins, including cytochrome P 450 2E1 (CYP2E1), causes swelling of the hepatocytes, and triggers the immune response. It also induces peroxidation of the lipid membranes and, at high and constant concentrations, reduces the ability of the mitochondria to metabolize it, damaging the membranes and resulting in the release of cytochrome c and activation of the caspase system (cell death by apoptosis). Finally, acetaldehyde interacts with cellular DNA with possible effects on carcinogenesis. An extended review of the pathogenetic mechanisms of liver injury from ethanol goes beyond the aims of this treatise. In general, alcohol-related liver injury is closely linked to oxidative stress, which perpetuates the production of ROS (oxygen reactive species), lipid peroxidation, antioxidant depletion, and cell damage as a vicious circle. Furthermore, ethanol activates genes that regulate lipogenic enzymes such as the sterol regulatory element-binding protein-1c (SREBP-1c), which favours the synthesis of triglycerides from fatty acids and their accumulation in the cytoplasm of hepatocytes, resulting in steatosis. Oxidative stress and ATP depletion cause hepatocyte death by necrosis or apoptosis. Cellular death also contributes to the increased production of proinflammatory cytokines, including interleukin 1 (IL-1), IL-6, IL-8, tumour necrosis factor (TNF)-α, and transforming growth factor (TGF)-β. These molecules are produced directly by the hepatocyte under the stimulation of lipid peroxidation products and by Kupffer cells activated both by the same lipoperoxidation products and by endotoxins from the intestine. In fact, alcohol in the intestine induces alterations in the bacterial flora (dysbiosis) and increases the permeability of the barrier, thus favouring the passage in the portal and systemic circulation of bacteria and endotoxins such as lipopolysaccharide (LPS). The perpetuation of these phenomena, especially in the presence of continued use of ethanol and already triggered damage, progressively leads to the structural subversion of the hepatic lobule and cirrhosis. At the same ethanol consumption, only 25-30% of drinkers develop severe liver disease. This suggests the role of possible cofactors able to interact with alcohol in the determinism and progression of liver injury. The main ones are: genetic predisposition, in particular to polymorphisms of the *patatin-like phospholipase domain-containing protein 3* (PNPLA3) which is able to influence the progression to cirrhosis; sex and age, particularly the harmful additive role of oestrogens; iron; malnutrition and obesity; hepatitis viruses; xenon biotic; and drugs.

DIAGNOSIS OF ALCOHOL-RELATED LIVER DISEASE (ALD)

ALD has a chronic progressive progression in relation to the prolongation of incongruous use of alcohol, however, it can be initiated or exacerbated in a sudden and dramatic way, giving rise to a clinical syndrome that is called "alcohol-related hepatitis". Therefore, two modalities of clinical presentation of ALD can be identified that require different management in terms of intensity and type of investigations and treatments: chronic, ranging from steatosis to cirrhosis, and the acute onset as alcohol-related hepatitis or acute alcohol intoxication or abstinence crisis. Finally, alcohol intake is one of the precipitating causes of the so-called acute on chronic liver failure.

ALD (Chronic)

Liver steatosis is present in 80-90% of habitual users of more than 30 g of ethanol/day. Histologically steatosis can be of the microvescicular type, or more frequently of mixed type, micro and macro-vesicular, characterized by small and large intrahepatocytic lipid vacuoles in more than 5% of hepatocytes, which move the nucleus laterally. Steatosis is asymptomatic, but on physical examination there may be painless hepatomegaly with a rounded edge, slightly increased consistency, and a smooth surface. On ultrasound examination, the liver appears to be hyperechoic, with a "shiny" appearance. Laboratory data, in most cases completely normal, may sometimes show mild-moderate hypertransaminaseemia and/or increase in γGT. The histological presence of necroinflammation characterizes alcohol-related steatohepatitis (ASH). The peculiar elementary lesions are: the neutrophil infiltrate, the swelling of the hepatocytes (ballooning), the Mallory bodies (perinuclear acidophilus apoptotic corpuscles, constituted by cytokeratin aggregates), the result of lipid peroxidation, and finally perivenular fibrosis, sometimes also perisinusoidal, with an unfavourable prognostic significance. The clinical presentation may not differ from that of steatosis and no biochemical or instrumental parameters are known to differentiate the two forms. However, the two pathologies have different prognoses and a patient with steatohepatitis has a 40% chance of developing cirrhosis in 5 years. Liver cirrhosis is often asymptomatic or oligosymptomatic. However, sometimes it presents with one of its complications: ascites, jaundice, hepatic encephalopathy, digestive haemorrhage due to rupture of oesophageal and/or gastric varices, or hypertensive gastropathy.

The diagnostic procedure for ALD is substantially common to other forms of liver disease and is aimed at: 1) recognizing the presence and defining the extent and duration of the incongruous use of alcohol; 2) recognizing existence and defining the evolutionary stage of liver disease; 3) identifying the presence of possible damage cofactors.

In the history of the patient with suspected ALD, drinking habits should be examined with accuracy (starting age of consumption, daily or concentrated daily intake, use at meals or outside meals). The interview with the patient is not always simple and reliable and sometimes an inquisitorial attitude can be counterproductive. An interview with family members or cohabitants can be useful. The Alcohol Use Disorders Identification Test (AUDIT) is the 'gold standard' screening test to establish incongruous use of alcohol and addiction. The patient can report episodes of tremors, morning vomiting, amnesia, traffic accidents or at work. If a history of hepatopathy is already present, the previous clinical, biochemical, and instrumental data must be acquired.

The objective examination must consider: a) the coexistence of alcohol-related pathologies affecting other organs or systems (Wernicke's encephalopathy, peripheral neuropathy, dilated cardiopathy, chronic pancreatitis); b) the clinical signs of ALD and of any cirrhosis. It is important to evaluate the breath (alcohol-related halitosis) as a possible sign of a recent ingestion of ethanol. No laboratory test is absolutely valid for defining the alcohol-related aetiology of liver injury, however, by combining the results of multiple investigations (e.g., γGT, MCV, AST) and some hepatic histological findings, adequate sensitivity and diagnostic specificity (**Table 31.1**), even if, in the presence of cofactors, it is difficult to establish in the individual case how much of the liver pathology is attributable to one or the other.

Biochemical and instrumental examinations should be used for the staging of chronic liver diseases and its complications. Although the presence of

Tabella 31.1 Major markers of ethanol consumption.

Recent Consumption Markers	
Dosage of ethanol concentrations	Limited utility (short half-life plasma of ethanol)
Indirect Markers of Chronic Abuse of Alcohol	
↑ γGT: induction effect	Sensitive but nonspecific index; progressive reduction with abstinence: 50% in 2 weeks, normalization in 5 weeks
↑ ALT: main centro-lobular location of th necrosisis; mitochondrial damage	Less specific but sensitive (also present in 53% drinkers without hepatic injury); indicative, but not specific, ALT/AST ratio <1.50% reduction after 1 week of abstinence
↑ MCV: indicative of a toxic effect on red blood cell differerentiation, reduced absorption, and use of folates	Present in 80-100% of drinkers but also in 1/5 of other non-alcohol-related liver diseases. Normalize after 3 months of abstinence
↑ Desialylated transferrin: direct effect of alcohol	Present in 40-100% of drinkers, poor specificity in the presence of hepatopathies, Fe ++, genetic variants
↑ Triglycerides: increased synthesis and reduced metabolism, mobilization from deposits	Present in the majority of drinkers, influenced by hepatic damage and presence of primitive disorders of lipid metabolism. Normalise after 1 week of abstinence.
↑ Uricemia: increased purine degradation, reduced renal excretion for the increase of the lactic acid	Present in 50% of subjects with inadequate use of alcohol
↑ IgA: immune response due to the effect of alcohol on the intestinal mucosa	Mitochondrial present in 30% of healthy drinkers, in 60% of the alcohol-related cirrhotic subjects. Poor specificity
Greater sensitivity and specificity are obtained by associating several determinations: e.g., γGT, AST, MCV, and desalted transferrin.	

ALD may be suspected on the basis of clinical, anamnestic, bio-temporal and instrumental parameters, histology is able to confirm the diagnosis and assess the severity and should be considered in patients with rapidly progressive forms in which there is a diagnostic doubt due to the presence of cofactors suspected of contributing to liver injury.

Alcoholic Hepatitis (Acute Onset)

Alcohol-related hepatitis is a clinical syndrome, that is represented by the recent appearance of jaundice and/or ascites in a patient with ongoing alcohol incongruous. The appearance of progressive jaundice is the main feature. It can be associated with fever, with or without infection, weight loss and malnutrition and hepatomegaly. In severe cases, progressive liver failure may occur with ascites, encephalopathy, and gastrointestinal bleeding. Regarding biochemical tests, AST levels are typically elevated to 2-6 times the upper limit of the normal range with an AST/ALT ratio greater than 2, associated with increased bilirubinemia and neutrophilic leucocitosis. Depending on the severity, serum albumin may be reduced, prothrombin time (PT) prolonged, and the international normalized ratio (INR) may be high. Clinical diagnosis of AH is determined in a patient with rapid development or worsening of jaundice and liver-related complications, with serum total bilirubin >3 mg/dL; ALT and AST elevated >1.5 times the upper limit of normal but <400 U/L with the AST/ALT ratio >1.5; documentation of persistent heavy alcohol use until 8 weeks before onset of symptoms; and exclusion of other liver diseases.

Patients with alcohol-related hepatitis are prone to developing bacterial infections and acute renal failure due to type 1 hepato-renal syndrome. Prognostic models have been designed to identify patients with acute alcohol-related hepatitis at high risk of early death. The discriminant function of Maddrey (DF) was the first score developed and remains the most used. The score is based on the values of PT and bilirubin. The severe forms of alcohol-related hepatitis are those with DF >32. In the absence of treatment, spontaneous 1-month survival of patients with a DF >32 ranges between 35%

and 45%. In these patients steroid therapy is indicated (**Figure 31.2**). Anther prognostic scores proposed in the context of alcohol-related hepatitis is MELD (model for end stage liver disease). Changes in liver function after the first week of diagnosis have a major impact on the patient's prognosis. The Lille score, which is carried out on day 7 from the start of steroid therapy, includes age, albumin, creatinine, PT, and the variation in bilirubin and gives indications on the patient's prognosis and the possible efficacy of the treatment. Patients with Maddrey DF >32 who do not respond to steroid therapy (7 days) based on the Lille score have a 6-month mortality of 75%.

Acute alcohol-related hepatitis can arise on a previously healthy liver. However, it is not always easy to clinically define the presence of pre-existing chronic liver disease in subjects with acute alcohol-related hepatitis, especially in the severe form that can manifest itself with ascites, jaundice and severe liver function impairment. More frequently,

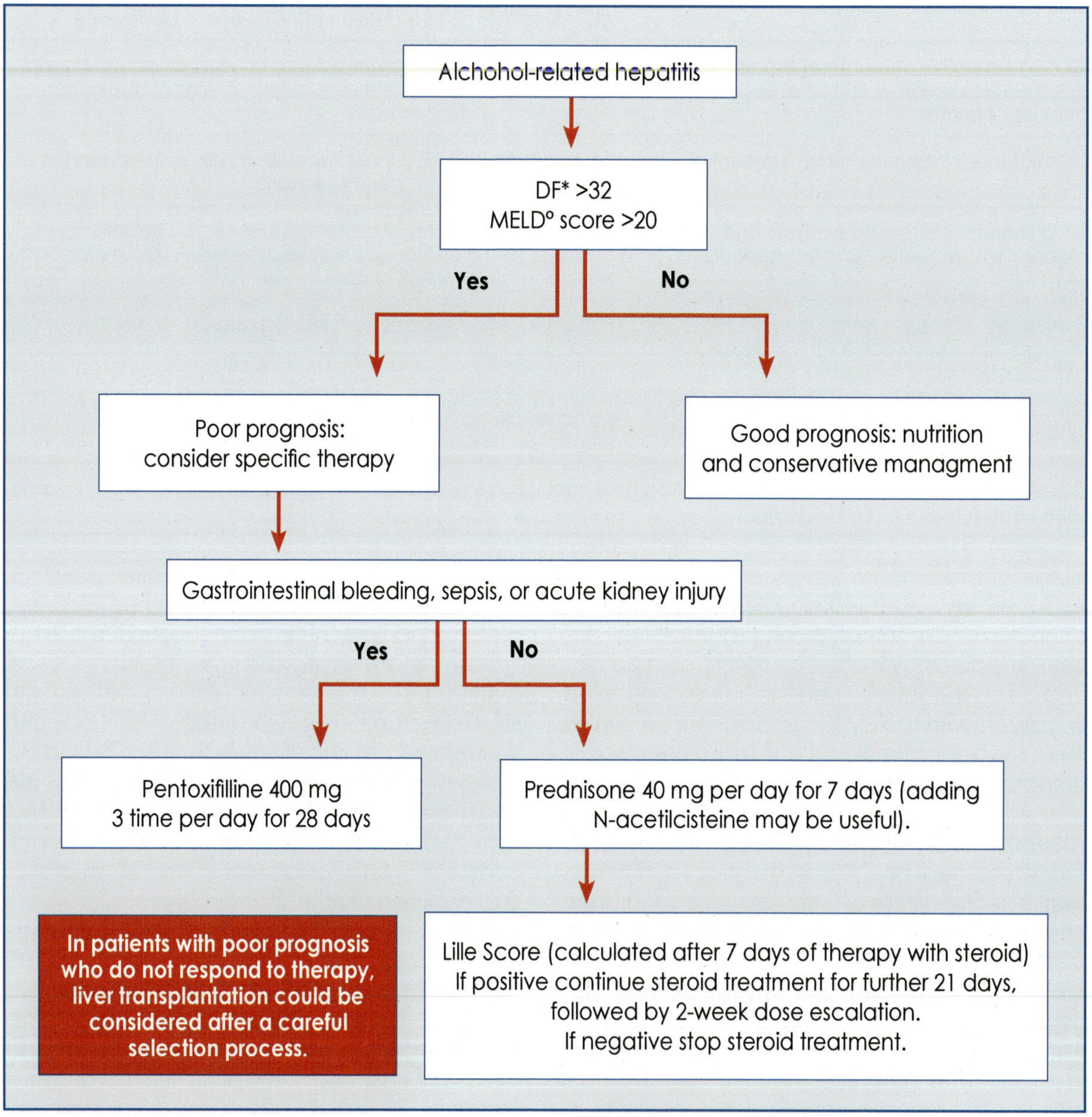

Figure 31.2 Algorithm for the management of patients with alcohol-related hepatitis.
Legend: DF is calculated as follows: 4.6 (prothrombin time - control prothrombin time) + bilirubin (in mg/dL). ° The MELD score is based on serum levels of bilirubin, INR, and serum creatinine. DF, Maddrey discriminating function; MELD, model for end stage liver disease. Modified from Sleisenger and Fordtran's Gastrointestinal and Liver Disease di: Mark Feldman, Lawrence S. Friedman, Lawrence J. Brandt. Editore: Saunders (W.B.) Co Ltd Edizione: 10 (2015).

in Mediterranean countries, alcohol-related hepatitis can occur in a patient already suffering from an underlying alcohol-related liver cirrhosis (doi: 10.1038/ajg.2017.469). In this case, alcohol-related hepatitis is one of the precipitating causes of the so-called acute on chronic liver failure, which determines a worsening systemic inflammatory process leads to multi-organ involvement and has a high mortality at 28 days from its onset.

An alcohol-related patient can present with a condition of ethyl coma, and this requires the differential diagnosis of the cause of the encephalopathy: severe cerebral alteration from acute intoxication; hypoglycemic, ketoacidose, hepatic encephalopathy in cirrhotic patients or severe alcohol-related hepatitis; post-traumatic; or mixed.

Abstinence syndrome is triggered in a chronic alcohol-related by abrupt withdrawal or reduction of alcohol intake. The clinical picture is characterized by tremors, nausea, vomiting, diarrhoea, cramps, insomnia, psychomotor agitation, and epileptic crisis in the so called 'minor abstinence syndrome'. In contrast, the most severe forms are characterised by auditory hallucinations with accusatory and threatening content that can last up to 1-3 weeks. Sometimes the clinical picture can progress into the so called 'major abstinence syndrome' in which there are hallucinations, convulsions up to the picture of delirium tremens (state of increasing mental confusion, sleep disorders, profuse sweating, deep depressive state).

THERAPY

ALD Treatment

Phosphatidylicolin, silybin and vitamin E have been proposed as possible treatments for steatosis and steatohepatitis; s-adenosyl methionine, colchicine and propylthiouracil for cirrhosis. On the other hand, other drugs are being tested and their validity has yet to be confirmed (anti-TNF-α antibodies and probiotics). None of these has been shown to improve survival. The clinical management of cirrhosis for both screening of hepatocellular carcinoma, early diagnosis and treatment of complications related to portal hypertension, is the same as cirrhosis from other aetiology and therefore refers to the specific chapter. Liver transplantation confers a survival benefit in patients with alcohol-related cirrhosis classified as MELD $\geq$15. A withdrawal period of 6 months before entering patients on the list is recommended in most centres as it eliminates the need to transplant patients who will spontaneously improve and selects patients with a lower risk of recurrence.

Treatment of Alcohol-Related Hepatitis

The medical treatment of alcohol-related hepatitis consists of a few drugs with proven efficacy: corticosteroids (associated with N-acetylcysteine) and pentoxifylline are used in severe alcohol-related hepatitis. As reported in Figure 31.2, the subject with alcoholic hepatitis must be immediately evaluated to establish the severity. In subjects with severe alcohol-related hepatitis, therapy with prednisone 40 mg for 7 days is indicated (the addition of N-acetylcysteine may be useful). After 7 days of steroid therapy, if the Lille Score is positive, continuation of the steroid for a further 21 days is indicated, followed by a 2-week taper; if negative, the treatment must be terminated. Infections are frequent and difficult to diagnose in these patients since the criteria of the Systemic inflammatory response syndrome (SIRS) are common at the time of admission and could reflect either the inflammatory state associated with acute hepatitis or an ongoing bacterial infection. For the early diagnosis of the infection, systematic sampling of body fluids and careful clinical monitoring on admission and during hospitalization are recommended repeatedly. In the absence of scientific evidence, criteria for initiating empirical antibiotic administration, although widely used, remain debated. Severe forms of ASH should be considered as a risk factor for kidney disease. The management of patients with alcohol-related hepatitis is proposed in the flowchart inserted in Figure 31.2. In this regard, it should be considered that the most recent guidelines identify transjugular liver biopsy as a useful tool for confirming the diagnosis of alcohol-related hepatitis, identifying possible alternative diagnoses, and therefore being able to better manage the therapy. Acute alcohol-related hepatitis has long been considered a contraindication to liver transplantation due to the high risk of relapse of alcoholism and therefore of loss of the transplanted organ. Recently, two retrospective multicentre studies (one European and one American) have shown that an early liver transplant in patients with severe acute alcohol-related hepatitis who do not respond to steroid therapy, respecting strict selection criteria, improves the survival of these patients. comparison with the non-transplanted.

The recommended selection criteria include the positive opinion of the staff of the transplant centre and the reference alcohol centre, the absence of comorbidities and the presence of a condition of social integration and family support.

Treatment and Prevention of Incongruous/ Dependence and General Measures

In patients with ALD, persistent alcohol intake is associated with disease progression; therefore the most effective recommendation for these individuals is the complete and persistent suspension of alcohol intake. Abstinence is the only treatment that clearly improves survival in patients with alcohol-related cirrhosis. There are many psycho-socio-therapeutic supports that can be used to achieve this goal, a multidisciplinary approach provided by first-line territorial structures is important for long-term counselling. Collaboration with self-help groups such as Alcohol-related Anonymous or similar has proved particularly useful. Motivational interventions should be routinely used in the medical management of alcohol incongruous disorders. In alcohol-dependent patients without advanced ALD, disulfiram, naltrexone or acamprosate, combined with counselling, reduce alcohol consumption and prevent relapse. These drugs cannot be recommended in patients with advanced ALD because of potential side effects. In patients with advanced ALD, recent studies suggest that baclofen is safe and effective to prevent relapse. Malnutrition is frequent and nutritional status should always be considered and corrected. Nutritional support should provide a balanced diet with about 30 Kcal/Kg of body weight in less severe forms and 40-50 Kcal/kg in severe ones. Regardless of hepatic encephalopathy, a daily protein intake of 1.5 g/kg of body weight should be ensured. Considering the potential risk of Wernicke encephalopathy, thiamine administration is recommended. Lack of fat-soluble vitamins must be compensated. In patients with acute withdrawal syndrome and ALD, benzodiazepines are the treatment of choice.

KEY CONCEPTS

- The organ damage from alcohol is influenced by several cofactors. The acceptable daily intake limit is a maximum of 20 g/day for females and 30 g/day for males.
- Incongruous use of alcohol can cause a spectrum of hepatic damage ranging from mild steatosis to established cirrhosis to hepatocellular carcinoma.
- Alcohol-related injury is associated with several mechanisms: ethanol metabolism and toxic metabolites (acetaldehyde), other metabolic mechanisms (methionine, folate), oxidative stress, mitochondrial dysfunction, hypoxia, immune and inflammatory mechanisms, gut-liver axis and dysregulated cytokine production, gender and genetic factors, endoplasmic reticulum stress response, malnutrition, fibrosis
- ALD has a chronic progressive progression in relation to the prolongation of incongruous use of alcohol, however, it can be initiated or exacerbated in a sudden and dramatic way, giving rise to a clinical syndrome that is called 'alcohol-related hepatitis'.
- In patients with ALD, persistent alcohol intake is associated with disease progression; therefore the most effective recommendation for these individuals is the complete and persistent suspension of alcohol intake.
- Corticosteroids (potentially associated with N-acetylcysteine) and pentoxifylline are used in severe alcohol-related hepatitis (DF >32; MELD score >20). Liver transplantation may be considered in selected cases.

REFERENCES

- EASL Clinical Practical Guidelines: Management of Alcoholic Liver Disease. J Hepatol. 2012;57:399-420.
- AISF e SIMG. Alcol ed Epatopatie: Indicazioni pratiche per una gestione condivisa tra medico di medicina generale e specialistica (2017).
- Burra P, Belli LS, Ginanni Corradini S, et al. Common issues in the management of patients in the waiting list and after liver transplantation. Dig Liver Dis. 2017;49(3):241-53.
- Singal AK, Bataller R, Ahn J, Kamath PS, Shah VH. ACG Clinical Guideline: Alcoholic Liver Disease. Am J Gastroenterol. 2018;113(2):175-94.

NON-ALCOHOLIC FATTY LIVER DISEASE AND NON-ALCOHOLIC STEATOHEPATITIS

Elisabetta Bugianesi, Gianluca Svegliati Baroni

LEARNING OBJECTIVES

- Summarize the most important aspects of the definition, aetiopathogenesis, epidemiology, management, and therapy of NAFLD/NASH.
- Focus attention on the main problems in NAFLD/NASH management.
- Discuss the problems related to non-invasive diagnosis of NAFLD/NASH and the most appropriate therapeutic approach.

DEFINITION AND AETIOLOGY

The term NAFLD (non-alcoholic fatty liver disease) defines a spectrum of histological liver damage characterized by an excess of fat (steatosis, consisting of intracellular accumulation of triglycerides in >5% of hepatocytes) in the absence of significant alcoholic consumption (cut-off of alcohol intake for NAFLD is 20 g/day in women, 30 g/day in men, corresponding, respectively, to 2 or 3 drinks/day) and other known causes of liver disease (e.g., hepatitis B, hepatitis C, autoimmune, genetic, etc).

Simple steatosis has a negligible risk of progression to cirrhosis, but in a significant percentage of persons with NAFLD (10-15%) the histological features are indistinguishable from ASH (alcoholic steatohepatitis), characterized by steatosis, necroinflammation, and balloniform degeneration, i.e., NASH (non-alcoholic steatohepatitis) (**Figure 32.1**).

Unlike simple steatosis, NASH can progress to in fibrosis, cirrhosis and related complications, including hepatocarcinoma (HCC).

From an etiopathogenic point of view, NAFLD is a complex and multifactorial pathology, whose onset and severity are conditioned by a combination of genetic and environmental factors.

In most cases, NAFLD is considered as the hepatic expression of the "metabolic syndrome", i.e., a cluster of conditions characterized by abdominal obesity, high-density lipoprotein (HDL) hypocholesterolemia, hyperglycemia, and arterial hypertension (**Table 32.1**).

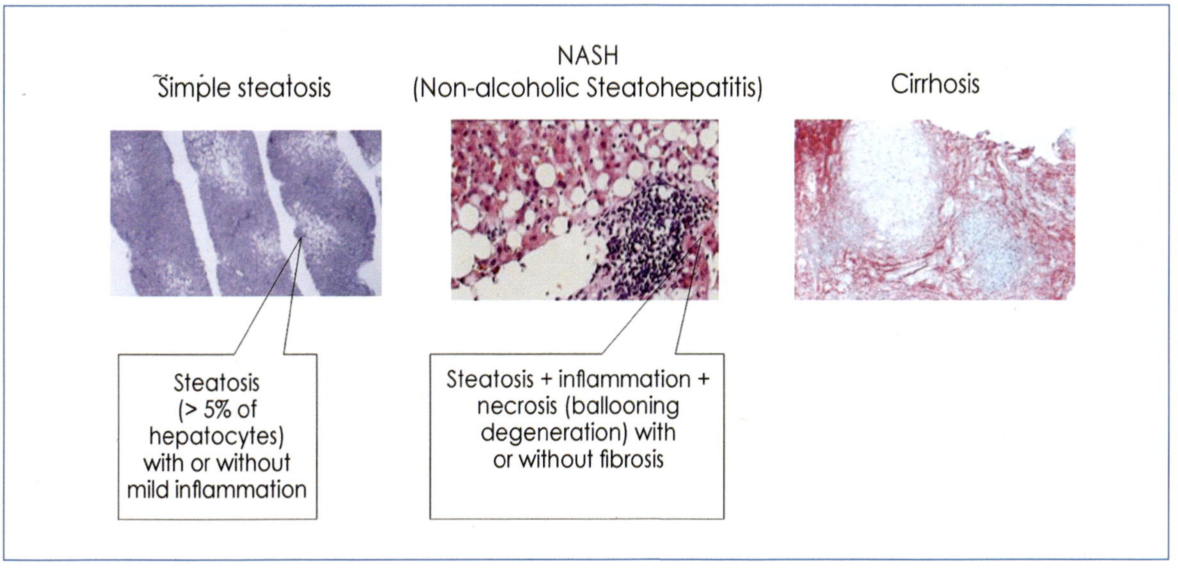

Figure 32.1 Histological spectrum of liver damage in NAFLD.

Table 32.1 Components of the metabolic syndrome.

Components of the Metabolic Syndrome (≥3)	Criteria
Visceral (abdominal) obesity	Waist circumference*
Triglycerides	≥150 mg/dL
HDL-C	<40 mg/dL in males; <50 mg/dL in females
Blood pressure	≥130/≥80 mm Hg
Fasting glucose	≥110 mg/dL

* Males > 102 cm; females > 88 cm

In more rare cases, fatty liver may also arise from other causes (i.e., secondary hepatic steatosis) such as: a nutrient-poor diet, hypothyroidism, ovarian polycytosis, intestinal bypass surgery for morbid obesity, and drugs, such as anti-estrogens in breast cancer (e.g., tamoxifen) or corticosteroids (**Table 32.2**).

Given the multiple clinical conditions that can potentially cause liver steatosis, the term MAFLD (Metabolic dysfunction-associated fatty liver disease) was recently coined by an international panel of experts. According to the new terminology, the sole presence of metabolic risk factors can define liver steatosis as MAFLD, irrespective of potential concomitant aetiologies of liver disease (e.g. HCV infection, high alcohol intake).

EPIDEMIOLOGY

The progressive change in lifestyle and eating habits of the last decades has significantly influenced the epidemiology of NAFLD. Given the treatment possibilities of the most common causes of chronic liver injury (HBV and HCV), epidemiological studies have shown that NAFLD is currently the most common cause of chronic liver injury, in close association with the obesity and diabetes epidemic.

The prevalence and incidence of hepatic steatosis in epidemiological studies on the general population cannot be estimated, for obvious ethical reasons, with an invasive but very precise method (the goldstandard), such as liver biopsy. This implies that the real prevalence and incidence of NAFLD, but especially of NASH, will remain unknown until a non-invasive but accurate method is available that allows to quantify the degree of inflammation, necrosis, and fibrosis within the liver.

The prevalence of NAFLD in the general population, estimated by liver ultrasound or autopsy studies, varies by geographical area. In the European Union, the prevalence of NAFLD has been estimated between 20% and 30% of the general population (about 116 million people), with about 3% of NASH (about 10 million people). In Italy, the prevalence of NAFLD varies between 4.0% and 49.6%,

Table 32.2 Causes of secondary steatosis.

Liver Diseases	Drugs	Nutritional	Systemic Diseases	Genetic Diseases
Viral Hepatitis (HCV, HBV)	Tamoxifen	Cachexia	Inflammatory Bowel Disease (IBD)	Hypobetalipoproteinemia
Alcoholic Hepatitis	Amiodarone	Total Parenteral Nutrition	Coeliac Disease	Familial and acquired lipodystrophies
Autoimmune Hepatitis	Synthetic Estrogens	Extended Intestinal Resection	Nephrotic Syndrome	Turner Syndrome
Wilson Disease	Glucocorticoids	Jejunoileal bypass	Thyroid Diseases	Cystic fibrosis
Haemochromatosis	Methotrexate		Polycystic ovary syndrome	
Alpha 1 antitrypsin deficiency	Valproic Acid		Obstructive Sleep Apnea Syndrome	
	HAART (HIV)		Hypogonadism	
	Calcium Channel Blockers		Hypopituitarism	
	NSAIDs			

with an average of 25%. Data on the prevalence of NASH are even scarcer. It is thought that a percentage from 10 to 15% of NAFLD evolves towards steatohepatitis, which will therefore have a prevalence of 2-3% in the general population.
The prevalence of NAFLD increases with body-mass index (BMI), from 25% in normal weight to 67% in overweight (BMI 25-30 kg/m^2) and 91% in obesity (BMI ≥30 kg/m^2).

PATHOGENESIS OF NAFLD

The main mechanism in the pathogenesis of NAFLD is insulin resistance, which is the main cause underlying the metabolic syndrome. Insulin, produced by the β cells in the pancreatic insula in response to postprandial hyperglycemia, is also the most powerful physiological anabolic hormone, promoting the deposition and synthesis of lipids, proteins, and carbohydrates, and inhibiting their release into systemic circulation.
Insulin resistance is defined as the inability of normal insulin levels to promote the use of glucose, but at abnormal level it acts diversely: in muscle it reduces the use of glucose (peripheral or muscular insulin resistance); in adipose tissue it increases the production of glycerol and non esterified fatty acids (NEFA) due to the lack of insulin capacity to effectively block lipolysis; finally, in the liver it causes an uncontrolled production of glucose, despite the high levels of insulin, associated with an increase in the production of very low-density lipoprotein (VLDL) triglycerides against low levels of HDL cholesterol (hepatic insulin resistance). The pathogenetic mechanism underlying the onset of insulin resistance is complex and includes genetic factors (for example, familiarity) and environmental factors, primarily sedentary lifestyle and a high-calorie diet rich in simple carbohydrates and lipids. The accumulation of lipids in hepatocytes resulting from an increase in lipolysis and de novo lipogenesis promotes, in genetically predisposed person, the onset of chronic liver injury, with activation of Kupffer cells and stellate hepatic cells, leading to the development of fibrosis and cirrhosis of the liver.

NATURAL HISTORY

Liver steatosis was once considered a benign condition, but current evidence indicates that NAFLD may evolve in NASH, which, in turn, may lead to liver fibrosis over time in 40% of patients or even cir-

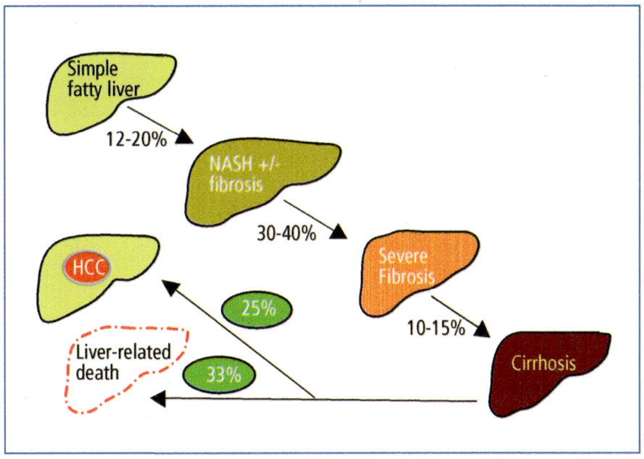

Figura 32.2 Natural history of NAFLD.

rhosis in 10-15% (**Figure 32.2**). It is not known why some patients with NASH progress towards cirrhosis while others do not.
The data available on the natural history of NAFLD are very variable.
The natural history of the evolution of steatosis to NAFLD/NASH, cirrhosis and ultimately hepatocellular carcinoma (HCC) is unknown, because once cirrhosis has been established (usually classified as cryptogenic) steatosis disappears and NASH cannot be retrospectively recognised. Data extrapolated from clinical studies have extimated that about 20% of individuals with NASH progress to cirrhosis, and about 20% of cirrhotic patients develop systemic complications induced by portal hypertension.
However, two important aspects in the evolution of NASH towards hepatocellular carcinoma must be considered:

- given the epidemiology of NAFLD and related factors (obesity, diabetes and dyslipidemia), hepatocellular carcinoma linked to NASH is becoming one of the main indications for liver transplantation in the Western world;
- hepatocellular carcinoma (HCC) linked to NASH occurs, in at least one third of cases, in a non-cirrhotic liver, and therefore not subjected to surveillance such as in cirrhotic patients.

In the United States, NASH is the second most common indication for liver transplantation, second only to HCV cirrhosis, and it is progressively increasing. It is likely that this trend will be seen in Europe, considering the new therapeutic options for HCV. However, the main causes of mortality in patients with NAFLD are cardiovascular and neoplastic diseases, because NAFLD is associated with insulin resistance and metabolic syndrome, known risk factors for cardiovascular disease and neoplastic complications.

GENETICS

Recent advances in NAFLD and NASH research have mainly derived from GWAS (genome-wide association studies), which search for polymorphisms associated with NAFLD. The PNPLA3 gene (patatin-like phospholipase domain containing 3), located on chromosome 22, has been identified as the main genetic factor of NAFLD, independent of both insulin resistance and body mass. It encodes the enzymatic protein adiponutrine (triacylglycerol lipase), involved in triglyceride hydrolysis within adipocytes and in lipid mobilization and storage. The rs738409 variant of the PNPLA3 gene, determining an amino acid substitution - isoleucine-methionine on codon 148, is associated with an increased hepatic triglyceride content. It has a consensual inter-ethnical distribution according to NAFLD prevalence (greater among Hispanics and lower among Blacks). A second polymorphism, the rs6006460 variant, was also associated with reduced levels of intrahepatic triglycerides, with an opposite geographical distribution compared to the above-mentioned variant. Subsequent studies confirmed a prominent role of PNPLA3 in determining the severity of steatohepatitis, the evolution to fibrosis, and the risk of HCC.

The identification of the PNPLA3 genetic variant has two main consequences:

- identification of a PNPLA3-NAFLD phenotype, characterized by accumulation of hepatic fat in the absence of metabolic alterations. This is typical of lean person, although an overlap with the insulin-resistant population is possible;
- development of genetic screening tests able to select person at risk for advanced disease and HCC.

The TM6SF2 (transmembrane 6 superfamily member 2) located on chromosome 19 is another gene involved in NAFLD progression. The rs58542926 polymorphism, leading to a loss of function of the encoded protein, promotes reduced secretion of lipoproteins (VLDL, triglycerides and APO-B) and intrahepatic retention and hyperaccumulation of triglycerides. It is associated with the entire spectrum of NAFLD hepatic manifestations, from necroinflammation and balloniform degeneration to fibrosis progression.

FInally, the rs641738 variant of MBOAT7 (Membrane Bound O-Acyltransferase Domain Containing 7) gene, encoding for a transmembrane protein invovled in the phospholipid metabolism, is associated with increased intrahepatic fat accumulation and a major susceptibility to develop liver fibrosis.

DIAGNOSIS OF NAFLD

NAFLD is rarely perceived by patients as a medical concern, but early diagnosis of NASH is particularly important as the disease may have an asymptomatic course towards severe liver disease. Nevertheless, this is a difficult task due to the absence of a serological marker for NAFLD and NASH, and because of the poor reliability of transaminase levels, which are normal in 80% of patients, despite significant histological damage.

In recent years the diagnosis of NAFLD passed from an "in-negative", i.e., the exclusion of other hepatopathies and secondary causes of hepatic steatosis (Table 32.2) to an "in-positive", i.e., the identification of metabolic risk factors. In this regard, the EASL-EASD-EASO Clinical Practice Guidelines for the management of non-alcoholic fatty liver disease suggest screening of the population at risk (i.e., persons with multiple components of the metabolic syndrome).

However, the need for generalized screening of NAFLD is still questionable, given the high direct and indirect costs of diagnostic tests, the low predictive value of surrogate markers of hepatic injury (transaminases and non-invasive tests), and the risks related to liver biopsy and the lack of effective treatments. However, it is desirable that the progressive form of NAFLD (NASH), particularly when associated with advanced fibrosis, be correctly identified in patients at risk (age >50 years, type 2 diabetes or metabolic syndrome), due to prognostic implications.

The most common NASH presentation is an incidental finding of hyper-transaminasemia and/or ultrasound hepatic steatosis. Most patients are asymptomatic or have nonspecific symptoms, such as asthenia, sleep abnormalities or a "heaviness" sensation in the right hypochondrium.

Diagnostic workup includes calculation of the body-mass index (BMI) and measurement of waist circumference, in addition to scrupulous collection of the physiological, diet, family, and pharmacological history. Given the well-known association with the metabolic syndrome, many NAFLD/NASH patients present a pattern of visceral obesity. All the remaining metabolic syndrome parameters (arterial hypertension, total cholesterol, HDL, fasting glucose) should be assessed. In young women, changes in the menstrual cycle and hirsutism may suggest a polycystic ovary syndrome that is frequently associated with hepatic steatosis.

Physical examination does not generally provide significant clinical findings but should always be

carefully performed to rule out signs of advanced liver disease. Hepatomegaly is the most common finding; splenomegaly may also be present, but it is not always associated with portal hypertension.
Liver function tests show a moderate increase (2-5-times) in transaminases (AST, ALT) and gamma-glutamyltranspeptidase (GGT), but indices of necroinflammation may be normal even in severe hepatic injury. The ALT/AST ratio is generally >1; an inverted ratio is observed in alcoholic steatohepatitis (ASH) or high-grade fibrosis. GGT levels are not a key criterion for ASH, as they are commonly found in metabolic disorders and indicate a predisposition to type 2 diabetes. HBV and HCV serology should be performed to rule out any association of steatosis with viral hepatitis.
The lipid profile typically shows high triglyceride levels and low HDL-cholesterol levels. When triglyceride and cholesterol levels are low, it is useful to dose apolipoprotein B levels, as hypobetalipoproteinemia is a rare but possible cause of NAFLD. Ferritin is frequently increased, but a real martial overload is found only in 5-10% of patients. Low or mild levels of autoantibody titer (ANA and SMA) can be found in 15-20% of persons with NAFLD and is generally associated with advanced liver disease. In very rare cases it may be associated with autoimmune damage.
Finally, glucose metabolism assessment should be performed using basal glucose determination. In non-diabetic person, insulin sensitivity should be assessed using surrogates (i.e., HOMA-R, homeostatic model of insulin resistance, derived from glycemia and fasting insulinemia); owing to the high risk of NAFLD-associated type 2 diabetes in selected cases it may be useful to estimate glucose tolerance by an oral glucose tolerance test. In addition to partial apolipoprotein B deficiency, another possible genetic cause is the LAL (lysosomal acid lipase) deficiency.
Among diagnostic imaging studies, both ultrasound and magnetic resonance can detect steatosis but not NASH or fibrosis. Ultrasonography is always used as a first-level survey and identifies steatosis as a hyper-reflective liver, with or without posterior attenuation of the ultrasound beam or skip areas, especially around the gallbladder. However, abdominal ultrasound has a poor sensitivity for identifying mild forms id (<20-30% of fat infiltration).
An interesting method of hepatic fat quantification, derived from the ultrasound investigation, is the "CAP" (controlled attenuation parameter), which is a quantitative measurement of hepatic fat, and is calculated along with the liver stiffness by Fibroscan (see below). Magnetic resonance imaging is a well-characterized alternative to ultrasound and is able to quantify hepatic steatosis with the PDFF technique (proton density fat fraction) together with photonic spectroscopy magnetic resonance. However, the latter is available only in a limited number of centers.

DIAGNOSIS OF NASH

The aim of the diagnostic workup is to identify patients with NASH among individuals with NAFLD. The reason for this approach is based on data demonstrating that the risk of progression to cirrhosis is in patients with NASH only.
To date, liver biopsy is the only reliable diagnostic tool, but high costs and the non-negligible risk of complications limit its use on a large scale. In recent years, one of the main research objectives is the identification and validation of non-invasive biomarkers of liver disease progression for the selection of high-risk persons.
While there are still no non-invasive markers for the diagnosis of NASH (which is based on steatosis, necroinflammation, and ballooning), the predictive scores of liver fibrosis are more useful, especially for the discrimination of more advanced disease stages. The main scores are: NAFLD Fibrosis score (NFS), FIB-4, BARD, FibroTest, FibroMeter, Enhanced Liver Fibrosis test (ELF), and APRI.
Among the non-invasive fibrosis scores, the latest European EASL Guidelines recommend the use of FIB-4 as first-line tool for the risk stratification of advanced liver fibrosis in high-risk groups (obese and diabetic individuals). In particular, FIB-4 values equal or above 1.30 identify those patients that require specialist referral for hepatological evaluation.
Among non-invasive tools for fibrosis quantification, hepatic elastography (Fibroscan) is the most widely used.
Potential limitations include poor sensitivity for mild stages of fibrosis and technical difficulty in the detection and interpretation of data in obese patients due to abundant subcutaneous adipose tissue. Recent studies have shown encouraging results regarding the application of the elastographic technique to magnetic resonance (TE-MRI).
This tool provides a quantification of liver stiffness, deduced from the mechanical properties of the tissue, with better diagnostic accuracy than standard hepatic elastography (Fibroscan).
However, the necessary equipment and costs preclude its wider use. A diagnostic algorithm is presented in **Figure 32.3**.

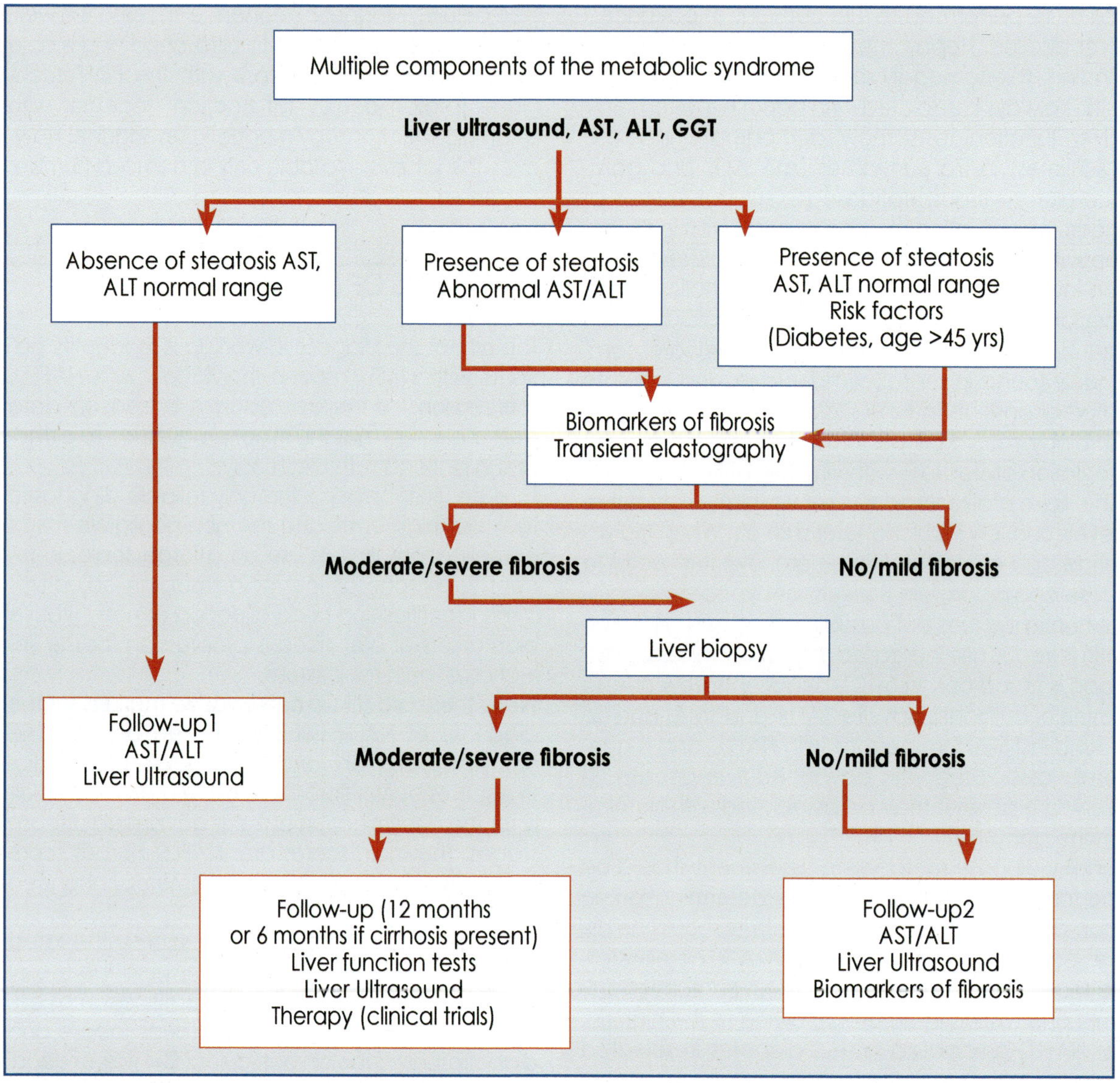

Figure 32.3 Diagnostic algorithm for NAFLD.
* Biomarkers of fibrosis: Fatty Liver Index, NAFLD Liver Fat Score; ° NAFLD Fibrosis Score, FIB-4;

HEPATIC COMPLICATIONS

Hepatocarcinoma (HCC) is the most feared hepatic NASH complication. It may occur both in the cirrhosis stage and in pre-cirrhotic NASH. To date, NASH is the second transplant indication in Europe for HCC and accounts for 13-38% of HCC in individuals with cryptogenic forms of liver disease. Obesity and type 2 diabetes are additional risk factors for HCC development, with a probable synergistic effect.
HCC screening in the cirrhotic population is performed as reccomended by the guidelines, while screening for HCC in non-cirrhotic patients is not currently recommended by any guideline.

EXTRA-HEPATIC COMPLICATIONS

The main cause of morbidity and mortality in the NAFLD population is cardiovascular complications. The prevalence – as estimated by instrumental diagnosis, of atherosclerosis, valvular calcifications or early subclinical alterations, such as increased intimal arterial thickness, is higher among patients with NAFLD than in the general population, regardless of the presence of type 2 diabetes and other risk factors. This suggests the need for targeted and anticipated cardiovascular screening in individuals with NAFLD, independent of the presence of other risk factors.

The same mechanisms involved in increased cardiovascular risk seem to play a role in the development of chronic renal damage, likely mediated by the renin-angiotensin-aldosterone system. A higher prevalence of renal impairment in patients with NAFLD was confirmed in large population studies and does not appear to be influenced by confounders such as arterial hypertension, type 2 diabetes, and obesity.

THERAPY

While simple steatosis therapy is based on the correction of metabolic risk factors, NASH therapy requires drugs able to act on liver injury. Although there are no medications specifically for NASH treatment, advances in therapeutic options have been made in recent years. Many new molecules are currently under study in international multicentar trials.

First-line therapy is non-pharmacological. It is recommended in all patients with NAFLD and is aimed at containing cardiovascular risk. Weight loss by lifestyle modification (i.e., increase in physical activity and healthy diet changes), showed an improvement in hepatic histology when weight loss is >7-10% of initial weight.

In a study involving 261 NAFLD patients in a 12-month diet and physical activity program, with biopsy assessment at the beginning and at the end of treatment, weight loss was proportional to NASH histological regression (25% of cases) without worsening of fibrosis. Individualized and pragmatic approaches combining dietary restriction with progressive increase of aerobic/resistance exercise are recommended.

Despite the dietary approach not being standardized for NAFLD individuals, due to the high cultural and geographical differences, as well as different food accessibility, Mediterranean Diet represents the best paradidm for the improvement of both cardiovascular risk and insulin resistance.

The Mediterranean Diet is a balanced diet (60% carbohydrates, 30% lipids and 10% proteins) and includes low glycemic index foods, daily fiber intake, consumption of poli-insaturated fats (vegetable origin) with minimum consumption of saturated fats, reduced intake of red meat and high intake of fish and legumes.

In addition to diet, some dietary habits, like snacking or consumption of sweetened beverages, need to be properly identified and discouraged.

Pharmacological therapy for the treatment of concomitant metabolic disorders (lipid-lowering, anti-hypertensive, and anti-diabetic drugs) is recommended in all NAFLD patients to prevent and contain extra-hepatic comorbidities. Statin administration is recommended by current guidelines on dyslipidaemias, and, in retrospective studies, showed a reduced incidence of HCC in patients with NASH.

Pharmacological treatment specifically addressed to liver disease is indicated only in the advanced stages of NASH.

Insulin-Sensitizing Agents

PPAR (Peroxisome proliferator-activated receptors) are a nuclear receptor superfamily that exert multiple regulatory effect on glucose and lipid metabolism.

Thiazolidinediones (TZD) are a alpha-delta PPAR agonists that have strongest pathogenetic rational of use in NASH among currently approved drugs and are recommended by current hepatological guidelines. They promote adipocyte differentiation into smaller cells, thus increasing insulin sensitivity.

Through lipoprotein-lipase induction, TDZ also increase fatty acid synthesis and uptake in adipose tissue and reduce its storage in liver and muscle. Metformin, another widely used drug in diabetes, is not recommended as a specific therapy for NASH due to the lack of evidence of histological improvement, although it has an insulin-sensitizing function mediated by the inhibition of hepatic glucose production and the increase in peripheral uptake. Pioglitazone is recommended by international guidelines for the treatment of diabetic patients with NASH. In addition, Lanifibranor, a pan-PPAR agonist, has shown a benefit on NASH without worsening of fibrosis and is currently under investigation in a large phase 3 trial. GLP-1 (glucagon-like peptide 1) receptor agonists, a physiologically produced post-prandial hormone with glucose modulatory action, are prescribed in the diabetic population and offer another promising treatment option for NASH patients. In particular, in a recent clinical trial liraglutide showed inhibitory action on de novo hepatic lipogenesis and an improvement in histological features.

Antioxidants

Vitamin E belongs to this category. It is a cell membrane component and protects it against oxidative damage. Two large randomized studies conducted on adults and children investigated a possible role of vitamin E in liver disease. Data showed a reduction in necroinflammation and balloniform degeneration, with NASH resolution in a non-negligible percentage of cases. Vitamin E at high doses (800 IU/day) is recommended by international guidelines for the treatment of non-diabetic patients with NASH.

Another therapeutical strategy is to address the mechanisms of hepatic fibrosis (the so-called antifibrotic drugs). The most promising medication is obethicolic acid, a Farnesoid-X nuclear receptor agonist, currently in use as second-line treatment for Primary Biliary Cholangitis. In a large phase 3 trial, obethicolic acid has shown efficacy in the liver fibrosis regrssion, without worsening of NASH.

Bariatric surgery is another therapeutic option; however, it is reserved for patients with severe obesity or co-morbidities. In this regard, some preliminary studies showed an improvement in necroinflammation and postoperative hepatic fibrosis, but further studies are needed to confirm these results. Among surgical procedures, gastric bypass and gastric band have given promising results, while bilio-pancreatic diversion should be avoided due to the risk of fibrotic evolution.

Finally, NAFLD/NASH will become the main indication for liver transplantation in the near future, given the advent of new anti-HCV therapies. Liver transplantation in NASH patients is invariably followed by post-transplantation steatosis recurrence and NASH can relapse within 2-5 years. However, organ function is maintained 5-10 years after transplantation. Although 5-year overall survival is comparable to patients transplanted for other aetiologies, they are at higher risk for cardiovascular- and infectious disease-related mortality.

KEY CONCEPTS

- NAFLD includes a wide spectrum of histological damage characterized by fatty infiltration of the liver: from simple steatosis to non-alcoholic steatohepatitis or NASH, characterized by steatosis, inflammation, necrosis (balloning degeneration), with or without fibrosis, and cirrhosis (evolved from NASH).
- The prevalence of NAFLD in the general population depends on the geographic area and in Europe it is about 25%; 10-15% of persons with NAFLD present NASH. The long-term prognosis of NAFLD depends on the extent of histological damage. Hepatocellular carcinoma (HCC) is a potential complication of NASH, even in non-cirrhotic liver.
- NAFLD is commonly associated with metabolic syndrome components and is the result of a complex interaction between genetic and environmental factors, having insulin resistance as an underlying pathogenetic mechanism. Lipotoxicity plays a key role in the progression of hepatic damage.
- NAFLD is often asymptomatic and diagnosed after the incidental finding of high levels of transaminases or steatosis on ultrasound, in the absence of other known causes of chronic liver disease.
- Liver biopsy is the most reliable diagnostic tool for the identification of NASH, but no non-invasive tests for severe liver fibrosis are currently available. None of the non-invasive tools can be considered "gold standard" for the diagnosis of NASH.
- NAFLD therapy includes treatment of metabolic syndrome components according to their respective guidelines, in particular balanced diet and regular physical activity. Insulin-sensitizing drugs (pioglitazone), antioxidants (vitamin E) are recommended by international clinical practice guidelines, but to date there is no drug with a specific indication for NASH.
- Patients with NAFLD, and particularly with NASH, have a significantly increased risk of type 2 diabetes and cardiovascular events.

REFERENCES

- Younossi ZM, Koenig AB, Abdelatif D, et al. Global epidemiology of nonalcoholic fatty liver disease-Meta-analytic assessment of prevalence, incidence, and outcomes. Hepatology. 2016 Jul;64(1):73-84.
- European Association for the Study of the Liver (EASL); European Association for the Study of Diabetes (EASD); European Association for the Study of Obesity (EASO). EASL-EASD-EASO Clinical Practice Guidelines for the management of non-alcoholic fatty liver disease. J Hepatol. 2016 Jun;64(6):1388-402.
- European Association for the Study of the Liver (EASL). EASL Clinical Practice Guidelines on non-invasive tests for evaluation of liver disease severity and prognosis - 2021 update. J Hepatol. 2021 Sep;75(3):659-689.
- Kleiner DE, Brunt EM, Van Natta M, et al. Design and validation of a histological scoring system for non-alcoholic fatty liver disease. Hepatology. 2005;41:1313-21.
- Eslam M, Newsome PN, Sarin SK, et al. A new definition for metabolic dysfunction-associated fatty liver disease: An international expert consensus statement. J Hepatol. 2020 Jul;73(1):202-209.

CHAPTER 33

AUTOIMMUNE HEPATITIS

Nora Cazzagon, Maria Grazia Rumi

LEARNING OBJECTIVES
- To know the diagnostic criteria of AIH.
- To acquire the tools for differential diagnosis with acute and chronic liver diseases.
- To know the therapeutic strategy with first- and second-line immunosuppressant drugs.

Autoimmune hepatitis (AIH) is a relatively rare heterogeneous liver disease, and a major clinical challenge; although is the first disease for which an effective therapeutic intervention was demonstrated. AIH is a non-resolving chronic liver disease that affects mainly women and is characterized by hypergammaglobulinemia, autoantibodies, interface hepatitis (severe necroinflammation and plasmacells on liver histology), and favorable response to immune-suppression. If left untreated, the disease often leads to cirrhosis, liver failure, and death.
The prevalence of AIH ranges from 17.3-18.3 per 100,000 persons and an incidence of 1.1-2.56 apparently increasing, with a female to male ratio of 3:1. AIH has been diagnosed in all ethnic and age groups, although the age at presentation typically presents two peaks, the first during childhood and the second in middle age. Recent studies have shown that the number of persons with AIH diagnosed at older age is increasing.

PATHOPHYSIOLOGY

The precise aetiology of AIH remains unknown, while pathophysiological mechanisms and risk factors have been described. Current knowledges suggest that a complex interplay between genetic predisposition, environmental and epigenetic factors is involved in disease occurrence and progression. The dominant hypothesis supports that AIH develops in a genetically predisposed individual after being exposed to one or certain environmental factors resulting to loss of self-tolerance and the activation of immune response against liver cells.
Genetic predisposition to AIH is mostly associated with HLA genes, in particular HLA-DR3 and HLA-DR4 and specifically DRB1*0301 and DRB1*0401. Moreover, a significant number of single nucleotide polymorphism (SNPs) concerning immunological pathways of T cell activation and response and cytokines production has been identified and linked to the clinical phenotype of AIH. Several environmental factors such as xenobiotics, drugs, viruses, herbals have been associated with loss of self-tolerance through neoantigens productions, as well as initiation and perpetuation of the immune response. Lastly, epigenetic modifications triggered by environmental factors influences gene expression and confer to immune dysregulation and disease pathogenesis. In AIH epigenetic studies were mainly engaged to the investigation of the role of micro-RNA (miRNAs) in disease pathogenesis and the implication of DNA methylation modifications.

DIAGNOSIS

There is no single diagnostic test for AIH and diagnosis is based on a combination of clinical, biochemical, immunological and histological indices, and the exclusion of other known causes of liver disease that may share serological and histological features with AIH (e.g. hepatitis B, C and E, Wilson disease, non-alcoholic steatohepatitis and DILI). According to both European and American guidelines liver biopsy is mandatory in the diagnostic work up of AIH, moreover it is useful to drive therapeutic choice.
A practical and useful tool for AIH diagnosis is the Simplified International AIH Group (IAIHG) Scoring System published on 2008 which is based on four parameters: presence of autoantibodies, IgG levels, histology, and absence of viral markers, for a definite or probable diagnosis of AIH (**Table 33.1**).
AIH can be characterized by ALT increase from near normal to more than 50 times the limit of normal, while cholestasis enzymes remain normal or only moderately elevated. Increased serum gam-

Table 33.1 Simplified diagnostic criteria of the International Autoimmune Study Group (Hennes et al., 2008).

High IgG	Score
IgG > upper limit of normal	+1
IgG >1.1 x upper limit of normal	+ 2
Autoantibodies	
ANA or ASMA >1:40	+ 1
ANA or ASMA >1:80	+ 2
LKM >1:40	+ 2
SLA/LP positive	+ 2
Liver Histology	
Compatible with AIH	+ 1
Typical of AIH	+ 2
Absence of Viral Hepatitis	+ 2
≥6: Probabile AIH	
≥7: Definite AIH	

ma-globulins, in particular IgG levels, are found in approximately 85% of patients, but this prevalence tends to be lower in patients with an acute onset in which a higher proportion of cases show normal IgG levels. The most important diagnostic finding is the presence of non-organ specific autoantibodies, which are the hallmark of AIH. On the basis of autoantibodies reactivity, AIH can be classified as type 1, more frequently diagnosed in adults, characterized by antinuclear antibody (ANA) directed against double-stranded DNA or ribonucleoprotein, and anti-smooth muscle antibody (SMA) directed against cytoskeletal elements. The anti-soluble liver antigens antibody (anti-SLA) is rarely detected but is highly specific for the diagnosis of type 1 AIH. Type 2 AIH, more frequently diagnosed during childhood, is characterized by the detection of anti-liver kidney microsomal antibody (anti-LKM) and by less common antibodies against liver cytosol (anti-LC1). Indirect immunofluorescence performed on frozen rodent substrate is the preferable technique for autoantibodies detection; positive sera should be titrated up to extinction of positivity (**Figure 33.1**). In adults, significant titers are >1: 40 dilution, while a titer of 1: 20 is diagnostic in children.

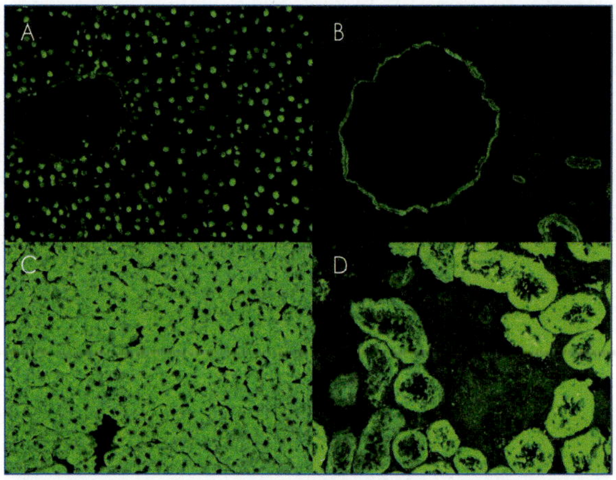

Figure 33.1 Indirect immunofluorescence showing auto-antibody positivity on mouse liver or kidney frozen sections. A: antinuclear antibodies (ANA, mouse hepatic section). B: anti-smooth muscle antibodies (ASMA, mouse hepatic section). C: anti-liver/kidney microsomal antibodies (LKM, mouse hepatic section). D: anti-liver/kidney microsomal antibodies (LKM, mouse kidney section).

Liver biopsy is considered an essential procedure in the diagnosis of AIH and it is generally used to guide treatment decision making, although there are no morphological features pathognomonic of AIH. Interface hepatitis with moderate to severe infiltrate characterized by the presence of plasmacells among lymphocytes, emperipolesis with a lymphocyte in the cytoplasm of a damaged hepatocyte, and the arrangement of hepatocytes in rosette formation are typical histologic features (**Figures 33.2, 33.3**). Panlobular hepatitis with bridging necrosis is characteristic of acute onset AIH or disease flare of chronic AIH. Liver biopsy is also useful for disease grading and staging and to assess histological remission.

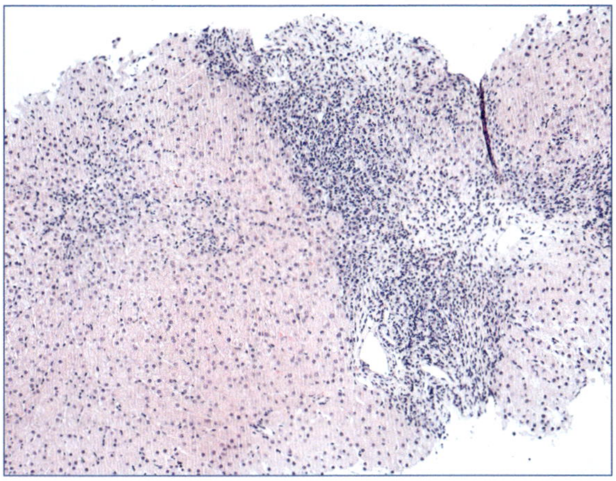

Figure 33.2 Interface hepatitis (hepatitis at the portal-parenchymal interface).

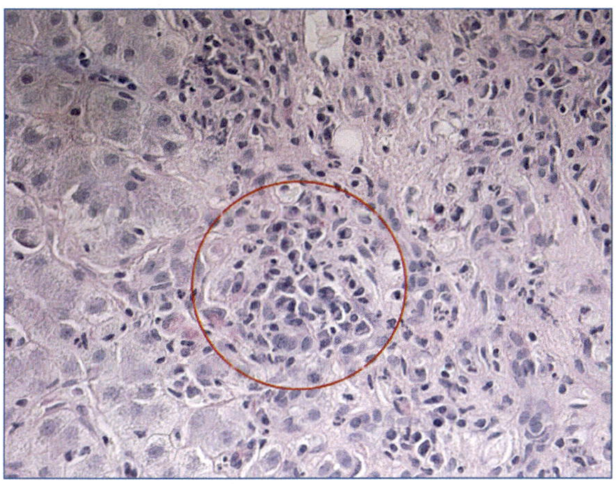

Figure 33.3 Plasmacells in the inflammatory infiltrate.

CLINICAL FEATURES

AIH is characterized by a large heterogeneity of clinical, biochemical, and histological manifestations. Clinical manifestations can vary from no signs or symptoms to severe chronic hepatitis or to an acute episode of hepatitis, almost identical to acute viral hepatitis. As a consequence, diagnosis of AIH should be considered in any patient with acute and chronic liver disease, particularly if hypergammaglobulinemia is concomitantly present and if the patient shows features of other autoimmune diseases.

More in detail, in about two thirds of patients the onset is insidious with gradual progression of liver damage with or without non-specific symptoms such fatigue, arthralgias, malaise, anorexia, weight loss and/or amenorrhea in young women. The diagnosis of AIH is usually established during investigations for unexplained elevation of ALT levels or during routine testing or testing performed for other reasons. Approximately one third of these patients, at initial diagnosis, have already developed advanced disease or cirrhosis, confirming a picture of unrecognized, asymptomatic but progressive liver disease.

One third of patients have an acute onset of AIH characterized by jaundice and symptoms such fatigue, nausea, abdominal pain and prolonged INR. However, acute presentation may disclose two different clinical entities. The first is a true acute onset of AIH without chronic pre-existing hepatitis, sometimes followed by jaundice. This pattern of presentation often has a severe course with rapid progression of liver damage and development of cirrhosis. Acute severe AIH is defined by the presence of jaundice and INR within 1.5 and 2. In some cases acute onset can also have a fulminant course leading to rapid liver failure. The second type is acute exacerbation of chronic AIH or acute exacerbation of an undiagnosed or misdiagnosed AIH. In most cases evidence of histology compatible with chronic damage in patients with acute presentation implies that they probably have had subclinical disease for a long time. In summary, AIH constitutes an important diagnostic challenge because a subclinical course often precedes the clinical onset of the disease, whereas long periods of subclinical disease may persist after presentation. AIH is associated with a wide variety of other autoimmune diseases. Therefore, in patients with a diagnosis of AIH, screening for other autoimmune diseases should be done.

THERAPY

The standard therapy for AIH relies on immunosuppressive drugs: predniso(lo)ne as initial therapy followed by the addition of azathioprine after two weeks is the first-line treatment of AIH. Current guidelines suggest the use of predniso(lo)ne 1 mg/Kg/day as monotherapy or 30 mg/die in combination with azathioprine 1-2 to mg/Kg/day followed by predniso(lo)ne tapering 10 mg/week. However, a recent study has suggested that the initial steroid dose is not decisive, and that 0.5 mg/Kg body weight predniso(lo)ne is probably sufficient in the majority of patients. Budesonide is an alternative steroid to predniso(lo)ne since it can induce remission with less steroid-specific sides effects, however caution should be used in patients with advanced disease for the increased risk of systemic effects due to a reduced hepatic drug metabolism.

Therapy is aimed to obtain complete biochemical and histological remission. Biochemical remission in AIH is defined as normal transaminases as well as normal IgG levels and should be assessed at 6 months to evaluate the response to therapy. Only a small proportion of patients do not achieve biochemical remission by using standard therapy, and, before considering second line therapies as mycophenolate mofetil, it's mandatory to assess compliance, re-exclude alternative diagnosis and increase dosage of standard therapy. Third line therapies include several possible immunosuppressive agents including calcineurin inhibitors, methotrexate, cyclophosphamide, biologic agents (i.e. infliximab, rituximab) which should be administered only in specialized hepatology centers. For the future, research epigenetics, immune pathways and changes in the intestinal microbiota may provide novel drugs for a better cure.
Patients with AIH should undergo semiannual lab and clinical examination, semiannual/annual ultrasound surveillance (depending to the presence/absence of cirrhosis) and transient elastography for monitoring disease progression. A careful prevention and assessment of immunosuppressive agent side effects need to be provided to AIH patients, along with a careful clinical evaluation during the transition from childhood to adolescence and during pregnancy.

LIVER TRANSPLANTATION

Liver transplantation is a life-saving option for patients who progress to end-stage liver disease or in case of acute liver failure although AIH can recur or develop de novo after liver transplantation (see Chapter X).
AIH accounted for 2% of all liver transplantation (LTs) and 5% of cirrhotic indications registered in the Europe between 1988 and 2016. According to a recent study based on the European Liver Transplant Registry (ELTR) including 2515 patients receiving LT for AIH over 30.970 LTs between 1998 and 2017, patients' survival after LTs for AIH was 79.4%, 70.8% e 60.3% after 5, 10 and 15 years of follow-up.

KEY CONCEPTS

- AIH is a non-resolving chronic liver disease that occurs in all age groups, but affects mainly women.
- The disease, if untreated, may lead to cirrhosis.
- The diagnosis of AIH is based on clinical, biochemical (elevated IgG levels), serological (presence of autoantibodies), and histological criteria.
- The simplified scoring system of AIH can be helpful in diagnosing difficult cases.
- Immunosuppressant therapy aims to obtain complete biochemical and histological remission.
- Steroids and azathioprine are first-line drugs for treating AIH.

REFERENCES

- Mieli-Vergani G, Vergani D, Czaja AJ, et al. Autoimmune hepatitis. Nat Rev Dis Primers. 2018;4:18017.
- European Association for the Study of the Liver. EASL Clinical Practice Guidelines: Autoimmune hepatitis. J Hepatol. 2015;63:971-1004.
- Mack CL, Adams D, Assis DN et al. Diagnosis and management of autoimmune hepatitis in adults and children: 2019 practice guidance and guidelines from the American Association for the Study of Liver Diseases. Hepatology 2020;72:671-722.
- Terziroli Beretta-Piccoli B, Mieli-Vergani G, Vergani D. The clinical usage and definition of autoantibodies in immune-mediated liver disease: A comprehensive overview. J Autoimmun. 2018;95:144-58.
- Zachou K, Arvaniti P, Lyberopoulou A, Dalekos GN. Impact of genetic and environmental factors on autoimmune hepatitis. J Transl Autoimmun. 2021;4:100125.
- Lohse AW, Sebode M, Jørgensen MH, et al. Second-line and third-line therapy for autoimmune hepatitis: a position statement from the European Reference Network on Hepatological Diseases and the International Autoimmune Hepatitis Group. J Hepatol 2020; 73: 1496-506.
- Heinemann M, Adam R, Berenguer M, et al. Longterm survival after liver transplantation for autoimmune hepatitis: results from the European Liver Transplant Registry. Liver Transpl. 2020;26:866-77.

CHAPTER 34

STORAGE LIVER DISEASES

Marco Carbone, Lorenzo Ridola

LEARNING OBJECTIVES

- To know the definition and classification of disease.
- To know the epidemiology.
- To understand the pathophysiological mechanisms.
- To recognize clinical manifestations.
- To know the diagnostic approach.
- To know the therapeutic strategies.

WILSON'S DESEASE

Definition

Wilson disease was first described in 1912, by Kinnear Wilson, as a familial disease characterised by progressive, lethal neurologic dysfunction with liver cirrhosis and a corneal abnormality, the Kayser-Fleischer ring.

Wilson's desease is a rare, autosomal recessive inherited disorder of copper metabolism, caused by mutation of the ATP7B gene. This gene encodes the homonymous protein, an ATPase with a predominantly hepatic expression, which couples the hydrolysis of ATP to the transfer of copper from the cytosol to the vesicular lumen of the trans-Golgi. Hereditary structural defects are associated with protein dysfunction and progressive copper accumulation, first in the liver and then throughout the system.

Epidemiology

The incidence of the disease is estimated at 1 in 30,000 individuals. More than 600 mutations have been described, most of which are missense mutations. Although some amino acid substitutions are relatively frequent and account for 10-40% of ATP7B defects within a given population (e.g., the H1069Q mutation in Caucasian and African-American populations), most are rare. For this+ reason, and due to the resulting high rate of composite heterozygosis, genetic studies are difficult to achieve; to date it has not been possible to identify a clear correlation between genotype and phenotype.

Pathophysiology

Copper is an indispensable element for the correct functioning of numerous metabolic pathways, its accumulation may be deleterious to the cell. For this reason, in its metabolic stages numerous mechanisms of homeostatic regulation control copper levels. The Western diet has an average copper content of 1.5-2.5 mg/day. The stomach and duodenum are the main sites where copper is absorbed by a high affinity transporter (CTR1, copper transporter 1).

The density of CTR1 on the luminal membrane is regulated by the concentration of copper in the body: reduced serum copper (cupremia) levels increase receptor exposure on the membrane and, therefore, increase intestinal absorption of the element. Copper flows into the portal circulation mainly linked to albumin. When it enters the liver, it is re-transposed by the hepatocyte CTR1 transporter and, within the cell, it is bound to the ATP7B protein.

ATP7B, located in the trans-Golgi vesicles, releases it in the blood, bound to ceruloplasmin, a cytoplasmic ferroxidase that contains about 95% of the copper in the circulation, or to remove excess copper from the liver, secreting it in the bile (**Figure 34.1**).

In Wilson's Disease ceruloplasmin is secreted in a copper-deficient form that rapidly degrades in the bloodstream, causing the low levels of ceruloplasmin typical of the disease. The copper that is not eliminated with the bile accumulates in the hepatocyte, ultimately causing its destruction. The liver also releases copper in the blood that is not bound to ceruloplasmin, which travels throughout the body and accumulates in certain organs, such as the eyes, kidneys, and basal ganglia. Furthermore, high levels of circulating copper not bound to ceruloplasmin may have adverse effects on erythrocytes and lead to in haemolysis.

Clinical Features

The clinical presentation of Wilson's disease can be extremely variable. The most frequent onset is

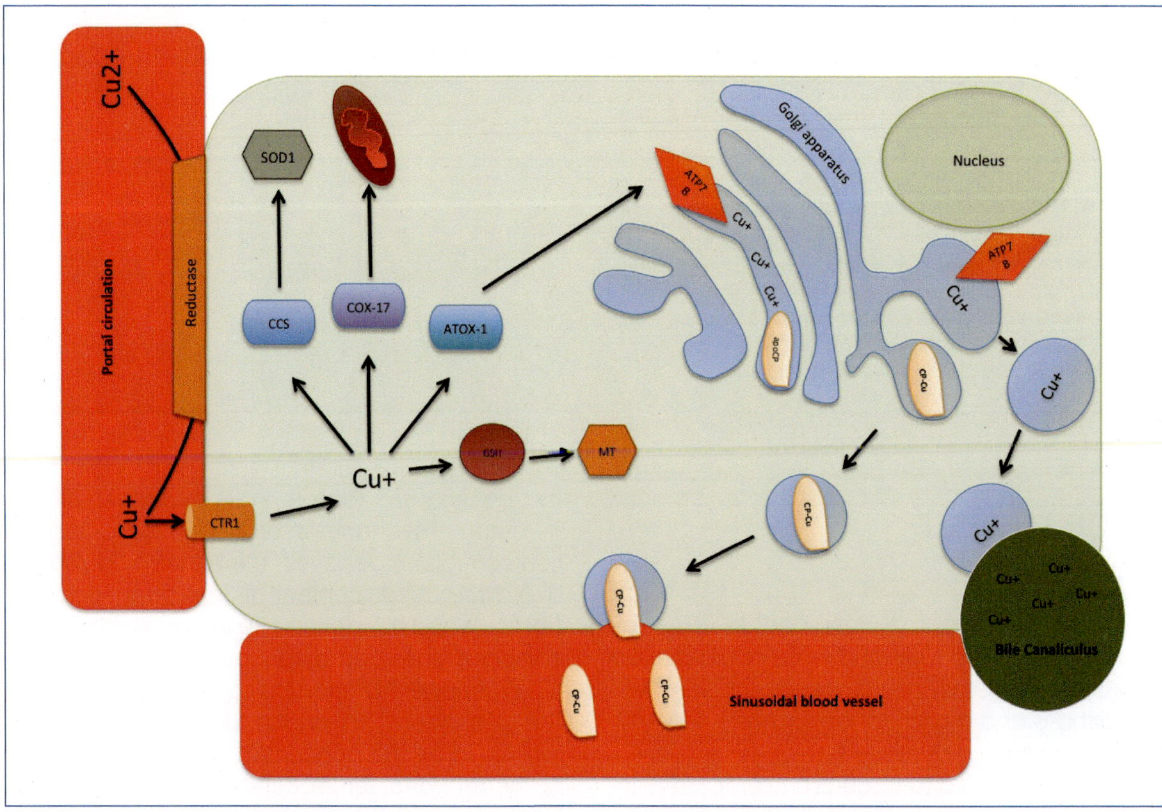

Figure 34.1 Copper circulates in the blood bound to albumin. In the liver it binds with the copper transporter. In the liver, hepatocytes are responsible for the uptake and storage of copper, as well as its excretion into the bile. In the hepatocyte many chaperons bind copper and transfer it to compartments for cellular functions. The cytoplasmic copper chaperone ATOX1 is needed for copper delivery to ATP7B in the hepatocyte secretory pathway. Copper can be bound to the aceruloplasmin or secreted into the bile.
Abbreviations: ATOX 1, antioxidant 1 copper chaperone; ATP7, adenosine triphosphate; CCS, copper chaperone for SOD; Cox 17, cytochrome c oxidase; Cp, ceruloplasmin; CTR1, Copper Transporter 1; GSH, glutathione; SOD, superoxide dismutase.

in childhood, with hepatic manifestations. The late onset form after age twenty, is more frequently associated with neurological manifestations. However, the two clinical entities often overlap. The disease may remain asymptomatic for years and begin in late age, with cases diagnosed even in the sixth decade of life.

Liver Disease

The spectrum of hepatic manifestations is very broad and ranges from acute liver failure to chronic forms that can progress to cirrhosis. The acute hepatic onset of Wilson's Disease mimics that of acute viral or autoimmune hepatitis, with malaise, loss of appetite, nausea, elevated transaminases, jaundice, and altered coagulation. Some patients may already have signs of advanced liver disease at the onset with portal hypertension. Wilson's Disease can also occur with fulminant hepatitis, severe coagulopathy, and hepatic encephalopathy.This can be further complicated by acute renal failure and acute intravascular haemolysis, due to the massive flow of copper released by hepatocyte lysis. The fulminant onset of Wilson's Disease affects predominantly young women (female to male ratio: 4:1), transaminases are generally <1500 U/L at onset, alkaline phosphatase is with in the normal range, and total bilirubin is high due to concomitant liver failure and haemolysis. Moreover, a greatly increased serum immunoglobulin (Ig)G concentration, and detectable nonspecific autoantibodies, such as antinuclear antibodies and smooth muscle (anti-actin) antibodies can be observed. Finally, compared with other chronic liver diseases, Wilson disease is infrequently complicated by hepatocellular carcinoma; however, patients may have an increased risk for abdominal malignancies.

Neurologic and Psychiatric Disease

About half of patients with Wilson's Disease have neurological and/or psychiatric problems. The

majority of adult patients initially exhibit a slight deterioration in cognitive abilities, associated with behavioral changes. With progression of unrecognized disease, symptoms of extrapyramidal syndrome may occur, with increased stiffness and slowing of movements, with or without the typical hand trembling, masked facial expressions, defects in articulation of speech, ataxia or dystonia. Seizures are uncommon, and intellect is not impaired.
Behavioral disorders and psychiatric symptoms may affect about 20% of patients at presentation and may precede liver and neurological involvement. In children there is often a drop in academic performance, with changes in personality and inappropriate behavior, attitudes that are often mistakenly pubertal. In adults, however, the symptoms take on characteristics of psychosis and anxiety-related disorders.

Ocular Signs

The ocular signs include the Kayser-Fleischer (KF) ring, a brownish-greenish ring that arises at the periphery of the cornea caused by the granular deposition of copper at the Descemet membrane and the bright sunflower cataract, which is caused by deposits of copper in the center of the lens. Both manifestations are generally observed with the slit lamp, although sometimes, in the most severe forms, the K-F ring is also visible to the naked eye.
K-F rings, present in 95% of cases with neurological involvement, can be absent up to 50% of patients with only hepatic involvement. Moreover, they are not pathognomonic of disease but may be present in other disorders caused by copper retention, particularly in cholestatic diseases such as primary biliary cholangitis, primary sclerosing cholangitis, and familial cholestasis.
Importantly, their absence does not exclude a diagnosis of Wilson's Disease and their presence is not the only diagnostic criterion.

Involvement of Other Organs

The disease can also affect the kidney, mainly as Fanconi syndrome. The most common alterations are proteinuria, glycosuria, and phosphaturia. In these patients there seems to be an increased incidence of tubular type I and type 2 acidosis. It is also possible to find hypercalciuria with increased formation of kidney stones. Osteopenia and osteoporosis are also frequently associated with Wilson's Disease, whereas cardiomyopathies are less frequent.

Diagnostic Approach

The diagnosis of Wilson's Disease is often complicated by the lack of pathognomonic signs or symptoms. This often results in diagnostic delay and worsening of symptoms. Chronic hepatopathy, associated with K-F rings and tremors or dystonia, are highly specific to the disease; however, this picture is quite rare and, in most cases, the disease has a subtle onset.
A diagnostic score has been proposed and, although it has never been validated, it is a useful tool in daily practice; this includes histologic, clinical and laboratory variables (**Table 34.1**).

Serum Levels of Ceruloplasmin

The impossibility of copper to reach the trans-Golgi vesicles and support the synthesis of ceruloplasmin, causes its deficiency and its circulating levels are therefore clearly reduced.
Low serum levels of ceruloplasmin raise the suspicion of Wilson's Disease, although this is not sufficient to make a diagnosis.
In fact, about 20% of patients heterozygous for the ATP7B defect have reduced levels of ceruloplasmin without an accumulation of copper.
In addition, various disorders reduce the plasma levels, such as renal or intestinal protein losses, malabsorption syndromes or advanced chronic liver disease. A complete absence of ceruloplasmin is observed in aceruloplasminemia, a genetic defect due to mutation of the ceruloplasmin gene.
In contrast, a percentage of patients with the disease (in some studies even >30%) may show normal levels of ceruloplasmin. This is probably due to the role of acute phase protein of ceruloplasmin that, with systemic inflammation, can increase to normal levels.

Serum Copper

Although a disease of copper overload, the total serum copper (which includes copper bound to ceruloplasmin) in Wilson's Disease is usually decreased in proportion to the decreased ceruloplasmin in circulation.
In patients with acute liver failure due to Wilson's Disease, serum copper levels may be markedly elevated due to its sudden release from liver tissue stores. An increase in cupremia, concomitant with low levels of ceruloplasmin, indicates an increase in the free share of copper, not bound to ceruloplasmin, but to albumin with a link with less affinity. The free copper can be calculated by subtracting from the total levels of cupremia the amount of copper associated with ceruloplasmin, estimated by multiplying total ceruloplasmin x 3.15 (quantity of copper in mg per mg of ceruloplasmin). The

Table 34.1 Scoring system developed at the 8th International Meeting on Wilson's Disease, Leipzig, 2001.

Signs and Symptoms	
Kayser-Fleischer Ring	
- Absent	0
- Present	2
Neurologic Symptoms [a]	
- Absent	0
- Mild	1
- Severe	2
Coombs-Negative Haemolytic Anemia	
- Absent	0
- Present	1
Serum Ceruoplasmin	
- Normal (>0.2 g/L)	0
- 0.1-0.2 g/L	1
- <0.1 g/L	2
Urinary Copper (in the Absence of Acute Hepatitis)	
- Normal	0
- 1-2 x ULN	1
- >2 x ULN	2
- Normal, but >x5 ULN after D-penicillamine	2
Liver Copper	
- normal (<0.8 umol/g)	-1
- 0.8-4 umol/g	1
- Rhodanine-positive granules*	1
- >5x ULN (>4umol/g)	2
Mutation Analysis	
- No mutation detected	0
- On one chromosome detected	1
- On both chromosomes detected	4

Total Score
- 4 or more → **diagnosis established**
- 3 › **diagnosis possible, more tests needed**
- 2 or less → **diagnosis very unlikely**

§ or typical abnormalities at brain magnetic resonance imaging; * if no quantitative liver copper available.
Abbreviation: ULN, upper limit of normal.

levels of free copper can be increased in acute hepatitis of other aetiology, in chronic cholestasis, and in copper intoxication.
Cupremia dosage is a valid test in monitoring the effectiveness of therapy.
However, one limitation of free copper assay as a diagnostic test for Wilson's Disease is the adequacy of the method for measuring copper and ceruloplasmin.

Urinary Copper Excretion
Copper excreted in the urine in untreated patients reflects the levels of free serum copper. The values considered diagnostic for Wilson's Disease is > 100 µg/24 hours.
However, at presentation, 16-23% of patients, especially children or family members of still asymptomatic patients, present lower values than those diagnosed. Therefore, in order to increase the sensitivity of the test, a cut-off reduction of 40 µg/24 hours has been proposed, which is suggestive of disease, particularly in children.
Another valuable tool in assessing children is the 24-hour cupruria after stimulation with D-penicillamine, a chelating drug that, through mobilization of iron from the tissues, increases urinary excretion of copper.
This test can be used to differentiate Wilson's Disease from other diseases characterized by accumulation of serum copper, such as cholestatic diseases, in which the pharmacological stimulus does not lead to a significant increase in urinary copper.
This test is more accurate than liver biopsy. However, stimulus testing is not recommended in adults

and is not effective in the diagnosis of asymptomatic patients.

Hepatic Parenchymal Copper Concentration

Hepatic copper accumulation is the hallmark of Wilson's Disease. However, specific stains like rhodamine or orcein reveal focal copper stores in less than 10% of patients because they detect only lysosomal copper depositions. Therefore, measurement of hepatic parenchymal copper concentration is the method of choice for the diagnosis of Wilson's Disease. Hepatic copper content >4 Imol/g dry weight is considered as the best biochemical evidence for Wilson's Disease.

The major problem with hepatic parenchymal copper concentration is the uneven distribution of copper in the liver in later stages of Wilson's Disease.

The concentration can be underestimated due to sampling error. Markedly elevated levels of hepatic copper may also be found in idiopathic copper toxicosis syndromes such as Indian childhood cirrhosis.

About half of patients are already cirrhotic at the onset. Histochemical stains (rhodamine for copper and orcein for proteins associated with copper) give rather variable outcomes and are useful for identifying only lysosomal copper. In fact, especially in the early stages of disease, copper is mostly cytosolic, linked to metallothionein and undetectable by histochemical analysis. One of its negativities does not exclude, therefore, the diagnosis.

In contrast, the dosage of copper on dry tissue with levels ≥250 µg of copper per gram of dry liver tissue (gts) confirms Wilson's Disease. However, the uneven distribution of copper in the liver leads to frequent false negatives. Furthermore, high levels of intrahepatic copper can be found in cholestatic diseases and in Indian infant cirrhosis (Indian childhood cirrhosis).

Genetic Testing

Genetic testing of the ATP7B gene is indicated in doubtful diagnosis for diagnostic confirmation and for facilitating family screening.

Direct molecular-genetic diagnosis is difficult because of the more than 600 possible mutations. Also, the majority of patients are compound heterozygotes (i.e., carry two different mutations). Comprehensive molecular-genetic screening takes several months, which makes this an impractical method. Nevertheless, it is reasonable to perform molecular analysis of the ATP7B gene in any patient who has a provisional diagnosis of Wilson's Disease, both for confirmation purposes and to facilitate the subsequent screening of family members.

Therapy

A number of drugs are available for the treatment of Wilson's Disease, including agents and zinc salts. Among the chelating agents, the most commonly used is penicillamine, which works mainly by mobilizing the copper from the hepatic tissue and from the other sites of deposit, resulting in its excretion with the urine. Therapy is usually monitored by 24-hour cupruria, a useful tool for therapeutic compliance and treatment efficacy. Response to treatment is very slow and the effects become clinically evident only after 2-6 months. Resolution of neurological symptoms, which can take up to 3 years, is even slower. Worsening of neurological symptoms in the early treatment period is described in 10-50% of patients. Penicillamine is associated with numerous side effects. The earliest are hypersensitivity reactions with fever, rash, neutropenia, and thrombocytopenia.

The drug can have a real myelotoxic action and lead to medullary aplasia. Furthermore, there is a risk of renal toxicity, both short-term and long-term, which usually manifests with proteinuria. Lupus-like autoimmune reactions may occur in the long term, together with dermatological reactions such as sputum elastosis.

Because of the numerous cases of intolerance to penicillamine, another agent was introduced, trientine. This drug also belongs to the class of chelators and, although it has a cupruric effect inferior to that of penicillamine, it has shown excellent efficacy in clinical outcomes and has a better toxicity profile. The most recent is zinc salts, which interfere with copper uptake by the gastrointestinal tract. They work by metallothionein synthesis in the enterocytes which, by binding the copper with high affinity, causes it to be lost with the cellular turnover.

Zinc salts have few side effects, the most common is dyspepsia. The neurological deterioration observed with chelators is not common with zinc. This therapy is currently indicated only as maintenance or as an attack therapy in still asymptomatic patients, as it has less efficacy than chelators on liver disease.

Among the future pharmacological agents is tetraiodiomolybdate. It acts on two sites: the intestinal lumen, where it creates complexes between copper and proteins, preventing absorption; the circulation, where it makes copper inaccessible for hepatocyte uptake. Its pharmacological action is very powerful and is faster than that of other chelating agents.

Therapy is monitored by evaluating ceruloplasmin, cupremia, liver enzymes, plus physical and neurological examination at intervals of about 6 months.

Patients with acute liver failure secondary to Wilson's disease or with decompensated cirrhosis unresponsive to chelation therapy should be promptly referred for liver transplantation (see liver transplant chapter). The effect of transplantation on neurological involvement is controversial and, to date, there are no criteria or prognostic evaluations that make it possible to predict the impact of transplantation on these symptoms. Psychiatric symptoms, on the other hand, do not regress after transplantation and represent a relative contraindication. Dietary treatment alone is ineffective, but most patients should eliminate copper-rich foods from their diet. These foods include organ meats, shellfish, nuts, chocolate, and mushrooms. Vegetarians require specific dietary counseling.
Wilson's Disease, if left untreated, inevitably leads to death, especially due to liver disease. The prognosis depends on the severity of symptoms at onset and adherence to prescribed treatment. Usually, hepatic disease is controlled in about 1-2 years of therapy and, with proper compliance, does not progress further. Neurological symptoms, on the other hand, shape a longer life expectancy, but can be disabling and only partially reversible with therapy. Patients who stop treatment have a poor prognosis. In fact, new neurological manifestations, such as dysarthria, can develop. Liver failure usually develops within 3 years of stopping treatment and these patients require liver transplantation.
The quality of life of patients with Wilson's disease can be compromised by drug toxicity. Patients should be encouraged to maintain a healthy lifestyle, including abstaining from alcohol and avoid obesity.

HAEMOCHROMATOSIS

Definition and Classification

Iron overload, also known as haemochromatosis, is a clinical entity associated with different hereditary or acquired conditions. They all share the same pathogenetic mechanism: increased intestinal absorption of dietary iron, excessive release of iron deposited in the cells of the reticuloendothelial system, and accumulation in the parenchymatous organs, with the development of organ damage.
HFE-related haemochromatosis (type 1, HFE gene) is an autosomal recessive condition and is the most common form of haemochromatosis. Juvenile haemochromatosis (type 2) is due to mutations in the HFE2 gene or the HAMP gene; that of type 3 is due to mutation of the TFR2 gene; that of type 4 to mutations of SLC40A1 (ferroportin disease); the latter is the only one with an autosomal dominant form of transmission.
Secondary causes of iron overload, unrelated to genetic defects, include ineffective erythropoiesis, chronic liver disease, increased iron intake.

Epidemiology

In the Caucasian population the most frequent form of haemochromatosis (80% of cases) is associated with the C282Y polymorphism. The allele frequency (the frequency with which a certain gene occurs in a population) of C282Y homogeneity is about 6%, which translates into a genotypic frequency (the frequency in the population of each possible allelic combination) of 1/250-300 individuals.
In Italy, the frequency of HFE-related haemochromatosis is very variable, from 1 out of 500 individuals in some areas of the North to 1 out of 2,000 or 3,000 individuals in the Center-South.
Despite the high prevalence of C282Y homozygosity, which represents the "major" polymorphism, disease penetrance is basically low (10-30%). Furthermore, additional environmental and/or genetic factors can modify phenotypic expressivity and disease progression. Men are at greater risk for developing organ disease than women of child-bearing age who are protected by monthly blood loss.
The H63D amino acid substitution, which is the "minor" polymorphism of HFE-related haemochromatism, has been reported to have an allelic frequency of 14%, with less geographic variation.
C282Y/H63D compound heterozygosis was detected in approximately 5% of patients with haemochromatosis. However, It appears that this form manifests disease only in the presence of other cofactors (alcohol abuse, steatohepatitis). Finally, the S65C polymorphism has been described with an allelic frequency of about 0.5%.

Pathophysiology

Haemochromatosis, in its variants, is characterized by the same pathogenetic mechanism: increased intestinal (mainly duodenal) absorption of iron from foods and excessive release of the iron deposited in the reticulo-endothelial system cells, both caused by reduced synthesis or function of hepcidin, the hepatic hormone that negatively regulates such processes.
Iron can be accumulated in enterocytes as ferritin and eliminated by cell death; or transferred via the basolateral membrane of enterocytes into the blood. The latter process takes place thanks to ferroportin.
Hepcidin is secreted by the liver, once in circulation it binds to ferroportin and degrades it, causing iron

retention in these cells and reduces its absorption in the bloodstream.

Hepcidin deficiency in haemochromatosis leads to uncontrolled release of iron from enterocitary and macrophage ferroportin in the blood; once the binding capacity of serum transferrin is saturated, this translates into tissue overloading of the liver, pancreas, genital system, heart, joints, and skin (**Figure 34.2**).

The expression of hepcidin is regulated by various factors including the amount of iron bound to transferrin, the body's iron stores, inflammatory states, hypoxia/ anemia, and erythropoietic activity.

Under conditions of iron deficiency, hepcidin expression is reduced; this increases the intestinal expression of ferroportin, which results in increased intestinal absorption of iron. Under conditions of iron overload, hepcidin expression increases; this reduces the intestinal expression of ferroportin, resulting in reduced intestinal iron absorption.

Clinical Features

Haemochromatosis should be suspected in young adults with chronic liver disease, diabetes, impotence or amenorrhea, cardiomyopathy, arthropathy, and skin hyperpigmentation. Hyperpigmentation is characterised by either a bronze discoloration due to predominant melanin pigmentation or a gray pigmentation resulting from iron deposition in the basal layers of the epidermis. However, isolated hyperferritinemia is the most frequent clinical presentation, in the absence of clinical manifestations.

In such patients the transferrin saturation will be evaluated, which will be increased. The set of these elements justifies the execution of the genetic test for the research of the C282Y polymorphism of HFE.

Diagnosis

Serum ferritin is a sensitive index of body iron stores; however, it is not very specific. Ferritin, in

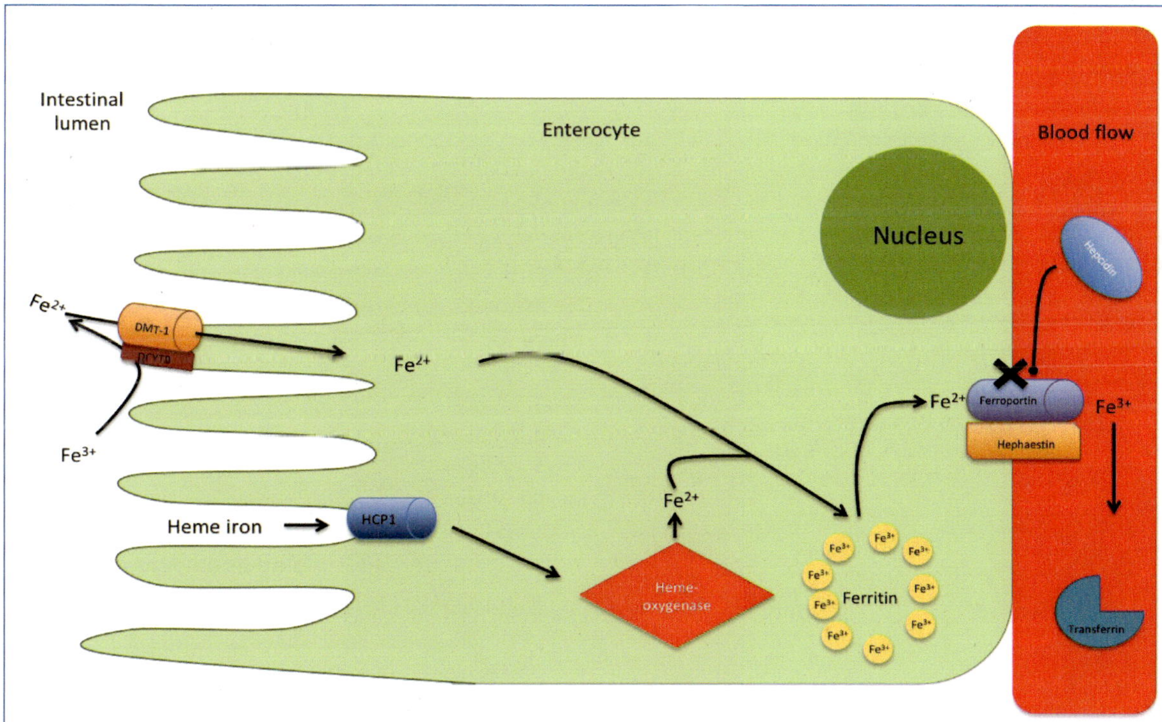

Figure 34.2 The iron is absorbed in the duodenum by enterocytes. To be absorbed, dietary iron can be absorbed as part of a protein, such as heme protein, or iron must be in its ferrous Fe2+ form. A ferric reductase enzyme on the enterocytes' brush border, duodenal cytochrome B (DDCYTB), reduces ferric Fe3+ to Fe2+. A protein (divalent metal transporter 1 (DMT1), which can transport several divalent metals across the plasma membrane, then transports iron across the enterocyte's cell membrane into the cell. These intestinal lining cells can then either store the iron as ferritin, which is accomplished by Fe3+ binding to apoferritin (in which case the iron will leave the body when the cell dies and is sloughed off into feces), or the cell can release it into the body via the iron exporter ferroportin. Hephaestin, a ferroxidase that can oxidize Fe2+ to Fe3+ and is found mainly in the small intestine, helps ferroportin transfer iron across the basolateral end of intestine cells. In contrast, ferroportin is post-translationally repressed by the hormone hepcidin. The body regulates iron levels by regulating each of these steps. For instance, enterocytes synthesize more Dcytb, DMT1 and ferroportin in response to iron deficiency anemia. Abbreviations: DDCYTB, duodenal cytochrome B; DMT-1, divalent metal transporter.

fact, can increase as an acute phase protein in different conditions: acute and chronic inflammatory states, chronic alcohol abuse, cancer, metabolic syndrome, cellular necrosis (hepatic and not). Once these conditions have been excluded or treated, transferrin saturation should be evaluated which, if >45% on at least two measurements, the search for polymorphisms with genetic analysis is initiated for differential diagnosis between various hereditary forms of martial overload. The most common is HFE-related haemochromatosis, then ferroportin disease. In general, biopsy is not necessary for diagnosis. However, in patients with very high ferritinemia (>1000 mg/L) and hypertransaminasemia, liver biopsy for the quantification of tissue iron and staging of organ damage is indicated. In the event that the genetic test is negative, after having confirmed tissue fibrosis by liver biopsy or MRI, the search begins for non-HFE haemochromatosis forms.

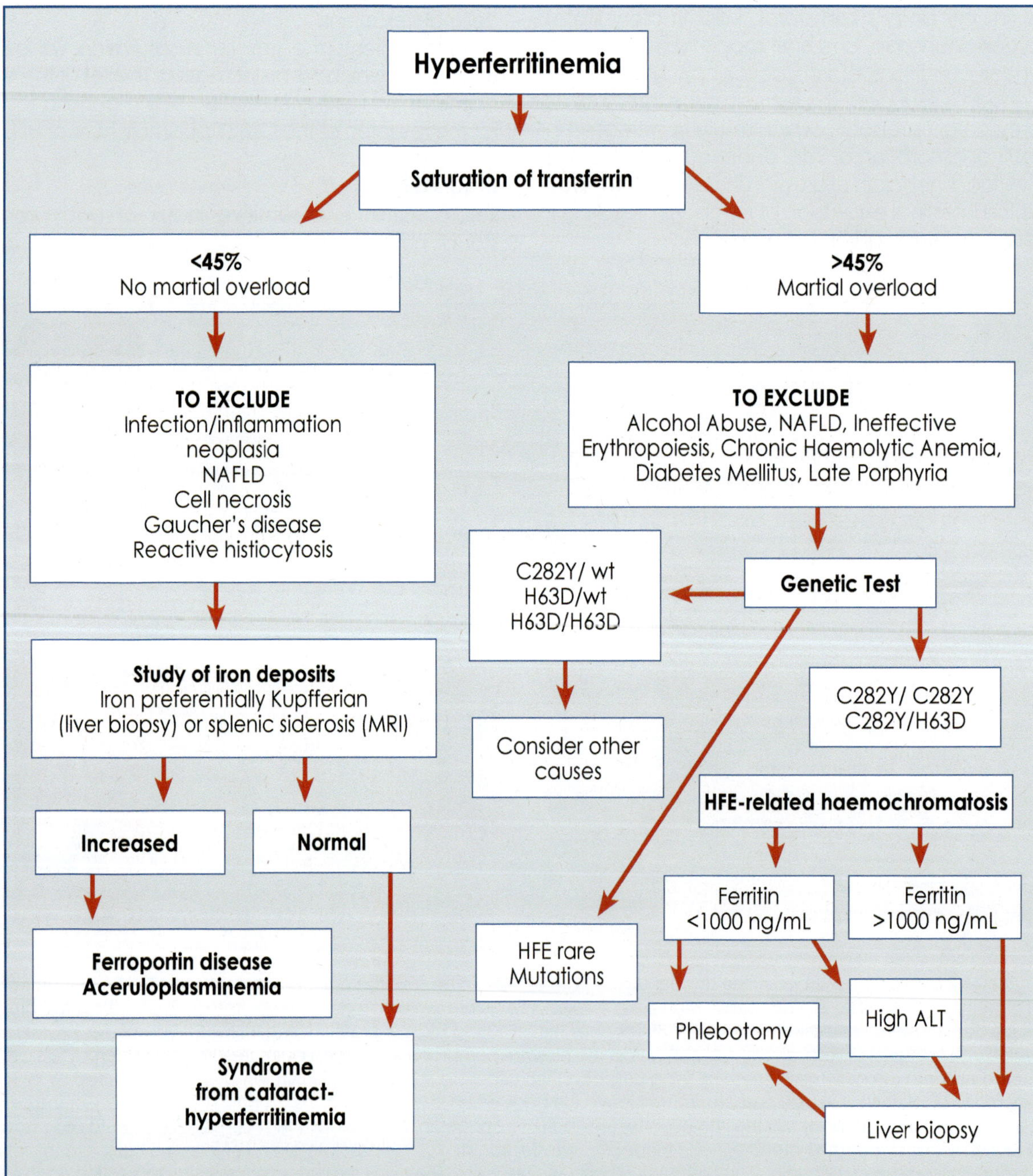

Figure 34.3 Algorithm for managing hyperferritinemia.

In hyperferritinemia associated with normal-low transferrin saturation, ferroportin disease should be considered. The early accumulation of iron in Kupffer cells on liver biopsy or accumulation of iron in the abdomen is pathognomonic for this condition (**Figure 34.3**).

The low penetrance of HFE C282Y is the main argument against the use of genetic screening in the general population. However, biochemical screening with ferritin dosage and transferrin saturation, followed by genetic testing if appropriate, are justified in individuals with a high number of such polymorphisms (patients with chronic liver disease, hepatocellular carcinoma, cutaneous porphyria tarda, chondrocalcinosis, type 1 diabetes mellitus, family members of patients with haemochromatosis).

Therapy

The therapy of choice is bloodletting which, through the removal of excess iron, can prevent or limit organ damage. The therapy entails draining 450-500 ml once a week until a serum ferritin of 50 ng/ml is reached and transferrin saturation <30%. Depletion is usually achieved within 1-2 years. The maintenance regimen involves assumption of salts, based on serum ferritin levels (2-4 drops per year). While hypertransaminasemia, liver fibrosis, skin hyperpigmentation, and asthenia improve after salassotherapy, arthropathy, diabetes and hypogonadism are irreversible. Chelation drugs should be reserved for patients in whom saliva therapy is contraindicated (e.g., heart failure, anemia).

The most common causes of death were infections, cardiovascular complications, and recurrence of hepatocellular carcinoma. When diagnosis and treatment are delayed complications of end-stage liver disease may be develop. Indications for liver transplantation, which can be considered a life-saving strategy, are the development of liver cirrhosis and/or hepatocellular carcinoma (see liver transplant chapter).

KEY CONCEPTS

- Wilson's disease is suspected in persons aged 6 to 40 years, with liver changes and/or neurological changes of uncertain origin.
- Older age is not a criterion for excluding Wilson's Disease.
- The diagnosis of Wilson's Disease is based on the presence of some or all of these signs: low serum ceruloplasmin and copper levels; increase in basal cupruria in 24 hours; presence of Kayser-Fleischer rings; neurological signs. Cupruria in the 24 hours after stimulation with penicillamine is the most specific test for Wilson's Disease and allows differential diagnosis with cholestatic diseases.
- Liver biopsy findings are key for definitive diagnosis of Wilson's Disease (tissue copper >250 μg/gts) and for the study of disease severity.
- Penicillamine is the drug of choice in Wilson's Disease both in monotherapy and combined with zinc salts.
- In patients presenting with high levels of ferritinemia and transferrin saturation >45%, it is necessary, before genetic testing for HFE-related haemochromatosis, to exclude forms of secondary haemochromatosis, such as chronic alcoholism, acute or chronic inflammatory status, non-steatohepatitis alcoholic in a metabolic syndrome.
- In view of the variable penetrance of the polymorphism, diagnosis of HFE-related haemochromatosis should not be based only on genetic testing but will include evidence of tissue iron overload (hyperferritinemia).
- In hyperferritinemia associated with other confounding factors (e.g., metabolic syndrome), liver biopsy, which is normally not necessary to obtain certainty, may be useful for confirming iron overload.
- Early diagnosis and prompt treatment increase survival of patients with haemochromatosis.
- Hypogonadism, diabetes mellitus, cardiomyopathy, and arthropathy secondary to haemochromatosis are generally irreversible even after salassotherapy.

REFERENCES

- Bandmann O, Weiss KH, Kaler SG. Wilson's disease and other neurological copper disorders. Lancet Neurol. 2015 Jan;14(1):103-13.
- European Association For The Study Of The Liver (EASL). Clinical Practice Guidelines: Wilson's disease.
- European Association For The Study Of The Liver (EASL). Clinical practice guidelines for HFE hemochromatosis. J Hepatol. 2010 Jul;53(1):3-22.
- Ferenci P, Roberts EA. Defining Wilson disease phenotypes: from the patient to the bench and back again. Gastroenterology. 2012 Apr;142(4):692-6.
- J Hepatol. 2012 Mar;56(3):671-85.
- Pietrangelo A, Caleffi A, Corradini E. Non-HFE hepatic iron overload. Semin Liver Dis. 2011 Aug;31(3):302-18.
- Pietrangelo A. Mechanisms of iron hepatotoxicity. J Hepatol. 2016 Jul;65(1):226-7.

CHAPTER 35

DRUG-INDUCED LIVER INJURY

Salvatore Petta, Alessio Michele Aghemo

LEARNING OBJECTIVES

- To learn the patho-physiological mechanism of drug-induced liver injury.
- To learn the most important clinical conditions associated with potentially liver toxic drugs.
- To learn about herbal toxicity.

EPIDEMIOLOGY

Drug-induced or toxic-induced liver injury (DILI) is defined as liver injury during pharmacologic treatment or intake of herbal product or dietary supplements in the absence of a known liver disease. The incidence is variable and suffers from under reporting in national and international registries. In France DILI occurs with an estimated incidence of 14/100,000 inhabitants per year, while In Spain according to the Spanish Registry of DILI the incidence is 34.2 per million, whereas mortality is 16.6 per million/year. The North American prevalence of DILI has been estimated as 1-2 cases per 10,000 inhabitants in the general population. There are, however, heterogeneous rates of incidence/ prevalence within Europe and within the United States. Paracetamol is responsible for 50% of acute liver failure in Northern Europe and the United States and is the commonest cause for liver transplant due to fulminant hepatocellular necrosis.

PATHOGENIC MECHANISMS

DILI can be classified into 2 subtypes on the basis of the underlying pathogenetic mechanisms of liver damage: Intrinsic DILI or idiosyncratic DILI. Intrinsic DILI is typically dose related, appears after a short period of time from drug intake (hours or days), and its incidence is directly linked to higher doses of the suspected drug. On the other hand, idiosyncratic DILI is often not dose related, is extremely rare, usually develops after a relatively long period of time from the drug intake (several days-weeks) and is associated with systemic symptoms such as fever, itching, purpura, and eosinophilia. In both cases peculiar chemical characteristics of the suspected drug such as lipophilicity and biotransformation, expose hepatocytes to reactive metabolites which lead to oxidative stress and derangement of key cellular pathways, which consequently impair cellular function or cause necrosis/apoptosis. Less frequently idiosyncratic DILI is the direct consequence of innate immune response activation which leads to liver damage. Reactive metabolites can indeed cross link with cellular proteins creating neo-antigens which will stimulate cytotoxic T-Cell Lymphoctyes targeting hepatocytes. **Figure 35.1** provides a schematic representation of DILI. **Table 35.1** shows examples of drugs associated with Intrinsic or Idiosyncratic DILI. The most common cause of Intrinsic DILI is paracetamol which in US is responsible for 40% of all causes of acute liver failure. Paracetamol is readily esterified to glucuronides and/ or sulphates unless the capacity for esterification is saturated; in that case, a secondary pathway comes into play, leading to the formation of N-acetyl-p-benzoquinone imine (NAPQ1) which can be detoxified via glutathione. However, once glutathione is saturated, NAPQ1 directly binds cell proteins, leading to hepatocellular disruption.

Several risk factors have been associated to DILI, including:

- age over 55;
- female gender;
- assumption of concomitant medications;
- alcohol intake;
- malnutrition;
- recent surgery;
- pregnancy.

Individual genetic factors (HLA-related and non HLA-related) are very important as well. **Table 35.2** present some examples of DILI in which genetic factors play a major role in the development of DILI. Besides the conventional medications, herbal products and dietary supplements can cause liver damage. The complex compositions, and the lack of quality control of contaminants, either

*The Authors would like to thank Dr. Vincenzo Carviotto (Humanitas University) for his assistance.

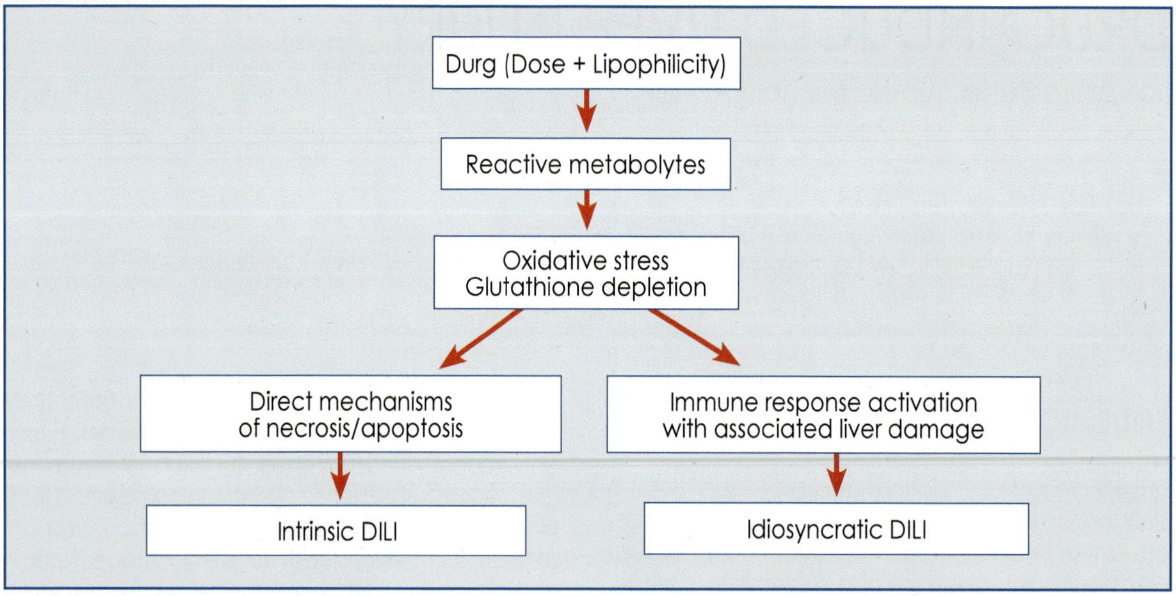

Figura 35.1 ?????

Tabella 35.1 Drugs associated with Intrinsic or Idiosyncratic DILI.

Intrinsic DILI
Paracetamol
Amiodarone
Anabolic-androgenic Steroids
Ciclosporine
Valproic Acids
Highly Acting Anti Retro Virals
Heparin
Statins
Idiosyncratic DILI
Allopurinol
Amiodarone
Amoxicilline-Clavulanic Acid
Diclofenac
Disulfiram
Fenofibrate
Flutamide
Alotane
Isoniazide
Ketoconazol
Nimesulide
Lisinopril
Metildopa
Minocicline
Nitrofurantoine
Pirazinamide
Statins
Ticlopidine
Quinolones Antibiotcs

microbiologic or chemical, makes evaluation of liver toxicity difficult. Case reports do not always document causation or association, thus liver toxicity of herbs is underestimated, and case reports are fewer than in real life. Moreover, the lack of standardized commercial regulations for dietary supplements needs to be taken into account to explain the potentially increasing role as causative agents of liver damage. Dietary supplements include vitamins, calcium, fish oil, laxatives, herbs (Chinese herbs, ayurvedic compounds used in Indian medicine). These compounds are thought to be safe as exemplified by natural science medicine; indeed, they have been associated with a higher rate of liver failure, liver transplant need, and in rare cases, death. This emerging problem is due to increasing use of these compounds in the general population and the lack of rigorous policy for their manufacturing and marketing, in the absence of a rigorous safety profile, which is compulsory for traditional medicine. There are no rules for recommended of maximum dosage or side effect warnings. Without a patient package insert, customers have no in- formation about side-effects, even in cases of documented toxicity.

CLINICAL FEATURES

Usually, DILI is asymptomatic and can be discovered only after an increase in serum transaminases, with resolution after drug or toxic discontinuation.

Table 35.2 Examples of drug-induced liver damage correlated with genetic susceptibility.

HLA-Related Genetic Factors

Drug	Allele at Risk
Amoxicillin + Clavulanic acid	HLA-DRB1*1501
Carbamazepine	HLA-B*1502
Ticlopidine	HLA-A*3303
Flucloxacillin	HLA-B+5701

Non HLA-Related Genetic Factors

Drug	Genetic Variant
Diclofenac	Structural variability of CYPC8*4
Diclofenac	Polymorphisms of MRP2 (multidrug resistant protein)
Hormones	Polymorphisms of bile salt export pump (BSEP)
Valproic acid	Polymorphisms of mitochondrial polymerase γ

In 12% of cases symptoms associated with DILI include fatigue, anorexia, subicterus or jaundice. In rare cases a massive liver necrosis may results in liver failure and death. Negative prognostic factors include elevated serum transaminases (>10 times the normal) and jaundice (Hy's law). In clinical practice, when suspecting DILI physical examination and accurate medical history should yield information about: drug assumption, over-the-counter products, herbs like green tea extracts, multi-ingredient dietary supplements, anabolic steroids, time of exposure and discontinuation. An international group of experts has proposed the following classification for DILI based on the patter of liver test abnormalities:

- hepatocellular pattern (ALT ≥5 times above normal or ALT value/Normal ALT values and Alkaline Phosphatase value/Normal Alkaline Phosphatase values ratio of >5);
- cholestatic pattern (alkaline phosphatase ≥2 times above normal or ALT value/Normal ALT values and Alkaline phosphatase value/Normal Alkaline phosphatase values ratio of <2);
- mixed pattern (ALT ≥5 times above normal or ALT value/Normal ALT values and Alkaline Phosphatase value/Normal Alkaline Phosphatase values ratio of >2 and <5). In hepatocellular damage with jaundice, the case-fatality rate or liver transplant is 10% (Hy's law).

The major symptoms of massive liver necrosis within acute liver failure include: encephalopathy (sleepwake rhythm disorder, confusion, lethargy), coagulation disorders (impaired synthesis of coagulation proteins). In these cases, if liver transplant is not performed mortality can reach 75%.

Hepatocellular Damage

In most cases DILI presents with a moderate asymptomatic hepatocellular pattern. Severe hepatitis symptoms may mimic an acute viral hepatitis: with anorexia, nausea, sometimes vomiting, moderate pain in the epigastrium and right hypochondrium the most common features reported by patients. Alkaline phosphatase is normal or slightly elevated. Bilirubin may be normal or elevated in the presence of severe disease. Differential diagnosis includes cholecystitis with gallstones, acute viral hepatitis, autoimmune hepatitis, ischaemic liver injury, Budd-Chiari syndrome, and fulminant Wilson disease. The most common histologic feature is acute necrosis in zone 3 of Rappaport's acinus and in zone 2 in severe necrosis. Inflammatory infiltrate with eosinophils and polymorphonuclear cells can be found in portal tracts. Some agents can cause steatosis, first in zone 3 and subsequently in other zones with the typical features of steatohepatitis. In most cases there is prompt amelioration of symptoms and biochemistry after drug discontinuation. Hepatocellular damage is typical of DILI related to intake of herbal and dietary supplements like green tea extracts and multi-ingredient dietary supplements.

Cholestatic Damage

Cholestatic pattern includes jaundice and itching. In severe liver damage symptoms such as anorexia, nausea and vomiting can occur. Biochemistry reveals a cholestatic syndrome with an increase in serum alkaline phosphatase (two times above normal) and in bilirubin (both total and direct component). In pure cholestatic injury, serum transaminases are within the normal range or only slightly elevated. Ultrasound does not reveal biliary tree dilatation or abnormalities in the pancreas; liver morphology is usually normal. Differential diagnosis includes gallbladder biliary obstruction, malignancy, pancreatic diseases, autoimmune cholangiopathies such as primary biliary cholangitis or primary sclerosing cholangitis. Liver biopsy shows bile within the hepatocytes and biliary casts in the canaliculi. Biliary sludge or other features of extrahepatic obstruction and signs of acute cholangitis or pericholangitis are absent. The outcome of cholestatic hepatitis is generally prolonged, with gradual amelioration; restoration of clinical and biochemical alterations in general takes several months. DILI related to anabolic steroids is responsible of a cholestatic damage characterized by long-duration jaundice with mild increase in liver enzymes.

Mixed Damage

Hepatocellular and cholestatic features coexist. Clinical presentation includes jaundice, itching, nausea, vomiting, and anorexia. Biochemistry is characterized by elevated serum transaminases (3 times above normal), in alkaline phosphatase and bilirubin (2 times above normal). Differential diagnosis is more complex and comprises all causes of both acute and chronic damage.

SPECIFIC TYPES OF DILI

Drug-Induced Liver Damage and Autoimmunity

A drug may trigger autoimmune hepatitis or cause DILI with "autoimmune-like" features. The main characteristics of this latter syndrome are:

- onset within 3 months of drug assumption;
- jaundice is rarely present at onset;
- improvement under steroids which can be discontinued without relapse; liver histology undistinguishable from classical AIH.

Two main pathogenic factors have been identified for "autoimmune-like" DILI:

- Metabolic pathway: The toxic agent is metabolised, leading to the formation of a neo antigen presented to T cells; in re-exposure to the drug, cytotoxic damage occurs;
- Immunologic pathway: A drug can by-pass the formation of a metabolite and can bind to T-cell receptors and/or major histocompatibility (MHC) molecules. The MHC mediates antigen presentation to T cells (immunogenic hapten). The MHC-peptides are present on the Kupffer cell surface; T-helper activation and cytotoxic T-lym- phocyte activation then occur. Various pro-inflammatory cytokines are synthesised, including TNFα, FasL, IFNγ, which contribute to the development of "allergic" symptoms such as rash, fever, pruritus, peripheral eosinophil increase, and an eosinophilic infiltrate within the liver.

DILI Associated with Immune Check Point Inhibitors

Immune check point inhibitors (ICI) are a new class of drugs which have revolutionized the treatment of several tumour types and currently represent the standard of care of treatment. This class includes drugs that target cytotoxic T-lymphocyte-associated protein4 (CTLA-4), programmed cell death receptor-1 (PD-1) or the programmed cell death receptor ligand 1 (PD-L1) with the ultimate aim to activate an immune response directed towards neoplastic cells. ICIs are associated with several Immune-related adverse events (irAEs), which result from an excessively activated immune system, and that can include DILI. An increase in Transaminases values has been reported in up to 5% of cases with rates that vary on the basis of the agents used but also on the specific characteristics of individual patients. Transaminases elevations are usually mild without any associated symptom, rare is the development of acute hepatitis with jaundice and systemic symptoms such as fever and asthenia. Histologically most cases show lymphocyte infiltration with hepatocellular injury, however cholestatic liver injury characterised by elevations in serum Alkaline Phosphatase (with or without serum bilirubin elevation) has also been reported with ICIs. Strict monitoring of liver blood tests is recommended in all patients receiving ICIs, with specific guidelines defined "Common Terminology Criteria for Adverse Events" (CTCAE) available to manage DILI. In case of ALT values <3 times the upper limit of normal (ULN) with bilirubin levels <1.5 times ULN, ICIs should not be discontinued but strict monitoring is mandatory. If grade II toxicity defined as ALT between 3 and 5 times ULN is demonstrated steroids need to be rapidly started and ICIs should be discontinued and restarted only after liver tests improvement. If ALT is higher than 5 times ULN ICIs need to be promptly and indefinetely suspended and steroids need to be started.

Microvesicular Steatosis

Drug-related steatosis is common and often transient and mild, asymptomatic or associated with slight liver enlargement. The exception is microvesicular steatosis which is a rare feature caused by drugs determining mitochondrial toxicity. Mitochondria damage is characterized both by a defect in the mitochondrial β-oxidation of free fatty acids and a major decrease in ATP mitochondrial production. Patients complain of anorexia, nausea, and vomiting or symptoms related to hepatic encephalopathy which can progress to coma with severe hyperammoniaemia; often accompanied by lactic acidosis due to a defect in mitochondrial respiration and oxidative phosphorylation pathways. Biochemistry shows a moderate or severe increase in serum transaminases; alkaline phosphatase levels are usually normal or slightly increased; bilirubin levels are variable, according to the severity of damage. Liver ultrasound is normal. Liver biopsy shows a widespread infiltration of lipids in the cytoplasm of hepatocytes without nucleus dislocation, sometimes the vesicle size is minimal, thus difficult to be recognized with optical microscope; inflammation is present, whereas fibrosis is absent. After discontinuation of the drug there is rapid amelioration; in some particularly severe cases liver transplant is needed. In general, resolution is not associated with chronicity.

Macrovesicular Steatosis

In general, macrovesicular steatosis is asymptomatic. In severe fatty infiltration, an enlarged liver develops with pain in the upper right abdomen (with mostly a sensation of weight). Symptoms are roughly absent; liver enzymes are normal or slightly altered. Liver ultrasound shows hyperechogenicity of the liver due to fatty infiltration. Liver histology is similar to alcoholic steatosis or non-alcoholic steatosis/steatohepatitis associated with metabolic syndrome. In some cases microvesicular steatosis coexists (mixed steatosis). Examples of drugs which can cause macrovesicular steatosis are amiodarone, methotrexate, tamoxifen and chemotherapy agents such as irinotecan.

DIAGNOSIS

Given the wide spectrum of clinical features, and in the absence of specific diagnostic tests, diagnostic tools for DILI include clinical suspicion, accurate pharmacological history including intake of herbal and dietary supplements, and the exclusion of other causes of liver damage. Assessment of aetiology includes:

- Latency time between exposure to drug, herb or dietary supplement and the onset of the adverse event (challenge): regarding idiosyncratic DILI, the latency period between the assumption of the drug and the occurrence of symptoms or biochemistry abnormalities is variable. For hypersensitivity reactions, the liver damage may occur after a brief period (24-72 hours), especially after rechallenge. The latency period can last 2-8 weeks in sulfamide-induced damage, or as a consequence of fluoroquinolon, penicillin, clozapine, anticonvulsants, minocyclin, protease inhibitors, pentoxyphilin, Chinese herbs, up to 20 weeks in toxicity from isoniazide, dantrolene, and troglitazone. Sometimes liver toxicity may occur after drug discontinuation; for example, oxypenicillinand amoxicillin/clavulanic acid induced DILI.
- Time of resolution after discontinuation (dechallenge): after discontinuation of drug, herb, or dietary supplement there is a variable period of days and weeks characterized by progressive amelioration of clinical features and biochemistry. Liver toxicity from ketoconazole, troglitazone, and amiodarone can be an exception, taking several months for complete resolution.
- Eventual recurrence after rechallenge: rechallenge with the suspected drug/toxic recorded in the medical history is considered the gold standard for diagnostic confirmation. Voluntary rechallenge is potentially dangerous and cannot be recommended in clinical practice.
- Extrahepatic manifestations and symptoms due to hypersensitivity: the symptoms due to hypersensitivity are specific for DILI but rare. Symptoms include: fever, rash, mucositis, eosinophilic reaction, lymph node enlargement, mononucleosis-like syndrome, immune suppression, vasculitis, renal failure, pneumonia, and pancreatitis (drug reaction with eosinophilia and systemic symptoms syndrome, DRESS).
- Exclusion of other causes of liver damage: assessment of suspected DILI should rule out other potential causes of liver damage together with an accurate medical history including risk factors for viral hepatitis, alcohol intake, associated medical conditions, in particular au-

toimmune disorders, heart failure, metabolic conditions, and infections. Standard diagnostic procedures include testing for serology for major and minor hepato- tropic viruses (HAV, HBV, HCV and HEV, herpes viruses, Epstein-Barr, and cytomegalovirus), autoantibodies (ANA, SMA, LKM), iron and copper metabolism tests, and accurate imaging for gallbladder, biliary tree, and liver parenchyma (liver ultrasound, abdominal magnetic resonance).

- The presence of Risk factors: alcohol intake, pregnancy, and age above 55 years.
- Scientific publications supporting the side effect of the suspected drug, herb, or dietary supplement: it is good medical practice to perform online searches for case reports or case series of DILI for a suspected specific drug/toxic.

Liver biopsy, which in general is unspecific for DILI, is not always necessary for diagnosis but may be helpful in complex cases. Liver biopsy is indicated when the timing between drug/herb/dietary supplement assumption and the onset of liver injury is unclear, when differential diagnosis is complex (i.e., positivity for autoantibodies suggesting autoimmune hepatitis after assumption of potentially hepatotoxic drugs) or when a rapid diagnosis is needed (i.e., after bone marrow transplantation or in paracetamol-induced acute damage, or chronic damage from methotrexate or amiodarone) (**Figure 35.2**).

THERAPY

In most cases patients are asymptomatic or oligosymptomatic, presenting with only elevated transaminases at blood tests.
Treatment entails removal of the offending drug. In asymptomatic hepatitis, in which elevated serum transaminases are associated with jaundice (Hy's law) the patient should be referred to a specialized facility for diagnosis and monitoring with liver function tests. In few cases with acute liver failure the patient should be evaluated for liver transplant and referred to a third level centre (see Chapter N. "X"). Paracetamol overdose should be kept in mind because stratification risk for liver damage is mandatory (high risk if >10 g assumption or serum levels of paracetamol >150 mg/mL at 4 hours; in N-acetylcystein infusion with a loading dose of 150 mg/kg, followed by 50 mg/kg over 4 hours for a total of 300 mg/kg over 24 hours. Steroids are often utilized when signs and symptoms of hypersensitivity are present, although data on efficacy and safety of steroids in DILI are rather limited. Finally, supportive care treatment can be necessary in prolonged cholestasis with coagulopathy due to deficient absorption of vitamin K, which should be administered parenterally, and pruritus which is managed with cholestyramine, antihistamines, sertraline, or cycles of UVA light therapy.

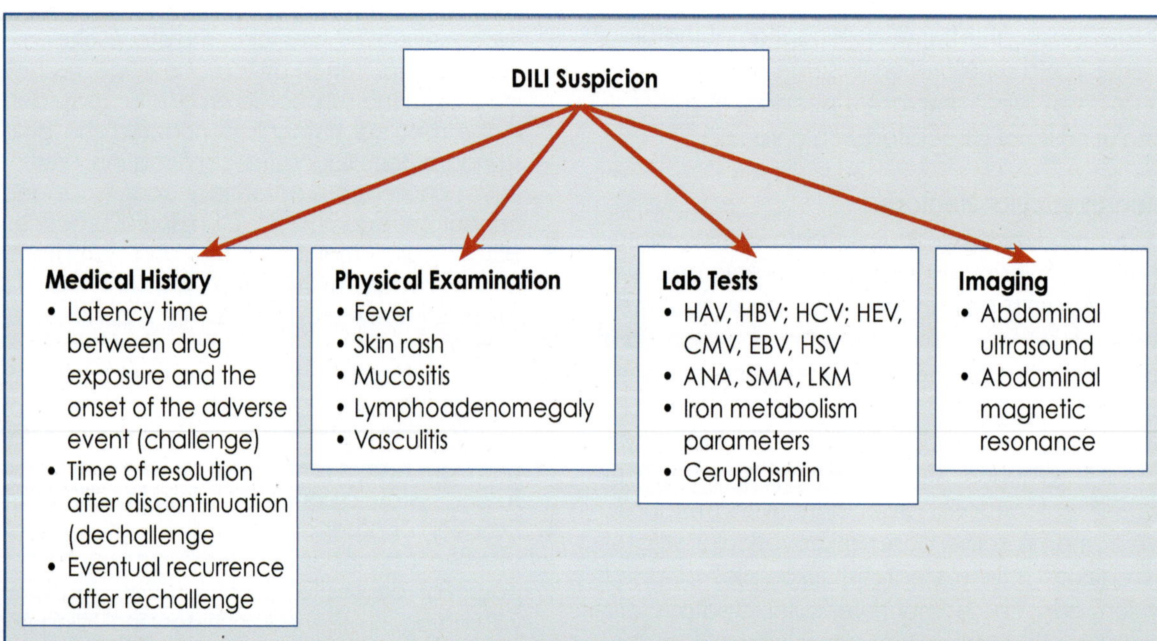

Figure 35.2 Diagnostic algorithm for drug-induced liver damage (DILI).

KEY CONCEPTS

- Drug-induced liver damage (DILI) has an undefined (underestimated) incidence).
- DILI occurs after intake of any drug or herbal product or dietary supplements even in small amounts and after a single administration.
- DILI may be associated with a wide spectrum of liver damage with an acute or chronic condition and is the main cause of acute liver failure.
- Differential diagnosis of DILI in patients with concomitant liver diseases is complex.

REFERENCES

- KullaK-Ublick GA, Andrade RJ, Merz M, et al. Drug-induced liver injury: recent advances in diagnosis and risk assessment. Gut. 2017;66:1154-64.
- Tujios SR, Lee WM. Acute liver failure induced by idiosyncratic reaction to drugs: challenges in diagnosis and therapy. Liver Int. 2018;38:6-14.
- Visentin M, Lenggenhager D, Gai Z, et al. Drug-induced bile duct injury. Biochim Biophys Acta Mol Basis Dis. 2018;1864 (4 Pt B):1498-506.
- Chalasani NP, Maddur H, Russo MW, et al; Practice Parameters Committee of the American College of Gastroenterology. ACG Clinical Guideline: Diagnosis and Management of Idiosyncratic Drug Induced Liver Injury. Am J Gastroenterol. 2021;116(5):878-98.
- European Association for the Study of the Liver. Electronic address: easloffice@easloffice.eu; Clinical Practice Guideline Panel: Chair; Panel members; EASL Governing Board representative: EASL Clinical Practice Guidelines: Drug-induced liver injury. J Hepatol. 2019;70(6):1222-61.
- Dougan M, Wang Y, Rubio-Tapia A, Lim JK. AGA Clinical Practice Update on Diagnosis and Management of Immune Checkpoint Inhibitor Colitis and Hepatitis: Expert Review. Gastroenterology. 2021;160(4):1384-93.
- Personeni N, Pressiani T, D'Alessio A, et al. Hepatotoxicity in Patients with Hepatocellular Carcinoma on Treatment with Immune Checkpoint Inhibitors. Cancers. 2021;13(22):5665.
- Navarro VJ, Khan I, Björnsson E, Seeff LB, Serrano J, Hoofnagle JH. Liver injury from herbal and dietary supplements. Hepatology. 2017;65(1):363-73.

CHAPTER 36

LIVER CIRRHOSIS AND ITS COMPLICATIONS

Giorgio Maria Saracco, Antonio Facciorusso

LEARNING OBJECTIVES

- To know the prevalence, incidence, and most frequent causes of cirrhosis.
- To know the pathophysiological bases of cirrhosis and its complications.
- To know the main clinical signs and tools for diagnosis and clinical staging.
- To know the natural history and the main therapeutic end points to treat liver cirrhosis.

Liver cirrhosis is a slowly progressive disease characterized by fibrosis and deposition of connective tissue in the liver which modify its normal architecture and impair normal function over time.
Histology of liver cirrhosis is characterized by the concomitant presence of fibrosis and regeneration nodules (**Figure 36.1**).
These anatomic alterations result from hepatocellular damage due to viruses, alcohol, metabolic factors which lead to necrosis of hepatocytes with subsequent inflammation, followed by regeneration, fibrosis and – at a later stage – structural alteration of parenchyma.
According to morphological classification, cirrhosis is divided into micronodular cirrhosis and macronodular cirrhosis; the distinction is based upon the size of nodules on the liver surface (< or > 3 mm). An example of micronodular cirrhosis is alcohol-related cirrhosis, while viral cirrhosis is more frequently macronodular.
The main consequences of cirrhosis are progressively impaired parenchymal function and microvascular disturbances that induce portal hypertension and create arterial-venous shunts and venous collaterals.

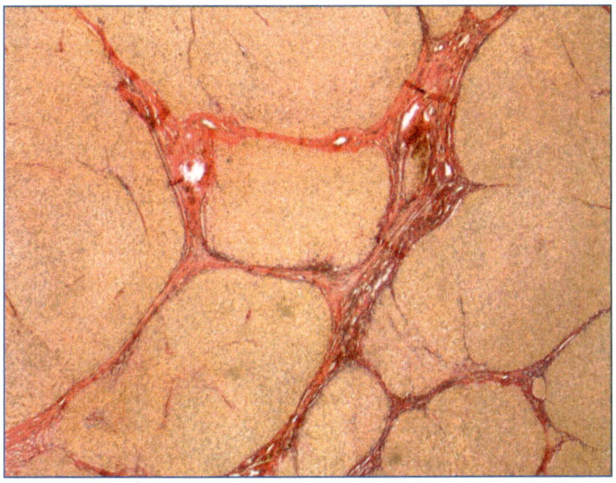

Figure 36.1 Histological aspect of the cirrhotic liver showing regeneration nodules separated by fibrous septa (courtesy of Prof. Maria Guido).

EPIDEMIOLOGY

Liver cirrhosis is a common chronic disease in Italy with elevated social impact. According to Istat Annual Report 2018, mortality due to liver cirrhosis in Italy is 19.5/100.000 inhabitants and is among the 10 leading causes of death. Prevalence is higher among males.
Alcohol-related liver cirrhosis is prevalent in the Northern Italy, particularly in the Northeast, whereas while viral cirrhosis is prevalent in Central and Southern Italy. According to Istat Annual Report 2018, its incidence is 30-60/100000 inhabitants/year, with about 26,000 new cases/year. The epidemiology of liver cirrhosis is shifting, reflecting implementation of large-scale hepatitis B vaccination and hepatitis C effective treatment programs, the increasing prevalence of the metabolic syndrome, and increasing alcohol misuse.
The temporal trend of the last 20 years shows that cirrhosis-related mortality in Italy is progressively decreasing, while mortality due to hepatocellular carcinoma (HCC) is increasing. The latter finding is probably due to better and earlier diagnosis; moreover, the mean age has increased as has the risk of developing cancer.
Finally, liver cirrhosis – particularly when complications occur – has a negative impact on quality of life and is a significant cause of medical care and hospital referral.

AETIOLOGY

Liver cirrhosis is the final product of chronic liver diseases of various aetiology (**Table 36.1**). In about 90% of cases, liver cirrhosis is caused by alcohol and

Table 36.1 Main causes of liver cirrhosis.

Viral
HBV, HCV, HDV
Alcohol-related liver disease
Autoimmune and cholestatic liver disease
Autoimmune Hepatitis
Primary Biliary Cholangitis
Primary Sclerosing Cholangitis
Metabolic liver disease
Hereditary Haemochromatosis
Wilson Disease
Alpha-1 antitrypsin deficiency
Cystic fibrosis
Porphyria
Vitamin A deficiency
Iatrogenic
Drugs: Methotrexate, Amiodarone, α methyldopa
Secondary biliary cirrhosis
Intestinal bypass in bariatric surgery
Vascular disease
Right heart failure
Constrictive pericarditis
Budd-Chiari syndrome
Hepatic veno-occlusive disease
Non-alcoholic fatty liver disease
Cryptogenic cirrhosis

chronic viral diseases; in particular, liver cirrhosis is due to:

- hepatitis B Virus (HBV) when serological markers of HBV infection are found (HBsAg, HBV-DNA);
- hepatitis D Virus (HDV) when the antibody against HDV is detectable in serum;
- hepatitis C Virus (HCV) when the antibody against HCV (anti-HCV) or the viral genome (HCV-RNA) is present in the serum.

Liver cirrhosis is probably caused by alcohol when a daily intake of alcoholic beverages >30 g in males and >20 g in females is established over 10 years in the absence of other possible causes of liver damage.
A mixed aetiology (alcohol + virus) is not infrequent. Other causes of liver cirrhosis (metabolic, cholestatic, autoimmune, iatrogenic, vascular) are less frequent but should be investigated in patients with liver disease without viral markers or a history of significant intake of alcoholic beverages. When no aetiological factor can be found, liver cirrhosis is defined as cryptogenic. A recent hypothesis suggests that cryptogenic cirrhosis may be the evolution of a non-alcoholic steatohepatitis (NASH).

PATHOPHYSIOLOGY

The three mechanisms leading to liver cirrhosis are hepatocellular necrosis, fibrogenesis, and vascular changes.
The alteration of the vascular pattern progressively reduces the liver mass because the hepatocyte has to maintain the space relationship with microvascular flow and the biliary system in order to work properly.
Moreover, these alterations induce portal hypertension, which is the main complication of liver cirrhosis.

Fibrogenesis

In liver cirrhosis, the chronic damage of hepatocytes induces proliferation of inflammatory cells, Kupffer cells, and platelets which produce cytokines (tumour necrosis factor-α, TNF-α), IL-2 and IL-6, growth factors such as platelet derived growth factor-β (PDGF-β) and transforming growth factor–β (TGF-β). The inflammatory cytokines activate the Ito cells, which lose and vitamin A-containing droplets and acquire the capacity to synthetize actin, becoming similar to fibroblasts and produce collagen. The progressive deposition of connective tissue (type I and III collagen, fibronectin, and proteoglycans) leads to complete alteration of the normal liver architecture over time. The abnormal deposition of collagen is also due to its decreased degradation usually exerted by Kupffer cell collagenases.
Initially, collagen deposition occurs in the subendothelial space (space of Disse) and "capillarization" of sinusoids, with consequent loss of elasticity and fenestrae; necrotic areas are then substituted by fibrosis with the formation of porto-portal and porto-central septa embedding the hepatocytes in irregular nodule structures, so-called "regeneration nodules".
Liver cirrhosis was long considered an irreversible diseasee; however, the exact moment when cirrhosis or advanced fibrosis become irreversible has not yet been identified.
The recent advances in therapy, with the advent of DAAs in chronic viral hepatitis, suggest that medical therapy may be of benefit even in cirrhotic patients; there is evidence that in some cases liver fibrosis may be reduced and reverted by antivirals.
The deposition of extracellular matrix during chronic liver disease is not a steady and unidirectional phenomenon but can be counterbalanced by fibrolysis. In fact, fibrolysis is induced by matrix ex-

cess and by metalloproteases (MMP). Current and future therapies may enhance endogenous mechanisms by eliminating the causal agent, degrade the extracellular matrix, and revert the fibrosis.

Portal Hypertension

The portal system of the normal liver is a high-compliance, low-resistance system that carries capillary blood from the abdominal organs to the liver; after flowing through the sinusoids and the hepatic veins, the blood reaches the inferior vena caval and the systemic circulation.

Portal inflow is about 1000-1200 mL/min. Normal portal pressure is 7 mmHg while hepatic venous pressure is 3-5 mmHg (similar to the right atrium) with a pressure gradient of 2-4 mmHg between the portal vein and the hepatic veins.

When the portal-hepatic venous pressure gradient is >10-12 mmHg, a clinically significant portal hypertension is present.

The clinical consequences of portal hypertension are presented in **Table 36.2**. The classification of causes of portal hypertension is based on the site of increased resistance to portal blood flow – namely, prehepatic, intrahepatic, and posthepatic (**Table 36.3**).

In Italy, the most frequent cause of portal hypertension is liver cirrhosis. There are several mechanisms involved in inducing portal hypertension. A crucial role is played by the increase in intrahepatic resistance to blood flow. The increased portal resistance occurs as a result of mechanical factors that reduce vessel diameter (regeneration nodules, fibrous septa, and sinusoid capillarization due to collagen deposition) and haemodynamic factors (hepatic vasoconstriction due to Ito cell activation by local vasoconstrictor factors such as endothelin).

Another relevant haemodynamic factor contributing to portal hypertension in liver cirrhosis is the increase in portal venous flow due to splanchnic vasodilatation induced by mediators such as nitric oxide. Splanchnic vasodilatation is one aspect of the generalized haemodynamic alteration present in liver cirrhosis known as hyperdynamic circulation syndrome.

The syndrome is characterised by peripheral and splanchnic vasodilatation with reduced peripheral vascular resistance and increased cardiac venous input and cardiac output. Vasodilatation induces a relative hypovolemia because total blood is not sufficient to fill an abnormally dilated vascular bed and activates vasoconstrictor (norepinephrine, vasopressin, etc.) and sodium-retentive hormones (renin, angiotensin, aldosterone). This hormonal cascade results in significant water and sodium retention, with secondary volume overload that

Table 36.2 Clinical consequences of portal hypertension.

Oesophageal and gastric varices
Congestive gastropathy
Hepatic encephalopathy
Ascites
Opening of collateral circulation
Splenic enlargement

Table 36.3 Conditions that can cause portal hypertension.

Pre-hepatic:	Portal vein thrombosis §
Hepatic	Pre-sinusoidal Schistosomiasis, sarcoidosis, toxic (arsenic and polyvinylchloride) Non-cirrhotic idiopathic portal hypertension Sinusoidal Liver cirrhosis, alcohol-related hepatitis Post-sinusoidal VOD (Veno-occlusive disease)*
Post- hepatic	Budd-Chiari syndrome Constrictive pericarditis

§ Portal vein thrombosis can occur after umbilical vein infection tumour invading the portal vein, cirrhosis of the liver, congenital thrombophilia, chronic inflammatory diseases of the intestine.
* The veno-occlusive disease, also called sinusoidal obstruction syndrome, affects the sinusoids in patients undergoing bone marrow transplantation and in the Budd-Chiari syndrome; it may be associated with myeloproliferative diseases, congenital thrombophilia, and oestrogen-progestin therapy.

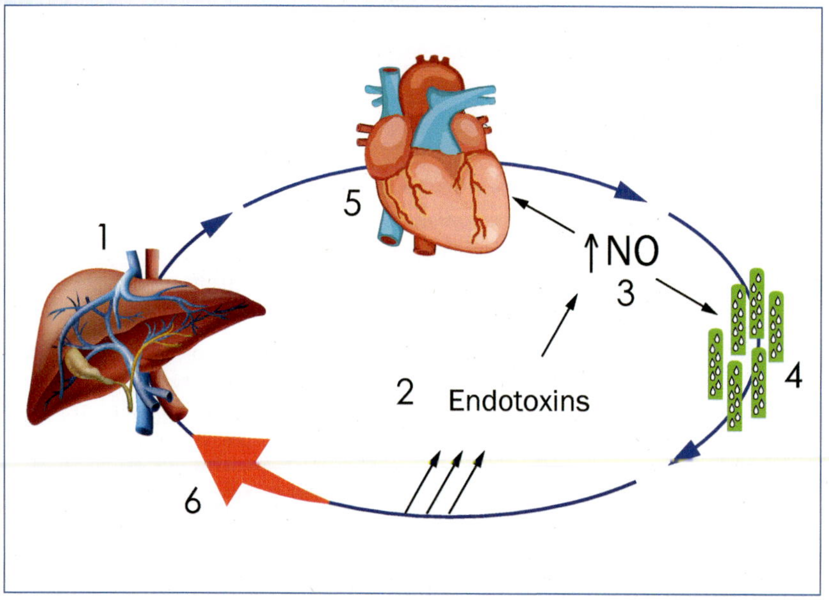

Figure 36.2 Sequential role of pathogenic factors involved in portal hypertension in liver cirrhosis. Cirrhosis increases intrahepatic resistance, leading to portal hypertension (1). Portal hypertension causes the opening of collateral circulation (2). Due to the shunts, vasoactive substances (endotoxins, nitric oxide) are increased in systemic circulation (3) and cause vasodilation predominantly in the splanchnic circulation (4). Vasodilatation increases venous return with elevated cardiac index and establishment of a hyperdynamic syndrome (5). Vasodilation increases blood flow from the splanchnic towards the portal circulation

worsens portal hypertension by increasing the portal venous inflow without completely counterbalancing vasodilatation (**Figure 36.2**).

CLINICAL ASPECTS

Patients with compensated liver cirrhosis usually do not show relevant clinical symptoms. Sometimes, when a viral aetiology is present, they complain of fatigue or fever if the disease is due to an autoimmune cause. In the cholestatic forms, pruritus may be the only symptom. This asymptomatic or low-symptomatic phase of liver cirrhosis may persist for many years; diagnosis is made incidentally during routine biochemical tests or pre-surgery exam.

When liver cirrhosis is compensated, the signs are similar to those usually found in chronic hepatitis (liver enlargement and mild elevation of transaminases). If final diagnosis is difficult, a liver biopsy is recommended to assess fibrosis staging and regeneration nodules. Recently, transient elastography has substituted liver biopsy in many cases, providing a non-invasive evaluation of fibrosis stage.

As cirrhosis progresses, the clinical features merge due to the reduction in functional liver mass and the severe portal hypertension.

As a consequence of the reduced liver function, the synthesis of clotting factors, albumin, and cholinesterase is impaired. Jaundice may occur early in the cholestatic forms such as primary biliary cholangitis (PBC) with a vanishing bile ducts pattern. In the non-cholestatic forms, an increase of >3 mg/dL of bilirubin carries an unfavorable prognosis.

Portal hypertension is the cause of complications: oesophageal varices, portal hypertensive gastropathy, ascites, and encephalopathy.

The progressive increase in spleen volume induces elevated intra-splenic drainage of leukocytes and platelets (leuko-thrombocytopenia secondary to hypersplenism); thrombocytopenia contributes to impaired haemocoagulation. In this phase, findings from history, clinical assessment, and altered biochemical tests make the final diagnosis easy (**Table 36.4**).

Not unfrequently, patients become aware of the disease due to the sudden onset of one of the cirrhosis complications: ascites, variceal bleeding, encephalopathy. Differential diagnosis is usually facilitated by clinical and biochemical evidences of the underlying chronic liver disease.

COMPLICATIONS

Liver cirrhosis is defined as "decompensated" when one or more complications occur. Liver cirrhosis complications are presented in **Table 36.5**.

About 10% of patients with "compensated" liver cirrhosis progress towards a "decompensated" status yearly. The major complications in the natural history of liver cirrhosis are gastrointestinal bleeding (Chapter 49), ascites, hepatic encephalopathy, and hepatocellular carcinoma (Chapter 37). Less frequent complications (but equally feared) are spontaneous bacterial peritonitis, hepatorenal syndrome, and portal thrombosis.

Table 36.4 Main history, clinical, and biochemical signs in hepatic cirrhosis.

History	Alcohol abuse, previous hepatitis infection, chronic use of hepatotoxic drugs, weight loss and asthenia, anorexia and reduced appetite, pruritus
Physical examination	Sub-jaundice or rarely jaundices, palmar erythema, spider nevi, petechiae, ecchymosis, purpura rash on the legs, gynecomastia and testicular atrophy, itching and scratch wounds, malnutrition, ascites or edema, collateral abdominal circulation, increased or reduced liver volume with increased consistency, uneven surface, and thinned margins, splenic enlargement, altered level of consciousness, flapping tremor
Main biochemical alterations	Necrotic markers: mild increase in transaminases (GOT and GPT) Synthetic markers: reduction of total protein, albumin, cholinesterase, prothrombin activity, hypofibrinogemia due to decreased hepatic function Cholestatic markers: moderately elevated, very high in biliary forms: Bilirubin, alkaline phosphatase, gamma-glutamyltranspeptidase
Further blood tests alterations	Anemia: Normochromic (hypersplenism), hypochromic (iron-deficiency) or macrocytic or ''spur cell'' (Vitamin B deficiency) Leukopenia (hypersplenism) (leukocytosis when associated with alcohol-related hepatitis) Thrombocytopenia (hypersplenism) Polyclonal hypogammaglobinemia Hyperammonemia (with hepatic encephalopathy) Hepatitis markers (positive in viral disease) ANA, AMA, AML, LKM, ENA (positive in autoimmune disease) Blood iron, ferritin, ceruloplasmin, alfa-1-atitripsin (altered in metabolic disease) Decreased cholesterol and triglycerides

Table 36.5 Complications of cirrhosis.

Digestive Haemorrhage
- oesophageal varices
- gastric varices
- congestive gastropathy

Ascites
- non-complicated
- recurrent
- refractory

Spontaneous Bacterial Peritonitis
Porto-Systemic Encephalopathy
Hepatorenal Syndrome
Hepatopulmonary Syndrome
Portal Vein Thrombosis
Hepatocellular Carcinoma

Oesophageal and Gastric Varices

The gastrointestinal manifestations of portal hypertension include oesophageal varices, gastric, and isolated intestinal varices. About 5-15% of cirrhotic patients develop oesophageal varices yearly. Most, will develop varices during their life.

Early diagnosis of oesophageal varices before the first variceal bleeding is crucial. Studies conducted on primary prophylaxis clearly show that the risk of bleeding can be significantly reduced. Endoscopy of the upper gastrointestinal tract is the gold standard for screening, but it is an invasive procedure. Unfortunately, current clinical, biochemical, and radiological parameters are not sufficiently accurate to substitute endoscopy, however, systemic haemodynamic evaluation and other serologic markers may play a role in the future. Oesophageal and gastric varices should be staged; Bopp's classification divides varices into 3 groups (F1, F2, and F3) according to size (< or >1/3 of the oesophageal lumen),and shape (linear or tortu-

ous); gastric varices are defined as IGV1 (isolated gastric varices 1) if transcardial, IGV2 (isolated gastric varices 2) if located in the gastric fundus, and IGV3 (isolated gastric varices 3) if located in the remaining regions of the stomach.
This classification allows to stratify the bleeding risk and to determine the appropriate prophylactic approach (medical and/or endoscopic).
Variceal rupture is influenced by Laplace's law: increase in wall tension is due to augmented intravascular pressure and variceal diameter, and to reduced wall thickness. Wall thickness can be assessed by red marks on the varices. These marks are the areas where the wall is particularly thin. Varices rupture occurs usually at the gastro-oesophageal junction where the varices have a particularly thin wall.
There is a debate about whether endoscopy can directly detect varices, evaluate their size, and identify high-risk marks of impending bleeding.
The best approach (medical or endoscopic) to prevent the first haemorrhagic episode is controversial; both interventions are effective in reducing the bleeding risk in cirrhotic patients with large varices, irrespective of the presence of red marks. Further details on variceal bleeding are reported in Chapter 49 on digestive bleeding.

Ascites and Spontaneous Bacterial Peritonitis

Ascites is a consequence of portal hypertension in more than 50% of cirrhotic patients during their life time; together with digestive bleeding, it is one of the most frequent causes of hospital referral and is associated with decreased survival rate. The mechanisms by which portal hypertension induces ascites have been reported. Moreover, renal retention of sodium induces the expansion of extracellular fluid, resulting in ascites and edema. Liver cirrhosis causes ascites in about 75% of patients in Western Europe and the United States. Causes of ascites are: malignant neoplasia's, heart failure, tuberculosis, pancreas diseases, and other infrequent causes (fulminant hepatitis, Budd-Chiari syndrome, etc.).
Each patient with ascites should be initially evaluated by means of appropriate history, physical examination, abdominal ultrasound, liver and kidney function tests, serologic and urine electrolytes, ascitic fluid analysis. In fact, a diagnostic paracentesis with appropriate ascetic fluid analysis is crucial in the evaluation for ascites, before adopting treatment, to exclude non-cirrhotic causes of ascites and spontaneous bacterial peritonitis (SBP). Differential diagnosis between the different types of ascites can be performed by the serum-ascites albumin gradient (SAAG). If the SAAG is 1.1 g/dL (11 g/L) or greater, diagnosis of portal hypertension has an accuracy of about 97%. Moreover, total protein value should be assessed in the ascitic fluid to evaluate the risk of a concomitant SBP as patients with total protein level <15 g/L have a higher risk of SBP.
Ascites is classified in 3 stages:

- 1st stage: mild, visible only by ultrasound;
- 2nd stage: detectable by physical examination assessing flank dullness by percussion and checking for shifting;
- 3rd stage: directly visible at physical examination, confirmed by shifting.

The onset of ascites carries an unfavorable prognosis. Mortality is about 40% at 1 year and 50% at 2 years. The most accurate unfavorable prognostic factors are: low sodium level, hypotension, increased creatinine, and low urinary sodium concentration.
Refractory ascites is defined as unresponsive ascites or rapidly relapsing after a sodium-restricted diet and high-dose diuretic treatment.
Ascites untreatable with appropriate dosage of diuretics due to the rapid onset of side effects such as hypovolemia, hypotension, electrolytes alteration, cramps and secondary renal failure is also considered refractory. The most frequent complication of ascites is SBP. SBP is the spontaneous infection of ascitic fluid usually due to bacterial translocation from the gut (*E. Coli*, *Klebsiella* etc.) to the intestinal mucosa, mesenteric nodes, enteric circulation, and hepatic sinusoids; this infection is favored by portal hypertension, impaired reticulo endothelial system, and lack of antimicrobial activity in the ascitic fluid. It is a potentially dangerous complication because s associated with elevated mortality unless recognized and treated promptly.
Clinical symptoms are extremely variable: some patients show fever and abdominal pain, others are asymptomatic, and still others report aspecific symptoms. SBP should always be suspected in worsening of general conditions, onset of hepatic encephalopathy, renal failure, hyponatremia or hypotension without apparent cause.
Diagnosis of SBP is based upon polymorphonuclear (PMN) cell count in the ascitic fluid and its culture; patients with an ascitic fluid PMN count of ≥250 cells/mm^3 can be considered carriers of SBP and should immediately receive antibiotic treatment. Ascitic fluid culture is not essential for diagnosis, however, if positive, it is useful for a targeted medical approach.

Hepatorenal Syndrome and Dilutional Hyponatremia

Another complication of portal hypertension is dilutional hyponatremia, defined as serum sodium level <130 mEq/L occurring in cirrhotic patients in the presence of marked sodium retention.

In fact, retention of solute-free water leads to the dilution of body fluids and a fall in serum sodium concentration, even in the presence of marked sodium retention.

The pathogenesis of solute-free water retention in cirrhosis seems to be related mainly to the increased secretion of arginine vasopressin (AVP), the antidiuretic hormone. In fact, the aforementioned reduced effective intravascular volume secondary to splanchnic vasodilation elicits the baroceptors of the neurohypophysis with consequent release of AVP in response to the perceived hypovolemia. Final result of AVP secretion is the reabsorption of solute-free water in the distal collecting duct of the kidney.

Spontaneous dilutional hyponatremia is associated to poor survival among cirrhotic patients with ascites and this represents a strong negative prognostic factor, hence the need to combine serum sodium concentration levels with the Model for End-Stage Liver Disease (MELD) score to increase the prognostic accuracy of MELD (Na-MELD) in patients listed for orthotopic liver transplantation.

Clinical manifestations of dilutional hyponatremia range from absence of symptoms to neurological disease, that often cannot be distinguished by hepatic encephalopathy.

The hepatorenal syndrome (HRS) is characterized by severe renal insufficiency that usually arises in the cirrhotic patient with ascites in the absence of other identifiable causes of renal injury (in the absence of shock, infection, nephrotoxic drugs, etc.).

In fact, in the cirrhotic patient usually with ascites, an acute renal impairment may occur due to pre-renal causes (infections, dehydration, diuretic abuse) in 27-50% of cases, to intra-renal causes (Acute Kidney Disease, AKD) in 14-35%, and to Hepato Renal Syndrome (HRS) associated with functional Acute Kidney Injury (AKI) in 15-43%. Therefore, the first diagnostic issue is to assess whether the patients has a Chronic Kidney Disease (CKD), a AKD or HRS-AKI. The diagnosis of HRS-AKI is based on an increase in serum creatinine of >0.3 mg/dL from baseline within 48 hours or a percent increase ≥50% from baseline within 7 days or an urinary output <0.5 mL/kg after 6 hours. Moreover, no improvement in serum creatinine after at least 48 hours from suspension of the diuretic and volume expansion with albumin should be observed and other confounding causes of kidney impairment (shock, current or recent treatment with nephrotoxic drugs, parenchymal kidney disease) should be excluded. Recently, the definition of HRS has been updated; specifically, the old definition of HRS type 1 has been reclassified as HRS-AKI while HRS type 2 is now referred to as HRS-NAKI (non-AKI) and includes those types of functional renal impairment that do not fulfill the criteria for HRS-AKI.

HRS-AKI is frequently associated to rapid worsening of liver function and encephalopathy and the prognosis is poor. Therapy is based on albumin infusion and terlipressin administration.

Hepatic Encephalopathy

Hepatic encephalopathy (HE) is a neurological syndrome characterized by alterations in consciousness, personality, and neuromuscular function. It occurs in about 20% of patients during the natural history of cirrhosis and it is particularly frequent (over 50%) in patients who, due to complications of portal hypertension, have undergone surgical or angiographic systemic shunt.

The typical symptoms of HE are listed in **Table 36.6**. Based on severity of symptoms, HE is defined as grade I, II, III or IV. A milder form, referred to as subclinical HE, is defined as a condition with quantifiable neuropsychological defects, even if patients appear to have a normal mental and neurological status on clinical examination. Based on presentation and clinical course, HE is classified as episodic, recurrent or chronic (**Table 36.7**).

Because HE often arises as a result of "precipitating factors", it is important to recognize these signs for treatment and to prevent any episodes. The most common causes of HE are constipation, digestive bleeding, infections, electrolyte imbalances, high protein diet, use of benzodiazepines or excess diuretics.

HE is a reversible neurological disorder and is therefore classified as a metabolic cause for coma. The exact pathophysiological mechanism underlying the syndrome has not yet been clarified and it is possible that its genesis is multifactorial.

However, there some concepts are shared by the various pathogenic theories. A try to explain the following observations:

- in HE, brain function is compromised by the accumulation of one or more toxic substances normally eliminated by the liver;
- these substances are of a nitrogenous nature and come from the intestine;

Table 36.6 Criteria for clinical evaluation of hepatic encephalopathy.

Grade I	Changes in behavior with minimal change in level of consciousness. Alterations in sleep-wake rhythm, difficulty in writing, slow and clumsy word formation. Sporadic hand flapping tremor.
Grade II	Gross disorientation, drowsiness, possibly asterixis, inappropriate behavior
Grade III	Marked confusion, incoherent speech, sleeping most of the time but arousable to vocal stimuli
Grade IV	Comatose, unresponsive to pain

Table 36.7 Classification of hepatic encephalopathy based on presentation and clinical course.

Sporadic	One or more sporadic episodes that generally recognize a clear precipitating cause and are interspersed with periods of complete well-being.
Recurrent	Recurring episodes, often without a triggering cause.
Chronic or permanent	Stable alterations of consciousness, which do not regress with therapy, sometimes associated with neurological symptoms of the extrapyramidal system. It concerns a minority of patients but seriously interferes with quality of life.

- the accumulation of these substances is determined by reduced functioning of the liver mass and by the opening of the porto-systemic shunts (PSS) that divert the blood outside the hepatic filter.

Ammonia was the first substance identified as responsible for HE. It is produced mainly in the intestine by deaminases in the intestinal wall or the bacterial flora. The liver eliminates ammonia through the synthesis of urea. Blood levels of ammonia are frequently elevated in HE. Moreover, alkalosis increases the amount of gaseous ammonia (NH_3), diffusible across the blood-brain barrier, and decreases the ionized quota (NH_4^+), non-diffusible. In the brain, ammonia reduces the ATP available for the Krebs cycle and prevents Cl-leakage, thus maintaining the hyperpolarized neuronal fibre. Patients with liver failure show an increase in aromatic amino acid levels (e.g. tyrosine, phenylalanine, or tryptophan) and a decrease in branched-chain amino acid levels (e.g. valine, leucine, or isoleucine). This imbalance with consequent passage of aromatic amino acids into the brain seems to induce the synthesis of false neurotransmitters (e.g. octopamine, phenylethanolamine) and serotonin thus with a prevalent inhibitory function.

Recently, it has been proposed that the main mechanism by which ammonia exerts its cerebral toxicity is astrocytic damage. Astrocytes are cells of the central nervous system that occupy about a third of the cortical volume and play a role in supporting the action of neurons. Since these cells are the main site of cerebral metabolism of ammonia, excess ammonia seriously alters their function and neuronal function. Swelling of astrocytes occurs in hepatic encephalopathy. Therapies considered effective for encephalopathy decrease ammonia.

The diagnosis of hepatic encephalopathy is mainly clinical. While in grades III-IV the problem may be differential diagnosis with other types of coma, in the initial stages, before diagnosis of underlying liver disease, these patients may be categorized as having a psychiatric or neurological disorder. Early diagnosis of encephalopathy is very important to initiate appropriate treatment and avoid unnecessary administration of drugs. The search for signs of motor incoordination (through the signature test or asterisk) and the determination of ammoniemia can be useful to confirm the diagnosis. A typical symptom is flapping tremor or "wing beat tremor" in the hands.

Coagulopathy

The term haemostasis comprises the physiological mechanisms that intervene to prevent blood loss. It takes place through the synchronized interaction of numerous physiological systems. Haemostatic mechanisms include four main systems: the vascular system, platelets, the coagulation system, and the fibrinolytic system.

Coagulopathies are congenital or acquired plasma coagulation disorders. Acquired disorders are more frequent and more complex because they derive from the lack of several factors and simultaneously affect primary and secondary haemostasis (Table 36.8).

Coagulation factors are proteins that circulate in the blood. Many are produced by the liver and are denoted in various ways, very often with Roman numeral that indicate the order in which they were discovered. They work to keep the blood in conditions of normal "fluidity", together with other circulating molecules: their increase can cause excessive coagulation (with risk of thrombosis), while their decrease can predispose to bleeding.

An example of acquired clotting disorder is advanced liver disease, characterized by haemostasis abnormalities due to hepatic synthesis dysfunction. In fact, cirrhosis of the liver is characterized by a reduced synthesis of procoagulant proteins II, VII, IX, X, as well as of factor V and factor XI. These deficiencies of coagulation factors directly affect the standard laboratory evaluation in clinical practice, in particular for the evaluation of prothrombin time (PT) and its standardization, the INR, and to a lesser extent for activated partial thromboplastin time (aPTT).

Despite decreased levels of procoagulant factors and altered INR values, patients with liver cirrhosis generally do not have spontaneous bleeding, unlike patients with congenital deficiencies of coagulation factors. In fact, there is strong scientific evidence showing that in the presence of an adequate platelet count and thrombomodulin, a cofactor derived from the endothelium and belonging to the anticoagulant system, cirrhotic patients have a normal ability to generate thrombin and the fundamental components of fibrin formation. The reason for this normal pro-coagulant potential is the diminished synthesis of protein C, a potent anticoagulant, along with an increased production of factor VIII derived from the endothelium. Therefore, compensatory mechanisms in the patient with advanced liver disease effectively rebalance the haemostatic system. Despite this compensatory mechanism, there are a variety of events that can induce a patient with advanced liver disease to bleeding or thrombotic episodes. As the disease progresses, the activity of procoagulant proteins decreases by up to 20-46%.

Although compensation mechanisms are active, the ability to adapt to pathological insults is diminished, and in some cases minimal events are able to overcome these compensatory mechanisms. Some patients with advanced liver disease have a pro-coagulant tendency, resembling clinically patients with congenital C-protein deficiency and, conversely, other patients are clearly more prone to bleeding. These trends are not static and may change with the patient's clinical status, even within hours of hospitalization due to decompensation. Acute events such as infection and bleeding from oesophageal varices can lead to changes in coagulative tendency, partially reversible with adequate treatment, and not well described by conventional laboratory examinations, such as INR.

Portal Vein Thrombosis

The portal vein thrombosis (PVT) is undoubtedly the most common thrombotic event in patients with liver cirrhosis, with an incidence of 7-12%. The prevalence of PVT is influenced by the diagnostic approach and by inclusion in the case histories patients with hepatocellular carcinoma. In fact,

Table 36.8 Acquired coagulation disorders.

Homeostasis	Pro-Haemostatic Factors	Anti-Haemostatic Factors
Primary homeostasis (platelet-vessal wall interactions)	• Von Willebrand Factor • ADAMTS 13	• Platelets
Blood coagulation (thrombin generation and inhibition) • Pro-coagulant factor:	• Anticoagulant factors: antithrombin, protein C Factor VIII	• Pro-coagulant factors: fibrinogen, Factors II, V, VII, IX, X, XI
Fibrinolysis (dissolution of the clot)	• Plasminogen • PAI	• t-PA, • TAFI • Plasmin inhibitor

ADAMTS 13 denotes disintegrin and metalloprotease with thrombospondin type 1 motif 13, PAI plasminogen activator inhibitor, TAFI thrombin-activatable fibrinolysis inhibitor, and t-PA tissue plasminogen activator.

in patients awaiting liver transplantation, the presence of hepatic neoplasia constitutes a statistically significant risk factor for the onset of PVT, which is why the prevalence is around 4-16%.
The onset of PVT is determined by altered regulation of pro- and anti-coagulant, and pathological changes in one of the components of Virchow's triad (venous stasis, endothelial injury, and hypercoagulability). In patients with advanced liver disease, venous stasis is the result of vasodilation of the splanchnic and hepatic architecture rearrangement, characteristic of the cirrhotic liver.
Neoplastic PVT is frequently observed in HCC patients and due to tumour macrovascular invasion that represents a major prognostic factor.
In the clinical practice it is important to distinguish between non-neoplastic PVT, which may also occur in cirrhotic patients with HCC, and neoplastic HCC due to direct macrovascular invasion of the tumour, which has different prognostic and therapeutic implications. Contrast-enhanced imaging techniques can distinguish portal vein thrombosis from tumoural portal vein invasion with high accuracy.

EVALUATION OF THE CIRRHOTIC PATIENT

The specialist who diagnoses liver cirrhosis must set the following end points:

- define the cause of disease;
- stage its severity;
- study the main complications.

Regarding aetiology it is important to investigate for possible alcohol abuse and to know the patient's serological pattern with regard to hepatitis viruses, as these elements are the most frequent causes of liver cirrhosis in Italy. Further investigations will be reserved for patients in whom alcohol-related and viral aetiology have been excluded.
For staging disease severity, the Child-Pugh classification is commonly used based on the values of liver function tests and on the presence of ascites and/or encephalopathy (**Table 36.9**).
More recently, a new score (model of end-stage liver disease - MELD) has been proposed based on calculation of the values of bilirubinemia, creatinine and INR (Table 36.9). Both indices were developed to predict survival expectancy of the cirrhotic patient; the second was initially developed for evaluating survival at three months after placement of a transjugular intrahepatic portosystemic shunt (TIPS) and, subsequently, to evaluate the prognosis and priority in candidates for liver transplantation.
In a newly diagnosed cirrhotic patient, it is always important to include oesophagogastroduodenoscopy for the investigation of oesophageal varices and assessment of their degree of haemorrhagic risk, with a follow-up at 1 or 3 years depending on the size of the varices.
Among the diagnostic investigations it is also important to include a liver ultrasound to rule out focal lesions almost always indicative of hepatocellular carcinoma, with subsequent semi-annual follow-up (see Chapter 37).
Since cirrhosis can evolve over time, some investigations must be repeated periodically to detect the onset of complications in the initial stages. Patient follow-up should be adjusted based on the degree of compensation or decompensation of disease and the need to change therapeutic prescriptions. To achieve optimal surveillance of the possible

Table 36.9 Child-Pugh score for staging severity of cirrhosis of the liver.

Score Assigned in Proportion to Increasing Degree of Abnormality

	1	2	3
Encephalopathy	Absent	Grade I-II	Grade III-IV
Ascites	Absent	Responsive to therapy	Refractory
Bilirubin (mg/dl)	<2	>2<3	>3
Albumin (gr/dl)	>3.5	>28<35	<28
Prothrombin activity (%)	>70	<70>40	<40

Score between 5 and 6: grade A; score between 7 and 9: grade B; score between 10 and 15: grade C

Formula for MELD calculation (evaluation of the probability of short-term survival in cirrhosis of the liver).
MELD = 0.957 x Ln (creatinine mg/dL) + 0.378 x Ln (bilirubin mg/dL) + 1.120 x Ln (%INR) + 0.643

Ln= Natural logarithm

development of hepatocellular carcinoma, ultrasound and alfa-fetoprotein dose should be repeated every six months.

THE NATURAL HISTORY

The average life of a cirrhotic patient naturally depends on the time of diagnosis. When the disease is diagnosed at a preclinical stage, survival can also be much longer than 10 years. A factor influencing the rate of disease progression is the persistence or not of hepatitis (for example, the persistence of viral replication or continuing alcohol abuse can accelerate the course of cirrhosis). The Child-Pugh classification is still used today to predict the average survival of a cirrhotic patient (see Table 36.9). Based on the score, patients are divided into three classes: the 5-year survival of patients in class A is around 75%, that of patients in class B is 40%, and that of patients in class C around 20%.
Cirrhosis increases the risk for the development of hepatocellular carcinoma (an estimated incidence of 2-3 new cases/year per 100 cirrhotic patients) and the onset of liver cancer can obviously accelerate the course of disease. The most frequent causes of death in patients with cirrhosis of the liver are terminal hepatic insufficiency (often associated with hepatic encephalopathy), gastrointestinal haemorrhage, hepatorenal syndrome, and spontaneous bacterial peritonitis.

THERAPY

There is no treatment of cirrhosis that resolves liver fibrosis and structural alterations. When possible, it is important to intervene early, removing the cause of liver necrosis. In this regard, the cessation of intake of alcoholic beverages in alcohol-related cirrhosis is of fundamental importance, as this can prevent further progression of disease with considerable improvement in the patient's prognosis. The possibilities of intervening on viral replication have been discussed in Chapter 30. Hepatitis B- and C-related liver cirrhosis represents an indication to the antiviral therapy as this treatment decreases the decompensation rate and delays the progression of the liver disease although it does not determine the regression of cirrhosis. Copper chelating therapy in Wilson's disease and phlebotomy in haemochromatosis (see Chapter 34) are further examples of aetiological therapy that can lead to satisfactory therapeutic results. When aetiological therapy is not feasible, prevention of episodes of decompensation or complications will be the end point. Among general recommendations, the patient will have to lead a healthy and balanced life, follow a varied diet, eating everything in moderation while avoiding hyponutrition. Intake of alcoholic beverages should also be strongly discouraged in cirrhotic disease with viral aetiology. Constipation will be corrected. Any infections or febrile episodes will be treated early. Drugs should be carefully evaluated and those with hepatic metabolism or hepatotoxic action avoided to prevent accumulation or hepatocyte damage.
For ascites therapy, in about 10-20% of cirrhotic patients with uncomplicated ascites, mobilization of the ascitic effusion can be obtained simply by observing a hyposodic diet and bed rest (spontaneous diuresis). Spontaneous diuresis occurs more frequently in cirrhotic patients with early-onset ascites. Patients presenting the first episode of grade 2 (moderate) ascites must receive an aldosterone antagonist such as spironolactone, at a dose of 100 mg/day, gradually increased every 7 days (100 mg) up to a maximum of 400 mg/day. In patients who do not respond to aldosterone antagonists, as defined by a body weight reduction of less than 2 kg/week, or in patients who develop hyperkaliemia, a loop diuretic (furosemide) should be added gradually, starting with a dose of 40-50 mg/day for up to 150-160 mg/day (depending on whether administered intravenously with 20 mg vials or orally with 25 mg tablets). All patients on diuretic therapy should undergo frequent clinical and biochemical monitoring particularly during the first month of treatment. Patients with recurrent ascites should be treated with a combination of an aldosterone antagonist plus furosemide, with a sequential increase in doses as previously described. During diuretic therapy the maximum weight a patient should lose is 0.5 kg/day in patients without edema and 1 kg/day in patients with edema. The goal of long-term treatment is to keep patients without ascites on the minimum dose of diuretics. Once the ascites has resolved, the dose of diuretics should be reduced and stopped whenever possible.
All diuretics should be discontinued in severe hyponatremia (sodium plasma concentration <120 mmol/L), progressive renal failure, worsening of hepatic encephalopathy, or disabling muscle cramps. Furosemide should be discontinued in severe hypokalemia (<3 mmol/L), whereas aldosterone antagonists should be discontinued if severe hyperkalemia (serum potassium >6 mmol/L) develops.
Given the high mortality rate and the risk of developing hepatorenal syndrome, prophylaxis of spon-

taneous bacterial peritonitis is indicated in three high-risk populations: patients with acute gastrointestinal haemorrhage, patients with low total protein content in ascitic fluid and advanced cirrhosis, and patients with a previous history of spontaneous bacterial peritonitis (secondary prophylaxis). In patients with gastrointestinal bleeding, prophylaxis should be started at the occurrence of the bleeding episode and continued for up to 7 days with intravenous ceftriaxone (1 g/day) or oral quinolones such as norfloxacin (400 mg twice a day for 7 days). In patients with low total protein content in the ascitic fluid (<1.5 g/dL) and deteriorated liver function (Child-Pugh score ≥B9, serum bilirubin level ≥3 mg/dL) or impaired renal function (creatinine ≥1.2 mg/dL blood urea nitrogen level ≥25 mg/dL or hyponatremia ≤130 mEq/L), norfloxacin 400 mg per day is recommended although ciprofloxacin might represent a valuable option. Lifelong administration of norfloxacin is recommended also in the setting of secondary prophylaxis.

Patients who develop SBP should be treated promptly. In fact, early therapy reduces the risk of hospital mortality by over 50%. In practice, a neutrophil leukocyte count in ascitic fluid >250/mmc, even in the absence of symptoms, is an absolute indication to initiate antibiotic treatment, without waiting for culture results. The latter will be useful only to modify the therapeutic regimen in the event of non-response. Treatment failure is the deterioration of the patient's clinical condition after initiation of antibiotic therapy or the non-reduction in the number of polymorphonuclear cells in ascites 48 hours after the start of treatment. As in about 70% of cases the responsible bacteria are *Escherichia coli* and *Klebsiella pneumoniae*, the antibiotics of choice are active against gram-bacteria:

- The first choice antibiotic is cefotaxime. The recommended dose, with normal renal function, is 2 g every 8-12 hours. Five days of therapy ensure results similar to a 10-day treatment.
- Other second or third generation cephalosporins (ceftriaxone, cefocid, etc.) or amoxicillin/clavulanic acid are possible alternatives.
- In patients with good general conditions, oral quinolone (ofloxacin, 400 mg every 12 hours) was as effective as cefotaxime.
- Aminoglycosides are contraindicated because they cause nephrotoxicity in a large number of cases.

In HE, the first-line therapy is to treat the triggering cause (constipation, infections potentially harmful drugs, hydroelectrolytic imbalance and anemia).

HRS, by definition, is not corrected by plasma expansion alone (for example, 1.5 l infusion of physiological solution). The therapeutic approach to this morbid condition can be summarized as follows:

- Ascites volume control: the use of diuretics is unable to induce a negative sodium balance. Evacuative paracentesis associated with adequate plasma expansion is the first choice approach.
- Modification of renal function: the haemodynamic context of HRS is the rational substrate for use of vasoconstrictors that, by acting on peripheral vascular resistance, can improve effective volemia and, therefore, renal perfusion. Studies evaluating the effectiveness of treatments based on vasoconstrictive drugs and human albumin, have reported very encouraging results. Among the different protocols, combined norepinephrine and albumin deserves particular attention, which induced the resolution of the syndrome in 86% of treated patients, the combination of midodrine, octreotide, and albumin, and terlipressin and albumin.

Liver transplantation is a highly effective therapeutic option in terminal hepatic failure. In view of the limited availability of organs for transplantion, it is reserved for precise indications (for indications for liver transplantation in cirrhosis of the liver see Chapter 38).

KEY CONCEPTS

- Liver cirrhosis is the common result of chronic injury factors (the most frequent are viral hepatitis and alcohol) that cause necrosis of hepatocytes and inflammation and subsequently activate mechanisms of liver repair/fibrosis and regeneration.
- Liver cirrhosis causes changes in the hepatic microcirculation responsible for portal hypertension. Portal hypertension is involved in the pathogenesis of the major complications of cirrhosis.
- Liver cirrhosis is the end stage of chronic liver disease; with a high impact as a cause of death and the frequent need for hospitalization.
- In liver cirrhosis it is appropriate to define the cause of disease, the severity stage, the presence and risk of bleeding oesophageal varices, and the presence of possible nodules of hepatocellular carcinoma.
- The major complications of cirrhosis are gastrointestinal haemorrhage, ascites, spontaneous bacterial peritonitis, hepatorenal syndrome, coagulopathy, hepatic encephalopathy, and hepatocarcinoma.

REFERENCES

- Bosch J, Groszmann RJ, Shah VH. Evolution in the understanding of the pathophysiological basis of portal hypertension: how changes in paradigm are leading to successful new treatm ents. J Hepatol. 2015 Apr; 62(1S):S121-S130.
- Italian Association for the Study of the Liver (AISF). Portal Hypertension and Ascites: Patient-and Population-centered Clinical Practice Guidelines by the Italian Association for the Study of the Liver (AISF). Dig Liver Dis. 2021;53(9):1089-104.
- de Franchis R; Baveno VI Faculty. Expanding consensus in portal hypertension: Report of the Baveno VI Consensus Workshop: Stratifying risk and individualizing care for portal hypertension. J Hepatol. 2015;63(3):743-52.
- Senzolo M, Garcia-Tsao G, García-Pagán JC. Current knowledge and management of portal vein thrombosis in cirrhosis. J Hepatol. 2021;75(2):442-53.

CHAPTER 37

HEPATOCELLULAR AND VASCULAR TUMOURS

Edoardo Giovanni Giannini, Andrea Galli

LEARNING OBJECTIVES
- To understand the role and modalities of hepatocellular carcinoma surveillance.
- To know the diagnosis and the stage of hepatocellular carcinoma.
- To discriminate and to select the best therapeutic option for various stages of hepatocellular carcinoma.
- To know the diagnosis and management of hepatic benign tumours.

HEPATOCELLULAR CARCINOMA

Epidemiology

Hepatocellular carcinoma (HCC) is the fifth most common cancer worldwide and the second most common cause of cancer related mortality, the leading cause of death in patients with compensated cirrhosis. The age-standardised incidence rate of HCC is high in geographic areas such as the Far East, South-east Asia, and Sub-Saharian Africa (9.4 cases/100,000 inhabitants/year), low in Northern Europe, the Unites States, and South America (4 cases/100,000 inhabitants/year), and intermediate in North America and Southern Europe. Italy ranks at intermediate HCC incidence, with a reported incidence of approximately 12,000 cases/year. The geographic distribution of the incidence of HCC is closely related to the distribution of the main risk factors for chronic liver disease, such as infection with hepatitis B and C viruses. HCC has a higher incidence in males (male-to-female ratio 2-3:1) due to a greater prevalence of risk factors in males, as well as a putative role played by oestrogens in cell damage and prolife- ration. In Western countries, the median age of HCC incidence is approximately 65 years, and in Italy the incidence of HCC peaks at 70-74 years of age.

Risk Factors

The presence of liver cirrhosis, of any aetiology, is the main risk factor associated with the development of HCC, being present in more than 90% of patients with this condition, although in patients with non viral chronic liver diseases this association is less frequent. The most common causes of chronic liver disease in patients with HCC are infection with hepatitis B or C virus, alcohol abuse, and non-alcoholic steatohepatitis, while less common causes are autoimmune liver diseases, hereditary haemochromatosis, α1-antitripsin deficiency, and Wilson's Disease.

In Italy, between 2014 and 2018, hepatitis C virus-related cirrhosis was responsible for approximately 40% of HCC cases, with a progressive increase – up to one-third of cases – attributed to nonviral causes, in particular to non-alcoholic steatohepatitis. This temporal trend is secondary to active implementation of measures of primary prophylaxis for the most common causes of liver disease (e.g., blood donor screening, hepatitis B virus (HBV) vaccination, use of disposable sanitary devices) and to the improvement in treatment of chronic viral hepatitis. Hepatitis B virus may be responsible for the development of HCC even in non-cirrhotic patients due to direct carcinogenic properties secondary to its capacity to integrate viral DNA into the host genome, thus determining a direct modulation of gene expression. Likewise, also hepatitis C virus (HCV) and non-alcoholic steatohepatitis (NASH) can, although less frequently, induce HCC in patients without cirrhosis through mechanisms related to oxidative stress, altered lipid homeostasis, and insulin-resistance. Lastly, exposure to aflatoxin, a mycotoxin causing a mutation in the p53 oncosuppressor gene, is responsible for HCC in South-east Asia, and Sub-Saharian Africa where chronic HBV infection is also endemic.

Genetic Alterations and Hepatocarcinogenesis

The new methods of genetic sequencing have identified new important molecular pathways involved in hepatic carcinogenesis and their correlation with specific risk factors. More than 50 different somatic mutations are shown in HCC and are correlated with different steps of tumour transformation. Based upon mutation analysis of β-catenin and p53, studies have subclassified hepatic tumours. β-catenin (CTNNB1) mutation is present in 30-40% of HCC and less associated to

HBV infection. On the contrary, TP53 mutations are present in 50% of HCC and correlated with HBV-induced carcinogenesis. A specific mutation at 249 codon (R249S) of TP53 is linked to aflatoxin B1 intoxication. Mutations of TERT promoters are frequent and correlated with telomerase reactivation that is essential for cell proliferation. Genetic alteration of ARID1A and ARID2 genes involved in chromatin remodelling have been recently identified and correlated with chronic alcohol consumption, while amplification of the chromosomal region 6p21.1 where CULLIN7 gene is located, is common in NASH carcinogenesis. Expression signatures found via global gene expression profiling can stratify HCCs into several clinically relevant groups that have a different progression and a specific prognostic evolution.

Surveillance

HCC surveillance relies on the availability of methods that can identify early tumoural lesions potentially amenable to curative intention, and where treatment is associated with a decrease in liver-related mortality, in patients at increased risk for primary liver cancer. As far as this last issue is concerned, chronic HBV carriers and patients with compensated cirrhosis, independently of aetiology of liver disease and in the absence of comorbidities dictating patient prognosis, are the ideal candidates for HCC surveillance. Surveillance for HCC can also be considered in patients with advanced fibrosis (F3), in particular those with chronic viral hepatitis or NASH, especially in patients with cofactors such as diabetes, advanced age, and use of alcohol. The yearly incidence of HCC in these patients (0.2% in chronic HBV infection, 1.5% in cirrhotic patients) justifies the cost/ benefit ratio of surveillance. From practical point of view, surveillance in these at-risk categories is by means of liver ultrasonography every 6 months to detect liver nodules <2 cm in diameter – as the probability of micro vascular invasion and satellite lesions significantly increases in larger lesions – in patients with compensated liver disease and therefore amenable to curative treatment. Assessment of serum alphafetoprotein alone is not recommended as a surveillance tool since, in this setting, this onco-marker is burdened by low sensitivity and inadequate specificity for the detection of early HCCs, while it still has a role – together with liver ultrasound surveillance – in patients with virusrelated chronic liver disease after cure of HCV infection and in patients with chronic HBV who are virus-suppressed on nucleos(t)ide analogues treatment. Lastly, determination of serum alphafetoprotein can be useful in patients with HCC when elevated levels of this oncomarker are used to monitor treatment efficacy or tumour recurrence.

Natural History

The size of HCC at diagnosis does not accurately predict prognosis since, despite median tumour doubling time is approximately 180 days, tumoural growth cannot be predicted in the single individual. Elevated serum alpha-fetoprotein levels at diagnosis are associated with negative tumoural characteristics such as biological aggressiveness and worse prognosis. Microvascular invasion and satellite lesions, whose prevalence increases in lesions >2 cm in diameter, are histological features associated with worse prognosis. HCC typically has a tendency to macro vascular invasion (portal vein, supra hepatic veins), whose presence is a negative prognostic factor as it adversely affects therapeutic management. The presence of extrahepatic spread is not frequent in patients with HCC as compared to patients affected by other solid tumours even in patients with advanced cancer.

Diagnosis

The identification of a hepatic nodular lesion, either during surveillance or incidentally, not previously been identified and characterised, should lead to further instrumental evaluation to identify the nature of the lesion (recall policy). The final diagnosis of HCC is based on contrast-enhanced imaging techniques (spiral CT or MRI) or histology and is mainly a function of lesion size. Contrast-enhanced ultrasonography can be part of the diagnostic work-up of patients with suspected HCC although its sensitivity, as compared with contrast-enhanced CT and MRI, is lower since it cannot provide panoramic images of the whole liver and is associated with a higher risk of false positive results in patients with a final diagnosis of intrahepatic cholangiocarcinoma. The rationale behind the use of contrast-enhanced imaging, with the use of intravascular contrast medium, resides in the anatomical characteristics of HCC whose blood supply is mainly provided by arterial vasculature, typical behaviour, as compared with non-tumoural hepatic parenchyma during the dynamic phases (arterial, venous, late phase) of contrast-enhanced imaging techniques. In cirrhotic patients, HCC can be diagnosed in no- dules ≥1cm showing arterial hypervascularity (wash-in), followed by rapid elimination of the contrast medium in the equilibrium and portal phases (wash-out) during a contrast enhanced imaging (spiral CT or MRI) evaluation. In nontypical findings at the first imaging exam, another alternative imaging technique can be applied so as to verify the presence of typical vascular findings. Should even this latter technique not allow a definite diagnosis of HCC, the diagnosis can be made by means of ultrasound-guided biopsy of the lesion and histological examination. Lastly, in the case of inconclusive instrumental and histological results, it is suggested to perform a (3-montly interval) ultrasonographic follow-up with repetition of contrast enhanced imaging in the case of lesion growth. In the case of identification of nodular lesions < 1cm, it is advised to carry out a (3-monthly interval) follow-up until the lesion eventually grows to allow contrast-enhanced imaging with a higher likelihood of obtaining a final diagnosis (**Figure 37.1**). MRI techniques using contrast medium with hepato-biliary excretion may be of help in supporting the diagnosis of HCC in the absence of hypointensity in the hepato-biliary phase. Biopsy of the nodule and histological evaluation are indicated as the first diagnostic approach in patients without cirrhosis. At histological examination, stromal invasion of hepatocytes can differentiate very early HCCs from macro regenerative nodules with dysplasia. Supraexpression of immunohistochemical markers may help differentiate early HCCs from high-grade dysplastic nodules (glypican-3) and in the identification of mixed HCC-cholangiocarcinoma type tumours (cytokeratin 19). Histological

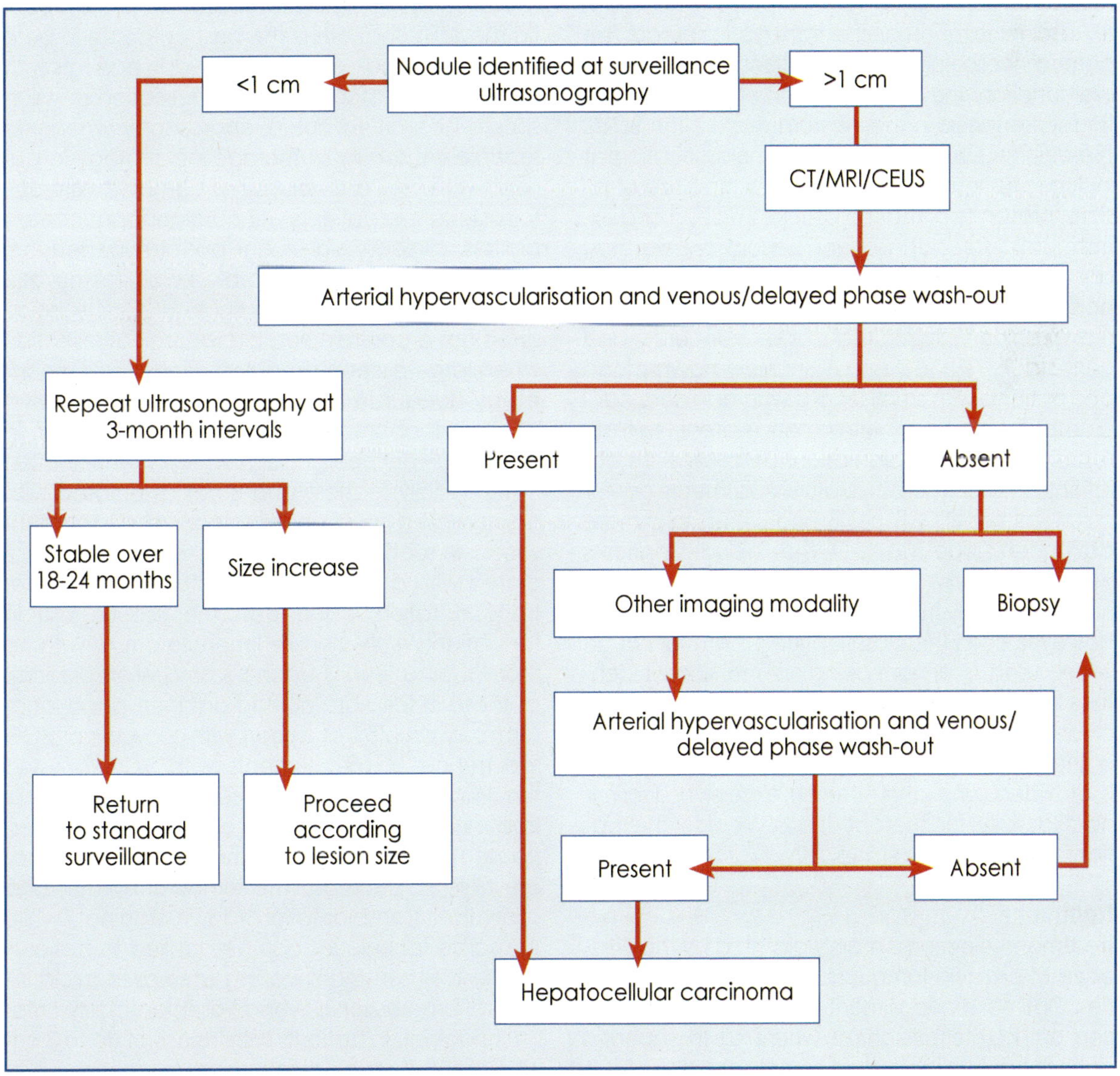

Figure 37.1 Diagnostic algorithm for hepatocellular carcinoma.

diagnosis becomes mandatory when it influences the choice of therapeutic option, particularly liver transplantation.

Staging

An adequate staging system for patients with HCC should define their prognosis and guide the most appropriate therapeutic option for each stage. The peculiarity of HCC, often arising in patients affected by chronic liver disease, makes the common staging criteria for patients with other solid cancers (TNM staging system: tumour, lymph nodes, metastasis) inadequate to predict survival and to guide treatment decisions, as the TNM staging system does not take into account the role played by residual liver function. The best staging systems for HCC combine assessment of number of lesions, their size, the presence of macro vascular invasion and extrahepatic spread, the general wellbeing of the patient, and residual liver function. The most commonly used classification system used in the Western world is the BCLC (Barcelona Clinic Liver Cancer) classification; it includes tumour variables (number and size of lesions, presence of macrovascular invasion and extrahepatic spread), patient performance status, and stage of liver disease (presence of significant portal hypertension, Child-Pugh class). The BCLC classification includes five stages: very early and early stages (stage 0 and A) including asymptomatic patients with small lesions who are ideal candidates for treatment with curative intent (surgical resection, liver transplantation, percutaneous ablation), stages where palliative treatments confer a survival benefit (stages B and C), up to a more advanced stage (stage D) that includes patients with terminal disease and where supportive care is often the only treatment available (**Figure 37.2**). However, even this classification system, although widely used, is far from being optimal since it identifies some stages (e.g., stage B and C) that include heterogeneous patients populations where a single treatment indication for each HCC stage is provided, and attributes an excessive discriminant activity for therapeutic choice to the patient's performance status.

Treatment

Treatment selection is mainly dictated by the presence of cirrhosis, tumour staging, and comorbidities. Optimal management of HCC should be carried out in referral centres where all therapeutic options are available, and where selection of the most appropriate treatment can be established with a multidisciplinary approach including specialists dealing with (gastroenterologist, surgeon, transplant surgeon, interventional radiologist, oncologist) so as to identify the best individualized therapeutic approach.

Hepatocellular Carcinoma in Patients without Liver Disease

Surgical liver resection is the main therapeutic option for HCCs arising in patients without liver disease, as they are able to tolerate large liver parenchymal resections with minimal risk of post-surgical liver decompensation and can obtain 5-year survival rates above 50%.

Very Early and Early Stages (BCLC 0 e A)

Surgical approach, either by means of surgical resection or liver transplantation, is the therapeutic modality that offers the best outcome in both oncological radicality and survival in patients with HCC at these stages. Surgical resection – which should be carried out in laparoscopy whenever feasible – is the main therapeutic strategy in patients with very early or early-stage HCC with unifocal lesion, in patients without significant comorbidities, clinically significant portal hypertension, and increased serum bilirubin levels (≥1mg/dL). Moreover, in patients with single HCC, the lesion size is not a contraindication to surgical resection when large parenchymal resections are supported by adequate residual liver function. Likewise, a surgical approach can be indicated even in multifocal, peripheral HCCs where liver resection is technically feasible and is not associated with an increased risk of post-surgical liver decompensation. In such patients, surgical resection is associated with a 5-year survival rate over 70%. Liver transplantation is the best therapeutic option for patients with a single lesion ≤5 cm or with no more than 3 lesions each ≤3 cm (Milan criteria), as these criteria are able to balance good long-term survival (75% at 5 year) with a low risk of HCC recurrence (<10%). Patients with HCC beyond the Milan criteria may benefit from locoregional treatments (percutaneous ablative techniques, transcatheter arterial chemoembolisation) that are able to decrease the tumoural burden and allow liver transplantation (down staging), while the same techniques can be applied to patients on the liver transplant waiting list so as to avoid tumoural progression beyond transplantability criteria (bridging). In patients with lesions of up to 3 cm who are not candidates surgical resection or liver transplantation, the use of percutaneous radiofre-

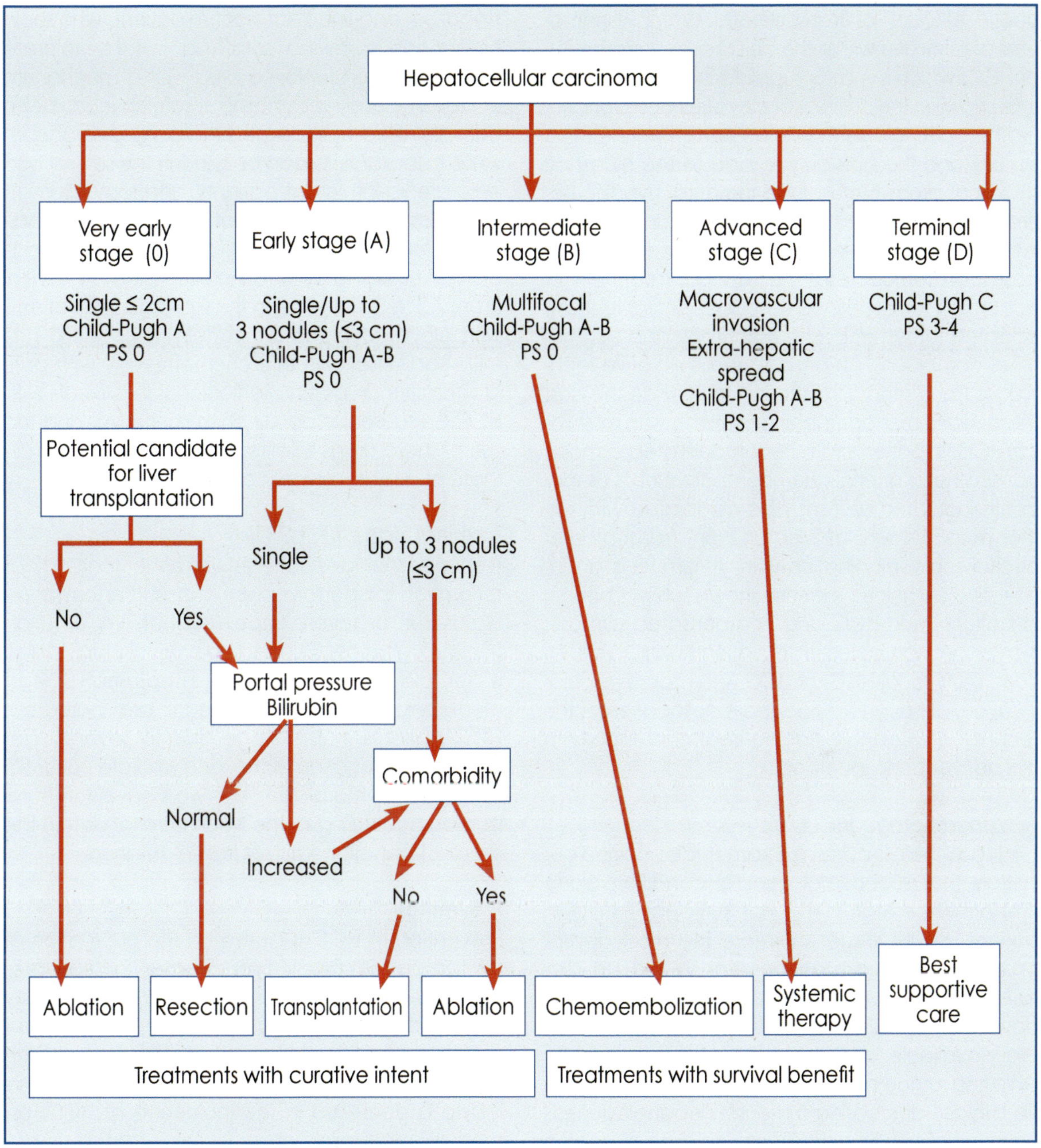

Figure 37.2 BCLC staging system and therapeutic indications.

quency ablation is associated with survival rates up to 50% at 5-year follow-up. In patients with small (i.e., <2 cm) lesions, the use of percutaneous radiofrequency ablation allows ablation of both the tumour and creation of a "safety margin" of non-tumoural liver parenchyma surrounding the lesion. The use of percutaneous radiofrequency ablation is not indicated for tumours close to large vessels, or to hollow organs and sub-capsular lesions, because of the risk of incomplete ablation due to the "heat sink" effect of blood flow and to the risk of local complications, respectively. The efficacy of percutaneous radiofrequency ablation is significantly reduced due to technical reasons (maximum ablation range) in lesions larger than 3-3.5 cm.

Intermediate Stage (BCLC B)

Transcatheter arterial chemoembolisation is a palliative treatment that increases survival in selected patients and is the treatment of choice for patients at this stage. The rationale underlying the therapeutic efficacy of transcatheter arterial chemoembolization lies within the peculiar vascularization of HCC, which is mainly supplied by arterial blood, thus allowing the delivery of elevated doses of chemotherapeutic agents with no or minimal systemic toxicity and the possibility to add to the cytotoxic action of drugs that induce tumoural hypoxic necrosis by transiently blocking blood supply to the lesion. This technique can be repeated over time based on tumour response to initial treatment or according to predefined schedules similar to those adopted for systemic chemotherapy and is sometimes combined with percutaneous ablative techniques (multi modal treatment) to provide the best therapeutic management for patients with multi focal HCC. In patients with decompensated cirrhosis, transcatheter arterial chemoembolization is usually contraindicated as it may be associated with further derangement of liver function. Transcatheter arterial radioembolisation with yttrium-90 is an innovative technique that has shown survival benefit in patients with HCC and compensated cirrhosis; it may be administered to patients with large lesions, multi focal HCC, or HCC with macrovascular invasion, although an adequate collocation of this technique within the staging-treatment algorithm has not yet been identified.

Advanced Stage (BCLC C)

Clinically, there is evidence from studies carried out in Italy that suboptimal general condition alone (Performance Status 1) is not sufficient to assign patients to this stage; therefore the most appropriate therapeutic management should be dictated by tumour and liver staging. In patients with advanced HCC, administration of sorafenib – an orally-available, multikinase inhibitor that acts by inhibiting tumoural growth and inducing its apoptosis, besides decreasing tumoural neoangiogenesis – is associated with a significant increase in median survival versus placebo (from 8 to 11 months in a Western study), while the administration of lenvatinib – another orally available multikinase inhibitor – has recently shown non inferiority versus sorafenib in previously untreated patients with compensated disease. More recently, the association of atezolizumab – an immunotherapic that acts on the receptors that inhibit lymphocyte T-mediated antitumour immune response – and bevacizumab, a monoclonal antibody that blocks the activity of vascular endothelial growth factor (VEGF), was able to determine an overall median survival of approximately 19 months to patients with this tumoural stage. Second-line treatment, in patients who show progression following sorafenib but ho tolerate the drug, regorafenib - a drug with a mechanism of action closely resembling sorafenib - has been demonstrated to increase survival versus placebo, while cabozantinib can be used in this setting also in sorafenib-intolerant patients, and ramucirumab represents the first drug that in this setting is indicated for a population enriched according to a biomarker, being able to increase median survival (from 7.3 to 8.5 months) in the sub-group of patients with elevated alpha-fetoprotein levels (≥400 ng/mL). Traditional systemic chemotherapy with antiproliferative drugs is not efficacious in patients with HCC because it is poorly chemosensitive, and the use of these drugs is limited by the presence of cirrhosis and by its clinical correlates.

Terminal Stage (BCLC D)

This stage includes patients with either marked deterioration of performance status (Performance Status 3-4) or severe impairment of liver function (Child-Pugh class C). Median survival in this stage is approximately 3-4 months, symptomatic treatment and best supportive care are indicated. HCC patients in this stage due to severely deranged liver function alone, and who are free from significant comorbidities but who have tumoural burden according to the Milan criteria, obtain the greatest benefit from liver transplantation.

Prevention

Prevention of HCC is based on the prevention of risk factors for chronic liver diseases (primary prevention) or on their early treatment (secondary prevention), with the aim to reduce the rate of tumour development. Compulsory HBV vaccination is the primary preventive measure that primarily led to a decrease in the incidence of HCC, especially in endemic areas for this infection. In patients with chronic HBV infection, treatment with nucloes(t)ide analogues is associated with a significant decrease, but not with elimination, of the risk of HCC development, and this finding is especially evident in patients with cirrhosis. Also in patients with chronic HCV infection, viral clearance is associated with a significant decrease in risk of HCC development, although risk is not completely abolished, thus mandating the need of continuous surveillance in both these categories of patients and in those who are virus suppressed or after viral clearance if in at-risk categories before cure or functional cure, of hepatitis virus infection.

BENIGN HEPATIC TUMOURS

Benign hepatic tumours are a heterogeneous group mostly asymptomatic, often incidentally discovered during ultrasound exams, posing a significant challenge in differential diagnosis. They usually develop in a normal liver and can originate from any hepatic cellular subtype, classified as epithelial and nonepithelial tumours (**Table 37.1**).

Hepatocellular Adenoma

Hepatocellular adenoma is a rare form of benign neoplasia, characterized by benign proliferation of hepatocytes.

Hepatocellular adenoma is more frequent among females, especially in reproductive age, and it is closely related to estroprogestinics use. Regarding males there is a frequent correlation with anabolic steroids use, in particular methyltestosterone and noretrandolone. Other associations are Kleinfelter Syndrome, type 1a glycogen storage disease, frequent therapy cycles with clomiphene and danazole. Hepatocellular adenoma often occurs as a solitary lesion, but in 30% of cases, it can be multifocal; hepatic adenomatosis is characterized by ≥10 adenomas a distinct nosological entity. These lesions are predominantly capsulated and vascularized; vascular proliferation and subsequent haemorrhage risk are closely related to pregnancy and estroprogestinic use. Reduction or interruption of estroprogestinic treatment often leads to regression of the lesion. It was recently established that hepatocellular adenomas are monoclonal neoplasms characterized by specific molecular aspects related to clinical and anatomopathological characteristics of 5 subtypes of adenoma.

HA-H subtype (40% of adenomas) is characterized by inactivating mutations of the TCF1 gene, which encodes transcriptional factor HNF1A. HNF1A mutation leads to increased lipogenesis through synthesis of fatty acids, related to a characteristic steatosis that is not found in other subtypes of adenomas. Lipid accumulation is due to reduced expression of liver fatty acid binding protein (LFABP). This mutation is frequently observed also in familiar hepatic adenomatosis, which is frequently associated with a particular form of adultonset diabetes (MODY3) related to a deficit of insulin secretion.

HA-B subtype (15% of adenomas) is characterized by mutations of β-catenin (CTNB1) and associated with malignant transformation. This mutation frequently occurs in well differentiated hepatocarcinoma, leading to a more difficult differential diagnosis. There are various types of CTNB1 mutation; one is located on exon 3 and is considered a canonical mutation related to higher risk for malignant evolution; other non canonical mutations on exons 7 and 8 seem to be unrelated to malignant transformation.

HA-I subtype is characterized by abundant inflammatory infiltration and is frequently associated with mutations of the IL6ST gene, which encodes gp-130 protein, a subunit of the interleukin 6-receptor. This mutation modulates typical inflammatory response and C-reactive protein increase associated with this form of adenoma. A fourth subtype (HA-sh) was recently identified and is associated with a constitutive activation of the sonic hedgehog system; this subtype is strongly associated with high haemorrhagic risk due to widespread telan-

Table 37.1 Benign Tumour Classification.

Hepatocellular tumours	Regenerative lesions (nodular regenerative hyperplasia, focal nodular hyperplasia) Neoplastic lesions (hepatocellular adenoma, familiar hepatic adenomyosis)
Biliary tumours	Bile duct adenoma Bile duct microhamartomas Bile duct cystoadenoma Biliary papillomatosis
Vascolar tumours	Haemangioma Infantile haemangioendothelioma Hereditary haemorrhagic telangiectasia (HHT)
Mesenchymal tumours	Leiomyoma Lipomatous tumours Mesenchymal hamartoma

giectasia. Finally, a fifth subtype, HA-U, includes forms without definite morphological and genetic characterization, in contrast to the other subtypes.

Clinical Findings

Hepatic adenoma is frequently asymptomatic, it rarely presents with acute and sporadic abdominal pain, which is consequent to haemorrhagic events. Tumour size, shHCA and, b-catenin mutation on exon 7/8 subtype are identified risk factors of clinical bleeding. A rare complication is rupture of the adenoma, with consequent haemoperitoneum.

Diagnosis

Hepatic adenomas are usually identified during ultrasound examinations as hyperechoic masses presenting anechoic cyst like areas of variable dimension, caused by frequent haemorrhagic and necrotic phenomena. CT scan does not provide further information and hepatic biopsy is not useful because of lack of peculiar elements of the lesion compared to the surrounding parenchyma; biopsy has a high haemorrhagic risk due to the vascularization of the lesion. Magnetic resonance imaging with hepato-specific contrast medium is a useful diagnostic tool: adenomas present well defined margins and characteristic parallel vascular structures penetrating the lesion from the peripheral area, giving them the typical wagon wheel aspect.

Treatment

The best strategy for patients under estroprogestinic treatment in whom a small adenoma (<4 cm) is casually identified is to stop hormonal treatment and to frequently monitor the lesion by ultrasound. Regression of the adenoma allows surgical resection to be deferred. Surgical resection may be indicated in large adenomas (>10 cm), associated with symptoms or lack of response to estroprogestinic treatment suspension.

Surgical treatment should be considered also when estroprogestinic treatment cannot be suspended for medical reasons, in women wanting to become pregnant, and in genotypes of adenoma strongly associated with malignant transformation. Transarterial embolization is useful for treating bleeding large lesions; this treatment can reduce the volume of adenomas. Liver transplantation should be considered in adenomas associated with type-1a glycogen storage disease or familiar hepatic adenomatosis due to the high risk of malignant transformation.

Nodular Regenerative Hyperplasia

Nodular regenerative hyperplasia (NRH) is a benign condition characterized by nodules of proliferating hepatocytes within a liver with a structure free of fibrous septa. Since the lesion is frequently located near the hepatic hilum or around large portal areas, it can lead to portal hypertension or cholestasis (2.5% of cases). NRH was described in patients under antiretroviral treatment and those affected by portal hypertension or portal vein thrombosis. It is frequently associated with systemic diseases, such as rheumatoid arthritis, CREST syndrome, Felty syndrome, polyarteritis nodosa, myeloproliferative disorders, and chronic intake of anabolic steroids. NRH is considered an adaptive process to heterogeneous distribution of blood flow. Some experts consider NRH a proliferative disease with potential for transformation into hepatocarcinoma, given its frequent association with hepatocellular dysplasia.

Clinical Findings

NRH is characterized by a slow and asymptomatic course. Hepatomegaly and splenomegaly occur in at least half of patients. Hepatic function is usually preserved despite a slight increase in transaminases. In rare cases of hepatic dysfunction, hepatic failure slowly occurs. The most frequent clinical complication is haemorrhage due to rupture of oesophageal varices in a context of portal hypertension.

Diagnosis

Hepatic function tests are normal in most patients. One third of cases is characterized by a slight increase in alkaline phosphatases. Ultrasound examination shows isoor hyperchoic nodules that can become hypo- or anechoic intralesional haemorrhages. CT scan shows hypervascularised lesions and nodules with isodense appearance compared to parenchyma; MRI shows lesions with isointense appearance in comparison to parenchyma at T1- and T2-weighted scans. Hepatic biopsy is frequently definitive for diagnosis.

Treatment

In most cases, evolution of the lesion is particularly slow, and it does not require any specific treatment. In rare cases characterized by symptomatic portal hypertension, associated with haemorrhage due to rupture of oesophageal varices, endoscopic treatment, portacaval shunt, and liver transplantation have proved effective.

Haemangioma

Haemangiomas are the second most frequent focal hepatic lesion following metastases (1-2% in the general population); they can be found at any age with an incidence peak between the third and fifth decade. Pathogenesis is unknown, though a potential role for sexual hormones is suspected, given cases of enlargement of lesions during pregnancy. Haemangiomas are characterized by cavernous type vascular areas separated by fibrous branches.

Clinical Findings

Haemangiomas are frequently asymptomatic and often incidentally found. They are mostly clinical benign and rarely tend to enlarge (10%) and eventually become symptomatic. Rupture is rare and occurs only in trauma to large lesions. In newborns, they can cause thrombocytopenia due to platelet entrapment in a context of Kasabach-Merrit syndrome.

Diagnosis

Haemangioma is usually diagnosed by ultrasound examination in patients without neoplasms or chronic liver diseases. In 70% of cases, haemangiomas are homogenously hyperechoic lesions versus surrounding hepatic parenchyma (typical haemangioma). Atypical haemangiomas (30% of cases) are hypoechoic lesions with a hyperechoic border or inhomogeneous structure. Contrast enhanced ultrasound shows peripheral hypervascularization during the early enhancement phase with progressive centripetal filling. MRI is necessary in suspected atypical haemangioma or in lesions with suspected high risk for malignant transformation.

Treatment

Surgical resection is indicated only in hepatic lesions of uncertain diagnosis or with a suspected malignant component, in progressive or disabling symptoms, which are possible with large haemangiomas characterized by high risk of rupture or haemorrhagic complication.

Focal nodular hyperplasia

Focal nodular hyperplasia (FNH) is the second benign liver tumour by frequency (0.4-0.8%). FNH is more common in women (female to male ratio between 2:1 and 26:1) and the median age at diagnosis is 35-50 years Focal nodular hyperplasia has rarely presented in children. Most paediatric cases have been reported in patients with a history of chemotherapy, malignancy, or haematopoietic stem cell therapy. FNH is characterized by a hyperplastic lesion of the hepatic parenchyma concentric to a scar with a stellate appearance containing an anomalous artery. Aetiology is unknown and the role of estroprogestinic treatment is uncertain. Patients who present FNH can also be affected by vascular or neuroendocrine alterations, such as cavernous haemangiomas, multiple neuroendocrine neoplasms, glioblastomas, and astrocytomas. Within a central stellate scar is an anomalous artery, inside of which turbulent flow leads to the development of a dynamic platelet thrombus, releasing growing factors that cause hyperplasia of hepatocytes.

Clinical Findings

Most patients present a single lesion, some (20%) present 2-5 hepatic nodules of variable size (between 1 mm and 19 cm). FNH in usually accidentally discovered; rarely, patients complain of symptoms related to hepatomegaly or abdominal mass. Tumour markers alphafetoprotein, CEA, and Ca 19-9 usually have normal values. FNH has a benign course, no cases of malignant evolution have been described.

Diagnosis

FNH is usually accidentally found at ultrasound examination, which shows a nodular lesion with hyperechoic or isoechoic appearance in comparison to the hepatic parenchyma. In small lesions, CT scan accuracy is low; MRI provides more accuracy thanks to liver-specific contrast agent. Hepatic biopsy is indicated in enlarged nodules without central scar and vascular patterns typical of FNH.

Treatment

Surgical resection is suggested in haemorrhage, disabling symptoms, and uncertain diagnosis.

KEY CONCEPTS

- Infection with HBV is the main aetiological factor associated with the development of HCC in Asia and Africa, while HCV infection and alcohol abuse are the dominant aetiological factors in Western countries. In the last decades the proportion of non-viral causes of HCC has increased, especially due to non-alcoholic steatohepatitis (NASH) and alcohol abuse.
- In patients with cirrhosis, bi-annual liver ultrasonography allows identification of early HCC, thus favouring initiation of treatment with curative intent, and associated with increased survival.
- Number and size of lesions, general health conditions, and residual liver function are the main factors determining the prognosis of patients with HCC. Staging of HCC using these parameters allows to select the most appropriate therapeutic strategy for each disease stage. In accurately selected patients, both surgical resection and liver transplantation are able to obtain 5-year survival rates >50%.
- Liver benign epithelial tumours for which surgery is necessary are rare. In most cases, diagnosis and follow up rely on imaging studies.

REFERENCES

- Garuti F, Neri A, Avanzato F, et al. The changing scenario of hepatocellular carcinoma in Italy: an update. Liver Int. 2021 Mar;41(3):585-97.
- Heimbach JK, Kulik LM, Finn RS, et al. AASLD guidelines for the treatment of hepatocellular carcinoma. Hepatology. 2018;67(1):358-80.
- Italian Association for the Study of the Liver (AISF). Position paper of the Italian Association for the Study of the Liver (AISF): the multidisciplinary clinical approach to hepatocellular carcinoma. Dig Liver Dis. 2013;45(9):712-23.
- Marrero JA, Ahn J, Rajender Reddy K; Americal College of Gastroenterology. ACG clinical guideline: the diagnosis and management of focal liver lesions. Am J Gastroenterol. 2014;109:1328-47.
- Ryerson AB, Eheman CR, Altekruse SF, et al. Annual report to the nation on the status of cancer, 1975-2012, featuring the increasing incidence of liver cancer. Cancer. 2016;122(9):1312-37.

LIVER TRANSPLANTATION

Patrizia Burra, Francesco Paolo Russo

LEARNING OBJECTIVES
- To learn the indications for and contraindications to liver transplantation according to aetiology of disease.
- To identify selection criteria for liver transplant.
- To describe the major complications after liver transplantation.
- To learn about liver transplant outcome according to aetiology of disease.
- To identify the issues related to alternatives to deceased donor liver transplant.
- To learn about future clinical applications of cell therapy in liver disease.

Liver transplantation is the therapeutic option for most acute and chronic liver diseases and in selected cases of fulminant hepatitis. Liver transplantation should be offered to patients in whom survival is affected by liver disease and liver disease complications, but also in cases in which quality of life is severely affected by the disease. The first liver transplant was performed by Thomas Starzl in Denver, Colorado, in 1963 and since 2013, 25.000 liver transplants have been performed worldwide every year. After more than 50 years of experience, this is "Transplant Medicine" with increasing indications for liver transplant, improved management of surgical and medical complications after surgery, and improved rates of graft and patient survival in the early and long term follow up. In Italy in 2022, there were 22 liver transplant centres. Between 2006 and 2015, there was a plateau effect of liver transplant in Italy, with nearly 1000 performed per year. In 2016 a 10% increased rate of liver transplantation was reported with 1213 liver transplants performed in 2016 and 1290 in 2017.
Unfortunately, due to the COVID-19 pandemic in 2020, the number of transplants decreased on average by 7.4% at the national level, reaching a decline of 14% in Lombardy, the region most affected by the pandemic. Five-year patient survival is 70-75% according to the aetiology of liver disease, patient's clinical status at the time of surgery, and donor features.

INDICATIONS FOR LIVER TRANSPLANTATION AND CANDIDATE SELECTION

Indications

Liver cirrhosis is the main indication for liver transplantation. The development of cirrhosis complications with the risk of reduced survival, indicates the right time for referral to transplant hepatologists working in a liver transplant centre. The most common indications are alcoholic cirrhosis, viral cirrhosis, non-alcoholic steato-hepatitis (NASH), cholestatic liver diseases, hepatocellular carcinoma, in selected cases, cholangiocarcinoma, and neuroendocrine tumours, some benign tumours and metabolic liver diseases (**Table 38.1**). Indications for liver transplant for acute hepatic failure are discussed in Chapter 50.

Contraindications

There are absolute contraindications to liver transplantation (**Table 38.2**):
- severe cardiac or pulmonary dysfunction due to high anaesthesiology risk during surgery;
- extra hepatic malignancies, since immunosuppression can favour the dissemination of cancer cells;
- dependence on substances of abuse including alcohol since the relapse after transplant will compromise function of the new graft.

Candidate Selection

The aim of liver transplantation is to enhance survival in patients with endstage liver disease. A multidisciplinary team of heptologist, gastroenterologist, surgeon, anaesthetist, radiologist, pathologist, toxicologist, psychologist, among others at liver transplant centres evaluates potential candidates and his/her priority in the waiting list. Candidates will be selected according to type of liver disease complications, severity of complications, evolution of liver disease, age, blood group, and anatomical shape. Patients should be referred to a liver transplant centre after the first episode of decompensation, or when signs and symptoms

Table 38.1 Liver diseases with indication for liver transplantation.

Chronic Liver Disease

- Viral cirrhosis (HBV, HCV, HDV, HEV)
- Alcoholic liver cirrhosis
- Non alcoholic steato-hepatitis (NASH)
- Cholestatic liver diseases (primary biliary cholangitis, primary sclerosing cholangitis, secondary biliary cholangitis, secondary sclerosing cholangitis, intrahepatic cholestasis, Alagille syndrome)
- Autoimmune liver cirrhosis
- Metabolic liver diseases (haemochromatosis, Wilson disease, alfa-1 antitrypsin deficiency)
- Vascular liver diseases (veno-occlusive disease, Budd-Chiari syndrome)
- Hepatic tumours (hepatocellular carcinoma, cholangiocarcinoma in selected cases, carcinoids, hepatoblastoma)
- Cryptogenic cirrhosis
- Congenital hepatic fybrosis, Caroli disease
- Hyperoxaluria type I, hypercholesterolemia type II, haemophilia

Acute Liver Failure

- Viral hepatitis (HBV, HAV, HDV, HEV and rarely HCV)
- Toxic ("drug-induced liver injury", amanita phalloides, hepatotoxic xenobiotics)
- Metabolic (Wilson's disease)
- Autoimmune
- Idiopathic
- Acute live failure in pregnancy

Rare Indications

- Epithelioid haemangioendothelioma
- Neuroendocrine tumours (well differentiated) metastatic to the liver
- Rendu Osler Weber syndrome
- Polycystic disease

Table 38.2 Indications for liver transplantation in patients with liver cirrhosis.

- Ascites
- Recurrent hepatic encephalopathy
- Oesophageal variceal bleeding/gastric variceal bleeding/gastric antral vascular ectasia/congestive gastropathy refractory to endoscopic treatments/medical therapy/interventional radiology
- Spontaneous bacterial peritonitis
- Hepatorenal syndrome
- Hepatopulmonary syndrome
- Intractable itching
- Severe osteoporosis
- Recurrent cholangitis in patients with Caroli disease or primary sclerosing cholangitis
- Hepatocellular carcinoma

would severely compromise the quality of life. Unfortunately, still quite often the referral of patients with end stage liver disease to the transplant hepatologist is too late and they arrive at the transplant hospital with too advanced liver disease and compromised clinical features, in which case liver transplantation is considered futile for the high risk of patient to die despite transplant. There are several scores that predict liver disease mortality and are used to select candidates for liver transplant.
For more than 20 years the Child-Pugh classification was used then the followed by Model for End-stage Liver Disease (MELD) since 2002. The Child-Pugh includes biochemical variables such as albumin, bilirubin, prothrombin time, and clinical features such as ascites and encephalopathy. The MELD score is derived from three biochemical variables bilirubin, creatinine, and INR. In Italy, patients are categorized as Child-Pu-gh ≥B7 or MELD ≥15. These scores are useful for the majority of liver diseases, but there are some exceptions. When the patient with cirrhosis develops hepatocellular carcinoma, the indication for liver transplant is driven by the cancer and not only by the severity of underlying liver disease, since the progression of cancer with vascular invasion, extra hepatic metastases, are contraindications to liver transplantation. The waiting list is updated every week in all liver transplant centres according to clinical changes, priority, and prognostic scores. In addition, patients may develop extra hepatic complications that need specific management, including hepatopulmonary syndrome, cardiomyopathy, due to shunts, hyperdynamic circulation, cirrhotic cardiopathy, hepatorenal syndrome, renal disease, encephalopathy, vascular damage, alcohol related injury, hypersplenism, anaemia, immunodepression. In fulminant hepatic failure, liver transplantation should be performed before the development of cerebral oedema and irreversible brain damage.

Outcome After Liver Transplantation

Graft and patient survival rates are excellent in Italy (**Figure 38.1 A-B**).
Early mortality (within 3 months after transplant) may be related to surgical complications, graft primary dysfunction, but very often infections are the cause of death, especially in very sick candidates. The long-term mortality is associated with late infections, cardiovascular complications, and de novo tumours, and in a limited proportion, with recurrence of primary liver disease.

SURGICAL ISSUES

Liver transplantation is based on the replacement of diseased graft with a new graft obtained from a deceased donor.
Usually, the whole liver is used for transplantation, however, the graft can be split (split liver, **Figure 38.2**) into two parts and transplanted in two different recipients. During living related liver transplantation, the split part of the graft is used for the recipient. It is called orthotopic liver transplant since the graft is transplanted in the same anatomic position as the explanted liver (**Figure 38.3**). Liver transplant surgery is very complex and should be performed by surgeons expert on hepatobiliary surgery; it is based on three steps:

- total hepatectomy;
- anhepatic phase, when the diseased liver is removed and anstomoses of portal vein and hepatic artery are performed, but the graft is not yet flushed with blood;
- the new graft is flushed with blood.

IMMUNOSUPPRESSION, ACUTE, AND CHRONIC REJECTION

After transplant, immunosuppression is life-long in all recipients, except in cases in which tolerance is induced. Immunosuppressive therapy will potentially avoid:

- hyperacute rejection, quite rare, due to an unexpected massive reaction from the immune system against the graft;
- acute rejection, very common event, usually within the first two weeks after transplant (10-30% of cases) that can be treated with steroid therapy;
- chronic rejection, nearly 5% of cases, usually late after transplant, which may progress; when rejection becomes irreversible, re-transplantation is the only curative treatment (**Figures 38.4, 38.5**).

Tolerance may be induced by minimizing and/or withdrawing immunosuppression without episodes of rejection, but this happens quite rarely. The major immune suppressive drugs are calcineurin inhibitors, namely, cyclosporine and tacrolimus. Moreover, azathioprine or mofetil mycophenolate (same drug class and therefore must not be used together) can be added on as

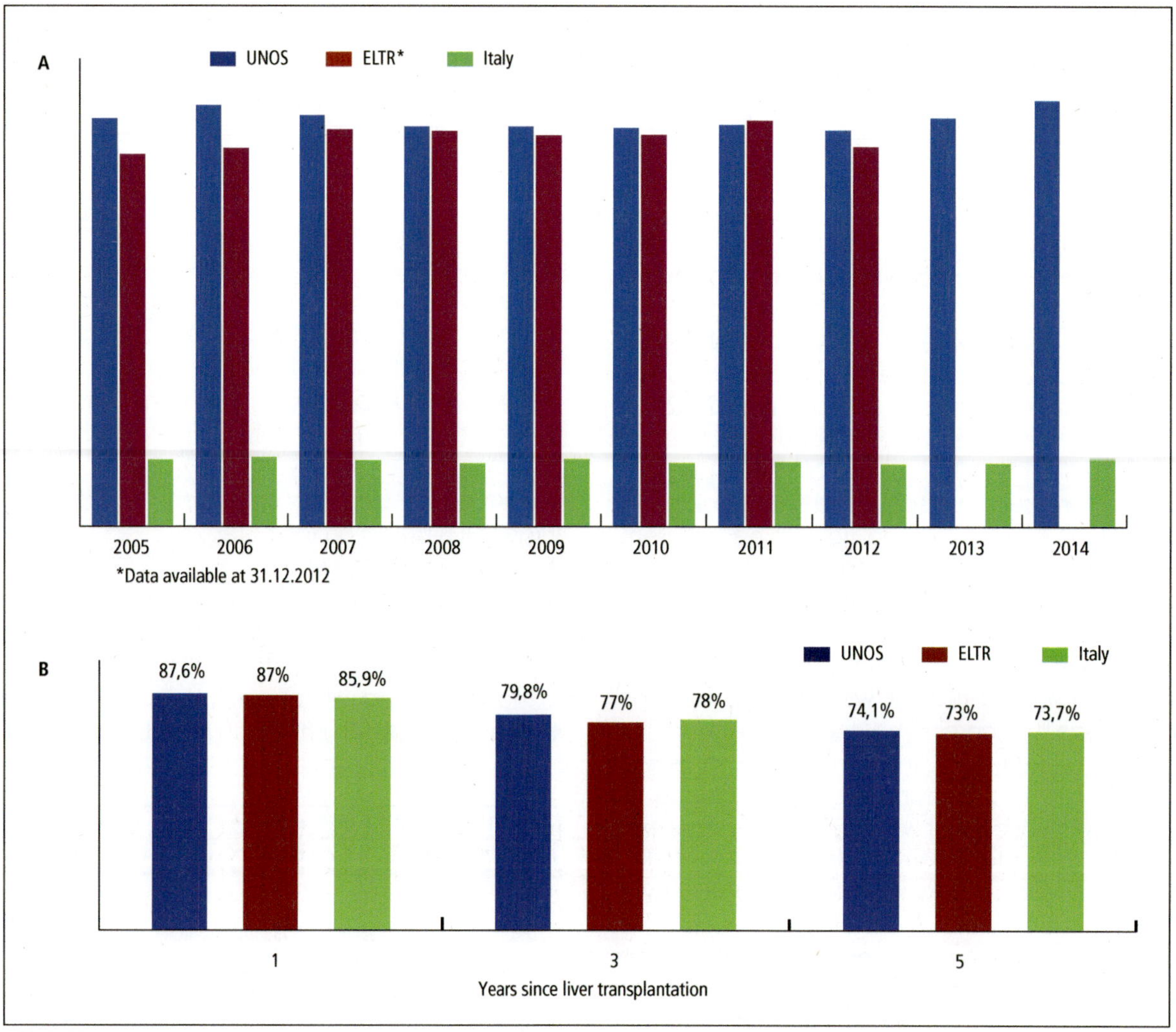

Figure 38.1 Panel A Liver transplantation between 2005 and 2014. Panel B One - three -,and five - years survival in liver transplant recipients in Italy, Europe (European Liver Transplant Registry – ELTR) and the United States (UNOS); www.trapianti.salute.gov.it; www.eltr.org; www.unos.org.

second agent, and also steroids can be part of immunosuppression. In recently years, mTOR (mammalian target of rapamycin) inhibitors, such as sirolimus and everolimus have been introduced as immune suppressants. There are also monoclonal antibodies induction immunosuppression therapy at the time of transplant or few days later, but their use is less common in clinical practice.

MEDICAL COMPLICATIONS AFTER LIVER TRANSPLANTATION

Infections

The liver transplant patient will continue on immunosuppressive therapy, with very few exceptions, throughout life. This inevitably leads to decreased immune defences and increased risk of infections. Immediately after surgery, bacterial infections are more frequent, while viral infections may develop within 3 months of transplantation; the risk of opportunistic or fungal infections cannot be ruled out, which can be so severe as become fatal.

Medical Complications

Renal Dysfunction

Immunosuppressive therapy causes renal dysfunction and increases serum levels of creatinine in 30-70% of cases. Several drugs are classified as renal sparing, such as mofetil mycophenolate, and everolimus.

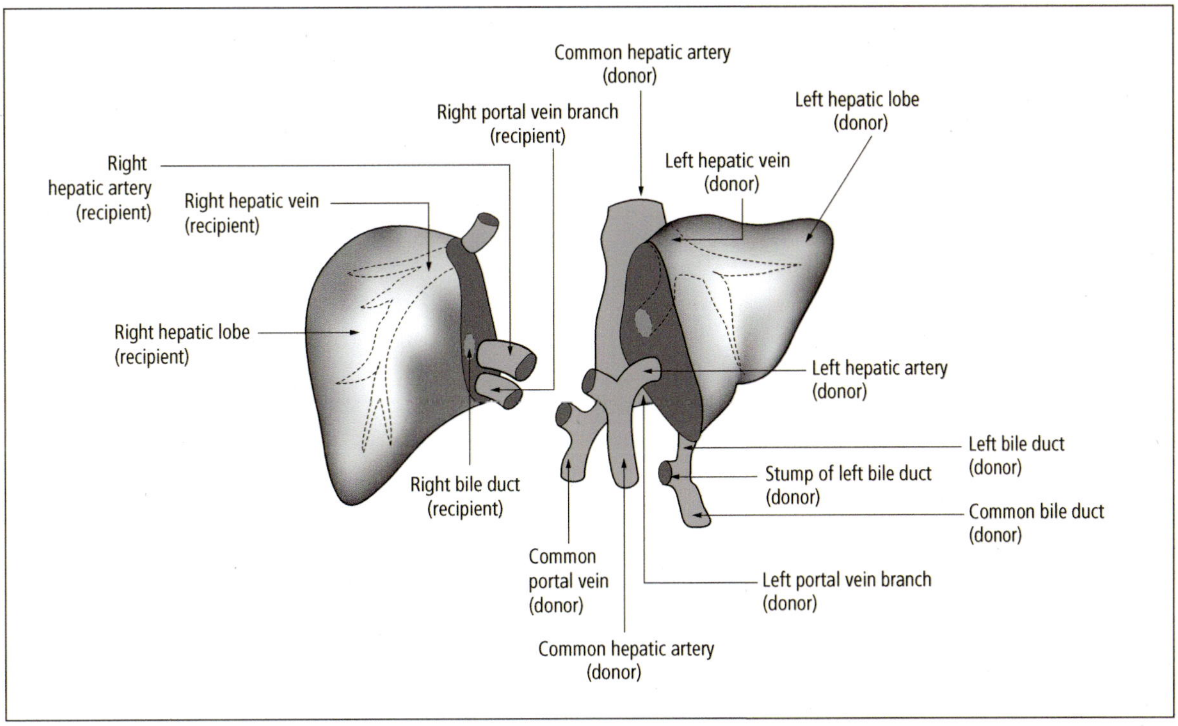

Figure 38.2 Split liver transplantation.

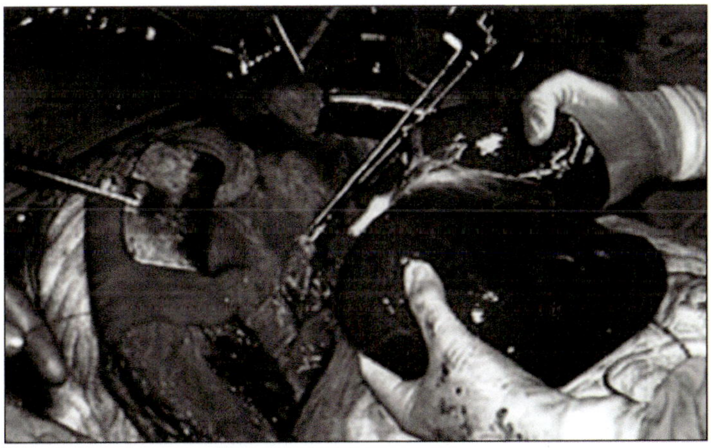

Figure 38.3 Orthotopic liver transplantation; classical technique.

Metabolic Complications

Immunosuppression may cause development of diabetes (20-30% of cases), dyslipidaemia (20% of cases), obesity (30-70% of cases). Arterial hypertension is a common complication due to immunosuppression and cardiovascular complications can lead to death in 10% of cases.

Neurologic Complications

Neurologic abnormalities (up to 60% of cases) may be mild (tremors, difficulty in concentration) or severe, ranging from headache to dysarthria.

Osteoporosis

Immunosuppression, mainly steroids, may impair of bone mineralization, with the risk of spontaneous fractures, especially in post-menopausal women transplanted for cholestatic liver diseases.

Surgical Complications

Early surgical complications include vascular and biliary anastomoses, such as portal veinvena cava and suprahepatic vein, hepatic artery, choledoco choledoco or choledo hepaticojejunum anastomosis. Acute hepatic artery thrombosis can cause

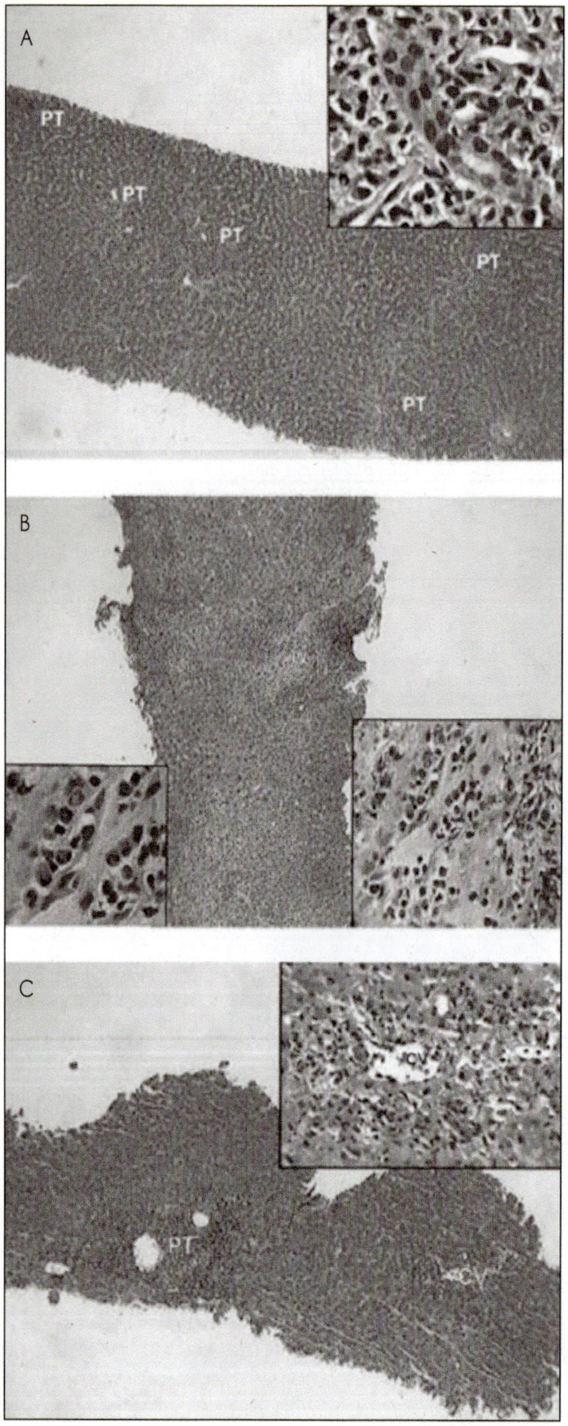

Figure 38.4 Acute rejection after liver transplantation.
a) Mild: portal inflammation characterized by mononuclear leukocytes infiltration (lymphocytes, neutrophils, and eosinophils).
b) Moderate: more severe inflammation.
c) Severe: portal inflammation with portal and/or subendothelial inflammation of terminal hepatic venules, inflammation and hepatocyte necrosis.

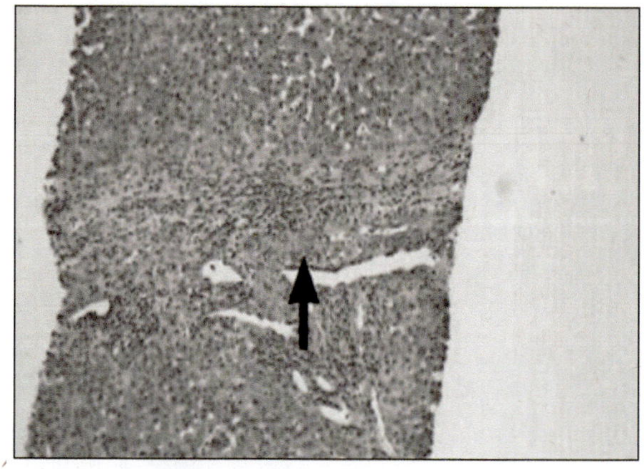

Figure 38.5 Chronic rejection after liver transplantation. Histological aspect of bile ducts.

severe graft ischaemic injury resulting in ischaemic biliary injury.

Portal vein anastomotic stenosis is rare, whereas portal vein thrombosis may occur less rarely. Biliary complications are frequent due to anastomotic or non-anastomotic strictures, usually in long term follow-up.

Technical, immune-mediated or recurrence of primary liver disease (primary sclerosing cholangitis) are the most common causes.

OUTCOME ACCORDING TO AETIOLOGY OF PRIMARY LIVER DISEASE

Alcoholic Liver Disease

Alcoholic cirrhosis is one of the most common indications for liver transplantation (about 20% of cases). Until the late 1980s, it was considered a controversial indication because patients were held accountable for their illness and unreliable in the post transplantation period (resumption of alcohol intake, failure to take immunosuppressive drugs, lack of adherence to follow-up controls). Transplant candidates must maintain complete cessation of alcohol intake for at least 6 months prior to inclusion on the list. Furthermore, a team of physicians, toxicologists, psychologists and/or psychiatrists must confirm that the patient has understood the importance of transplantation and has adequate psychosocial support from family members to address the intervention. In recent years the discussion has reopened on whether to reduce the abstinence interval, but expert opinion also international, is not yet universal. A pilot study in progress in Italy has proposed liver transplantation in selected cases of severe acute alcoholic hepatitis in young patients (a condition that has always represented a contraindication to transplantation in the past). Before this approach can be proposed at the national level, it is necessary to wait for the results of this extension of indications.

During selection of patients with alcohol related liver disease, it is necessary to exclude the coexistence of alcohol related pathologies (chronic pancreatitis, myocardial disease, chronic bronchopathy, cerebral atrophy, peripheral neuropathy), which would compromise the result of the transplant.

After liver transplantation, a return to the use of alcoholic beverages is described in 30-50% of cases. Survival, however, is completely overlaps with rates after transplantation in cirrhosis from other aetiologies.

Non-Alcoholic Steato Hepatitis

In the last 10 years the incidence of non-alcoholic steatohepatitis (NASH) and non-alcoholic fatty liver disease (NAFLD) has increased in Europe and other countries, leading to a rise in the overall rates of chronic liver disease. In the United States, NASH is one of the most common indications for liver transplantation due to complications of cirrhosis and the development of hepatocellular carcinoma.

In Europe, NASH is an indication for liver transplantation in nearly 5-10% of cases, according to individual countries. Patients with NAFLD/NASH have several cardiovascular comorbidities, therefore, evaluation is warranted not only for the preand post-transplant risk factors, but also for the impact those factors may have on long-term survival. Usually, graft and patient survival rates are similar to those reported for other indications, but patients can experience metabolic and cardiovascular events, as well as recurrence of NAFLD and NASH. The transplant hepatologist, together with the nutritionist, dietician, endocrinologist, diabetologist, among others, should follow-up patients for metabolic and nutritional aspects, physical activity, and body weight before and after transplantation.

HBV-Related Cirrhosis

HBV-related cirrhosis, with and without HDV infection, accounts for nearly 15-20% of indications for liver transplantation. HBV-related fulminant hepatitis is reported in 5 to 35% of cases of fulminant hepatitis. Since the virus can replicate in extra hepatic sites, the new graft can be infected. The risk is lower in fulminant hepatitis and HDV coinfection than in HBV cirrhosis. Antivirals are used before transplantation and the majority of patients will not be viraemic or will have mild viremia at the time of transplant. The same antivirals used before transplantation are administered after transplantation. Together with anti-HBs immunoglobulins, they achieve very efficient and safe control of HBV reinfection, with no more than 1-3% of cases reported after transplantation.

HCV-Related Cirrhosis

HCV-related cirrhosis until a few years ago, accounted for 30-40% of all indications for liver transplantation, and graft reinfection detected on histology occurred in 50-75% of cases.

Since 2014 new antivirals are available and HCV infection can be treated before or after transplantation. Drugs that can be used in compensated cirrhosis are:

- sofosbuvir/velpatasvir, contraindicated in Child-Pugh C patients;
- glecaprevir/pibrentasvir, not recommended in Child-Pugh B patients, contraindicated in Child-Pugh C patients;
- elbasvir/grazoprevir, contraindicated in Child-Pugh B-C patients.

The new antivirals are very effective drugs, much safer when compared to interferon-based therapies, with very mild side effects. Interferon-based therapies were associated with low rates of sustained virologic response (SVR); reported in 30-35% of cases. With new antivirals, SVR is reported in 60-70% of patients with compensated cirrhosis. Within just a few years, we have observed landscape changes in indications for liver transplantation, with a 25% reduction of patients with HCV-related cirrhosis on the waiting list. In patients who are transplanted for HCV-related cirrhosis, these new antiviral drugs can also be used early after surgery to avoid, in case of reinfection, evolution of the liver disease and development of fibrosis, as observed until a few years ago in almost all cases. The following drugs are currently available in post-transplantation:

- sofosbuvir/velpatasvir, which do not interfere with most immunosuppressive drugs;
- glecaprevir/pibrentasvir, which are not recommended in patients receiving cyclosporine.

Even in post transplantation, the use of these drugs has proven safe and effective; only measures are needed in patients who develop renal failure.

Cholestatic Liver Diseases

Primary biliary cholangitis (PBC) and primary sclerosing cholangitis (PSC) are the most common forms of cholestatic liver diseases that may represent indications for liver transplantation. Generally, PBC remains stable for years; when the first signs of decompensation appear, the progression of hepatic dysfunction is generally very fast. Bilirubin is the most important prognostic index. Survival after transplantation is very good and the risk of recurrence of primary disease is reported in 10-20% of cases. PSC is associated in 60-80% of cases with chronic inflammatory bowel disease, especially ulcerative colitis. The progression of liver disease is usually slow but can be accelerated by frequent episodes of cholangitis. The risk to develop cholangiocarcinoma should be carefully ruled out because it is often a contraindication to transplantation due to the high risk of recurrence and poor survival within 1-2 years after transplant. Survival after transplantation for PSC is good, with recurrence of the disease in 20-30% of cases.

Autoimmune Hepatitis

Liver transplantation is indicated in autoimmune hepatitis with evolution in cirrhosis. Autoimmune hepatitis may have a fulminant hepatitis onset, one of the most common causes of fulminant hepatitis. After transplantation, acute rejection is very frequent, seen in 60-70% of cases, with higher risk of chronic rejection (10-15% of cases). Recurrence after transplant is reported in 20-30% of cases.

De Novo Immune Hepatitis

De novo immune hepatitis after transplant is reported in 2.5-3.5% of cases. The first case was described in 1998. It is an unpredictable event; usually the diagnosis is made after having ruled out other causes of immune, mediated diseases. Patients are treated by increasing immunosuppression, but resolution of the injury is not always easy to achieve.

Metabolic Liver Diseases

Liver transplantation may be offered to patients with liver disease due to metabolic derangements caused by enzyme deficits underlying the disease. The new graft will replace the site of enzyme production. These diseases include Wilson's disease, haemochromatosis, $\alpha 1$ antitrypsin deficiency. Recurrence of these diseases is rarely reported.

Vascular Diseases

The Budd-Chiari syndrome is caused by suprahepatic vein occlusion, due to thrombi or other causes. The onset of disease may be acute or chronic, and liver transplantation is considered only in cases not responding to medical, radiological, or endoscopic therapy.

Hepatocellular Carcinoma

Hepatocellular carcinoma (HCC) as a complication of cirrhosis, is a common indication for liver transplantation.

The reference criteria as eligible candidates are called Milan criteria, based on the presence of a single nodule with diameter no larger than 5 cm or up to three nodules each with diameter no larger than 3 cm, without vascular invasion (neoplastic portal vein thrombosis), without spread of neoplastic disease outside the liver. Following these criteria, patient survival is similar to that reported in patients transplanted without HCC, and the recurrence rate is less than 10%. Waiting list registration is allowed in cases with HCC when cirrhosis is still compensated (Child-Pu-gh <7 or MELD <15), since these patients are at risk of drop out from the waiting list due to HCC extension, which is outside the criteria for transplant. However, in recent years, less rigorous criteria than the Milan criteria have been proposed, with acceptable survival and tumour recurrence rates, but this issue is still debated. The common aim is to extend criteria widely and homogeneously in liver transplant centres.

OPEN ISSUES

Transplant Oncology

In more recent years, also thanks to the significant decrease in patients on the waiting list for decompensated liver disease, criteria have been proposed for HCC that are less stringent than the Milan criteria with results, in terms of survival and cancer recurrence, acceptable, but the topic is still under discussion, even if there is an attempt to use more uniform criteria that are shared and applied by all transplant centres for patients with HCC. Another oncological indication that has been reconsidered in recent years is cholangiocarcinoma (CCA). In particular, the small unresectable perilar (pCCA) (Klatskin tumour) is now considered an indication for transplantation after neoadjuvant chemo-radiotherapy, while for the unresectable intrahepatic cholangiocarcinoma (iCCA) both on normal and cirrhotic liver is considered a possible indication for transplantation. Liver transplantation for neuroendocrine tumours (NETs) is well accepted with good results despite in small series. Finally, recently and with less evidence, liver transplantation has also been proposed in well-selected patients, with unresectable liver metastases from colorectal carcinoma. This provided the rationale for new prospective studies that are now underway.

Organ Donation

Despite the increasing number of patients with indications for liver transplantation, organ donations are still insufficient to meet the need of transplants. The donation rate in Italy rose in 2016, yet the waiting list mortality rate remains high.

Donors with Viral Hepatitis

Thanks to the advent of powerful antiviral therapies, one method of overcoming organ shortage is to use livers from donors that are positive for hepatitis C virus (HCV) or hepatitis B (HBV), and more recently organs from donors with human immunodeficiency (HIV) for positive recipients were also considered.

Machine Perfusion

Machine perfusion has been applied ex situ to liver grafts in the effort to improve static cold-storage preservation and also for defatting liver that without perfusion are usually discarged. If a more extensive application of this technology confirms the preliminary results, machine perfusion will become crucial in increasing the donor pool as well as improving recipients' outcomes.

Living Related Liver Transplantation

Living related liver transplantation is a procedure collateral to transplantation from a deceased donor. The living donor should be a healthy person, with good liver function, possibly with the same blood group as the recipient.

A partial liver resection is performed using the left lobe or sometimes also the right lobe of the liver that is transplanted into the recipient. Only liver transplant centres with hepatobiliary surgery and splitting experience are authorized to perform a living related liver transplant.

Hepatocytes and Stem Cells Transplantation

Liver transplantation is often the only therapy option in patients with end stage liver disease, but organ donation is still insufficient to meet the growing demand for organs. A therapeutic alternative to whole liver transplantation is regenerative medicine and more specifically by the cell therapy. Transplantation of hepatocytes and stem cells is a promising research area, developed initially to replace whole liver transplantation in selected cases of liver disease due to an enzymatic defect. In such cases the transplanted hepatocytes can restore the enzyme defect without the need for liver transplantation. The advantages of cell therapy are the lower costs compared to transplantation, a simple and less traumatic surgical procedure, the possibility to genetically modify hepatocytes before their use, and to obtain numerous hepatocytes from a single liver not suitable for transplantation. Hepatocytes are ideally considered the cells of choice for cell therapy in the liver, but the number of available cells is very limited. To overcome this obstacle, experts have searched for an alternative that has been identified in stem cells. Stem cells are non-specialised cells with the ability to transform potentially into any other type of cell in the body. The main source of stem cells is the bone marrow, but there are alternative sources such as the umbilical cord or the placenta. In recent years, clinical trials on the use of stem cells in patients with chronic liver disease were conducted in research centres in Italy and abroad. The results from these ongoing studies will improve knowledge on the applicability of stem cell therapy for the treatment of the major human liver diseases and may offer a possible alternative to liver transplantation in the future.

KEY CONCEPTS

- Liver transplantation should be proposed as therapeutic option to patients with end-stage liver disease in whom medical, surgical, endoscopic, radiologic therapy is not able to control progression of the disease and the development of complications with risk of death.
- Liver transplantation is a complex process that starts with the selection of the candidate, followed by waiting list management, donor graft assessment at the time of transplant, surgery, and post-transplant follow-up of the recipient.
- Transplant Medicine includes evaluation of the outcome, assessed by graft and patient survival, the prevention and treatment of post-transplant medical complications, and includes the ability to offer to recipients a good quality of life.

REFERENCES

- Burra P, Giannini EG, Caraceni P, et al. Specific issues concerning the management of patients on the waiting list and after liver transplantation. Liver Int. 2018 August;38(8):1338-62.
- European Association for the Study of the Liver. EASL Clinical Practice Guidelines: liver transplantation. J Hepatol. 2016;64:433-85.
- Sapisochin G, Hibi T, Toso C, et al. Transplant Oncology in Primary and Metastatic Liver Tumors: Principles, Evidence and Opportunities. Ann Surg. 2021 Mar 1;273(3):483-493.
- Hefler J, Marfil-Garza BA, Dadheech N, Shapiro AMJ. Machine Perfusion of the Liver: Applications Beyond Transplantation. Transplantation. 2020 Sep;104(9):1804-1812.

CHAPTER 39

THE PATHOPHYSIOLOGY OF BILE SECRETION

Stefano Ginanni Corradini, Gaetano Bertino

LEARNING OBJECTIVES

- To know the principles, cellular components, and transporters that regulate the synthesis, secretion and enterohepatic circulation of bile acids.
- To know the pathophysiology of the biliary secretion of bile acids, phospholipids, cholesterol, and bilirubin and the enterohepatic circulation of cholesterol and bilirubin.
- To know the principles that regulate the interactions between bile acids, intestinal microbiota, and nuclear receptors.

Bile is a micellar solution, isosmotic with respect to plasma, and composed primarily of water, inorganic electrolytes, and organic solutes such as bile acids (BA), phospholipids (PL, mainly phosphatidylcholine), cholesterol (CH), and bile pigments. The formation and secretion of bile is essential for digestion and intestinal absorption of lipids, for cholesterol homeostasis, and for the hepatic excretion of hydrophobic xenobiotics, drug metabolites, and heavy metals. BA are the driving force of bile formation.

The synthesis of the BA, starting from cholesterol, occurs through the classic pathway of 7α-hydrox ylase cholesterol or the alternative route of oxysterol 7α-hydroxylase, which leads to the formation of cholic acid and chenodeoxycholic acid, respectively, the two primary BAs. The BA are then conjugated with glycine or taurine and secreted in the biliary canaliculus. Hepatocytes have a fundamental role in the synthesis and the uptake of the BA from the portal blood and their secretion in the canalular lumen. In these processes, transport proteins are selectively localized in the basolateral or canalicular membrane of the hepatocytes, as described in **Table 39.1**, which illustrates cellular localization, functions, and involvement in cholestatic diseases.

These carriers are involved in cholestatic genetic diseases and acquired diseases, where their function can be compromised by drugs, hormones, alcohol or endotoxins. Thanks to these transport processes, BA reach in the bile canaliculus a concentration > 1000 fold (**Figure 39.1**) higher than serum concentration. This osmotic gradient recalls water through the hepatocyte tight junctions, thus generating the BA-dependent bile flow.

A genetic cholestasis (PFIC4) has been recently associated with mutation of the gene encoding the tight junction protein 2 (TJP2). A minor fraction of canalicular bile (BA-independent), however, is formed via the osmotic gradient generated by the active canalicular secretion of glutathione (GSH) and bicarbonate (HCO3-) operated, respectively, by MRP2 and AE2 (Cl-/HCO3- exchanger) to produce hepato-canalicular bile. Thanks to the phasic contractions of the bile canaliculus, bile flows downstream along segments of progressively increasing size of the intra- and extrahepatic bile duct system.

THE BILE DUCT SYSTEM AND THE CHOLHEPATIC SHUNT

The bile ducts are lined by cells, the cholangiocytes, that transform hepato-canalicular bile into the final secretion reaching the duodenum, through reabsorption and secretion carried out by transporters located on the apical or basolateral pole of cholangiocytes. Among the main ones are cystic fibrosis transmembrane regulator (CFTR) and Cl-/HCO3- exchanger for bicarbonate secretion and aquaporins, which facilitate water movement.

These transporters are genetically or functionally impaired in cystic fibrosis, thus explaining the formation of inspissated bile. The bile generated by cholangiocytes is called ductular/ductal bile and, in humans, contributes to about 30-40% of the bile reaching the duodenum.

However, cholangiocytes are also able to reabsorb hydrophobic substances secreted by the

*The Authors wish to thank Dr. Maria Consiglia Bragazzi for her assistance.

Table 39.1 Site and function of the transport proteins involved in bile formation and bile acid enterohepatic circulation.

Transport Proteins (Gene)	Site	Function	Cholestatic Disease (Protein and Gene Involved)
Hepatocyte	**Bile Acid-Dependent Bile Flow**		
NTCP (*SLC10A1*)	Basolateral membrane	Na^+-dependent absorption of bile acids and xenobiotics	
OATP1B1 (*SLCO1B1*)	Basolateral membrane	Na^+-independent absorption of bile acids and xenobiotics	
OATP1B3 (*SLCO1B3*)	Basolateral membrane	Na^+-independent absorption of bile acids and xenobiotics	
Na+, K+-ATPasi	Basolateral membrane	Secretion of $2Na^+$ in exchange of $3K^+$	
BSEP (*ABCB11*)	Canalicular membrane	ATP-dependent secretion of bile acids	Progressive familial intrahepatic cholestasis Type 2, Benign recurrent intrahepatic cholestasis Type 2, intrahepatic cholestasis of pregnancy BSEP (*ABCB11*)
MDR3 (*ABCB4*)	Canalicular membrane	ATP-dependent secretion of lecithin	Progressive familial intrahepatic cholestasis Type 3, Benign recurrent intrahepatic cholestasis Type 3, intrahepatic cholestasis of pregnancy, LPAC (cholelithiasis from low concentration of lecithin in the bile) MDR3 (ABCB4)
ABCG5	Canalicular membrane	ATP-dependent secretion of sterols	Sitosterolaemia ABCG5
ABCG8	Canalicular membrane	ATP-dependent secretion of sterols	Sitosterolaemia ABCG8
NPC1L1	Canalicular membrane	Import of sterols	
FIC1	Canalicular membrane	ATP- flippasis dependent of aminophospholipids	Progressive familial intrahepatic cholestasis Type 1, Benign recurrent intrahepatic cholestasis Type 1 FIC1 (ATP8B1)
	Bile Acid-Independent BileFlow		
MRP2 (*ABCC2*)	Canalicular membrane	Dependent ATP-transport of glucuronide, glutathione and sulphate conjugates	Dubin-Johnson Syndrome MRP2 (*ABCC2*)
OATP1B1, 1B3, 2B1	Basolateral membrane	Na^+-dependent transport of organic anions, cations and neutral steroids	Rotor Syndrome OATP1B1 (*SLCO1B1*) OATP1B3 (*SLCO1B3*)

Continue →

Continued ⟶

Table 39.1 Site and function of the transport proteins involved in bile formation and bile acid enterohepatic circulation.

Transport Proteins (Gene)	Site	Function	Cholestatic Disease (Protein and Gene Involved)
	Sinusoidal Export of Bile Acids		
MRP3 (*ABCC3*)	Basolateral membrane	ATP-dependent transport of bile acids and glycuron-conjugates	
MRP4 (*ABCC4*)	Basolateral membrane	ATP-dependent export of glutathione and bile acids	
OSTa-OSTb (*SLC51A1, SLC51A1BP*)	Basolateral membrane	Bile acid export	
	Ductular Secretion		
Colangiocytes Aquaporin 1 (*AQP1*)	Apical membrane	Water transport	
Acquaporin 4 (*AQP4*)	Basolateral membrane	Water transport	
AE2 (*SLC4A2*)	Apical membrane	Secretion of $HCO3^-$ in exchange for Cl^-	
CFTR (*ABCC7*)	Apical membrane	Secretion of Cl^-	
ASBT (SLC10A2)	Apical membrane	Bile acid absorption ("chole-hepatic shunt")	Primary malabsorption of bile acids (SLC10A2)
Ileal Enterocyte ASBT (*SLC10A2*)	Apical membrane	Na^+-dependent bile acid absorption	
NPC1L1	Apical membrane	Import of sterols	
OSTa-OSTb (*SLC51A1, SLC51A1BP*)	Basolateral membrane	Bile acid export	
MRP3 (*ABCC3*)	Basolateral membrane	Bile acid export	

hepatocytes or generated as a consequence of hepatocytic drug metabolism.
This system is a mechanism of protection against the secretion of hydrophobic substances and is the anatomo physiological basis of the chole-hepatic shunt (first described for BA protonated non-conjugated dihydroxylates secreted in the bile and activating the AE2 exchanger, with choleresis rich in bicarbonate).
In addition to passive absorption, the biliary epithelium expresses the apical transporter of sodium-dependent bile acids (ASBT, encoded by the SLC10A2 gene) and the transporter of the organic OSTα-OSTβ solutes (encoded by the SLC51A and SLC51B genes), thus providing the mechanism physiology for cholehepatic shunt of conjugated BA. In the biliary tree and in the gallbladder, the BA reach millimolar concentrations and micelles begin to form with a potential detergent action against cholangiocytes, but protective mechanisms are present, mainly phospholipids and bicarbonates. In some genetic disorders involving MDR3 (PFIC3), phospholipid deficiency creates the conditions in which BA damage cholangiocytes, generating progressive damage of the biliary tree.

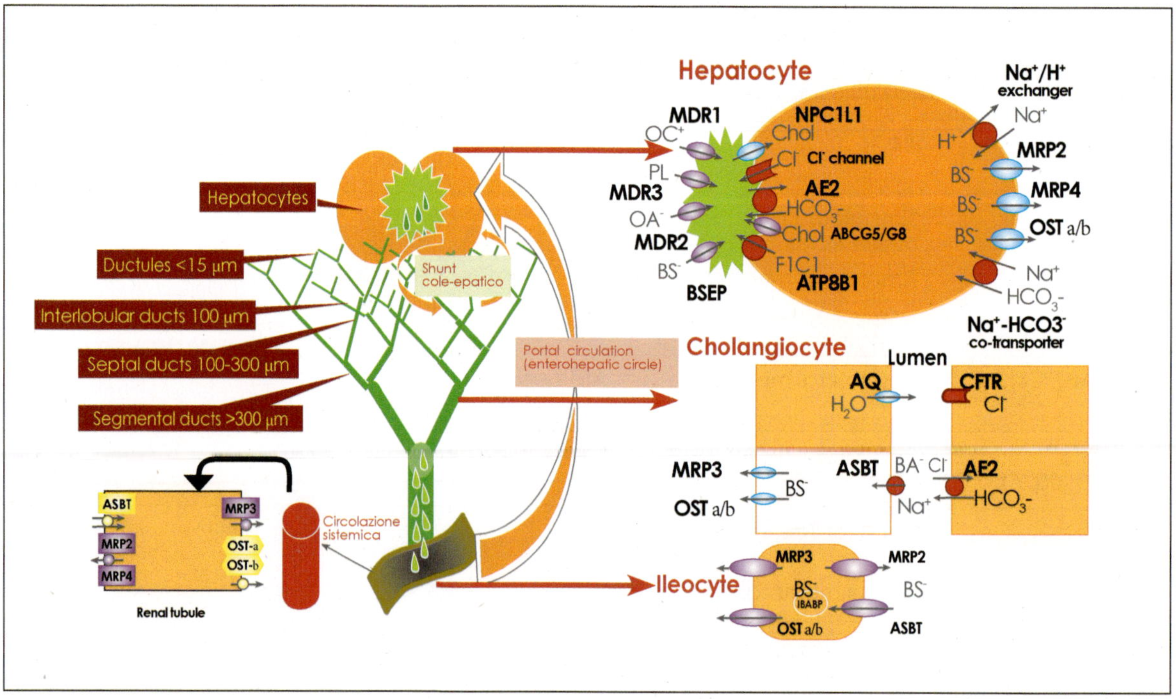

Figure 39.1 The formation and secretion of bile, the cholehepatic and enterohepatic circulation of bile acids.
NCTP= Sodium Taurocholate Cotransporting Polypeptide; MDR1= Multidrug Resistance 1, MDR3= Multidrug Resistance 3; MRP2= Multidrug Resistance Associate Protein 2; MRP2= Multidrug Resistance Associate Protein 3; MRP4= Multidrug Resistance Associate Protein 4; BSEP= Bile Salt Export Pump; NPC1L1= Niemann-Pick C1-Like 1; OST α/β = Organic solute transporter alpha and beta; Chol= Cholesterol; OC+= organic cations; AQ= acquaporins; CFTR= Cystic Fibrosis Transmembrane Regulator; ASBT= Apical Bile Salt Transporter; AE2= Anion Exchanger 2; BS= Bile salts; PL= Phospholipid; OA-= organic anions; ABCG5/G8= Active Heterodimers Transporters ABC5 e ABC8.

Under physiological conditions, an amount of bile equal to about 600-800 ml/day is secreted into the duodenum.

A sudden blockage of bile flow, caused, for example, by a stone in the main bile duct, results in acute distension of the biliary tree and stimulates of nervous fibers, leading to biliary pain, as well as fever and jaundice (Triad of Charcot), with accumulation of BA in the hepatocytes.

In contrast, when biliary flow in the small intrahepatic bile ducts is obstructed (i.e., in PBC) symptoms start with pruritus and fatigue but not jaundice, which occurs only in the terminal phases of the disease. Under cholestatic conditions, BA efflux at the hepatocyte basolateral membrane is an additional protective mechanism that reduces BA overload and is mainly driven by OSTα-OSTβ and members of the MRP family, including MRP3 (ABCC3 gene) and MRP4 (ABCC4 gene).

The down-regulation of the main carriers responsible for the hepatic uptake of BA, NTCP and members of the OATP family, also participates in this adaptive response to the intracellular accumulation of BA.

BA ENTEROHEPATIC CIRCULATION: GUT MICROBIOTA AND NUCLEAR RECEPTORS

Once secreted in the intestinal lumen, the BA facilitate the absorption of food lipids and fat-soluble vitamins. Intestinal absorption of BA is extremely efficient, about 5% of intestinal BAs escape reabsorption and are lost in the feces, being replaced by an equal amount of hepatic neo-synthesis (**Figure 39.2**). The BA are absorbed through a combination of passive absorption in the proximal small intestine and active absorption in the distal ileum. BA are deconjugated and dehydroxylated (secondary BA formation) by the bacterial flora in the distal small intestine and the colon, where they can be passively absorbed.

A fraction of the BA (from 10% to 50%, depending on the BA species) that returns to portal circulation escapes hepatic extraction at the first pass and enters into systemic circulation. Binding of BA to plasma proteins reduces glomerular filtration and minimizes urinary excretion. Generally, only 1-2 μmoles of BA are excreted in the urine, due to a highly efficient tubular reabsorption guided, as in

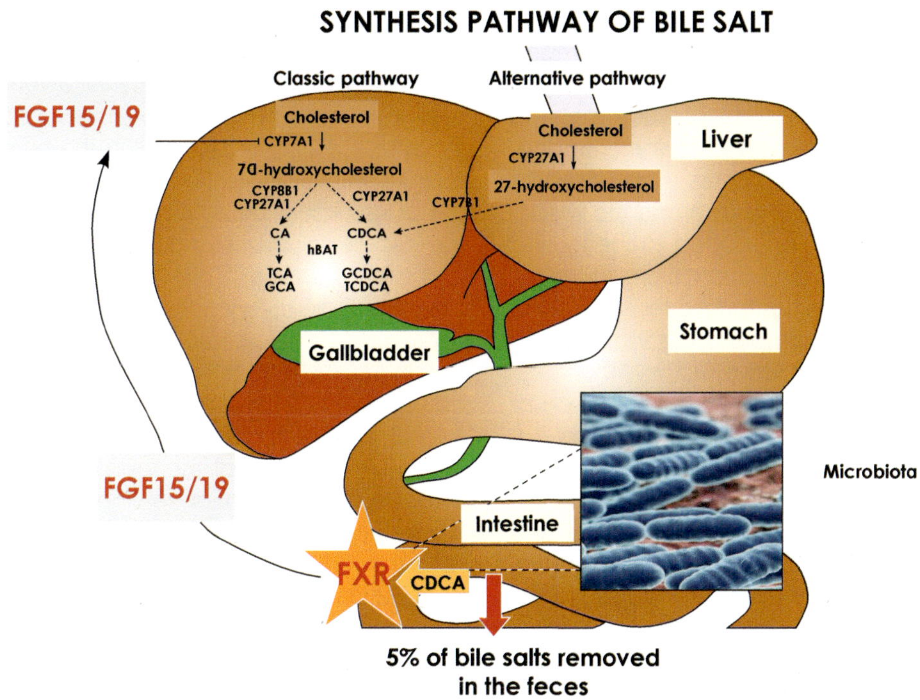

Figure 39.2 Synthesis pathway of bile salt in the liver, enterohepatic circulation.
5% of bile salts removed in the feces are replaced in enterohepatic circulation by equal amounts produced by hepatocytes. FXR, modulated by the most hydropobhobic bile salt (eg., CDCA), has a key role in reglulating the synthesis of bile salt through secretion in the portal circulation of FGF19.

the ileum, by ASBT (apical sodium-dependent BA transporter).
This efficient enterohepatic circulation of BA is regulated by negative feedback with tight control of their synthesis. BA not only regulate their own biosynthesis but also modulate important metabolic pathways that regulate lipoproteins, glucose, drugs, and energy metabolism through the activation of nuclear receptors such as FXR (farnesoid X receptor) and TGR5 (the G protein-coupled receptor). FXR is fundamental in the modulation of BA synthesis by regulationg the expression of key enzymes (CYP7A1 and CYP8B1). Specifically, intestinal FXR control of bile synthesis occurs through the secretion in the portal blood of FGF19, an entero-hormone.
In summary, the more that hydrophobic BAs (CDCA, DCA, LCA) come into contact with ileal FXR, the more FGF19 is secreted, which blocks the hepatic neosynthesis of BA and this is protective against the accumulation of BA. Conversely, the less BAs that arrive in the ileum, the more hepatocyte neosynthesis is stimulated. Activation of FXR also induces down-regulation of hepatocyte BA uptake and favors their elimination, thus reducing intrahepatic BA accumulation. Thanks to this new knowledge, several FXR agonists (obeticholic acid already in clinical use) are in an advanced stage of development with beneficial effects in cholestatic diseases. Recently, a genetic cholestasis (PIFC5) related to mutations of the NR1H4 gene that encodes FXR has been described. It is well known that intestinal microbiota has consistent effects on BA metabolism. Vice versa, BA reaching the intestine play a fundamental role in determining the quality and quantity of microbiota, exerting bacteriostatic and/or bactericidal effects. It is now evident that these interactions play a key role in glucose and lipid metabolism, with important implications for the control of body weight, the development of metabolic syndrome, and oncological risk. Therefore, the enterohepatic circulation of BA is of scientific interest in many pathologies and not only in those of the intestine and the liver.
The scientific literature is continuously enriched by discoveries of the relationships between intestinal microbiota and disease (GUT-LIVER-BRAIN axis), in particular the interactions between SA, microbio-

ta, intestinal nuclear receptors, and intestinal permeability. These interactions have a fundamental role in glucose and lipid metabolism, with important implications for the control of body weight, the development of the metabolic syndrome, and oncological risk. Our knowledge on the enterohepatic circulation of BA comprises many diseases and not only those of the intestine and the liver.

In the intestine, BA are transported to the lamina propria by passive or active absorption via the sodium-dependent bile acid transporter (ASBT) and also with the aid of a complex of alpha/beta organic solute transporters (OSTα/β).

Recent studies have shown that the presence of BA in the lamina propria is an adequate signal capable of suppressing the pro-inflammatory activity of Th1 and Th17 immune cells, through a reduced release of cytokines such as IL-6, IL-12, TNF-α and to promote the production of the anti-inflammatory cytokine IL-10. Furthermore, BA induce the restoration of the intestinal epithelial barrier.

These favorable functions of BA, which could be summarized in their ability to regulate intestinal inflammation and contribute to the balance between intestinal pro-inflammatory and anti-inflammatory factors, could be exploited to improve the therapeutic protocol of Chronic Inflammatory Bowel Diseases (IBD).

PHOSPHOLIPID AND CHOLESTEROL BILIARY SECRETION AND CHOLESTEROL ENTEROHEPATIC CIRCULATION

Whole-body cholesterol (CH) homeostasis is determined by cellular synthesis, uptake, and excretion and it is finely tuned to avoid excess or reduced CH content. Hepatocytes synthesize CH and take up most of the intestine-derived CH that enters the bloodstream in chylomicrons or HDL (see chapter 20).

Bile and the intestine are major routes for elimination of CH from the body because it is transformed into BA by hepatocytes or secreted as an intact molecule. CH is secreted into the bile at the canalicular membrane of hepatocytes mainly by the ABCG5/G8 transporter. The process is initiated by BA transported into the canalicular space between hepatocytes by ABCB11 (BSEP), followed by water osmotically, leading to BA simple micelle formation.

These micelles, in turn, recruit phosphatidylcholine (PC) via the canalicular transporter ABCB4 (MDR2/3), to form mixed micelles that have a high affinity for CH, which is then obtained from ABCG5/G8 or directly extracted from the canalicular membrane. SR-BI may also mediate secretion of CH into the bile, although to a minor extent. The formation of mixed micelles (bile salts, PC and CH) leads to the beneficial effect in the biliary tree of maintaining CH in solution. However, when excess CH or insufficient amount of PC is secreted in bile, the micelle solubilization capacity is reduced (CH supersaturated bile), CH crystallizes and gallstones develop. Gain-of-function mutations in ABCG5/G8 (increased CH secretion) and loss-of-function variants in ABCB4 (reduced PC secretion) are associated with an increased risk of CH gallstone disease. A second beneficial effect of mixed micelle formation is the reduction of the toxic detergent effects of bile salts on the biliary epithelium, by lowering the free (intermicelle) bile salt concentrations. Mutations in ABCB4 (MDR3) involving the reduction of PC secretion in bile are associated with genetic cholestatic diseases such as progressive familial intrahepatic cholestasis type 3, benign recurrent intrahepatic cholestasis type 3, and intrahepatic cholestasis of pregnancy (Table 39.1).

A further physiologically relevant function of biliary micellized CH takes place in the proximal small intestine, where it facilitates CH absorption and its enterohepatic circulation. CH enterohepatic circulation contributes to CH whole-body homeostasis, together with the recently discovered transintestinal CH excretion (TICE) pathway. With regard to CH intestinal absorption, the transmembrane protein Niemann–Pick type C1-like 1 (NPC1L1) is involved in the uptake of CH, of both biliary and dietary origin, from the intestinal lumen into the enterocytes. TICE is a CH excretion pathway from the blood across the enterocytes into the intestinal lumen of the proximal small intestine, resulting in CH removal from the body.

The mechanisms involved in TICE are not fully understood, however, it is clear that it is mostly mediated by ABCG5/G8 located on the apical membrane of enterocytes. Ezetimibe is a CH-lowering drug-targeting NPC1L1. This drug inhibits absorption of dietary and biliary CH, as well as reabsorption of CH excreted via TICE.

BILIRUBIN BILIARY SECRETION AND BILIRUBIN ENTEROHEPATIC CIRCULATION

Erythrocytes are broken down in the liver, spleen, and bone marrow by reticuloendothelial cells, causing the release of globin and heme. The heme ring is opened by heme oxygenase, releasing iron and carbon monoxide, and is converted to biliverdin, which is reduced to bilirubin by biliverdin reductase.

Bilirubin is insoluble in water and binds to albumin in the blood for transport to the liver. Bilirubin is transported into the hepatocyte by the basal membrane organic anion transporters OATP1 (SLCO1B1) and OATP2 (SLCO2B1). Within the hepatocyte, bilirubin is transported to the endoplasmic reticulum after binding in the cytosol to Y-protein (ligandin) and Z-protein.

In the endoplasmic reticulum, UDP-glucuronosyltransferase (UGT1A1) adds glucuronic acid to the unconjugated bilirubin, forming monoglucuronides and diglucuronides. These conjugated water-soluble bilirubin molecules are secreted into the bile through the canalicular membrane by the adenosine triphosphate–dependent efflux transporter multidrug-resistant protein MRP2 (ABCC2). Under physiological conditions, MRP3 (ABCC3) releases small amounts of conjugated bilirubin back into the blood at the sinusoidal hepatocyte membrane.

In the small intestine, bilirubin glucuronide can be excreted as such or deconjugated by b-glucuronidase and then absorbed or reduced by intestinal microbiota, resulting in various compounds. The main absorbed compound in portal blood is urobilinogen and stercobilin is excreted as the main pigment in feces. In the enterocytes, deconjugated bilirubin is glucuronidated again by UGT1A1. Recent data suggest that the bilirubin enterohepatic circulation could exert beneficial metabolic effects and increase antioxidant status and immune response. This is because mild hyperbilirubinemia associated with benign genetic (Gilbert Syndrome) and transient (physiological neonatal jaundice) conditions of reduced UGT1A1 activity have been shown to protect against different metabolic, infectious, allergic, and tumoural diseases.

KEY CONCEPTS

- The formation and secretion of bile is essential for digestion and intestinal absorption of lipids, for cholesterol (CH) homeostasis, and for the hepatic excretion of hydrophobic xenobiotics, drug metabolites, and heavy metals. Bile acids (BA) are the driving force of bile formation.
- BA, phospholipid (PL), and CH secretion by hepatocytes is finely regulated and allows micellar CH transport in bile, prevents cholangiocyte BA damage, and favors CH enterohepatic circulation.
- The efficient enterohepatic circulation of BA is regulated by negative feedback with tight control of their synthesis. BA not only regulate their own biosynthesis but also modulate important metabolic pathways regulating lipoproteins, glucose, drugs, and energy metabolism through the activation of nuclear receptors such as FXR (farnesoid X receptor) and TGR5 (G protein-coupled receptor).
- PL secretion in bile plays a key role in protecting the biliary epithelium from the detergent effects of BA.
- CH hepatic synthesis and secretion, proximal small intestine absorption, and transintestinal CH excretion are the main regulators of CH homeostasis.
- Bilirubin enterohepatic circulation is complex, and mild hyperbilirubinemia could be beneficial in the absence of underlying liver disease. BA reduce the activity of Th1 and Th17 lymphocytes and consequently the production of inflammatory cytokines. BA, together with the qualitative and quantitative improvement of the microbiota, play an anti-inflammatory role in Chronic Inflammatory Intestinal Diseases (IBD).

REFERENCES

- Boyer JL. Bile formation and secretion. Compr Physiol. 2013;3:1-44.
- de Boer JF, Kuipers F, Groen AK. Cholesterol transport revisited: a new turbo mechanism to drive cholesterol excretion. Trends Endocrinol Metab. 2018 Feb;29(2):123-33.
- Fujiwara R, Haag M, Schaeffeler E, et al. Systemic regulation of bilirubin homeostasis: potential benefits of hyperbilirubinemia. Hepatology. 2018 Apr;67(4):1609-19.
- Mertens KL, Kalsbeek A, Soeters MR, Eggink HM. Bile acid signaling pathways from the enterohepatic circulation to the central nervous system. Front Neurosci. 2017 Nov 7;11:61eb;65(2):722-38.
- Oduyebo I, Camilleri M. Bile acid disease: the emerging epidemic. Curr Opin Gastroenterol. 2017 May;33(3): 189-95.

CHAPTER 40

JAUNDICE (ICTERUS) AND CHOLESTASIS

Michele Barone, Luca Fabris

LEARNING OBJECTIVES

- To know the general principles of bilirubin metabolism.
- To recognize when hyperbilirubinemia has pathological significance.
- To distinguish the pathophysiological concept of jaundice from that of cholestasis.
- To develop a correct diagnostic approach to the patient with jaundice and/or cholestasis.

JAUNDICE

Jaundice is one of the main and most specific signs of liver disease; it is characterized by the yellowish color of the sclera, mucous membranes, and skin caused by an increase in plasma bilirubin concentration. Jaundice becomes clinically evident when the concentration of bilirubin in the blood exceeds 2.5 mg/dL, in contrast to normal values of up to 1-1.5 mg/dL and slightly higher in males than in females.

However, jaundice can be the expression not only of liver disease, but also of extrahepatic disorders that can lead to increased blood concentration of bilirubin.

Finally, there are some forms of familial hyperbilirubinemia in which increased bilirubin is an isolated finding, substantially devoid of pathological significance.

These conditions should be readily recognized to avoid unnecessary laboratory and instrumental investigations and to reassure the patient.

The main causes of jaundice can be grouped as: pre-hepatic, hepatic, and post-hepatic (**Table 40.1**).

1. Pre-hepatic: the increased blood concentration of bilirubin is produced almost exclusively by haematological disorders;
2. Hepatic: this form includes:
   - isolated familial disorders of hepatic bilirubin metabolism;
   - neonatal jaundice;
   - drug-related jaundice;
   - hepatic diseases (acute and chronic);
3. Post-hepatic: caused by obstructive diseases of the biliary tract (obstructive jaundice).

The dosage of bilirubin and, in particular, determination of the type of bilirubin (see next paragraph), constitute the first step in differential diagnosis of jaundice.

Table 40.1 Aetiopathogenic classification of jaundice

I. PRE-HEPATIC

increased production of bilirubin
- Haemolytic syndromes
- Ineffective erythropoiesis
- Transfusions
- Large haematomas

drugs that interfere with bilirubin transport

II. HEPATIC

isolated disorders of bilirubin metabolism

Familial hyperbilirubinemia
- Gilbert's syndrome, Crigler-Najjar syndrome type I, and II (unconjugated hyperbilirubinemia)
- Dubin-Johnson syndrome, Rotor syndrome (hyperconjugated bilirubinemia)

Hyperbilirubinemia of the newborn and infancy

drugs that interfere with hepatic bilirubin metabolism

acute diseases and cirrhosis of the liver

III. POST-HEPATIC

biliary tree obstruction
- lithiasis of the common bile duct
- inflammatory, traumatic, neoplastic stenosis
- ab extrinsic compression of the extrahepatic biliary tract (pancreas diseases, lymphadenopathy)

It should also be noted that serum bilirubin levels are an important parameter for the prognostic evaluation of the liver patient. In fact, the most widely used prognostic indices in hepatology, such as the Child-Pugh-Turcotte classification and MELD (Model for End-stage Liver Disease) score, include the values of bilirubin in their algorithms.

PATHOPHYSIOLOGY OF BILIRUBIN METABOLISM

Bilirubin is a tetrapyrrole compound predominantly formed in the reticuloendothelial system of the spleen and bone marrow mainly by the catabolism of the heme contained in the haemoglobin of senescent red blood cells (about 80% of the 250-300 mg of pigment produced in 24 hours). Its production strikingly increases in ineffective erythropoiesis, a disorder of heme or globin synthesis that is responsible for the destruction of developing erythroid cells in the bone marrow. Ineffective erythropoiesis can be caused by folate deficiency, iron deficiency, vitamin B6 deficiency, lead poisoning, and thalassemia. It also occurs in association with myeloproliferative and myelodysplastic disorders and congenital dyserythropoiesis.

A smaller proportion of bilirubin (<20%) derives from the heme component of haemoproteins, such as myoglobin, cytochrome, catalase, and peroxidase. The formation of bilirubin takes place in two steps, which leads to the formation and excretion of bilirubin from the heme (**Figure 40.1**):

- rupture of the ferriprotoporphyrin ring, with release of a biliverdin molecule, bivalent iron (Fe_{2+}) and carbon monoxide CO;
- transformation of biliverdin into bilirubin by the enzyme biliverdin-reductase, which requires NADPH as co-enzyme.

Figure 40.1 illustrates the pathogenetic mechanisms (in the boxes) underlying hyperbilirubinemia. The newly synthetized bilirubin, defined unconjugated bilirubin, is released into the plasma where it is covalently bound to albumin. This transport mechanism in the circulation is a protective factor of considerable importance, since unconjugated bilirubin is a toxic substance with marked lipophilicity, able to cross the blood-brain barrier and accumulate in the central nervous system (nuclear jaundice).

The unconjugated bilirubin is then captured by hepatocytes through an ATP-dependent transport mechanism mediated by membrane carriers. On the basolateral side of hepatocytes (in contact with hepatic sinusoids), the OATP2 (organic anion transporting polypeptide 2) carrier is expressed, which mediates the transport of organic anions, including bilirubin. Once inside the cytosol, biliru-

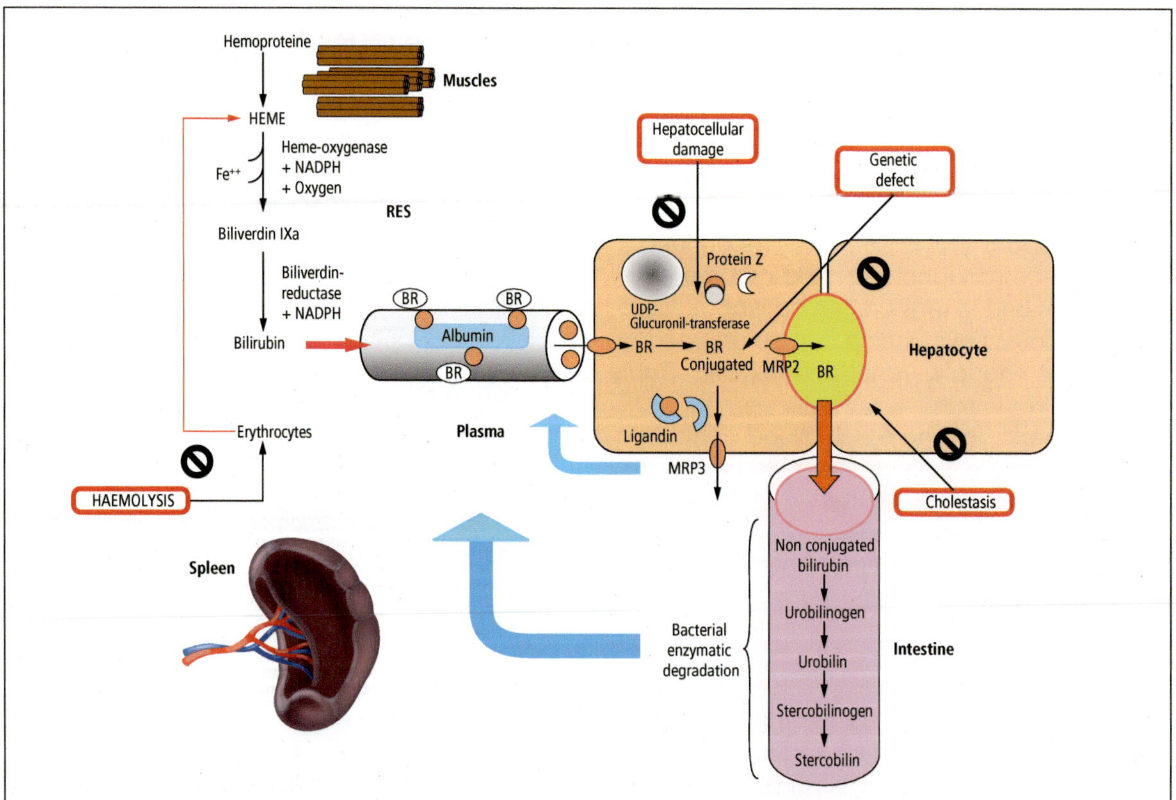

Figure 40.1 Pathophysiology of bilirubin metabolism and main causes of hyperbilirubinemia. RES = Reticuloendothelial System; BR = bilirubina; MRP3 e MDR" = multidrug resistance-associated protein 3 e 2.

bin binds to ligandins, structural storage proteins, and is then conveyed into the microsomes of the smooth endoplasmic reticulum. Here, conjugation with glucuronic acid in the form of mono- and di-glucuronide occurs by intervention of the UDP-glucuronyltransferase microsomal enzyme. Through this conjugation process, bilirubin becomes a water-soluble molecule susceptible to bile excretion. On the canalicular side of hepatocytes, a protein called multidrug resistance-associated protein 2 (MRP2) is responsible for the excretion of the conjugated bilirubin (and of other organic anions) via an ATP-dependent mechanism. A small amount of unconjugated bilirubin can also be excreted in the bile where it is solubilized by bile acids. However, only less than 1% of unconjugated bilirubin can be solubilized by this mechanism.

In humans, about 80% of bilirubin is excreted as diglucuronide. Once conjugated bilirubin reaches the terminal ileum and the colon, it undergoes deconjugation by bacterial glucuronidases and is transformed into urobilinogen. About 20% of urobilinogen is reabsorbed by the mucosa of the large intestine and excreted with the urine. The urobilinogens are colorless compounds that, in the presence of air, undergo oxidation to generate bilins, the pigments responsible for the usual color of feces.

Specific defects of the enzymes involved in the metabolism of bilirubin can cause familial hyperbilirubinemias. A reduced capacity of microsomal conjugation of bilirubin with glucuronic acid is responsible for Gilbert's syndrome and Crigler-Najjar syndrome, while Dubin-Johnson syndrome is caused by a defect in the MRP2 canalicular transporter of conjugated bilirubin.

In obstructive jaundice, there is a plasma regurgitation of bilirubin regularly conjugated by MRP3 in hepatocytes. Also, significant alterations of the expression of genes encoding membrane transporters can occur. In long-lasting obstructive jaundice, part of the conjugated bilirubin can be covalently bound to albumin, favoring the persistence of jaundice even after the resolution of obstruction.

As a consequence of the massive loss of functionally active hepatocytes, hepatic insufficiency can lead to hyperbilirubinemia. Nevertheless, in patients with advanced liver diseases, infectious events may precipitate hyperbilirubinemia, mainly due to the effect of endotoxins and pro-inflammatory cytokines that are able to down-regulate the expression of transporters involved in the metabolism of bilirubin, such as OATP2 and MRP2.

In addition to the assessment of bilirubinemia, the evaluation of urinary urobilinogen is another important indicator of morbidity. Urobilinogen is normally present in urine only in traces (up to 4 mg/24 hours). In the course of complete biliary obstruction urobilinogen is absent in the urine, because bilirubin does not reach the intestine, where the formation of urobilinogen occurs. Differently, in haemolytic jaundice, urobilinogen increases in urine. The increased production of bilirubin, which does not exceed the urinary filter, results in increased production of urobilinogen. The increase of urobilinogen in the absence of hyperbilirubinemia suggests haemolytic jaundice.

AETIOLOGY

Increased Production of Bilirubin

Several extrahepatic diseases are responsible for an increased production of bilirubin. One is the reduction of erythrocyte half-life, as can be seen in haemolytic anemia, ineffective erythropoiesis or reabsorption of a post-traumatic haematoma. Blood transfusion can also induce jaundice, due to the accelerated destruction of transfused red blood cells. In all these cases, jaundice is attributable to an excess of unconjugated bilirubin production in presence of normal function of the liver; however, bilirubin rarely exceeds 5 mg/dL.

Isolated Disorders of Bilirubin Metabolism: Familial Hyperbilirubinemias

This group of diseases includes a group of inherited conditions in which hyperbilirubinemia can be caused by the increase in both the unconjugated (more frequent) and the conjugated bilirubin fractions, in the absence of alterations of liver enzymes or other hepatic functional indices.

The forms of hyperbilirubinemia in which the unconjugated form is prevalent are characterized by reduced or absent bilirubin conjugation with glucuronic acid and may have different degrees of severity. Moderate hyperbilirubinemia occurs in Gilbert's syndrome, whereas serious hyperbilirubinemia is observed in the type I Crigler-Najjar syndrome.

In the type I Crigler-Najjar syndrome, jaundice appears between the first and third day of life. Bilirubin reaches very high serum levels between 25 and 45 mg/dL. The genetic defect responsible for this syndrome consists of complete inactivation of UDP-glucuronyltransferase (UDP-GT), which results in serious accumulation of unconjugated bilirubin. Since it cannot be eliminated in the bile, this pigment accumulates progressively in the circulation and the tissues. A nuclear jaundice frequently develops due to the deposition of unconjugated bilirubin in the central nervous system (CNS), especially in the caudate nucleus and the red nucleus (kernicterus). Bilirubin-induced neurotoxicity depends on the amount of circulating bilirubin that is not bound to albumin and the time of neuronal cell exposure. The prognosis is poor: these patients rarely live longer than 20-25 years. Several cases of good survival after liver transplantation have been reported. Transmission is autosomal recessive.

The type II Crigler-Najjar syndrome is characterized by the heterozygous mutation of the same locus, so that the residual activity of the enzyme, guaranteed by the presence of a normal allele, still allows partial conjugation of the bilirubin with glucuronic acid. In these patients, the plasma concentration of bilirubin is much lower than that observed in the type I syndrome, ranging from 6 to 20 mg/dL. The prognosis is relatively good, since patients typically survive for a long time without neurological manifestations. Both conditions are hereditary with autosomal dominant transmission.

Also in Gilbert's syndrome, a UDP-GT gene alteration has been demonstrated; patients with this syndrome are homozygous for mutations of the TATAA box, a gene promoter that controls glucuronyltransferase synthesis. These alterations, while necessary, are not sufficient to induce indirect hyperbilirubinemia that requires involvement of environmental factors, as demonstrated by the large phenotypic heterogeneity of these disorders.

Unlike the Crigler-Najjar syndromes, Gilbert's syndrome is a very common condition, with a prevalence of around 5-8% in the Italian population. The onset of jaundice is relatively late, around 15-18 years of age. Hyperbilirubinemia is almost always discovered by chance; the values of serum bilirubin range from 1.50 to 5 mg / 100 ml. Jaundice may intensify in relation to fasting, stress, physical exertion, alcohol abuse, and infections. In about 40% of persons with Gilbert's syndrome, there is also a slight decrease in erythrocyte half-life. The diagnosis requires the exclusion of other hepatocellular or biliary tract diseases that may cause jaundice. It is generally believed that two to three measurements of increased serum bilirubin, prevalently unconjugated, at intervals of several months, in the absence of other laboratory abnormalities (isolated hyperbilirubinemia), are sufficient to diagnose Gilbert's syndrome. However, a specific diagnosis can be obtained on blood samples using molecular biology analyses of single-strand conformation polymorphisms. The syndrome has an autosomal recessive transmission with incomplete penetrance and variable expressivity.

There are forms of familial hyperbilirubinemias due to the accumulation of conjugated bilirubin, such as the Dubin-Johnson and Rotor syndromes. These very rare forms are clinically characterized by an occasional appearance of jaundice, usually during pregnancy or estrogen-progestin therapy. Differential diagnosis with obstructive jaundice can sometimes be difficult, although cholestasis indices are typically normal in both syndromes. Bile pigments and increased amounts of urobilinogen may appear in the urine, while feces are normally colored. These syndromes are due to a genetic defect (mutation of MRP2 in Dubin-Johnson syndrome) involving the excretion of conjugated bilirubin through the biliary canaliculus. In Dubin-Johnson syndrome, unlike the Rotor syndrome, the liver tissue assumes a typically dark color, originally described as black liver, caused by the hepatocellular accumulation of pigment (brown granules visible at optical microscopy). Both conditions are hereditary and have an autosomal recessive mode of transmission.

Physiological Jaundice in the Newborn and Breast Milk Jaundice

These two benign conditions occur at birth. The former, due to a delay in the maturation of bilirubin metabolism, involves the non-conjugated fraction and it is observed from the 3rd to the 10th day of life. The second condition, also due to the accumulation of unconjugated bilirubin, is characterized by prolongation of physiological jaundice beyond ten days of life. It is determined by the presence in the breast milk of compounds that interfere with the function of UDP-glucuronyltransferase in predisposed subjects with genetic alterations similar to those found in Gilbert's syndrome. This form of jaundice immediately regresses with the suspension of breast feeding.

Drug-Induced Hyperbilirubinemia

Some drugs may interfere with the bilirubin transport by their competitive binding with albumin (sulphonamide - bacteriostatic). However, most drugs induce hyperbilirubinemia by their ability to specifically interfere with bilirubin metabolism at various levels (**Figure 40.2**), causing jaundice without cholestasis.

Some examples of drug-induced interference with bilirubin metabolism/excretion are uptake (tolbutamide - antidiabetic), intracellular transport to mi-

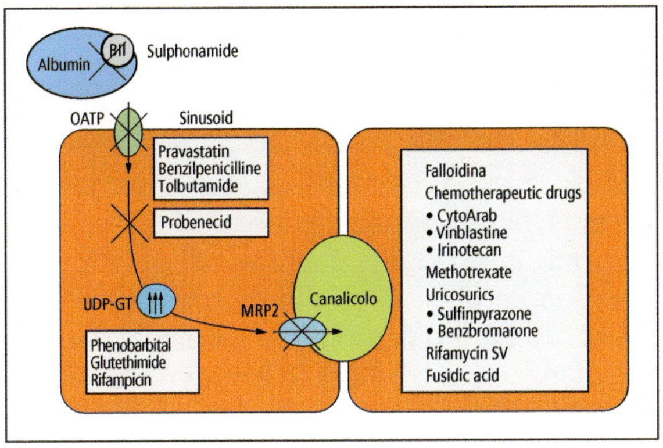

Figure 40.2 Pharmacological Interactions with Bilirubin Metabolism.

crosomes (probenecid, uricosuric) and canalicular excretion via MRP2 (fusidic acid).

It should be stressed that the key enzyme of bilirubin metabolism, microsomal UDP-GT, is responsible for the conjugation of glucuronic acid not only with bilirubin but also with numerous other xenobiotic and pharmacological compounds. Thus, different drugs can compete with bilirubin, reduce its conjugation, and lead to jaundice; vice versa, hyperbilirubinemia can increase drug toxicity by prolonging their half-life. Finally, there are drugs, such as barbiturates that ameliorate jaundice by inducing the same microsomal enzyme, an effect that is used in severe hyperbilirubinemia, as occurs in Crigler-Najjar syndrome.

Recently, drug-induced liver injury has been described in patients with familial hyperbilirubinemias, particularly with Gilbert's syndrome. Such patients should be closely monitored when under multidrug therapy or receiving with chemotherapy.

Acute and Chronic Liver Diseases

Jaundice is frequently found in various acute and chronic liver diseases.

Differently from other forms of familial hyperbilirubinemia, it is associated with liver function test alterations. In practice, all causes of hepatocyte and/or cholangiocyte damage due to hepatotropic viruses, drugs and toxic substances, vascular diseases, immunological and metabolic factors, can cause jaundice, whose degree correlates with the severity of damage. Clinically, we can distinguish two groups of liver damage associated with jaundice, hepatocellular and cholestatic damage, although not infrequently both mechanisms can coexist.

Biliary Tree Obstructions

There are multiple causes of biliary obstruction such as choledocholithiasis, intrinsic bile duct stenosis due to inflammatory (as in primary sclerosing cholangitis), traumatic or neoplastic conditions.

Extrinsic compression of the extrahepatic bile ducts is usually due to growth of neoplastic masses or inflammatory lesions of the surrounding organs (pancreas, lymph nodes). Finally, it should be noted that up to 17% of patients with major surgery or undergoing intensive care experience jaundice due to various causes.

CHOLESTASIS

Cholestasis is a complex clinical syndrome caused by multiple aetiologies, characterized by the retention in the liver and then the blood system of one or more substances normally excreted in the bile. Cholestasis is caused by the functional impairment of the regulatory mechanisms of bile secretion or by obstructive lesions affecting the intra- or extrahepatic bile ducts. The clinical manifestations of cholestasis derive from the retention in the blood of bile components and/or from the impairment of bile delivery to the duodenum.

From a pathophysiological point of view, the causes of cholestasis can be broadly classified into hepatocanalicular, where the functional defect affects the metabolic steps of bile formation in the hepatocyte, and ductular, where the secretory function of the cholangiocyte and/or the bile flow through the ductal system are compromised.

Several morphological lesions feature in cholestasis, including bile stasis into the bile canaliculi and proliferation of the smallest bile ductules at the periphery of the portal space (ductural reaction); ultrastuctural changes involve lumen dilation, with loss of microvilli and pericanalicular accumulation of microfilaments and small vesicles.

Clinical and Laboratory Characteristics of Cholestasis

The clinical and biochemical features of cholestatic syndrome (**Table 40.2**) derive from:

- accumulation in the liver, blood, and other tissues of substances usually secreted into the bile, such as bile acids, bilirubin, and enzymes normally expressed by the cellular membrane and the cytosol of the hepatocyte
- malabsorption of lipids and fat-soluble vitamins, A, D, E, and K).

Pruritus

Itching is one of the most invalidating and most difficult symptoms to treat in the management of cholestasis. It is often present in patients with cholestasis and is a more specific symptom than jaundice. It has been hypothesised that pruritus is caused by the accumulation of not yet well-identified "pruritogen" molecules usually secreted into the bile. This is supported by clinical observations that patients complaining of pruritus improved markedly following liver transplantation or after relief of biliary mechanical obstruction. A causative role of bile acids has been presumed for decades, but it remains unclear. In fact, in patients with cholestasis and pruritus, itching tends to disappear during liver failure, when serum levels of bile acids are elevated. In the last few years, strong evidence suggests a mechanism of impaired neurotransmission in the central nervous system, mediated by an increase in opioid receptor tone (m and d receptors), upon stimulation of endogenous opioids, such as enkephalins; their levels are increased in cholestatic disease, such as primary biliary cholangitis. In cholestasis, itching is usually diffuse, and it can be constant or intermittent, mild or severe. Of note, intractable pruritus may be an indication for liver transplantation. Pruritus is often associated with fatigue and daily drowsiness, particularly in cholestasis featuring primary cholangiopathies, such as primary biliary cholangitis and primary sclerosing cholangitis.

Table 40.2 Clinical manifestations of cholestasis.

Plasmatic retention of bile constituents and liver enzymes

Symptoms/signs
- Pruritus
- Fatigue
- Jaundice
- Xanthomas, xanthelasmas

Biochemical abnormalities
- Increase in bile acid serum levels
- Increase in alkaline phosphatase and GGT
- Hyperbilirubinemia (mostly from an increase in the direct fraction)
- Hyperlipemia
- Schistocytes and acanthocytosis

Malabsorption of lipids and fat soluble vitamins
- Steatorrhea, weight loss
- Osteopenia, osteoporosis
- Night blindness
- Haemorrhagic diathesis
- Peripheral neuropathy

Jaundice

Jaundice is not a common feature during cholestasis, and typically appears in the most severe forms or in the late stages of cholestasis, particularly when caused by obstructive lesions, where total serum bilirubin is a prognostic indicator of disease. Part of the serum conjugated bilirubin is covalently bound to albumin. This fraction accounts for 20-50% of total bilirubin in patients with cholestatic jaundice, whereas it is undetectable in patients with unconjugated hyperbilirubinemia. During resolution, more than 90% of serum bilirubin is still bound covalently to albumin. Disappearance of the bilirubin-albumin complex is dependent on albumin half-life (10-13 days) and not on normalization of bile secretion. This biochemical aspect can explain why, in the resolution of obstructive cholestasis, conjugated bilirubin disappears in urine more quickly than the total bilirubin in serum.

Serum Bile Acids

The bile acid pool (3-4 g) is recycled in the hepatic parenchyma about six times a day thanks to the high reabsorptive capacity of the ileal mucosa. Serum levels of bile acids are normally lower than 10 mmol/L.

During cholestasis, serum levels can increase up to 100 times above the normal range. Levels of bile acids are increased in the majority of hepatic diseases, including cirrhosis and acute and chronic hepatitis. Serum bile acids are a sensitive, but not specific, marker of cholestasis, unless intrahepatic cholestasis of pregnancy is suspected where serum bile acids are the most sensitive and specific biochemical markers.

Alkaline Phosphatase (ALP)

An increase in serum ALP is a common finding in cholestasis, often regarded as the earliest laboratory sign, and associated with a parallel increase in γ-GT, an inducible enzyme (induced, for example, by alcohol intake and by drugs assumption, such as diazepine), is less specific. Increased serum ALP levels are a sensitive cholestatic biomarker and are likely caused by the detergent effect of bile acids on the hepatocyte cell membrane.

Hyperlipidemia

Cholesterol and phospholipids are excreted into

the bile as micelles assembled by bile acids. Serum levels of total cholesterol and phopholipids are usually increased in chronic cholestasis, and serum triglycerides can be also elevated. However, in cholestatic diseases hyperlipidemia does not predispose to atherosclerotic disease.

Copper Storage
Bile is the main route of copper excretion. In chronic cholestatic diseases, such as primary biliary cholangitis or primary sclerosing cholangitis, the increase in hepatic copper content is similar to that observed in Wilson disease. However, unlike Wilson disease, serum levels of copper and ceruloplasmin are normal.

Malabsorption of Lipids and Fat-Soluble Vitamins
In long-standing cholestasis, the reduction of bile delivery to the bowel can lead to fat and fat-soluble vitamin malabsorption but it is not a frequent complication.

Overt malabsorption leads to steatorrhea, which is the production of pale, bulky, and malodorous stools, accompanied by weight loss. Furthermore, deficiency in vitamin A, K, and E may lead to loss of night vision, prolongation of prothrombin time, and neurological symptoms, including peripheral neuropathy, cerebellar ataxia, and retinal degeneration, respectively.

Cholestasis, can lead to altered blood clotting even in the short term, due to the scarcity in vitamin K storage (in fat and liver tissue). Unlike coagulopathy in liver failure, cholestasis-related coagulopathy can be corrected by parental supplementation of vitamin K.

Deficiency in vitamin D deserves particular consideration in clinical management, as it is the most frequent cholestasis-related vitamin deficit. Notably, the incidence of osteoporosis in chronic cholestatic diseases is relevant (13-35%), depending upon the severity and the duration of disease. However, additional factors besides vitamin D malabsorption can contribute further to osteoporosis, including hormones, low calcium intake, and lack of physical exercise.

Diagnostic Approach to Jaundice and Cholestasis

In the clinical work-up of the jaundiced patient, we need first to determine whether accompanying symptoms are present. In fact, jaundice in an asymptomatic patient strongly suggests a diagnosis of familial hyperbilirubinemia. Although aspecific symptoms can be present, the majority of these patients are asymptomatic. If hyperbilirubinemia is mainly indirect without signs of haemolysis (complete blood count, reticulocytes, haptoglobin, LDH), age at presentation is essential, as its onset in children coupled with total serum bilirubin values >5mg/dL suggests Crigler-Najjar syndrome, whereas onset at puberty or later in teens, together with bilirubinemia <6mg/dL, indicates Gilbert syndrome. Instead, preponderance of direct hyperbilirubinemia indicates Dubin-Johnson or Rotor syndromes (**Figure 40.3**). Otherwise, if jaundice is associated with clinical and laboratory signs of liver damage, we will next investigate the presence of chronic liver disease, and eventually its cholestatic behaviour (**Figure 40.4**).

The diagnostic approach to jaundice and/or cholestasis starts with thorough medical history and physical examination, and continues with appropriate planning of laboratory and instrumental tests. Medical history must investigate whether symptoms or risk factors for liver disease are present, such as potential exposure to risk of hepatitis virus infections, blood or blood product transfusions, alcohol abuse or ingestion of potentially contaminated food (i.e., seafood).

Abdominal pain with or without fever, previous abdominal surgery, in particular of the biliary tract, and old age should raise the suspicion of biliary obstruction. In this case, a smouldering clinical course, eventually associated with weight loss, typically occurring without pain (painless jaundice) may indicate a neoplastic origin, whereas a rapid onset, often accompanied by pain, suggests biliary stone disease complicated or not by acute cholangitis.

Drugs and xenobiotics merit special attention and deserve thoughtfulness when taking history, because their intake may not be necessarily recent. Several drugs, such as sedatives, chemotherapeutic agents and antibiotics, as well as sexual hormones (estrogens and testosterone), but also herbal remedies can frequently cause cholestasis. Generally, discontinuation leads to rapid clinical improvement and resolution; rarely, cholestasis can progress after the drug is discontinuated. At physical examination, detection of surgical scars, signs of chronic liver disease (such as spider nevi) or tenderness in the Chauffard-River area can lend further support to the diagnosis.

Depending upon the initial clinical suspicion, laboratory and instrumental investigations are then planned to confirm the diagnostic hypothesis. Serum biochemistry usually encompasses complete blood count, cholestasis indexes (bilirubin, ALP, γ-GT, bile acids), liver function tests (prothrombin time, albumin), hepatitis A, B, and C serology, specific markers for cholestatic and autoimmune diseases (non-organ specific autoantibodies, ANA and AMA above all), amylasemia.

At a first glance, assessment of routine laboratory tests usually discriminates between hepatocellular and cholestatic disease (**Table 40.3**). If a cholestatic pattern is present, detection of bile duct dilatation by ultrasound examination, indicating biliary obstruction, is the next step.

If ultrasound is not able to detect the nature of the obstruction, a magnetic resonance cholangiopancreatography (MRCP) is strongly recommended because of its high sensitivity (especially when bile ducts are dilated) and the accuracy to visualize bile duct stones or pancreatic lesions. Endoscopic ultrasound is useful for the detection of distal biliary tract or ampullary carcinomas.

If diagnosis is consistent with biliary obstruction, an endoscopic retrograde cholangiopancreatography (ERCP) should be performed to remove the stones or relieve obstruction of the bile ducts. If a pancreatic neoplasm or chronic pancreatitis has been detected, a spiral CT scan is needed for confirmation before taking the appropriate therapeutic decisions.

If the biliary system is not dilated (following assessment by ultrasound/MRCP) and laboratory findings are not clear-cut (for instance by revealing AMA-positivity), a liver biopsy should be performed.

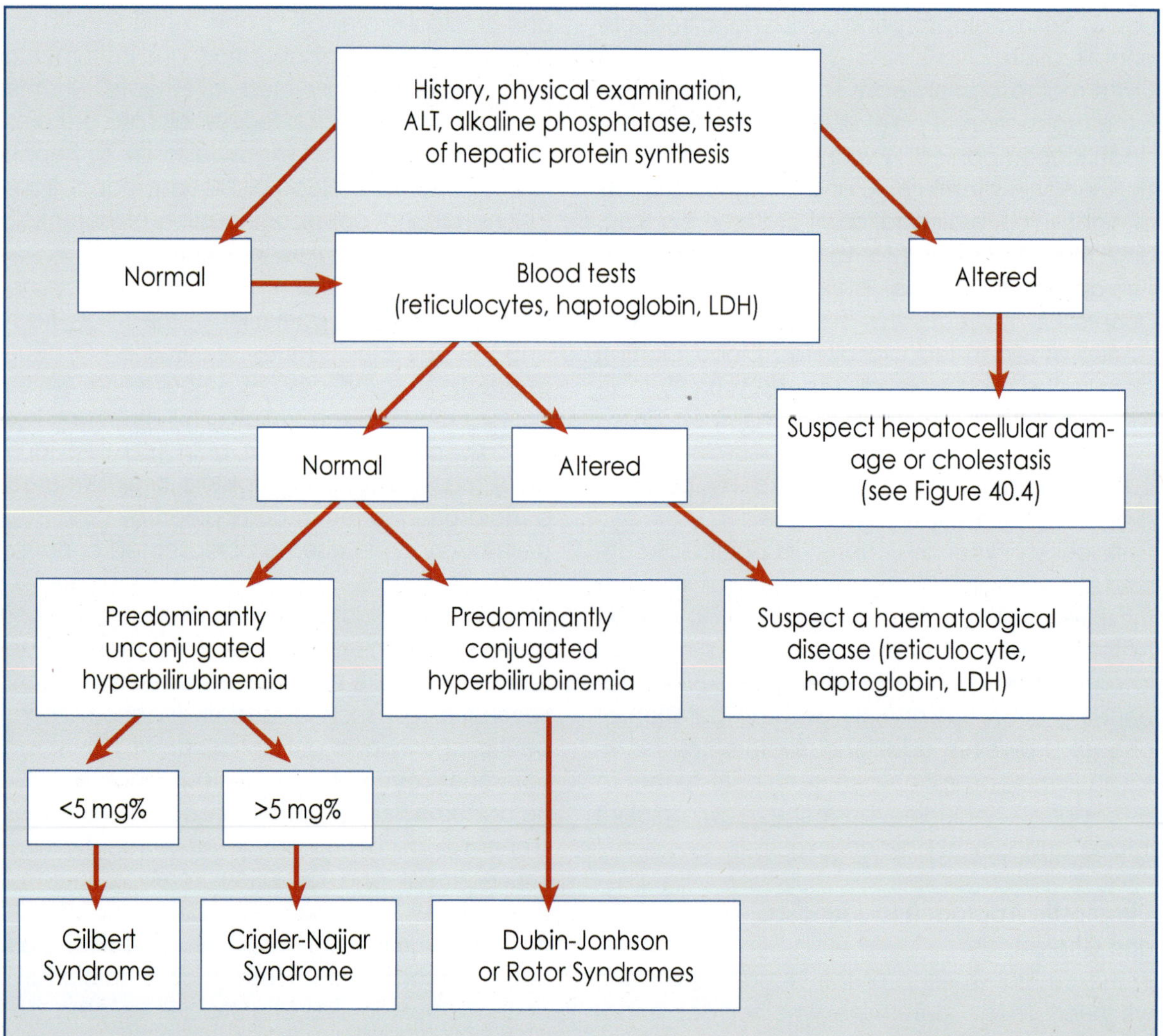

Figure 40.3 Diagnostic algorithm in isolated hyperbilirubinemias.

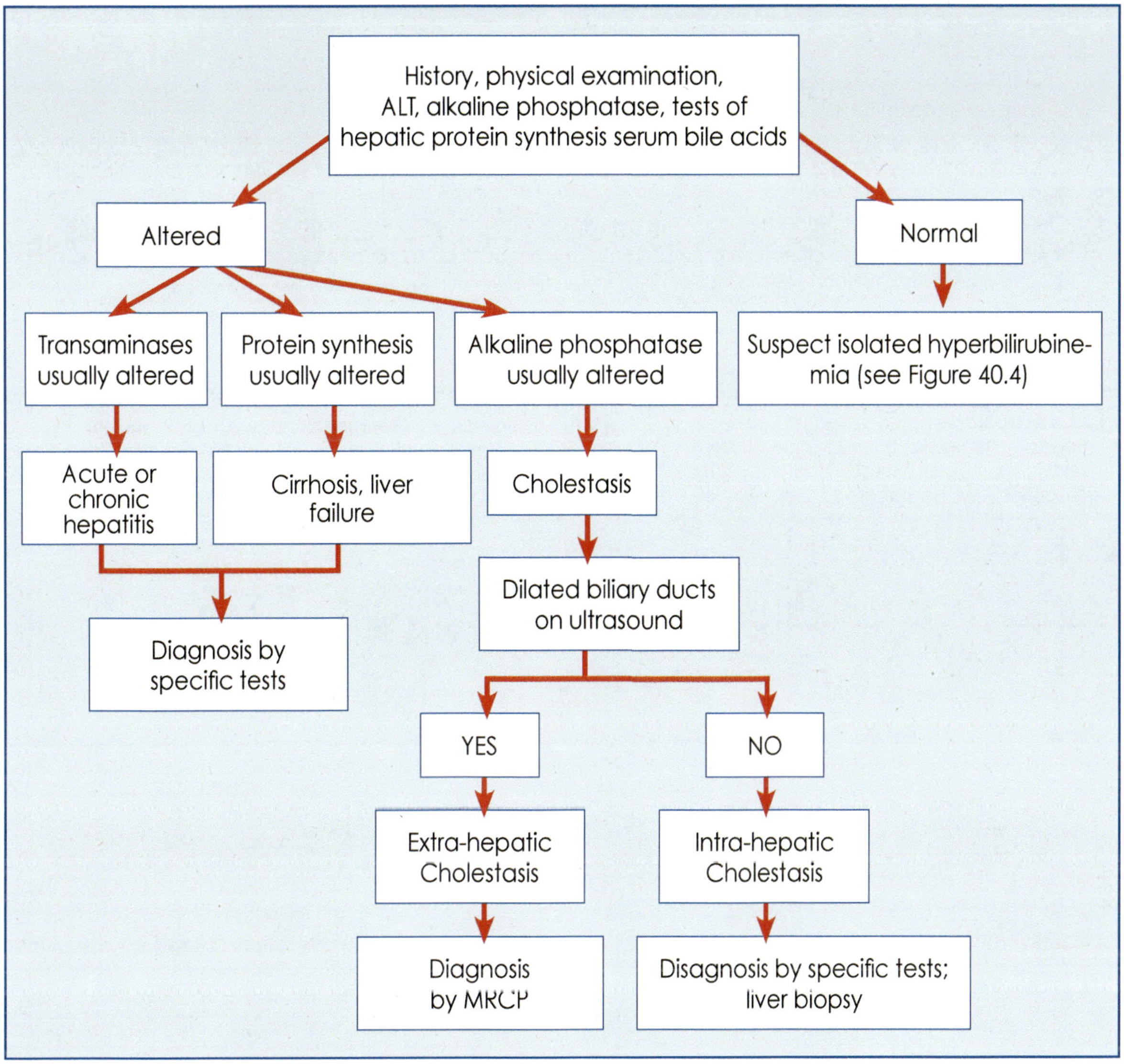

Figure 40.4 Diagnostic algorithm in hyperbilirubinemias and liver functions test abnormalities.

Table 40.3 Laboratory tests for differential diagnosis of jaundice.

Test	Hepatocellular Insufficiency	Cholestasis	Haemolysis
Bilirubin	↑ d/Unconjugated	↑ Conjugated	↑ Unconjugated
AST/ALT	↑↑ - ↑↑↑	n - ↑	n
Bille acids	n - ↑	↑↑ - ↑↑↑	n
Alkaline phosphatase	n - ↑	↑↑ - ↑↑↑	0
LDH	↑	↑ - ↑↑	↑↑↑
Aptoglobin	n - ↓	n	↓↓ - ↓↓↓
PT-INR	↑ - ↑↑ Vit. K ineffective	↑ Vit. K effective	n
Albumin	↓ - ↓↓↓	n	n

KEY CONCEPTS

- Jaundice can be a serious sign of liver disease or just a simple "cosmetic" sign of a familial hyperbilirubinemia, which may have scarce clinical significance.
- Jaundice should not be confused with cholestasis. In liver disease, jaundice could be an expression of hepatocellular insufficiency. Moreover, several extrahepatic conditions (mainly haematological) could be responsible for jaundice.
- Cholestatic liver diseases usually appear without jaundice, and may progress without jaundice for a long time.
- Pruritus and laboratory test alterations (increased serum levels of alkaline phosphatase and bile acids) are the most specific manifestations of cholestasis.

REFERENCES

- Beuers U, Kremer AE, Bolier R, Oude Elferink RP. Pruritus in cholestasis: facts and fiction. Hepatology. 2014;60:399-407.
- Hirschfield GM, Heathcote EJ, Gershwin ME. Pathogenesis of cholestatic liver disease and therapeutic approaches. Gastroenterology 2010;139:1481-96.
- Watchko JF, Tiribelli C. Bilirubin-induced neurologic damage – mechanisms and management approaches. N Engl J Med. 2013;369:2021-30.

CHRONIC CHOLESTATIC DISEASES

Marco Marzioni, Stefano Milani

LEARNING OBJECTIVES

- To know the general characteristics of the most common chronic cholestatic diseases.
- To understand the general principles of clinical management of patients with chronic cholestatic diseases.
- To identify the main differences between chronic biliary cholangitis and primary sclerosing cholangitis.

Chronic cholestatic diseases are heterogeneous disorders characterized by an impairment of bile formation and/or bile flow persisting for more than 6 months. They are associated with increased levels of serum alkaline phosphatase (ALP) and, at advanced stages, with conjugated hyperbilirubinemia. Some patients may present with persistent pruritus. Some of these diseases are associated with hepatocellular damage and may progress to cirrhosis and liver failure.

Effective therapies are limited and, at advanced stages, chronic cholestatic diseases may be an indication for liver transplantation.

In most cases, chronic cholestasis is caused by inflammatory obstruction of intrahepatic bile ducts. Progressive destruction of bile ducts associated with autoimmune inflammation, and particularly primary biliary cholangitis (PBC) and primary sclerosing cholangitis (PSC), are the most common chronic cholestatic diseases in the adult.

Less frequent causes may include direct inhibition of hepatocellular bile secretion, and either congenital or acquired damage of intrahepatic bile ducts (**Table 41.1**).

PRIMARY BILIARY CHOLANGITIS

Primary biliary cholangitis is a progressive inflammatory liver disease of unknown aetiology, leading to immune-mediated destruction of small and medium sized intrahepatic bile ducts. Formerly known as primary biliary cirrhosis, its name has been recently changed because the term "cirrhosis" identifies only the most advanced stage of the disease.

Epidemiology

Primary biliary cholangitis affects predominantly women (F/M ratio: 4/1) in the fifth decade, being rare before 25 years of age. Recent studies report an incidence between 0.3 and 5.8 per 100,000 population per year and a prevalence between 1.9-40.2 per 100,000. A north–south gradient has been reported as in other cholangiopathies, with higher incidence and prevalence in Northern Europe and the United States than in Mediterranean countries.

Pathogenesis

PBC pathogenesis is still unknown. It is believed that various environmental factors may lead to development of the disease in genetically predisposed individuals. Accordingly, PBC prevalence is particularly high in some familial clusters, and high concordance rates have been found in homozygous twins. Recent studies indicate that specific haplotypes of several human leukocyte antigen (HLA) genes may be protective against development of the disease.

The development of the disease has been attributed to a loss of immunological tolerance to biliary epithelial cells and mitochondrial pyruvate dehydrogenase complex E2 subunit (PDC-E2), with formation of specific autoantibodies against PDC-E2. These autoantibodies display a mitochondrial pattern at immunofluorescence (anti-mitochondrial antibodies, AMA) and can be demonstrated in more than 90% patients with PBC. It is not yet clear how the PDC-E2 antigen is exposed on the surface of biliary cells and the mechanism leading to AMA formation. It has been suggested that molecular mimicry with bacterial antigens, structural alterations induced by xenobiotics, and exposure of immunogenic epitopes in apoptotic cholangiocytes may be responsible for activation of the immune reaction.

Clinical Manifestations

Primary biliary cholangitis runs, for most of its course, asymptomatic or mildly symptomatic; the onset of symptoms may also arise several years after the onset of damage to the biliary tree. The most com-

Table 40.1 Vanishing bile duct diseases.

Diseases	Origin	Pathogenesis
Diseases with prevalent damage of small intra-hepatic bile ducts		
Primary biliary cholangitis	Acquired	Immune-mediated
Bile duct paucity (syndromic/non syndromic)	Congenital/Acquired	Genetic/Idiopathic
Transplant rejection	Acquired	Immune-mediated
Graft-versus-host disease	Acquired	Immune-mediated
Sarcoidosis	Acquired	Idiopathic
Adult idiopathic ductopenia	Acquired	Idiopathic
Vascular	Acquired	Ischaemic
Infections	Acquired	Viral/bacteric/parasitic
Drugs	Acquired	Toxic
Histiocytosis	Acquired	Immune-mediated
Diseases with prevalent damage of large intra- and extra-hepatic bile ducts		
Primary sclerosing cholangitis	Acquired	Immune-mediated
Biliary atresia	Congenital	Idiopathic
Cystic fibrosis	Congenital	Genetic
Caroli disease	Congenital	Genetic
Alagille syndrome	Congenital	Genetic
Fibropolycystic disease	Congenital	Genetic

mon symptom, but also nonspecific and difficult to interpret, is asthenia. A more specific symptom, which is common to all cholestatic diseases, is pruritus, whose pathophysiology is not yet clear. Generally, pruritus worsens in more advanced stages of disease, although patients suffering from this symptom from clinical onset are not infrequent. In the advanced stages, jaundice is manifested, which is an unfavorable prognostic factor. Symptoms due to deficiency in the absorption of fat-soluble vitamins may also occur in patients with long-term illness, consequent to reduced excretion of bile acids; among which osteoporosis (due to vitamin D deficiency) is the most frequent. When the disease progresses to cirrhosis, symptoms, signs and complications of cirrhosis are manifested, such as portal hypertension, ascites, oesophageal varices, hypersplenism, and hepatic encephalopathy. Monitoring of the onset of portal hypertension is of particular importance, since it may arise early compared to the degree of organic and functional impairment of the hepatic parenchyma. This places the patient with CBP at risk of early development of oesophageal varices than those with cirrhosis of other aetiologies. Not infrequently, CBP is associated with other autoimmune diseases (Sicca syndrome, Hashimoto's thyroiditis, Sjögren's syndrome), of which the patient may therefore complain of symptoms.

Diagnosis

The diagnosis of PBC should be suspected in patients, more frequently females in the 4th-6th decade of age, with persistent increase in ALP with or without pruritus and/or fatigue, after other causes of chronic cholestasis have been ruled out.

A prerequisite for diagnosis, in addition to high serum levels of AP for more than 6 months, is the demonstration of the absence of bile duct obstruction, as shown by the absence of bile duct dilatation at abdominal ultrasound. High serum titers of anti-mitochondrial autoantibodies (AMA) (≥ 1/40) are also required for diagnosis.

Serum AMAs are absent in 5-10% patients with PBC (AMA negative PBC). In these patients, high titers of anti-nuclear autoantibodies with a specific immunofluorescence pattern, nuclear dots (anti-nucleoprotein SP100) and perinuclear rims (anti-nucleoprotein gp210), may be useful to confirm diagnosis. Liver biopsy is not mandatory for diagnosis but it may be useful in patients without specific serum autoantibodies and in those with co-existent liver diseases such as non-alcoholic liver disease and autoimmune hepatitis.

Histological examination may be useful to identify typical lesions and stratify them into four histogical stages:

1. granulomatous inflammation of portal tracts with bile duct destruction;

2. periportal inflammation with reactive proliferation of bile ductules;
3. bridging (porto-portal or porto-central) necrosis with fibrotic septa;
4. cirrhosis.

Transhepatic fibroelastography may be a useful diagnostic test to assess significant liver fibrosis and cirrhosis. It has been shown that stiffness values above 9.6 kPascal identify PBC patients at high risk for decompensated cirrhosis, liver transplantation, and death.

Therapy

The aim of therapy in PBC is to prevent complications in advanced stages and ameliorate symptoms associated with the disease.
Long-time oral administration of ursodeoxycholic acid (UDCA), 13–15 mg/kg per day, is the recommended therapy.
It has been shown that UDCA can improve serum liver tests, (particularly AP can reverse to normal values), and decrease the progression of liver damage. Still unclear is the effect of UDCA treatment on survival. Patients responding to UDCA administration with an improvement in liver serum tests have 10-year and 20-year survival rates of 80% and 66%, respectively. Both are better than those observed in patients not treated with UDCA.
In most patients who do not respond to UDCA alone (about 30% of cases), the addition of either obeticholic acid (5-10 mg/day), a highly selective agonist of the Farnesoid X Receptor, or bezafibrate (400 mg/die) may improve serum liver tests.
Liver transplantation is a curative therapy in PBC with decompensated cirrhosis. It may also be indicated in precirrhotic patients with invalidating pruritus not responding to therapy.
Patient survival is 80-85% five years after liver transplantation. Disease recurrence after liver transplantation has been reported in 20% of patients.
There is no effective therapy for fatigue, whereas pruritus can be treated with oral administration of nonabsorbable resins such as cholestyramine (4 g/day) and oral administration of rifampicin (150-300 mg/day).

PRIMARY SCLEROSING CHOLANGITIS

Primary sclerosing cholangitis (PSC) is a chronic cholestatic disease characterised by multi focal bile duct strictures alternated with dilatations. Extrahepatic and intrahepatic bile ducts are both affected and progressive liver disease may ensue.

Epidemiology

Primary sclerosing cholangitis (PSC) has an incidence ranging from 0.4 to 1.3 per 100,000 per year, and a prevalence of 1.0 and 16.0 per 100,000 per year. Incidence and prevalence are higher in Northern Europe (particularly in Scandinavian countries) and the United States, whereas Mediterranean and Asian countries have low prevalence.
PSC affects mainly male patients (M/F ratio: 2/1), and clinical manifestations typically begin before 40 years of age. Signs and symptoms of inflammatory bowel disease, in most cases with the characteristics of ulcerative colitis, are present in 80% of patients, and the development of bowel disease may precede PSC for several years. PSC is formally included among the rare diseases recognized in the European Union.

Pathogenesis

The causes of PSC are still unknown; it is believed that several factors may contribute to its pathogenesis.
The immune system plays a crucial role, as suggested by a clear association with HLA and non-HLA haplotypes and the frequent finding of serum autoantibodies. Bacterial translocation across an inflamed bowel and localization in the liver of immune cells activated in the gut are also believed to participate in the pathogenic pathway. Some studies suggest that its pathogenesis may be influenced by damage of biliary tree vessels and altered of bile composition.

Clinical Manifestations

At diagnosis 50% patients are asymptomatic with persistent abnormality of liver tests. Symptoms, when present, are mainly aspecific (fatigue, abdominal pain). Signs and symptoms of biliary obstruction may occur and in some cases may indicate recurrent cholangitis (fever, abdominal pain, pruritus, jaundice).
A small number of patients may remain asymptomatic up to advanced stages of liver disease, when signs and symptoms of cirrhosis become evident.

Diagnosis

Primary sclerosing cholangitis should be suspected in young males, often affected by inflammatory bowel disease, with altered of serum liver tests, and persistent increase in ALP. In case of cholangitis, an increase of aminotransferases and bilirubin may also be observed. Normal bilirubin serum levels are present in 70% patients at the time of di-

agnosis. A progressive increase of bilirubin predicts an unfavourable outcome.
Serum autoantibodies are frequently found in patients with PSC. Perinuclear anti-neutrophil cytoplasmic antibodies (pANCA) are present in 26-94% patients. Antinuclear antibodies (ANA) and anti-smooth muscle antibodies (SMA) are less frequent. Altogether, their presence may support the clinical suspicion, but they are not specific for PSC.
Diagnosis is based on imaging of the biliary tree, with demonstration of alterations in the large bile ducts at magnetic resonance cholangiopancreatography (MRCP). In patients with contraindications to MRCP or ambiguous results, endoscopic retrograde cholangiopancreatography (ERCP) may also be used for studying biliary ducts.
Liver biopsy is not necessary to establish diagnosis. However, it may be useful for histological staging of disease.
The typical histologic lesion is the periductal concentric "onion skin" fibrosis, associated with lymphocyte infiltration of portal tracts and cholangiocyte proliferation. With disease progression, fibrosis and inflammation extend into the periportal areas (stage 2) and may form confluent fibrotic septa (stage 3). Finally, nodular regeneration and cirrhosis may occur (stage 4).
Liver biopsy may be useful for the diagnosis in patients with "small duct" PSC, in which inflammatory damage is confined to small caliber bile ducts and bile duct imaging is negative.
In addition, liver biopsy may also be useful for differential diagnosis of IgG4-associated sclerosing cholangitis, a bile duct disease often associated with type 1 autoimmune pancreatitis, that has a similar pattern of bile duct damage.

Therapy

There is no effective medical treatment for PSC. UDCA has been tested in several clinical trials, however, its effectiveness is controversial.
Its use for the management of patients with PSC cannot be recommended. Some studies have suggested that UDCA may decrease the risk of colorectal cancer in patients with PSC and ulcerous colitis, whereas the risk for the development of cholangiocarcinoma (CCA) is not modified.
A wide range of immuno-suppressive drugs (corticosteroids, budesonide, azathioprine, methotrexate, ciclosporin, mycophenolate mofetil, tacrolimus, anti-TNFa monoclonal antibodies) has been tested for the treatment of PSC, but a significant benefit has never been demonstrated.
Major strictures of large bile ducts ("dominant strictures") can be treated by either pneumatic dilatation or placement of endoluminal stents during ERCP, thus relieving obstructive symptoms and reducing the risk of recurrence of cholangitis.
Cytology specimens collected by "brushing" the bile ducts during ERCP may be useful for differential diagnosis of CCA.
Liver transplantation is recommended in PSC with decompensated cirrhosis, recurrent cholangitis or intractable pruritus. Disease recurrence is observed in 20-30% of patients after 5 years.

Surveillance

In western countries, PSC is the main risk factor for the development of cholangiocarcinoma (CCA). The risk of CCA is 161 times higher in patients with PSC than in the general population, and more than half of CCA are diagnosed within one year of PSC diagnosis.
Risk factors for the development of CCA in the setting of PSC are still not known.
The risk of colorectal cancer is higher among patients with PSC and ulcerous colitis than in patients with ulcerous colitis without PSC. Thus, a strict colonoscopy surveillance strategy is recommended for these patients.

IGG4-ASSOCIATED SCLEROSING CHOLANGITIS

IgG4-associated sclerosing cholangitis is a rare inflammatory disease of extrahepatic bile ducts with bioumoral and cholangiographic features very similar to those found in PSC.
It is often associated with type 1 autoimmune pancreatitis and other IgG4-associated diseases (orbital inflammatory pseudotumour. Mikulicz syndrome, retroperitonel fibrosis, lymphadenopaties). Unlike PSC, it is not associated with inflammatory bowel diseases and it may respond to corticosteroid treatment.
Diagnosis is based on the demonstration of at least two of the following conditions: high serum levels of IgG4, pancreatic imaging suggesting autoimmune pancreatitis, association with other diseases with infiltration of IgG4-positive plasmacells, more than 10 IgG4-positive plasmacells per high power field in biopsy specimens collected in bile ducts. In addition, a clear response to corticosteroids should be demonstrated.

KEY CONCEPTS

- Vanishing bile duct syndromes are the most frequent chronic cholestatic diseases. They may lead to chronic damage of biliary epithelia that may develop into cirrhosis and liver failure.
- Primary biliary cholangitis is an immune-mediated disease mainly found in female patients. The disease usually begins in the fourth to fifth decade of life and leads to progressive destruction of small and medium caliber bile ducts.
- Primary sclerosing cholangitis is an immune-mediated disease that mainly affects young males. It usually leads to fibrotic strictures of large intra- and extrahepatic bile ducts.

REFERENCES

- ACG Clinical Guideline: Primary Sclerosing Cholangitis. Am J Gastroenterol. 2015;110:646-59.
- European Association for the Study of the Liver. EASL Clinical Practice Guidelines: management of cholestatic liver diseases. J Hepatol. 2009;51:237-67.
- European Association for the Study of the Liver. EASL Clinical Practice Guidelines: the diagnosis and management of patients with primary biliary cholangitis. J Hepatol. 2017;67:145-72.
- Karlsen TH, Folseraas T, Thorburn D, Vesterhus M. Primary sclerosing cholangitis – a comprehensive review. J Hepatol. 2017;67:1298-323.

CHAPTER 42

CHOLELITHIASIS AND DISORDERS OF THE DUODENAL PAPILLA

Roberto Catanzaro, Maria Pina Dore

LEARNING OBJECTIVES

- To know the epidemiology, pathogenesis, and risk factors of the main forms of cholelithiasis.
- To know the clinical manifestations, complications and natural history of cholelithiasis.
- To know the diagnostic procedure and the current therapeutic guidelines for gallstones and cholelithiasis.
- To know the main pathologies of the papilla of Vater, the clinic, and diagnostic and therapeutic pathway.

GALLSTONE DISEASE

The term biliary lithiasis or cholelithiasis defines the presence in the gallbladder and/or in the biliary tree of solid bodies consisting of a mixture of cholesterol crystals, mucin, calcium bilirubinate and proteins. Biliary lithiasis can be considered a metabolic condition with a multifactorial pathogenesis. It has a high prevalence in Western countries, affecting 10-15% of the adult population, and among the gastroenterological disorders it is one of the most frequent causes of access to the emergency room.

Epidemiology

Cholelithiasis is rare in children, except in cases where haemolytic disorders are present. The formation of stones tends to increase with age in both sexes.

In the more developed countries, cholesterol stones prevail (75%), black pigmented stones (black stones) are about 20%, and brown pigmented stones (brown stones) 5%. The prevalence varies according to the population considered, being higher in whites Caucasians and Native Americans than in African Americans, Eastern Europeans and Orientals.

In Italy, at the end of the 1980s, the prevalence of the disease was 18.9% in the female population and 9.5% in the male population respectively, not diverging from the prevalence found in non-Hispanic white American males and females (8.6% and 16.6%, respectively).

The risk factors related to gallstones include:

- female sex (F/M = 2:1 due to female sex hormones that may increase the excretion of cholesterol, reducing biliary saturation), and the number of pregnancies (>2), associated with a slowing of the emptying of the gallbladder as well as qualitative changes in the composition of bile, both of which are involved in the formation of stones;
- age (5% prevalence around the age of 30 to over 25% after the age of 60);
- the ethnic group (high incidence rate among the Pima Indians of Arizona and Mexico and among the Chileans, in relation to the reduction in the secretion of bile acids);
- familiarity (and twinning) due to genetic predisposition. Among the genes involved in the pathogenesis of lithiasis are liths, involved in the regulation of hydroxymethylglutaryl-CoA (HMG-CoA)-reductase, a key enzyme in the cholesterol synthesis. The presence of mutations in the hepatic cholesterol transporter ABCG8 confers an increased genetic risk of developing gallstones;
- obesity (Body Mass Index >28 kg/m^2);
- repeated and low-fiber diets;
- rapid weight loss;
- lipid profile (high plasma levels of triglycerides and low cholesterol);
- other risk factors are truncular vagotomy resulting in gallbladder stasis, bariatric surgery, total parenteral nutrition, prolonged fasting, disorders or resection of the terminal ileum leading to increased faecal elimination of bile acids,

*The Authors wish to thank Dr. Morena Sciuto for her assistance.

use of octreotide, oestrogen-progestins and lipid-lowering drugs, which increase the secretion of biliary cholesterol, ceftriaxone and spinal cord injury;

There are also some conditions that predispose to stone formation such as Crohn's disease and ileal resection, liver cirrhosis, chronic haemolytic diseases, diabetes mellitus, peptic ulcer, ischaemic heart disease, chronic biliary tract infections.

Protective factors include diets rich in fibres and vegetable protein, mono- and polyunsaturated fats, nuts, coffee, statin therapy and physical activity.

Classification and Pathogenesis

The term gallbladder stones (or lithiasis) defines the asymptomatic presence of stones in the gallbladder. In the presence of symptoms, the diagnosis of lithiasic disease of the gallbladder is formulated, which is further divided into uncomplicated or complicated by the occurrence of acute cholecystitis, cholangitis, hepatitis, and pancreatitis. Rarer complications may be gallbladder cancer and mechanical obstruction of the ileum and/or ileocecal valve or cystic duct (Mirizzi's syndrome). Based on their main constituent, gallstones can be divided into (i) cholesterol stones (in which a small amount of calcium palmitate and bilirubinate salts may be present, (ii) black stones, composed mainly by bilirubinate and calcium phosphate, affecting subjects experiencing repeated haemolytic episodes; and (iii) brown stones, associated with bacterial or parasitic infections of the biliary tract or invasive procedures of biliary tract. Black stones are found more frequently in the gallbladder, brown stones can also be found in the bile ducts (**Figure 42.1**).

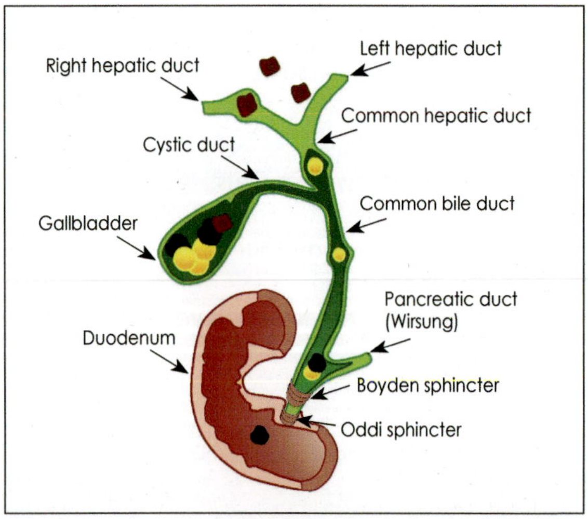

Figure 42.1 Stones distribution based on their composition.

Cholesterol Lithiasis

The aetiopathogenetic factors responsible for the formation of cholesterol stones are cholecystic hypocontractility/hypomotility and an altered qualitative/quantitative ratio of bile main components: cholesterol, bile acids and phospholipids. Cholesterol makes up over 25% of the dry weight of this type stones. Once synthesized in the hepatocyte, cholesterol is conveyed inside micelles and vesicles, whose formation involves bile acids and phospholipids which have the function of keeping cholesterol in solution. If this capacity exceeds a certain threshold, the bile is supersaturated with cholesterol, creating the conditions for its aggregation first as cholesterol crystals and subsequent formation of stones (**Figure 42.2**).

Biliary supersaturation can result from excessive secretion of cholesterol, from a reduction in the synthesis of bile acids and phospholipids or from both mechanisms. This ability is measure through the cholesterol saturation index.

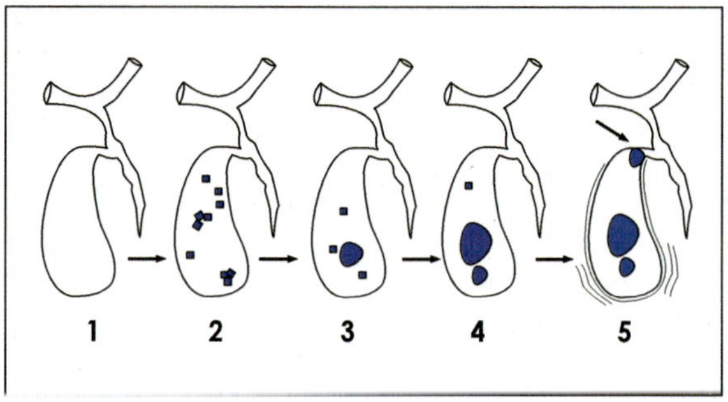

Figure 42.2 Pathogenesis of cholesterol stones (1: alitiasic gallbladder; 2: increase in cholesterol saturation index and crystal formation; 3: aggregation of crystals and formation of stones; 4: increase of stones; 5: wedging of the stone - arrow - and onset of the symptoms).

Role of Bile Acids

The hepatocyte synthesizes primary bile acids from cholesterol: cholic acid (CA) and chenodeoxycholic acid (CDCA). Both are metabolized by the intestinal microbiota and transformed into secondary bile acids: deoxycholic (DCA) by CA, lithocolic and ursodeoxycholic (UDCA) starting from CDCA. Bile acids are transported back to the liver via portal circulation, and here are conjugated with the amino acids glycine and taurine within the hepatocyte, thus becoming more stable and suitable for carrying out their intestinal functions. Bile acids, especially taurine conjugates, are in the form of anions at the pH of the bile and small intestine, and more specifically as bile salts of Na+

and K+. Their synthesis is regulated by the bile acids themselves (mainly by the CDCA), through a negative feedback on the activity of the hepatic enzyme CYP7A1. The latter promotes the transformation of cholesterol into bile acids. The production of fibroblast growth factor-19 by the intestine blocks the activity of CYP7A1.

Active transporters have also been identified in the enterocyte of the terminal ileum and in the hepatocyte, involved in the enterohepatic circulation of bile salts and responsible for a further limitation of their hepatic neosynthesis. In a person of normal weight, the absolute amount of bile acids (pool) contained in the bile is about 2 g, compared to the 12-16 g secreted daily in the intestine. In patients with cholesterol lithiasis, the total pool is decreased, while that of the DCA is increased. The type of diet could be the main cause of an increase in DCA concentrations in bile, although this increase appears more related to a prolonged intestinal transit that would favour the catabolism of CA by 7 α-dehydroxylation in DCA by the bacterial flora.

Other pronucleating factors are the inflammation proteins and the mucus in the bile, which favour an accelerated nucleation of cholesterol.

Pigmentary Lithiasis

Pigmentary lithiasis is present in about 25% of all cases of biliary lithiasis. These stones are often associated with chronic haemolysis phenomena, as observed in hereditary spherocytosis, beta-thalassemia, sickle cell anaemia, glucose-6-phosphate dehydrogenase deficiency and in general in all cases of increased haemocateretic processes and hyperbilirubinemia, as well as in alcoholics and elderly males. Brown stones can develop in any part of the biliary tree and can recur.

Clinical Features

Gallstones often remain silent throughout life and can be a casual finding during instrumental investigations carried out for other clinical indications. Only 15-25% of these patients will develop symptoms within 10-15 years and only 2-5% will require surgery due to the onset of symptoms and/or complications of the disease. Complications tend to recur with more serious complications in 30% of cases.

Lithiasic disease of the gallbladder. The specific symptom of biliary lithiasis is the biliary colic. The term 'colic' is used improperly, as the pain is continuous and not with poussées, like that typical of hollow organs. The pain is described as intense and deep, localised in the right upper quadrant, in the epigastrium, or more rarely in the cardial region, and can radiate dorsally and, more specifically, to the right scapular angle (probably due to stimulation of the posterior cutaneous branch of the phrenic nerve) or to the right shoulder. Sometimes, it can mimic the typical symptoms of gastro-oeasophageal reflux disease or angina pectoris. It is not exacerbated by movements and is not reduced following a change of position or with bowel movements. It can be associated with nausea, vomiting and generalized sweating. Generally, the pain occurs after meals, especially if high in fat, but also when fasting, although it can appear at night or early in the morning. The pain may persist for 1 to 4 hours, with a peak of about 30 minutes and then gradually disappears spontaneously. Its occurrence is quite low (0.5-1%/year), if we consider symptomatic and asymptomatic subjects overall, while the probability that a painful episode will recur is about 50%, and a complication of 0.5-1%/year.

Biliary colic is probably caused by the wedging of a stone in the cystic duct followed by contractions of the gallbladder with consequent increase in intracholecistic pressure that could trigger a condition of inflammation or be associated with it, and subsequent activation of the inflammatory cascade (cytokines, etc.).

Dyspeptic symptoms, such as postprandial fullness, early satiation, epigastric pain or epigastric burning, belching, etc., should not be considered symptoms of cholelithiasis, as they are equally present in subjects without biliary lithiasis. These symptoms usually persist, and sometimes worsen, after cholecystectomy.

Complications

Acute cholecystitis is the most frequent complication of gallbladder disease and can occur after 7-11 years in 6-11% of symptomatic patients. The suspicion of acute cholecystitis should be posed when the symptoms of biliary colic persist. The patient complains pain, with shallow breathing, may report persistent pain in the right upper quadrant and in the epigastric area, and tends to maintain a crouched position to relieve discomfort. The abdomen is poorly treatable and resistance to palpation in the right upper quadrant and epigastrium is appreciable (peritoneal pain due to stimulation of the anterior branches of the phrenic nerve, innervating the diaphragmatic peritoneum). Nausea and vomiting may be present as well, and there may be fever, mostly not elevated. Jaundice is rarely present; in this case bilirubin hardly exceeds 4-5 mg/dL. The gallbladder may be palpable and palpation of the right hypochondrium, during deep inspiration, the patient stops his or her breath (positive Murphy's sign). Laboratory tests may document neutrophilic leukocytosis and elevation of acute inflammation markers (C-Reactive Protein), liver cytolysis (transaminase) and cholestasis (gamma-glutamyltranspeptidase - γ-GT - and alkaline phosphatase). In 60-70% of cases, symptoms disappear spontaneously.

The aetiopathogenesis of acute cholecystitis is attributable to a number of factors: (i) reduced absorption of endocolecystic fluid due to parietal oedema; (ii) formation of lysolecithin from biliary lecithin by the action of phospholipases (chemical inflammation); (iii) coexistence of a bacterial infection.

Prolonged obstruction of the cystic duct by a wedged stone can determine a progressive accumulation of fluid and mucus within the gallbladder, resulting in a hydrops, often paucisymptomatic, with moderate pain in the right upper abdominal quadrant. Upon physical examination, the gallbladder is palpable as a mass of elastic consistency that can extend to the right iliac fossa.

If the contents of the gallbladder become infected, the clinical picture evolves towards a condition of empyema. The presentation is that of sepsis, with high fever, shaking chills, intense pain in the right hypochondrium or epigastrium, marked neutrophilic leukocytosis, elevation of the patient's inflammation indices and prostration. The bacteria most frequently involved belong to the genus *Escherichia coli, Klebsiella, Streptococcus, Staphylococcus and Clostridium*. During empyema of the gallbladder, the risk of perforation and septic shock is quite high, so the gallbladder must be urgently removed or drained (in cases of high surgical risk) and adequate antibiotic therapy provided.

Emphysematous cholecystitis occurs as an acute cholecystitis, but is later complicated with ischaemia or gangrene of the wall which can lead to organ perforation. The infection is sustained by gas-producing bacteria such as *Clostridium welchii or perfringens and Escherichia coli*. Comorbidities such as diabetes, vasculitis, and torsion of the gallbladder with arterial occlusion, may favour the onset of this complication.

The perforation of the gallbladder can be open in the peritoneum, or cause a fistula with the adjacent organs, more frequently with the duodenum. The event of perforation in the peritoneum is characterized by a high mortality (30%), due to subsequent peritonitis. Perforation in the adjacent small bowel, with consequent bilioenteric fistula, leads to the release of stones in the ileum; if these are large (>2.5 cm) can cause intestinal obstruction due to their impaction at the ileocecal valve (biliary ileus). Bilioenteric fistulas can be silent and develop in the presence of chronic cholecystitis, and found during surgery or diagnostic tests. It is not uncommon for biliary symptoms to disappear after fistulisation.

The presence of stones can cause inflammation that can be demonstrated by gallbladder wall thickening on ultrasound. Chronic cholecystitis is mostly asymptomatic for years and can progress to symptomatic disease or have a complication as the first clinical sign.

Diagnosis

Biliary colic is the typical symptom of cholelithiasis. In the course of biliary colic, transient changes in transaminases, γ-GTs, alkaline phosphatase and, less frequently, conjugated bilirubin are often observed. The diagnosis is confirmed by imaging techniques, primarily the transabdominal ultrasound.

Acute cholecystitis and its complications (empyema and perforation) are accompanied by an elevation of plasma leukocytes and neutrophils, inflammatory indices (ESR and CRP), transaminases, γ-GT, alkaline phosphatase and, to a lesser extent, bilirubin.

Ultrasound is the gold standard to confirm the clinical suspicion of lithiasis. It is a highly sensitive (>90%) and specific technique, widely available, non-invasive, of relatively low cost, able to visualize even stones of a few millimetres or biliary sludge. The accuracy of the method can be influenced by excessive abdominal bloating, obesity and failure to comply with fasting. In the presence of suggestive symptoms and a negative ultrasound or in the presence of an increased bile duct, second-level investigations are necessary.

In these cases, endoscopic ultrasound (EUS) can allow to visualize the gallbladder without the interference of meteorism, adipose tissue or liver, thus resulting more accurate. However, this is an invasive examination, susceptible to potential adverse events related to sedation and endoscopic examination.

Computed tomography (CT) is a technique less sensitive than ultrasound to identify stones.

Based on the tomographic density, information on the characteristics of the stone can be acquired: low-density stones are rich in cholesterol, high-density ones are rich in calcium. In the case of acute cholecystitis, CT provides information on the extent of inflammation of the gallbladder walls and the possible presence of abscess collections.

Therapy

Medical Therapy

Ursodeoxycholic acid (UDCA) is the only medical therapy currently available. The stones are dissolved by the UDCA through the solubilization of cholesterol from the surface and from the core. The remainder of the stone tends to disintegrate in the form of bile sand which is expelled with the bile. In addition, the UDCA improves the emptying of the gallbladder and reduces the intestinal absorption of cholesterol. The UDCA therapy is indicated in symptomatic patients with non-calcified, floating cholesterol stones less than 10 mm in size. The recommended dosage is 10 mg/kg/day, subdivided into 2-3 doses. Stones dissolution occurs in 70% of ideal candidates after one year of therapy; in 60% of these patients after ten years there is a relapse, frequently with multiple stones. Stone dissolution of around 20 mm in diameter is effective only in 30-50% of cases. Patients with radio-opaque or pigmented stones do not respond to UDCA therapy.

In case of biliary pain, the use of non-steroidal anti-inflammatory drugs is indicated, instead of antispasmodics.

Surgical Therapy

Laparoscopic cholecystectomy (LC), introduced in 1987, proved to be superior to laparotomic cholecystectomy, as it is less invasive, associated with less post-surgical pain, reduced length of hospitalization, fewer pulmonary complications in at-risk subjects, such as patients with liver cirrhosis, rapid mobilization, refeeding and shorter disability from work. Currently about 75% of cholecystectomies are performed laparoscopically, with a conversion rate to laparotomy in 6% of cases. The LC is also indicated in acute cholecystitis and empyema. The incidence of major and minor complications is respectively <1 and 5% if the intervention is carried out by an experienced operator. Major complications consist mostly in injury of the biliary tract, with leakage of bile into the peritoneum or stenosis of the common or intrahepatic right hepatic duct. These complications are easily managed by endoscopic retrograde cholangiopancreatography (ERCP), through the insertion of a biliary stent across the ampulla to decrease pressure in the proximal biliary system or by performing a sphincterotomy to promote free flow of bile across the ampulla.

The gallbladder empyema in patients at high surgical risk can be drained percutaneously or, more physiologically, by an endoscopic ultrasound-guided route, with the creation of a cholecysto-duodenum/gastro anastomosis, through the application of self-expandable removable metal stenting.

Lithiasis of Choledochus and Biliary Tract

Clinical Manifestations

The direct formation of stones in the biliary tree is a rare event due primarily to biliary stasis (e.g. in cystic fibrosis). Also, in people with periampullary diverticula or with bile ducts of increased diameter, as in the elderly, the risk of stones occurring in the ducts is greater. Primary gallstones are generally brown stones, consisting mainly of calcium palmitate derived by the hydrolysis of lecithin due to bacteria present in the biliary tract. Brown stones are more frequent in Eastern Asia due to the high incidence of parasitic infections of the biliary tract (Ascaris lumbricoides and Clonorchis sinensis). Stones can also occur in the intrahepatic biliary tract, upstream of stenotic segments (sclerosing cholangitis or post-surgical stenosis). The presence of stones in the biliary tract causes partial or total obstruction, mostly symptomatic, and is associated with a high risk of complications.

In 5-20% of patients with gallbladder stones, one or more stones may migrate from the gallbladder into the bile duct via the cystic duct.

Biliary obstruction causes colicky pain, sometimes intermittent, with abnormal liver function tests, mainly of cholestatic pattern (γ-GT, alkaline phosphatase and bilirubin), and moderate elevation of transaminases (mostly ALT), nausea and vomiting. In case of complete obstruction, itching and jaundice may develop. Gallstones can also be asymptomatic, especially in elderly patients, and be suspected in the presence of laboratory indices of chronic cholestasis, even in the absence of jaundice.

Complications

Possible complications of choledocholithiasis are:

- acute pancreatitis, due to the impaction of a stone in the papilla of Vater or by oedema of the latter following the passage of the stone/s into the duodenum and subsequent obstruc-

tion, even transitory, of the Wirsung duct. Oedema is more frequently mild and tends to spontaneous resolution, while the severe necrotic-haemorrhagic form can be associated with local or systemic complications;
- acute cholangitis, due to bacterial infection; presence of septic fever with chills, jaundice, and pain in the right hypochondrium constitute the Charcot's triad; it can be associated with systemic sepsis with shock and disseminated intravascular coagulation syndrome (DIC); or occurrence of multiple liver abscesses, a condition burdened by high mortality.

Diagnosis

In association with the biliary colic, transient changes in liver enzymes and cholestasis markers may be observed. In the case of acute cholangitis, neutrophilic leukocytosis and an increase in the inflammation indexes may be detected; if the pancreas is involved, a rise in amylases and lipases may be observed.
Ultrasound is the first-level diagnostic examination; in the case of gallstones it shows hyperechoic images in the biliary tract. The sensitivity of ultrasound in the diagnosis of common bile duct stones falls to 50%, since small stones located in the prepapillary area may not be identified.
Magnetic resonance imaging (MRI) uses bile as a contrast medium and allows the morphology of the biliary tract to be reconstructed in detail, although it is unable to identify stones smaller than 5 mm. The MRI is indicated when there is clinical suspicion of gallstones and a negative ultrasound, as well as for the morphological definition of the biliary tract in the presence of intrahepatic biliary tract stones.
The EUS permits to visualize the biliary tract in its retroduodenal tract, difficult to explore with conventional ultrasound, it has a high diagnostic power for choledocholithiasis being able to document in addition to small stones, also the biliary sludge in the prepapillary site, with a negative predictive value of 100%.

Therapy of Common Bile Duct and Biliary Tract Stones

The ERCP represents the method of choice in the management of stones of the choledochus and biliary tract. It is able to confirm the diagnosis and also allows treatment through the sphincterotomy of the papilla with stone removal, and clearance of the biliary tract. In the event of ERCP failure due to large stones or located in difficult to access locations, cholangioscopy during ERCP, and lithotripsy of the calculus by laser, or extracorporeal shock wave lithotripsy (ESWL) can be used. In the presence of biliary tract infection, placement of a nasal-biliary tube or removable stent may be indicated to drain and detach the biliary tract. The ERCP with biliary sphincterotomy is also the first-line treatment in case of severe acute biliary pancreatitis or associated with cholangitis. The therapeutic algorithm for choledocholithiasis is shown in **Figure 42.3**.

OTHER CHOLECYSTIC DISORDERS

Porcelain gallbladder: it is a rare manifestation of chronic cholecystitis, characterized by deposition of calcium in the gallbladder wall. It is associated with cholelithiasis in 95% of cases and an increased risk (2-3%) for gallbladder cancer. It can be diagnosed both with ultrasound and with a simple plain X-Ray of the abdomen, as the walls of the gallbladder are radio-opaque. Some authors suggest a prophylactic cholecystectomy.
Cholesterolosis of the gallbladder: is due to the accumulation of lipids (in particular, cholesterol esters) in the submucosa of the gallbladder wall, in diffuse form (strawberry gallbladder) or localized (cholesterol polyps). Cholesterolosis can be associated with cholesterol biliary lithiasis.
Gallbladder adenomyomatosis: most gallbladder polyps are benign. Most frequently they consist of cholesterol deposits or are hyperplastic or inflammatory. Malignant lesions are usually adenocarcinomas.
Polyps of the gallbladder are usually found incidentally during radiological examinations and are rarely symptomatic. No method is able to accurately distinguish a malignant polyp from a benign one. Prophylactic cholecystectomy (in order to prevent possible neoplastic evolution) is indicated in the presence of polyps > 10 mm, sessile, the patient's age over 50 years and in the presence of primary sclerosing cholangitis, while in other cases ultrasound surveillance is indicated.

Acalculous Cholecystitis

It is a condition related to a motility dysfunction of the gallbladder in the absence of lithiasis, characterized by:
- recurrent episodes of biliary pain in the absence of stones in the gallbladder;
- presence of contractile anomalies of the gallbladder, with reduced ejection fraction (<40%) on cholescintigraphy after i.v. infusion of chol-

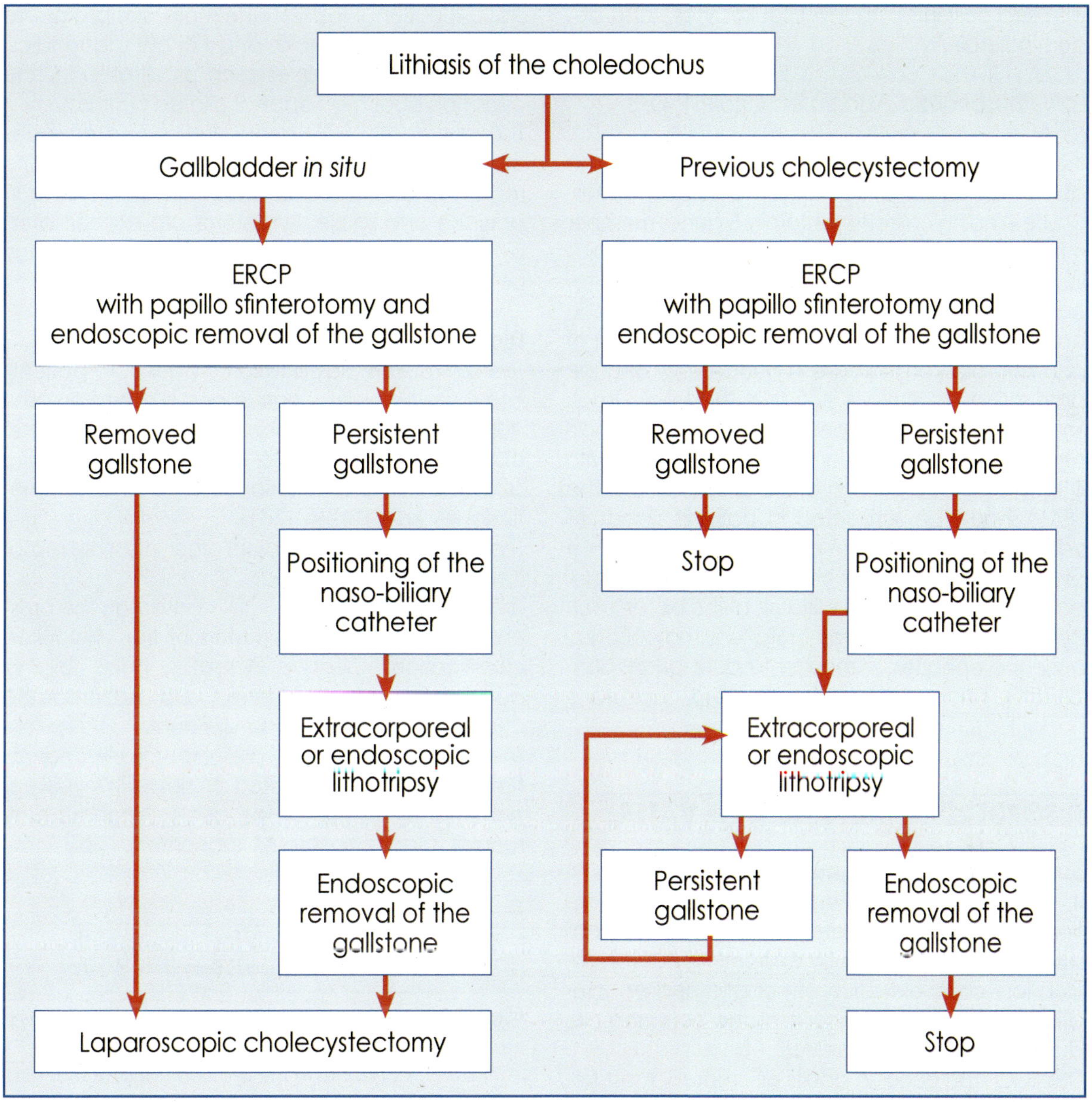

Figure 42.3 Therapeutic algorithm of choledochus lithiasis.

ecystokinin (CCK), a hormone that stimulates the contraction of the gallbladder;
- onset of painful symptoms after CCK infusion;
- abnormality of cytolysis and cholestasis enzymes during painful episodes.

However, it is believed that a large proportion of patients carry biliary sludge not detectable with imaging techniques. Cholecystectomy is the definitive therapy for acalculous cholecystitis and usually leads to symptoms disappearance.

Acute Acalculous Cholecystitis

In 5-10% of patients with acute cholecystitis, no stones are identifiable and in 50% of cases it is not possible to identify a specific aetiological cause. Symptoms are similar to those present in acute lithiasic cholecystitis. Predisposing factors include vasculitis, diabetes, torsion of the gallbladder at the level of the cystic duct, obstructing adenocarcinoma, bacterial and parasitic infections, systemic diseases, such as sarcoidosis, cardiovascular diseases, syphilis, actinomycosis and tuberculosis. The risk of acute cholecystitis is also increased in severe trauma or burns, major surgical interventions not involving the biliary tract and prolonged delivery (labour). It is a necroinflammatory disease associated with high morbidity and mortality. Clinical suspicion should be raised in critically ill hospitalized patients with fever, leukocytosis and abdominal pain.

Low Phospholipid-Associated Cholelithiasis (LPAC)

It is a rare congenital disease characterized by the association of mutations in the adenosine triphosphate-binding cassette subfamily B gene, member 4 (ABCB4) and low concentration of phospholipids in the bile, with symptomatic cholelithiasis and recurrent gallstones. The defect of ABCB4 function causes the formation of bile with a low content of phospholipids, an increase in lithogenicity and the production of primitive stones in the biliary tract. The high cleansing property of bile, poor in phospholipids, generates lesions in the biliary tract with a progressive destruction of the smaller ducts. The LPAC should be suspected in patients under 40 years of age at the onset of symptoms; recurrence of biliary symptoms after cholecystectomy, intrahepatic hyperechoic foci or lithiasis of the biliary tract. Patients with ABCB4 gene mutations may also experience episodes of recurrent acute biliary pancreatitis, biliary cirrhosis and fibrosing cholestatic hepatitis.

DISORDERS OF THE PAPILLA OF VATER

Sphincter of Oddi Dysfunction (SOD)

It is a benign clinical syndrome caused by functional (dyskinesia) or anatomical (mechanical) obstruction, characterized by abdominal pain similar to biliary colic, elevation of hepatic and pancreatic laboratory tests, dilation of the common bile duct and/or pancreatic duct.

The SOD can occur in adults or children, most frequently affects women between the ages of 20 and 50, and subjects who underwent cholecystectomy. The prevalence of SOD is 1.5% in the general population, while in subjects with idiopathic recurrent pancreatitis it can reach 72%. The real prevalence of the syndrome, however, is difficult to determine due to the scarcity of specific biomarkers or precise diagnostic criteria.

Clinical Manifestations

The SOD can affect the biliary sphincter, the pancreatic sphincter, or both. The biliary SOD is typically characterized by pain in the right upper quadrant and epigastrium, recurrent, lasting 30 minutes or several hours, not triggered by meals nor reduced by evacuation, it is not associated with diarrhoea, with or without elevation of the hepatic functional tests. Furthermore, symptoms are not relieved by antacids and / or antispasmodics. On imaging techniques such as ultrasound, the common duct may appear dilated (>8 mm).

The pancreatic SOD may cause acute episodes of pancreatitis or aching/pain in the epigastric region, radiating to the back with an increase in amylase and lipase. Symptoms are exacerbated by food intake. On X-rays investigations there may be evidence of pancreatic duct dilation.

Diagnosis

The Milwaukee classification divides SOD patients into three types (1, 2 and 3) and is based on clinical presentation and laboratory and / or imaging abnormalities related to biliary and pancreatic SOD. The Rome IV criteria classify SOD as a functional disorder (**Table 42.1**).

The coexistence of SOD with other intestinal motor disorders is also observed.

The diagnosis of type 1 SOD is based on the presence of the three parameters of the Milwaukee classification: biliary/pancreatic pain, biliary/pancreatic hyperenzymemia, and dilation of the choledochus and/or Wirsung's duct.

The SOD type 2 and 3, are respectively characterized by pain associated or not with hyperenzymemia or dilation of the ducts. Diagnosis may require Oddi's sphincter manometry (the gold

Table 42.1 Rome IV Criteria for Diagnosis of the Sphincter of Oddi Functional Disorders (SOD).

Biliary SOD
- Biliary pain
- Absence of stones in the bile ducts and/or structural abnormalities
- Elevated liver enzymes or presence of dilated bile ducts, but not both signs

Additional Criteria
- Normal levels of amylase/lipase
- Manometric alterations of the Oddi's sphincter
- Hepato-biliary anomalies on scintigraphy

Pancreatic SOD
- Documented recurrent episodes of pancreatitis (typical pain with amylase or lipase elevations >3 folds, and/or evidence of acute pancreatitis on imaging)
- Absence of other causes of pancreatitis
- Negative ultrasound examination
- Manometric alterations of the Oddi's sphincter

standard, although little used due to the risk of pancreatitis) or performing an MRI cholangiopancreatic stimulus. Secretin stimulates pancreatic secretion of water and bicarbonates, with increased secretory flow and dilation of the Wirsung duct, which tends to return to its original diameter after about 15 minutes. Persistent dilation due to slowed emptying of the pancreatic duct into the papilla of Vater is an indirect sign of SOD.

Treatment

The therapy consists of biliary and / or pancreatic sphincterotomy during the ERCP, which is successful in 90-100% of type 1 SOD cases. In type 2 and 3 SOD the efficacy is 85% and 50-60% respectively, in the presence of documented SOD (manometry or MRCP with secretin), while it drops to 35% and less than 10% in the absence of documented SOD.

Vater Papillae Adenoma/Carcinoma

Periampullary tumours are rare neoplasms that originate in the vicinity of the ampulla of Vater. Lesions can originate from the pancreas, duodenum, the portion of the common bile duct or the structures of the ampullary complex. The adenocarcinoma of the papilla is a rare condition, which develops within 2 cm from the distal end of the choledochus and Wirsung's duct and can also involve the duodenum, near the papilla.

The lesion can be sporadic and mainly affect the elderly, or develop in familial adenomatous polyposis (FAP), where the risk of developing a papilla adenoma / carcinoma in the course of life is nearly 90%. In both forms, progression is slow, while recurrence after excision is very low in the sporadic form, frequent in FAP.

Diagnosis

In majority of cases, the patient is asymptomatic and the finding is occasional, in the course of an endoscopic examination of the upper digestive tract or in the course of ultrasound or CT, which detect a dilation of the choledochus, the duct of Wirsung or both.

Additional signs or symptoms that may lead to the suspicion of the diagnosis are the presence of cholestasis or cholestatic jaundice, elevation of pancreatic enzymes, biliary or pancreatic pain, acute pancreatitis, weight loss, dyspepsia and positive stool occult blood.

Treatment

Resection is the only therapy available. Endoscopic staging of the lesion is mandatory for the choice of technique. In the presence of adenoma or intramucosal carcinoma or infiltrating the superficial submucosa, endoscopic removal Is recommended, regardless of the size of the lesion; in the presence of advanced carcinoma, surgical resection is indicated.

KEY CONCEPTS

- Biliary lithiasis is a metabolic disorder with multifactorial pathogenesis. Stones can be found both in the gallbladder and in the intra- and extrahepatic biliary tracts.
- The aetiopathogenetic factors include qualitative and quantitative alterations of the components of the bile (cholesterol, bile acids and phospholipids).
- Cholesterol lithiasis and pigmentary lithiasis are distinct. Probable risk factors of cholesterol lithiasis are: reduced gallbladder contractility, qualitative and quantitative changes in the bile components, presence of pronucleating factors, biliary stasis and hypomotility of the digestive system.
- The disease is more prevalent in Western countries and is more frequent in women, due to female sex hormones, which favour cholesterol excretion. The genes involved are the lith that regulate HMG-CoA-reductase.
- Clinically, a silent lithiasis and a symptomatic lithiasis are distinct. The specific symptom is biliary colic, characterized by pain in the right upper quadrant, epigastrium, and right angular-scapular region. Nausea and vomiting may be associated.
- Several imaging techniques, including ultrasound (the gold standard), MRI, EUS, CT are available for the diagnosis of biliary lithiasis.
- Medical treatment of gallbladder lithiasis involves the use of UDCA, surgical management includes laparoscopic or laparotomic cholecystectomy.
- Possible complications of choledochus lithiasis are acute pancreatitis and acute cholangitis, the latter associated with systemic sepsis and DIC.
- Lithiasis of the choledochus and biliary tract can be treated with a sphinterotomy of the papilla and lithotripsy during ERCP.
- The Oddi's sphincter can undergo functional (dyskinesias) or anatomical (mechanical) disorders that induce the onset of symptoms similar to the biliary colic.
- The treatment of the SOD requires biliary and/or pancreatic sphincterotomy during ERCP.

REFERENCES

- Williams E, Beckingham I, El Sayed G, et al. Updated guideline on the management of common bile duct stones (CBDS). Gut. 2017;66:765-82.
- Baiu I, Hawn MT. Choledocholithiasis. JAMA 2018;320: 1506.
- ASGE Standards of Practice Committee, Buxbaum JL, Abbas Fehmi SM, et al. ASGE guideline on the role of endoscopy in the evaluation and management of choledocholithiasis. Gastrointest Endosc 2019; 89:1075.
- Cotton PB, Elta GH, Carter CR, et al. Rome IV. Gallbladder and Sphincter of Oddi Disorders. Gastroenterology 2016; 150:1420-29.
- Lammert F, Gurusamy K, Ko CW, et al. Gallstones. Nat Rev Dis Primers 2016;2:16024.

CHAPTER 43

NEOPLASMS OF THE BILIARY TRACT

Stefano Brillanti, Gian Ludovico Rapaccini

LEARNING OBJECTIVES

- To provide elements on the site, nature, and progression of benign and malignant tumours of the gallbladder, intra and extra-hepatic biliary tract, and distal common bile duct.
- To provide guidance on the diagnostic techniques and principles of therapy for these types of cancers.

CLASSIFICATION

Neoplasms of the biliary tract are tumours of epithelial origin that may arise in the entire area of the biliary tree.
Benign tumours mainly affect the gallbladder and the periampullar region, while malignant tumours can affect all bile ducts. This chapter adopts a topographic classification (**Table 43.1**) according to the site of origin and development:

- neoplasms of the gallbladder;
- neoplasms of the intrahepatic biliary ducts;
- neoplasms of the perihilar region;
- neoplasms of the distal common bile duct.

This classification is based not only on the topographical distribution but also reflects different epidemiological and pathogenetic characteristics, clinical manifestations, and diagnostic techniques for the management of these tumours.
Unfortunately, the majority are malignant tumours and particularly aggressive, which frequently cause obstructive jaundice, altered liver function, abdominal pain and weight loss, often long before definitive diagnosis is made.

Table 43.1 Classification of tumours of the biliary tract.

Tumours of the Gallbladder	
Benign tumours	Cholesterol pseudo-polyps Adenomas
Malignant tumours	Carcinoma
Tumours of the Biliary Ducts	
Malignant tumours	Intrahepatic cholangiocarcinoma Extrahepatic peri-hilar cholangiocarcinoma Extrahepatic distal cholangiocarcinoma

Apart from a portion of tumours of the distal common bile duct, the majority carries a poor prognosis in the short-medium term.

TUMOURS OF THE GALLBLADDER

Benign Tumours of the Gallbladder

Benign tumours of the gallbladder are frequently asymptomatic and appear as small polypoid lesions of the gallbladder wall during diagnostic investigations such as ultrasonography of the abdomen. Among polyps of the gallbladder, the true neoplasm is the adenoma, which appears as a polyp of the gallbladder wall at diagnostic imaging (abdominal ultrasound, CT or MRI), hardly distinguishable from the more frequent cholesterol pseudo-polyps.
Polypoid lesions of the gallbladder wall are found in approximately 5% of patients who undergo abdominal ultrasonography. Of these, more than 50% are cholesterol pseudo-polyps, protrusions of the inner wall of the gallbladder filled with cholesterol. Generally, the pseudo-polyps of cholesterol are <10 mm in diameter do not change their position within the gallbladder lumen according to variation in the decubitus of the patient, and do not cast a shadow cone during ultrasound examination. These pseudo-polyps do not have potential for malignant transformation.
The adenomatous polyp (adenoma) of the gallbladder, instead, is much less common, reaching, however, a prevalence of 10% in some series of polypoid lesions. It is a true epithelial tumour, generally single and asymptomatic, and has the potential to evolve in adenocarcinoma. However, the majority of malignant tumours of the gallbladder arises without going through a stage of adenomatous polyp. It is not easy to distinguish adenomas from the pseudo-polyps cholesterol, because they have similar characteristics at imaging.

It is, therefore, important to establish criteria to identify adenomatous polyps "at risk" of malignant transformation, to refer patients to cholecystectomy. All polypoid lesions of the gallbladder wall >10 mm are at risk of malignant transformation and are an indication for cholecystectomy. If the polyp is >15 mm, it is at high risk of malignant transformation and prompt cholecystectomy must be performed.
Polyps <6 mm are benign and generally do not represent an indication for cholecystectomy.
More controversial is the management of polyps ranging between 6 and 10 mm. In first detection, a follow-up with ultrasound repeated every 3 months is indicated to determine whether the polyp remains stable or tends to grow. If the polyp remains stable <8 mm, periodic monitoring (every 6-12 months) is sufficient. If the polyp tends to grow rapidly, cholecystectomy should be considered even the polyp is <10 mm. Other factors associated with the potential risk of neoplastic transformation of adenoma are age > 50 years and the concomitant presence of gallbladder stones, which should be considered in the therapeutic decision.

Malignant Tumours of the Gallbladder

Carcinoma of the gallbladder is relatively rare in Europe and the Western world, with a frequently poor prognosis. The annual incidence is about 3 cases per 100,000 inhabitants. In Chile, India, Israel, and Japan the incidence is higher. It arises more frequently in females (F:M 3:1) and during the sixth or seventh decade of life.
The most frequent form (>80% of cases) is infiltrating adenocarcinoma that develops inside the wall of the gallbladder, gradually occupying the entire gallbladder lumen and extending to the liver. Less frequent is the papillary form, a polypoid type, which develops more slowly as a protrusion. Other rare forms are squamous cell, scirrhosus, and anaplastic carcinoma.
Carcinoma of the gallbladder that arises from the fundus of the gallbladder spreads by local extension to the adjacent organs, particularly the liver, omentum, colon, and duodenum, while carcinoma arising from the infundibulum infiltrates more frequently the common hepatic duct and duodenum. Lymph nodes draining the cystic duct, peri-choledochal and hepatoduodenal lymph nodes are rapidly involved (N1), then lymph node metastases may involve the retropancreatic nodes, celiac axis, aortocaval, and periaortic nodes (N2). The prominent site of metastasis by spread by venous route is the liver. Finally, dissemination on the peritoneal surface gives rise to carcinomatosis. About 85% of patients with carcinoma of the gallbladder have gallstones, a neoplastic risk factor, probably through the induction of chronic inflammation of the gallbladder mucosa. Only 1% of patients with gallstones develop carcinoma. The relative risk appears to be higher in patients carrying stones >30 mm.
Other possible risk factors are: obesity, choledochal cysts, anomalies of the pancreaticobiliary duct junction, occupational exposure to industrial carcinogens and Thorotrast, Salmonella infection, chronic cholecystitis with porcelain gallbladder, and polyps of the gallbladder. The diagnosis of carcinoma of the gallbladder does not generally occur at an early stage. This depends on the lack of precancerous lesions for screening and monitoring and the fact that the symptoms and clinical signs are the main expression of already advanced disease.
The most common symptom is abdominal pain in the upper right quadrant. Nausea and vomiting episodes and progressive loss of weight are often present. A palpable mass, sometimes painful, can be found at physical examination. Jaundice is more frequent in carcinoma arising from the fundus of the gallbladder and is a negative prognostic sign.
Laboratory tests do not reveal specific markers of carcinoma of the gallbladder: CEA and CA 19-9 have low diagnostic accuracy. Liver function tests can be altered, especially if there is an extension of the tumour to the liver or biliary tract.
Diagnostic imaging is based on: abdominal ultrasound, CT, and magnetic resonance cholangiopancreatography (MRCP). Ultrasonography and CT show a complex mass that fills the gallbladder lumen and asymmetric thickening of the gallbladder wall. CT is more accurate in identifying hepatic metastasis or neoplastic invasion of adjacent organs, lymph node metastases, and eventual vascular invasion or obstruction of the biliary tract. MRCP is, in expert hands, the best diagnostic investigation for the definition of tumour extension in the liver parenchyma, biliary tree, vascular structures, and lymph nodes.
Secondary diagnostic investigations are endoscopic ultrasonography (EUS), useful for precise definition of local extension of the neoplasm and positron-emission tomography (PET) for characterization of distant lymph node metastasis. There are no indications to perform biopsies.
The staging of carcinoma of the gallbladder is performed following the criteria of the American Joint Commission on Cancer (AJCC).

It is beyond the scope of this discussion to address in detail surgical and oncological therapy. In summary, in extensive neoplasms, precluding surgical resection, palliative interventions focus on the solution of complications (for example, placement of endoprostheses or internal-external stents in obstructive jaundice). If the neoplasm is potentially resectable, surgery, possibly followed by adjuvant chemotherapy, is the gold standard therapy. Unfortunately, the 5-year survival is < 10%. In the rare cases of complete resectability of early neoplasia confined to the gallbladder, the 5-year survival is 60%.

TUMOURS OF THE INTRA AND EXTRAHEPATIC BILIARY TRACT

Benign tumours of the bile ducts, unlike those of the gallbladder, are very rare and of limited clinical interest. The present discussion will focus on carcinoma of the biliary ducts (cholangiocarcinoma).
Cholangiocarcinoma (CCA) is an epithelial cell malignancy that may occur in any portion of the bile ducts, both intra and extrahepatic, and presents cholangiocyte differentiation. Over 95% of cases are adenocarcinoma, frequently the mucin-producing type, well, moderately or poorly differentiated. Depending on anatomical localization, three types of cholangiocarcinoma are distinguished: intrahepatic, peri-hilar, and distal. Intrahepatic cholangiocarcinoma (iCCA) arises from the intrahepatic bile ducts, the peri-hilar (pCCA) in the biliary tree between second-order bile ducts and the insertion of the cystic duct into the common bile duct, and distal (dCCA) in the section of the biliary tract below insertion of the cystic duct into the common bile duct until the ampulla of Vater. The most frequent is pCCA (approximately 50% of cases), followed by distal CCA, and the intrahepatic. In less than 10% of cases CCA is of the diffuse type or multifocal.
From an epidemiological point of view, CCA is distinct from gallbladder carcinoma. It is less frequent, with an annual incidence of 0.8-1.2 cases per 100,000 inhabitants and has a slight predominance of males (M:F=1.3:1). The onset mainly occurs in patients in the sixth and seventh decade of life.
The majority of CCA arises de novo without known risk factors. Liver cirrhosis of viral aetiology (HBV and HCV) is a risk factor for the development of iCCA. The main precancerous condition for CCA, especially pCCA, is primary sclerosing cholangitis (PSC). Chronic inflammation of the biliary ducts, characteristic of PSC, involves a relative risk of developing CCA that, depending on cases, ranges from 6 to 36%. CCA in the course of PSC generally occurs at an earlier age (fifth decade of life), often within the first two years after PSC diagnosis. In addition, in livers transplanted for PSC, CCA, not diagnosed before transplantation, is found in about 15% of cases.
Patients with PSC and ulcerative colitis have an increased risk of developing CCA, with a prevalence of between 0.2 and 0.9%, corresponding to an increased risk of over 100 times compared to the general population. The risk is greater in patients with pancolitis and a long history of the disease the onset of CCA occurs at a younger age compared to sporadic CCA.
Other risk factors for CCA are Caroli disease, choledochal cysts, biliary lithiasis complicated by episodes of bacterial cholangitis, exposure to Thorotrast, diabetes mellitus, and obesity, and in Asian countries parasitic infections from *Clonorchis sinensis* and *Opisthorchis viverrini*. Finally, in recent years, several associations between genetic polymorphisms and an increased risk of CCA have been identified.

Intrahepatic Cholangiocarcinoma (iCCA)

iCCA develops starting from the intrahepatic small biliary ducts and generally occurs as a focal lesion of the liver, which can be revealed in the course of ultrasound examination or CT. From a pathological point of view, this is an adenocarcinoma with rapid proliferation of the stromal cells, which contributes to the typical appearance of desmoplastic neoplasia. Some iCCA have a pattern of gene expression, clinicopathologic aspects, and molecular features of mixed neoplasia: hepatocellular carcinoma (HCC) and cholangiocarcinoma (HCC).
iCCA may arise in healthy and in cirrhotic liver, and may be related to infection with HBV or HCV. In the cirrhotic patient, in regular follow-up with ultrasonography, the discovery of the focal hepatic mass usually takes place during an asymptomatic phase. In patients without cirrhosis, diagnosis is generally late, when aspecific symptoms such as abdominal pain, asthenia, and weight loss are already present.
Abdominal CT and MRI are often sufficient to establish diagnosis of iCCA. In fact, unlike HCC, iCCA progressively takes up the contrast agent during the arterial and venous phases of the exam, maintaining contrast-enhancement in the venous phase. HCC, to the contrary, presents a characteristic wash-out of the contrast agent in the venous phase. iCCA in the CT scan has a typ-

ical heterogeneous uptake of contrast medium, with characteristic enhancement in the arterial phase of the margins of the lesion. However, in the rare cases of mixed neoplasia (iCCA + HCC) diagnostic imaging is not so easy. Contrast-enhanced ultrasonography is not accurate for iCCA. CT and MRI are important in defining the extension of the neoplasm and if potentially resectable.

In cases where CT and MRI are not able to define the diagnosis of the liver mass, PET with 18F-FDG is positive in approximately 80% of iCCA, and percutaneous liver biopsy can complete the diagnostic process, especially with immunohistochemistry for the identification of cytokeratin.

The determination in the serum of the tumour marker CA 19-9 is important: although the sensitivity of the test does not exceed 60%, values >100 U/mL, in the presence of a hepatic focal lesion, raises strong suspicion of cholangiocarcinoma.

Complete surgical resection, feasible in a minority of cases, is the treatment of choice. The survival at 3 years is about 45%. The high rate of relapse is a contraindication to liver transplantation.

Peri-Hilar (pCCA) and Distal (dCCA) Cholangiocarcinoma

Extrahepatic cholangiocarcinomas (pCCA and dCCA) account for the majority of CCA. pCCA arises in the region of the hepatic hilum and can grow as an exophytic mass or as intraductal neoplasia (**Figure 43.1**). Intraductal neoplasms are frequently well differentiated, have a better prognosis, and can be differentiated in nodular and periductal infiltrating. pCCA tends to spread via perineural and lymphatic invasion. dCCA develops in the portion of the common bile duct below the insertion of the cystic duct. This is an adenocarcinoma that may not be easy to differentiate from adenocarcinoma of the head of pancreas.

Clinically, 90% of patients have jaundice at the time of diagnosis, often not associated with pain but vague abdominal tenderness. Systemic symptoms such as nausea, weight loss, itching, asthenia, and malaise are present in 50% of cases. Laboratory tests reveal increased bilirubin and alkaline phosphatase values. CA 19-9 is generally high.

Diagnosis starts from abdominal ultrasound and CT showing dilation of the intrahepatic biliary ducts in pCCA, associated with dilatation of the extrahepatic biliary tract in dCCA. Ultrasound and CT also permit the definition of vascular invasion and lymph node metastases. MRCP completes the diagnostic process, defining with accuracy the level and spread of biliary cancer. More complex is the diagnosis of cholangiocarcinoma in patients with PSC and dominant stenosis detected at MRCP. In such patients it is often necessary to evaluate values of CA 19-9 (a cut-off of 129 U/mL was proposed) and perform ERCP with brushing for cytological examination and fluorescence in-situ hybridization (FISH). In unresectable cases with obstructive jaundice, ERCP can also serve to position a biliary stent. EUS can add information, but fine needle biopsy is associated with risk of dissemination of the neoplasm and is often not justified. Particular attention must be devoted to timing of diagnosis of dCCA, in so far as it has a better prognosis if early resected using pancreatoduodenectomy (25-40% survival at 5 years according to different series).

Staging of pCCA and planning the therapeutic approach has been reviewed in recent years. The most widely used system is that of the American Joint Commission on Cancer (AJCC), though different staging systems are used in some centers (classification of Bismuth-Corlette, Blumgart, De Oliveira).

The main purpose of staging is to identify resectable lesions. Unfortunately, the preoperative diagnosis often does not coincide with intraoperative staging that determines the radicality and complexity of resection. In unfortunately not very frequent cases where surgical resection has been radical, without microscopic evidence of residue of disease, the 5-year survival is 40%. Liver transplantation for pCCA is an option only in selected centers within protocols that provide for a meticulous staging and neoadjuvant therapy.

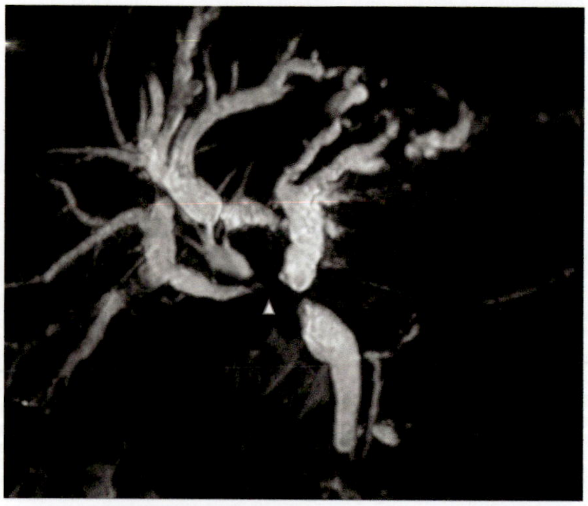

Figure 43.1 Imaging study of extrahepatic peri-hilar cholangiocarcinoma: magnetic resonance cholangiography showing biliary tree dilatation with peri-hilar obstruction and extension to the right hepatic bile duct (arrow) (courtesy of Dr. Matteo Renzulli).

KEY CONCEPTS

- Neoplasms of the biliary tract are categorized into neoplasms of the gallbladder and neoplasms of the bile ducts. Neoplasms of the gallbladder can be benign or malignant. Adenoma is the most frequent benign neoplasm and must be distinguished from frequent cholesterol pseudo-polyps, without malignant potential. Adenomas greater than 10 mm are at risk of malignant transformation and are indication for cholecystectomy.
- Carcinoma of the gallbladder is relatively rare, generally diagnosed in advanced phase, and often fatal. Controversial is the pathogenetic role of chronic inflammation due to gallstones.
- Biliary ducts are affected by cholangiocarcinoma. Three different types are distinguished: intrahepatic, extrahepatic peri-hilar, and extrahepatic distal cholangiocarcinoma. These are relatively rare and often fatal tumours.
- Primary sclerosing cholangitis is a precancerous condition for cholangiocarcinoma. It must be monitored and in dominant stenosis it requires a careful and complex diagnostic process.
- Intrahepatic cholangiocarcinoma develops as a liver focal mass and should be differentiated from hepatocellular carcinoma, especially in patients with chronic liver disease.
- If complete surgical resection is achieved, 5-year survival of peri-hilar cholangiocarcinoma can reach 40%. Liver transplantation may be indicated only in selected cases of peri-hilar cholangiocarcinoma, included in careful selection protocols with neoadjuvant therapy.
- Pancreatoduodenectomy is the surgical treatment of choice in patients with distal cholangiocarcinoma.

REFERENCES

- European Society of Gastrointestinal Endoscopy; European Association for the Study of the Liver. Role of endoscopy in primary sclerosing cholangitis: European Society of Gastrointestinal Endoscopy (ESGE) and European Association for the Study of the Liver (EASL) Clinical Guideline. J Hepatol. 2017; 66:1265-81.
- Razumilava N, Gores GJ. Classification, diagnosis, and management of cholangiocarcinoma. Clin Gastroenterol Hepatol. 2013;11:13-21.
- Rizvi S, Eaton J, Yang JD, et al. Emerging technologies for the diagnosis of perihilar cholangiocarcinoma. Semin Liver Dis. 2018;38:160-9.
- Valle JW, Borbath I, Khan SA, et al.; ESMO Guidelines Committee. Biliary cancer: ESMO Clinical Practice Guidelines for diagnosis, treatment and follow-up. Ann Oncol. 2016;27(suppl 5):v28-v37.
- Wiles R, Varadpande M, Muly S, Webb J. Growth rate and malignant potential of small gallbladder polyps. Systematic review of evidence. Surgeon. 2014;12: 221-6.

CHAPTER 44

PATHOPHYSIOLOGY OF PANCREATIC SECRETION

Giulia Martina Cavestro, Vito Domenico Corleto

LEARNING OBJECTIVES

- To know the anatomy and physiology of the pancreas.
- To know the pathophysiology of intrapanrceatic enzymatic activation.
- To know the pathophysiology of chronic pancreatic insufficiency.

EMBRYOLOGY AND ANATOMY

The pancreas develops cranially to the communication between the duodenum and the yolk sac, in an annular area immediately after the stomach where, from the fourth to the sixth week of gestation, epithelial buds originate that will form the dorsal pancreas and the ventral pancreas.

The ventral bud, from which the uncinate process originates, undergoes rotation during embryogenesis that allows it to approach the dorsal bud, which remains superior and gives rise to the upper portion of the head, the body, and the tail of the pancreas.

Fusion of the parenchyma with the two buds, takes place during the union of the two excretory ducts: the dorsal, which travels axially along the dorsal bud reaching the duodenum directly (duct of Santorini), and the ventral bud, which will accommodate the major pancreatic flow and, for this reason is called the "main pancreatic duct or Wirsung". Abnormalities in embryological development of the pancreatic gland include pancreas divisum, characterized by the lack of anastomosis between the ventral and the ductal duct.

The pancreas is 10-15 cm long, 4 cm high, 2 cm thick, weighs about 100 g, and is located in the retroperitoneal space, in front of the vertebral column and behind the stomach.

The head of the pancreas is the right end of the gland; it is flat and enveloped by the duodenal "C". The body extends to the left, crossing the vertebral column and ending with the tail at the splenic ailus. From the pancreatic head a strip of tissue called the uncinate process branches off inferiorly and to the left curves inferiorly to the body of the gland.

Pancreatic arteries are derived from the splenic artery and pancreatic-duodenal arteries; the veins flow into the portal, the superior, and the mesenteric veins. The nerves come from the celiac plexus and penetrate the organ with the branches of the arteries.

PANCREATIC PHYSIOLOGY

Exocrine Pancreas

The exocrine pancreas is composed of branched tubuloacinar glands divided into lobules separated by connective tissue. Pyramidal secreting cells line the acini and contain a Golgi complex in the cell's apical portion, surrounded by numerous granules containing inactive pancreatic enzymes. The pancreatic exocrine cells are organized in clusters, called acini in which the digestive enzymes are secreted and then conveyed to the intralobular ducts to the major pancreatic duct, which drains directly into the duodenum through the papilla of Vater.

The pancreatic juice is composed primarily of two substance: digestive enzymes and bicarbonate. The enzymes are synthesized and secreted by the exocrine acinar cells, while bicarbonate is secreted by the epithelium of cells lining the small pancreatic ducts. In humans, approximately 1500cc/day of alkaline (pH 7.0-8.3) pancreatic juice is secreted. These secretions contain a bicarbonate concentration of 115 mEq /L versus the 24 mEq /L typically found in plasma. Some 98% of the pancreatic juice is made up of water, bicarbonate, cations, and anions. The secretion of these fluids is controlled by secretin in the centroacinar cells and intercalated ducts.

The remaining 2% is made up of digestive enzymes, globulins, and albumin produced by acinar cells under the control of cholecystokinin.

Acinar Cells and Secretion of Digestive Enzymes

Pancreatic acinar cells synthesize and secrete almost all the digestive enzymes active in the lumen of the small intestine which are necessary for nutrient digestion. Both synthesis and secretion are highly regulated to ensure an appropriate supply of digestive enzymes.

In the acinar cells, digestive enzymes are synthesized in the ribosomes of the rough endoplasmic reticulum and then stored in the zymogen granules in the apical portion of the cell.

The zymogen granules are secreted into the ducts in response to hormonal stimuli controlled mainly by cholecystokinin. The composition of pancreatic enzymes in the zymogen granules may vary in response to diet or hormonal stimuli. It has been demonstrated that a low-protein diet increases proteases, with a concomitant decrease in amylase and lipase, irrespective of the carbohydrate content in the diet.

Proteases

The pancreas secretes a variety of proteases. The two most abundant are trypsin and chymotrypsin, secreted in the state of inactive proenzymes (trypsinogen and chymotrypsinogen). In the lumen of the small intestine, trypsinogen is transformed into the active enzyme trypsin by enteropeptidase. Trypsin, in turn, activates other proenzymes, including chymotrypsinogens in chymotrypsins. Trypsin, chymotrypsin, and elastase are endopeptidases that split specific peptide bonds adjacent to specific amino acids.

Other proteases, such as carboxypeptidase and hexopeptidase, split peptide bonds at the ends of proteins. Together with the proteases their inhibitoror is also secreted. This controller limits the potential damage from the release of small amounts of trypsin into the pancreas, with subsequent glandular self-digestion.

The function of pancreatic proteases is to reduce proteins into oligopeptides that, subsequently, will be further reduced in single amino acids able to be absorbed. Trypsin, once in the duodenum, activates a negative feedback mechanism mediated by cholecystokinin, which inhibits its further pancreatic secretion.

Amylases

Amylases, secreted in inactive form, hydrolyze the 1,4-glycosidic bonds of polysaccharides as starch and glycogen present in the diet. The products of the digestion of amylases (maltose, maltotriose) are then hydrolyzed to monosaccharides (e.g., glucose) by the enzymes of the brush border of enterocytes in the small intestine.

Lipases

Lipases are secreted in inactive form in a 1: 1 ratio together with colipase. Colipase is a coenzyme that optimizes the digestive action of lipase and provides for its anchoring to the lipid core of micella, promoting the hydrolysis of fatty acids in positions 1 and 3 of triglycerides and producing free fatty acids and monoglycerides.

Phospholipase A is a lipase activated in the duodenal lumen by trypsin it and hydrolyzes the fatty acid in position 2 of lecithin and phosphatidylalkonamine. Another lipase is carboxylesterase, for which bile salts are important; it breaks down cholesterol, fat-soluble vitamins, and triglycerides.

Ductal Cells and Secretion of Bicarbonate

The function of pancreatic ductal cells is to secrete sodium bicarbonate that neutralizes gastric acid in the duodenum. Bicarbonate is transported into the ductal cells by a basolateral Na+-HCO3- cotransporter then secreted in the ductal lumen by an HCO3-/ Cl- exchanger.

In pancreatic bicarbonate secretion, the CFTR (cystic fibrosis transmembrane regulator) in the chloride channel plays an important role because, if mutated, a lower concentration of chlorine is released in the ductal lumen.

Secretin, produced by the endocrine cells of the duodenal mucosa and the pancreas, is the major stimulus for bicarbonate secretion.

Islet Cells and Endocrine Secretion

The endocrine cells of the pancreas are grouped into spheroidal structures called islets of Langerhans and distributed in the exocrine pancreas parenchyma. The most numerous endocrine cells are type A (or alpha) secreting glucagon and B (or beta) secreting insulin. In humans, A cells tend to be disposed towards the periphery of the insulae, whereas B cells occupy a more central position. Two other hormones secreted by pancreatic endocrine cells are somatostatin and pancreatic polypeptide.

Regulation of Exocrine Function

Pancreatic exocrine secretion takes place to ensure efficient digestion of nutrients and adequate buffering of gastric acidity. Like gastric secretion, exocrine pancreatic secretion is subdivided into three phases:

- cephalic, caused by the smell or taste of food that can stimulate up to 50% of maximal pancreatic secretion;

- gastric, regulated by stimuli starting from the stomach as distension and content in peptides; this phase accounts for 10% of pancreatic secretion;
- intestinal, in which the gastric chyme in the small intestine stimulates the vagal fibers to secrete cholecystokinin and secretin.

Stellate Cells

Stellate pancreatic cells (SPC) are found neighboring pancreatic acinar structures. They maintain normal tissue architecture by regulating the synthesis and degradation of extracellular matrix proteins. They are differentiated from fibroblasts by the expression of numerous specific markers, such as desmin, glial fibrillary acidic protein, vimentin, nestin, growth factors, and neural cell adhesion molecules. Activated SPCs are usually found in areas of necrosis and inflammation. They are present in the periacin space with long cytoplasmic processes surrounding the base of the acinus. They can also be found in perivascular and periductal areas of the pancreas and participate in the pathogenesis of major exocrine pancreatic disorder, including chronic pancreatitis and pancreatic cancer after transformation from a quiescent state into an activated state known as myofibroblastic state.

Studies of animal models of experimental pancreatitis indicate that necrosis and inflammation of the parenchyma precede the activation of SPC, suggesting that a necrotic inflammatory process is a prerequisite for the activation of these cells. It has also been shown that SPCs have phagocytic activity in vivo and may be active as such during pancreatitis. In vivo CSP activators include paracrine factors, such as cytokines (IL-1, IL-6, IL-8, and TNF-α), growth factors (PDGF and TGF-β1), angiotensin II, and reactive oxygen species, released from damaged neighbor, cells and leukocytes recruited in response to pancreatic damage. Activated CSPs, in turn, can produce autocrine factors, such as PDGF, TGF-β1, cytokines (IL-1, IL-6 and TRAIL) and pro-inflammatory molecules (COX-2), which may maintain activation. Ethanol directly activates the SPC, most likely due to the oxidative metabolism that leads from ethanol to acetaldehyde through the enzyme alcohol dehydrogenase and the subsequent generation of oxidative stress within the cell.

Pancreatic adenocarcinomas are characterized by a notable increase in connective tissue that infiltrates and envelops the neoplastic tissue (desmoplasia). SPCs activated in pancreatic tumours are probably the main producers of extracellular matrix proteins that constitute desmoplasia. Furthermore, isolation and characterization of stromal cells from human pancreatic adenocarcinoma and chronic pancreatitis showed that cells from both sources had the same morphology, expression of cytofilament, and ability to synthesize extracellular matrix proteins.

This demonstrates that these two disorders share common stromal elements and suggests similar mechanisms underlying the development of fibrosis in chronic pancreatitis and in the desmoplasia in pancreatic adenocarcinoma.

PATHOPHYSIOLOGY

Pancreatic inflammatory diseases are characterized by two main events: intrapancreatic enzymatic activation and pancreatic insufficiency due to reduced secretion outflow.

Intrapancreatic Enzyme Activation

Intrapancreatic enzyme activation is a key element in the pathogenesis of pancreatic autodigestion in the course of acute pancreatitis.

Regardless of aetiology, intraparenchymal enzymatic activation results in anatomical damage to intracellular membranes of pancreatic cells, with a loss of intracellular compartmentalization of proenzymes. This activates trypsinogen (which seems to play a key role in the activation of all proenzymes), triggers the proteolytic cascade, and results in autodigestion of the pancreas.

The vascular endothelium and the interstitium are affected by self-digestion due to activation of the enzyme elastase, leading to digestion of the vessel walls, progressive ischaemia, amplification of pancreatic damage, and release of activated enzymes, free radicals, and pro-inflammatory cytokines into circulation. As a result, some patients develop systemic complications that involve the lung, kidney, and heart.

In acute pancreatitis, the release of digestive enzymes into the surrounding tissue and/or the systemic circulation causes various disease manifestations. The release of lipase in the pancreas, omentum, and mesentery provokes necrosis, and hydrolysis of triglycerides may lead to the liberation of fatty acids that can react with serum calcium to form "soaps", which are subsequently deposited within the fat tissue. More rarely, lipase may enter the bloodstream and cause gas necrosis, mediastinitis, and pericarditis.

Bradykinin, activated by pancreatic kallikrein,

causes vasodilation and increased vascular permeability, and hence, further spread of the enzyme.

The subsequent formation of transudate and exudate in the retroperitoneum may lead to the onset of hypovolemia and hypotension and result in shock. The action of proteases also activates coagulation factors and fibrinolysis via plasmin and factor XII, causing serious alterations in haemostasis, including disseminated intravascular coagulation (DIC).

Severe acute pancreatitis may be associated with renal and respiratory failure and acute respiratory distress syndrome (ARDS) as a result of changes in surfactant induced by circulating phospholipases or due to the damage of the renal basal membrane caused by enzymes or the deposition of immune complexes (**Table 44.1**).

In the pathogenesis of tissue and systemic damage during intrapancreatic enzyme activation, amylases and lipases play a marginal role, contrary to their diagnostic value in acute pancreatitis.

Pancreatic Insufficiency Secondary to Reduced Outflow of Secretions

A persistent obstacle to outflow, or changes in the composition of anions (particularly bicarbonate) that comprise pancreatic secretions represent the basis of chronic inflammation and fibrosis that lead to late impairment of the glandular endocrine component in the course of chronic pancreatitis.

Obstructed outflow (e.g., outcome of acute pancreatitis, pancreas divisum, sphincter of Oddi hypertension, stenosis of the papilla due to benign

Table 44.1 Systemic effects of intrapancreatic enzyme activation.

Effects	Cause
Hypovolemia, hypovolemic shock	Increased capillary permeability and vasodilation by: • activation of callicrein with bradykinin formation, peroxide formation • cellular hypoxic phenomena • destruction of blood vessels by activation of elastase
Increased leukocyte chemotaxis	Activation of the complement cascade Leukocyte release of elastase, phospholipase A2 and leukotrienes
Metabolic and electrolytic abnormalities	• Hypocalcemia (due to precipitation of calcium following the formation of soaps, hormonal alterations, calcium binding to acid-fat-albumin complexes, intracellular calcium translocation) • Hyperglycemia, hypoglycemia, keto-diabetic acidosis due to simultaneous impairment of the endocrine component
Cardiovascular insufficiency	• Hypovolemia • Primitive pump deficiency (from hypomagnesemia, inotropic effect negative of quinines, myocardial depression factor) • Reduced perfusion, DIC, mechanical compression
Kidney failure	
Acute respiratory failure (ARDS)	
Pleural effusion	• Pulmonary lipid surfactant lesion (by activation of phospholipase A2) • Interstitial hypothylation
Disseminated intravascular coagulation (DIC)	• Interaction of pancreatic enzymes with coagulation factors (thrombin activation)
Digestive bleeding	• Acute mucous injury from stress • Rupture of oesophageal varices by portal hypertension due to thrombosis of the splenic vein and leads.

or malignant tumours) or impaired viscosity of secretions (decreased bicarbonate, chloride, and water) results in increased pressure in the Wirsung duct, resulting in its dilatation, and finally the formation of calcium stones, and intraductal acinar cell atrophy.

Several exogenous factors have been associated with reduced outflow of secretions leading to pancreatic insufficiency:

- Alcohol. The pancreas metabolizes ethanol into acetaldehyde and esterified fatty acids that depolymerize membrane proteins, thus forming covalent bonds between phospholipids and membrane proteins and altering the membrane potential of lysosomes and zymogen vesicles.
- Cigarette smoking. The pathogenic mechanism of injury by cigarette smoke is not well known, however, decreased secretion of bicarbonate in the pancreatic juice, and decreased activity of the inhibitory protein of trypsinogen and α1-antitrypsin have been observed in smokers.
- Drugs: Often not considered adequately, they are among the causes of pancreatitis, either alone or in association with other factors. An updated list of drugs capable of causing acute pancreatitis is impossible due to the continued introduction of new substances and the many possible associations. Instead, it is useful to remember the mechanisms by which they can determine pancreatitis (**Figure 44.1**).
- Gene mutations. Numerous host-related factors contribute to parenchymal damage and the onset of pancreatic insufficiency by reduced or impaired pancreatic secretion. These factors include anatomical malformations and genetic alterations, directly or indirectly related to exocrine pancreatic secretion. The genetic susceptibility of pancreatitis revolves around the genes involved in controlling the activity of trypsin within the pancreas. So far, five genes have been shown to be able to cause and / or favor pancreatitis: cationic trypsinogen (PRSS1); secretory trypsin inhibitor (SPINK1); chloride channel mutation (CFTR); the chymotrypsinogen gene (CTRC); the calcium-sensitive receptor gene (CASR). PRSS1 mutations are inherited in an autosomal dominant manner, whereas SPINK1, CFTR and CTRC mutations can be inherited in multiple ways and are dependent on the transfer of mutations.

  Heterozygous mutation in the chloride channel CFTR. The heterozygous CFTR mutation in the Caucasian population has a frequency of 1 out of 25 healthy births, and determines the formation of a more viscous than normal pancreatic secretion due to the decreased efflux of chlorine and, consequently, of bicarbonate. Homozygous mutations in CFTR cause cystic fibrosis characterized by organic secretions that are far more viscous than normal. Homozygous mutations in the chloride channel may instead promote the onset of pancreatic insufficiency (chronic pancreatitis).

  Mutations of human cationic trypsinogen (PRSS1). Trypsinogen is capable of autoactivation into trypsin, which has an amino acid site responsible for self-inhibition. Familial chronic pancreatitis is associated with mutations in this self-inhibiting site, resulting in the formation of trypsin that is constitutively active.

  Mutations of the protein that inhibits trypsinogen (SPINK1). The inhibitory protein of trypsinogen physiologically inactivates 20% of the trypsin activated, which, if mutated, is no longer able to exerts its regulatory action.

  Chymotrypsinogen gene (CTRC). Digestive enzyme produced by the acinar cells, included in the zymogen granules and secreted by the pancreas with other digestive enzymes, the chymotrypsinogen destroys prematurely activated trypsin. Many functional polymorphisms have been associated with idiopathic or hereditary pancreatitis.

  Calcium-sensitive receptor (CASR). In the acinar cells, a low level of calcium limits activation of trypsinogen and its control is critical in preventing pancreatic damage. CASR plays a crucial role in maintaining calcium homeostasis through its action on the renal tubules and the parathyroid glands.

  Mutations in the CASR gene are associated with hypercalcemic syndromes and chronic pancreatitis, suggesting that these mutations are genetic factors that increase susceptibility to chronic pancreatitis.
- Human leukocyte antigen (HLA) system. In chronic pancreatitis, specific antigens of the HLA system are expressed which, under physiological conditions, are not expressed in pancreatic tissue.

  It is likely that some forms of chronic pancreatic

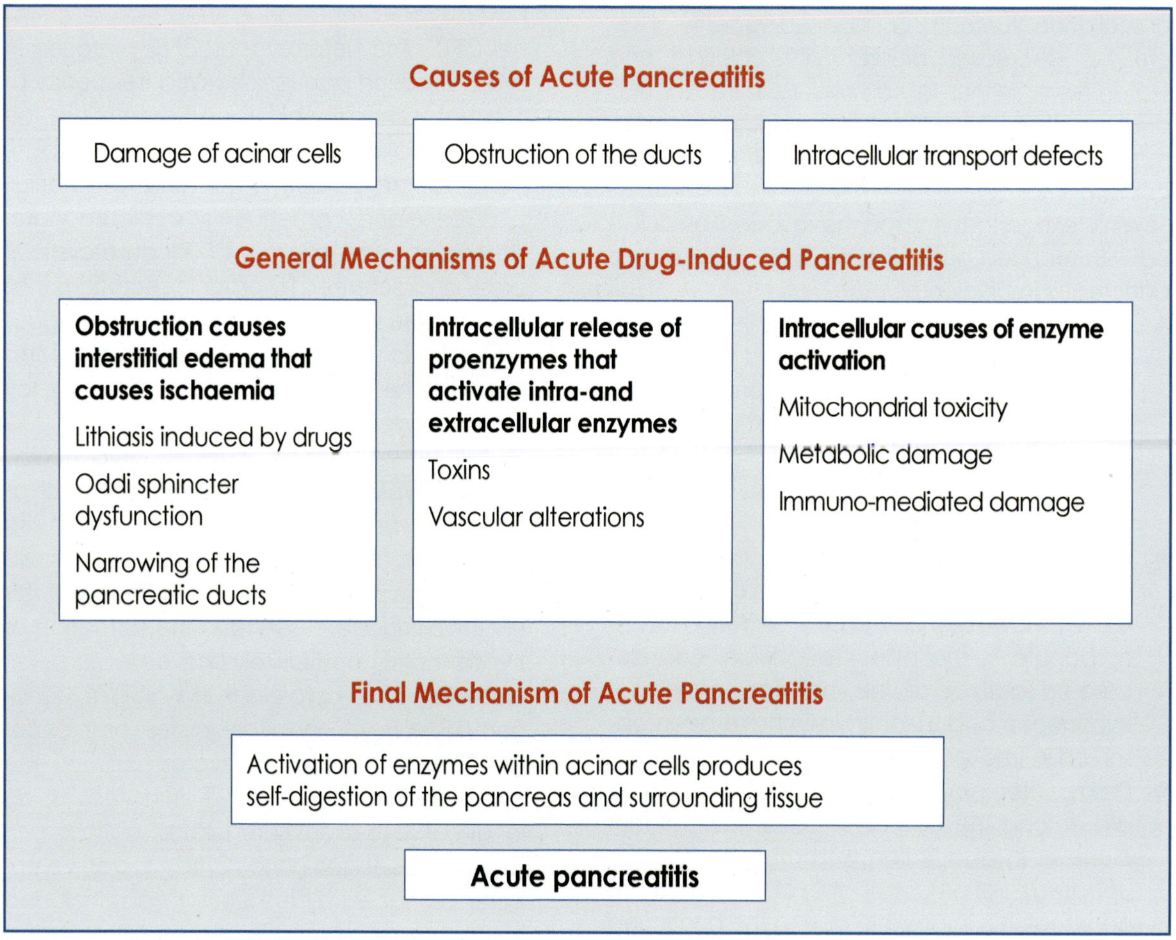

Figure 44.1 Main mechanisms of drug-induced acute pancreatitis.

insufficiency are immunomediated. In fact, the disease is sometimes associated with other immunomediate diseases, such as primary biliary cholangitis, sclerosing cholangitis, chronic inflammatory bowel diseases, Sjögren syndrome, systemic lupus erythematosus, and autoimmune pancreatitis recognized as a manifestation of IgG4-related disease.

- Pancreas divisum. During embryogenesis, the missed anastomosis of the ventral duct with the dorsal duct involves the drainage of most of pancreatic secretion through the duct (dorsal or of Santorini).
- Hypercalcemia. Hyperparathyroidism and multiple myeloma can cause calcium precipitation in the form of intraductal calculi.
- Familial dyslipidaemia type I and V. In these disorder, there is an increase in serum triglycerides with ischaemic lesions caused by vascular damage induced in microcirculation by the fatty acids produced by triglyceride metabolism.

Malabsorption and Pancreatic Pain

Atrophy of the acinar tissue, fibrotic reaction, and obstructed outflow of pancreatic secretion lead to a clinical syndrome characterized by abdominal pain of variable duration and intensity.

Abdominal pain, exacerbated by food intake, is caused mainly by:

- ductal hypertension;
- neuritis of sympathetic algogenic fibers; perineural accumulation of inflammatory cells dissolves the barrier between the surrounding connective tissue and the neural component, exposing it to the activated enzymes and the products of the inflammatory cells;
- pancreatic ischaemia resulting in increased vascular resistance and reduced intrapancreatic flow.

Lipid and protein malabsorption underlie the malnutrition observed in patients with advanced chronic pancreatitis. It is characterized clinically by weight loss, muscle hypotrophy, diarrhoea with steatorrhea and creatorrhea, lack of fat-soluble

KEY CONCEPTS

- Pancreatic exocrine cells secrete enzymes that make food digestion possible. Pancreatic secretions also contain water and bicarbonate for optimal enzymatic activation in the duodenum at an alkaline pH.
- Three phases are recognized in the regulation of exocrine pancreatic secretion: the cephalic phase - the smell and/or taste of food can stimulate up to 50% of maximal pancreatic secretion; the gastric phase - stimulation by distension of the stomach and the peptide content; intestinal phase - the gastric chyme in the small intestine, through neurohormonal stimuli, stimulates the secretion of cholecystokinin and secretin.
- Cellular and secretory factors, combined with specific enzyme synthesis, prevent premature activation in the pancreatic gland. Intrapancreatic enzyme activation is the key pathogenetic element in the development of pancreatic self-digestion during acute pancreatitis. The extent of cascade activation of enzymes and cytokines determines the severity of local and systemic damage and multi-organ dysfunction.
- A persistent outflow obstruction of secretions or alterations in the anion composition (especially bicarbonate) of pancreatic secretion underlie chronic inflammation, with fibrous substitution and late compromise of the endocrine glandular component, in chronic pancreatitis.
- Several exogenous factors associated with reduced pancreatic insufficiency or impaired secretion outflow have been identified; alcohol and tobacco consumption, but also drugs, although often these are not properly considered. Other factors contributing to parenchymal damage and onset of pancreatic insufficiency are related to the host and include anatomical malformations and genetic alterations directly or indirectly related to exocrine pancreatic secretion.
- The pain exacerbated by food intake is the basis of malnutrition during chronic pancreatitis and one of the symptoms in pancreatic disease. It is caused by obstructive ductal hypertension, neural inflammatory phenomena, and pancreatic ischaemia resulting in increased vascular resistance and reduced intrapancreatic flow.

vitamins (A, D, E, K).

REFERENCES

- Hung WY, Lanfranco OA. Contemporary review of drug-induced pancreatitis: a different perspective. World J Gastrointest Pathophysiol. 2014;15:405-15.
- Pandol SJ. Pancreatic secretion. In: Feldman M, Friedman LS, Brandt LJ, eds. Sleisenger and Fordtran's gastrointestinal and liver disease: pathophysiology, diagnosis, management. 10th edition. Philadelphia: Elsevier Saunders 2016;934-43.
- Solomon S, Whitcomb DC. Genetics of pancreatitis: an update for clinicians and genetic counselors. Curr Gastroenterol Rep. 2012;14:112-7.

CHAPTER 45

ACUTE PANCREATITIS

Giovanni Cammarota, Mirko Tarocchi

LEARNING OBJECTIVES

- To know the definition and classification of acute pancreatitis.
- To know its epidemiology.
- To know its aetiology.
- To know its main clinical manifestations.
- To define diagnostic criteria (laboratory data and imaging). Identify elements for diagnosis.
- To know the natural history of the disease and its complications. Acquire notions for clinical and therapeutic management.

DEFINITION AND CLASSIFICATION

Acute pancreatitis is an inflammatory condition of the pancreas characterized clinically by abdominal pain and elevated levels of pancreatic enzymes in the blood.

According to the Atlanta classification, acute pancreatitis can be divided into two broad categories:

- Interstitial edematous acute pancreatitis: acute inflammation of the pancreatic parenchyma and peripancreatic tissues, but without recognizable tissue necrosis
- Necrotizing acute pancreatitis: inflammation associated with pancreatic parenchymal necrosis and/or peripancreatic necrosis

According to its severity, acute pancreatitis is graded as:

- Mild acute pancreatitis: absence of organ failure and local or systemic complications
- Moderately severe acute pancreatitis: no organ failure or transient organ failure (<48 hours) and/or local complications
- Severe acute pancreatitis: persistent organ failure (more than 48 hours) that may involve one or multiple organs

EPIDEMIOLOGICAL DATA

Acute pancreatitis is the main gastrointestinal cause of hospitalization in the United States. Its incidence is increasing, especially in some European and Scandinavian countries, due to the relative increase in alcohol consumption and improved diagnostic capacity.

The reported annual incidence of acute pancreatitis ranges from 4.9 to 35 cases per 100,000 inhabitants; however, an accurate estimate of the incidence and mortality of acute pancreatitis is difficult, as a mild form of pancreatitis may present with very blurred clinical symptoms, and in severe and fulminant cases, deaths may occur before diagnosis is made.

Nonetheless, progress in diagnosis and treatment has led to a decrease in mortality, especially in severe acute pancreatitis.

In such cases, mortality in acute pancreatitis is usually due to systemic inflammatory response syndrome and organ failure in the first two-week period, while after two weeks it is usually due to sepsis and its complications. The overall mortality rate is 5% (1.5% in mild acute pancreatitis and 17% in severe pancreatitis).

AETIOLOGY

The aetiology of acute pancreatitis can be established in nearly 75% of patients.

Mechanical Vater's Ampullary Obstruction

Gallstones

Gallstones (including microlithiasis) are the most frequent cause, being responsible for acute pancreatic inflammation in 35-40% of cases and in most areas of the world. Only 3-7% of patients with gallstones develop acute pancreatitis. The risk is higher in men, although the incidence of biliary pancreatitis is higher in women due to a higher relative prevalence of gallstones.

Obstruction of the ampoule calculi can be transient, and favor reflux of bile into the pancreatic duct, or permanent, and associated with surrounding edema.

Biliary Sludge and Microlitiasis

Biliary sludge is a viscous suspension in the bile, which also contains microcalcules (<5 mm in diameter), which is formed due to changes in the hepatic bile within the gallbladder. Most patients with biliary sludge are asymptomatic. However, bile mud is present in 20-40% of patients with acute pancreatitis without an obvious cause. In such cases, biliary sludge should be suspected as the possible cause of pancreatitis.

Other

Other conditions that cause Vater's ampoule obstruction and have been associated with acute pancreatitis include biliary ascariasis, periampullary diverticula, pancreatic, and periampullary tumours. Intraductal papillary mucinous neoplasms (IPMN) of the pancreas are an occasional finding, especially in older males.

Alcohol

Alcohol is responsible for about 30% of cases of acute pancreatitis in the United States. About 10% of chronic alcoholics develop clinically acute pancreatitis attacks. The exact mechanism of pancreatic damage caused by alcohol and why only a small percentage of alcoholics develop pancreatitis are unclear.

However, it is believed that alcohol can act by causing inappropriate activation of the digestive and lysosomal enzymes produced by acinar pancreatic cells and alteration of the sphincter motility of Oddi. Initially, it was thought that alcoholics with clinically acute pancreatitis had a chronic underlying disease. However, long-term follow-up studies of patients with acute alcoholic pancreatitis have shown that not all patients progress to chronic pancreatitis, even with continued alcohol abuse.

Smoking

Cigarette smoking is an independent risk factor for acute and chronic pancreatitis, with mechanisms that are still unclear.

Hypertriglyceridemia

Acute hypertriglyceridemia pancreatitis is diagnosed when the serum triglyceride concentration is >1000 mg/dL (11 mmol/l) and accounts for 1-4% of cases of disease. Recent studies show, however, that the risk of disease and its severity correlate directly with the increase in serum triglyceride levels. The pathogenesis of inflammation in this peculiar clinical condition is not clear.

Post-Endoscopic Retrograde Cholangiopancreatography (ERCP)

Acute pancreatitis occurs in about 5% of patients undergoing ERCP. It should be kept in mind, however, that asymptomatic hyperamylasemia (non-pancreatitis) occurs in 35-70% of patients undergoing ERCP.

Hypercalcemia

Hypercalcemia from any cause can cause acute pancreatitis. The mechanisms appear to be the deposition of calcium in the pancreatic duct and activation of trypsinogen in the pancreatic parenchyma.

Genetic Mutations

Several genetic mutations, including those involving PRSS1 (cationic trypsinogen), CFTR (ion channel involved in cystic fibrosis), SPNK1 (inhibitor of pancreatic trypsin secretion), have been associated with pancreatitis. Hereditary forms of pancreatitis may present as recurrent pancreatitis, with frequent evolution in chronic pancreatitis.

Drugs

Pancreatitis due to drugs is rare (0.3-1.4%), albeit increasing. Several mechanisms of drug-induced pancreatitis have been proposed immunological reactions (6-mercaptopurine, aminosalicylates, sulphonamides); direct toxic effect (diuretics, sulphonamides); accumulation of toxic metabolites (valproic acid, didanosine, pentamidine, tetracycline); ischaemia (diuretics, azathioprine); intravascular thrombosis (estrogen); increased viscosity of pancreatic juice (diuretics and steroids). The time course depends on the drug involved. For example, pancreatitis may develop within a few weeks after taking a drug associated with an immunologically mediated adverse reaction; patients taking valproic acid, pentamidine or didanosine may not develop pancreatitis until after many months of medication use, presumably due to accumulation of toxic metabolites.

Infections

Pancreatitis has been associated with viruses (mumps, Coxsackievirus, HAV, HBV, HEV, cytomegalovirus, varicella-zoster, herpes simplex, HIV), bacteria (mycoplasma, legionella, leptospira, salmonella), fungi (Candida) and parasites (Toxoplasma, Cryptosporidium, Ascaris), although the incidence is very rare.

Abdominal Surgery or Extra-Abdominal

The mechanism appears to be linked to ischaemia-revascularization.

Idiopathic
In 15-25% of cases there is no certain cause of acute pancreatitis.

Other Causes
Uncommon causes of clinically significant pancreatitis may be trauma, pancreas divisum, ischaemia due to vascular disease (vasculitis).
Exposure to toxic substances is also known to cause activation of pancreatic damage: among them methanol, organophosphorus insecticides, and the poison of the Trinidad scorpion.

CLINICAL MANIFESTATIONS

Acute pancreatitis should be suspected in patients with severe acute upper abdominal pain but requires biochemical or radiologic evidence to establish a diagnosis. The diagnosis relies on findings of an increase in pancreatic amylasemia or lipaseemia, or radiological evidence of pancreatic inflammation.
Approximately 90% of patients have associated nausea and vomiting that may persist for several hours. Patients with a severe clinical picture may have fever, tachypnea, hypoxemia and hypotension, sometimes dyspnea (due to diaphragmatic inflammation secondary to pancreatitis), pleural effusion or respiratory distress syndrome.
About 5-10% of patients may have a very nuanced clinical picture, without pain or with an unexplained drop in blood pressure (especially in postoperative and critical patients). Patients may have abdominal distention and hypoactive bowel sounds due to an ileus secondary to inflammation, and/or may have scleral icterus due to obstructive jaundice due to choledocholithiasis or edema of the head of pancreas.
In 3% of cases, ecchymosis may be observed in the periumbilical region (Cullen's sign) or along the flank (Grey Turner's sign). These findings, although nonspecific, suggest retroperitoneal bleeding in the setting of pancreatic necrosis.

LABORATORY FINDINGS

In the early stages of acute pancreatitis, rupture of pancreatic acini, secondary to the inflammatory process, results in the release of digestive enzymes from the acinar cells into systemic circulation.
During an acute episode, serum amylase rises within 6 to 12 hours of the onset of acute pancreatitis. Amylase has a short half-life of approximately 10 hours. However, substantial elevation in serum amylase may not be seen in approximately 20% of patients with alcoholic pancreatitis due to the inability of the parenchyma to produce amylase, and in 50% of patients with hypertriglyceridemia-associated pancreatitis as triglycerides interfere with the amylase assay. Serum lipase rises within 4-8 hours of the onset of symptoms, peaks at 24 hours, and returns to normal within 1-2 weeks. Increases in lipase occur sooner and last longer than amylase; they are, therefore, particularly useful in patients who come to observation 1-2 days after the onset of symptoms.
Patients with pancreatitis may have leukocytosis, elevationed C-reactive protein and an elevated haematocrit from haemoconcentration due to extravasation of intravascular fluid into third spaces.

IMAGING

Imaging is important in the diagnosis of acute pancreatitis and its complications.

Abdominal and Chest Radiographs
Abdominal radiographic signs may be mild or indicative of a severe clinical picture, with demonstration, for example, of a localized ileum (sentinel loop) or of the colon "exclusion sign".
The latter reflects a scarcity of air in the distal colon with respect to the splenic flexure due to functional spasm of the descending colon secondary to inflammation of the pancreas. The ground glass sign may indicate, instead, an acute fluid collection in the peripancreatic area.
Approximately one third of patients with acute pancreatitis have abnormalities that are also visible on the chest radiogram, such as elevation of a haemidiaphragm, pleural effusion, baseline atelectasis, and pulmonary infiltrates.

Abdominal Ultrasound
In patients with acute pancreatitis, the pancreas appears diffusely enlarged and hypoechoic on abdominal ultrasound. Gallstones may be visualized in the gallbladder or the bile duct.
Peripancreatic fluid appears as an anechoic collection on abdominal ultrasound. These collections may demonstrate internal echoes in the setting of pancreatic necrosis. However, in approximately 25 to 35% of subjects with acute pancreatitis, bowel gas due to an ileus precludes evaluation of the pancreas or bile duct.

Abdominal Computed Tomography (CT)

The CT scan of the abdomen allows to determine focal or diffuse enlargement of the pancreas, and /or necrosis of the pancreatic tissue. This procedure should be performed 48-72 hours after the onset of symptoms, which is necessary for the development of pancreatic necrosis, which would not be visible if the examination were performed earlier. Contrast CT scans establish the presence and extent of pancreatic necrosis and/ or local complications, and disease severity.

Magnetic Resonance Imaging (MRI)

Magnetic resonance imaging can reveal diffuse or focal magnification of the pancreatic gland and the blurred edges of the parenchyma. Non-detection of parenchyma in contrast-enhanced MRI may be indicative of necrosis. MRI is more sensitive to early diagnosis of acute pancreatitis than contrast-enhanced CT and may better characterize pancreatic and biliary ducts and complications.
The use of MRI is limited, however, by less local availability and by the fact that it can not be urgently requested. Furthermore, MRI needs a longer scan time than CT, so it may be difficult to perform in critical cases with non-collaborating patients.

DIAGNOSIS

The diagnosis of acute pancreatitis is based on two of the following three criteria:

- acute onset of persistent, severe, epigastric pain often radiating to the back;
- elevation in serum lipase or amylase to three times or greater than the upper limit of normal;
- characteristic findings of acute pancreatitis on imaging (contrast-enhanced CT, MRI or transabdominal ultrasonography).

In patients with characteristic abdominal pain and increased lipase and/or serum amylase more than 3 times normal, no radiodiagnostic examination is necessary to confirm the diagnosis of acute pancreatitis. However, in patients with abdominal pain not characteristic of acute pancreatitis or with serum levels of amylase or lipase less than 3 times the normal limit, or in which the diagnosis is uncertain, abdominal imaging with CT or MRI may be useful for diagnosis.
Laboratory tests - complete blood count, electrolytes, alanine aminotransferase (ALT), aspartate aminotransferase (AST), bilirubin, calcium, and albumin - may also be useful to rule out other causes of acute abdominal pain.

A pregnancy test should be performed in all women of childbearing age. The diagnosis of a biliary cause of disease is based on stones or sludge within the bile duct, which can be documented by imaging studies (US abdomen, CT abdomen, MRI abdomen or echoendoscopy) or on elevated ALT with rapid normalization after a few days.

NATURAL HISTORY AND COMPLICATIONS

Most cases of acute pancreatitis (80%) are mild and patients recover within a few days without complications. However, about 20% of patients can have moderately severe or severe acute pancreatitis with local or systemic complications and/or organ failure (**Table 45.1**); such patients have a higher risk of mortality.
Some patients with acute pancreatitis may have recurrent disease attacks and develop chronic pancreatitis over time.

Local Complications

Local complications of acute pancreatitis include: acute peripancreatic fluid collection; pancreatic pseudocyst; acute necrotic collection; and walled-off necrosis (**Figure 45.1**).
Both acute necrotic fluid collections and walled off necrosis, usually, after 4 weeks from the beginning acute disease may become infected. Splenomesenteric thrombosis can be found in 50% of acute severe pancreatitis and is rare in the absence of necrosis.
Patients with severe pancreatitis have an increased risk for abdominal compartment syndrome (defined as sustained intra-abdominal pressure with new onset organ failure) due to tissue edema from aggressive fluid resuscitation, peripancreatic inflammation, ascites, ileus, and sometimes by a too aggressive therapeutic support.

Systemic Complications

According to the revised Atlanta classification of acute pancreatitis, systemic complication of acute pancreatitis is defined as an exacerbation of an underlying comorbidity (e.g., coronary artery disease or chronic lung disease).

Organ Failure

In the Atlanta classification, organ failure is a distinct entity, separate from a systemic complication. Pancreatic inflammation results in the activation of a cytokine cascade that manifests clinically as a

Table 45.1 Complications of acute pancreatitis.

Local	Systemic
Pseudocyst	Respiratory failure
Sterile Necrosis	Renal failure
Septic Necrosis	Shock
Abscess	Hyperglycemia
GI Bleeding	Hypercalcemia
Pancreatitis related	DIC
Pancreatitis unrelated	Adipose Necrosis
Spleen Complications	
Intestinal Fistulisation or Obtrusion	
Hydronephrosis	

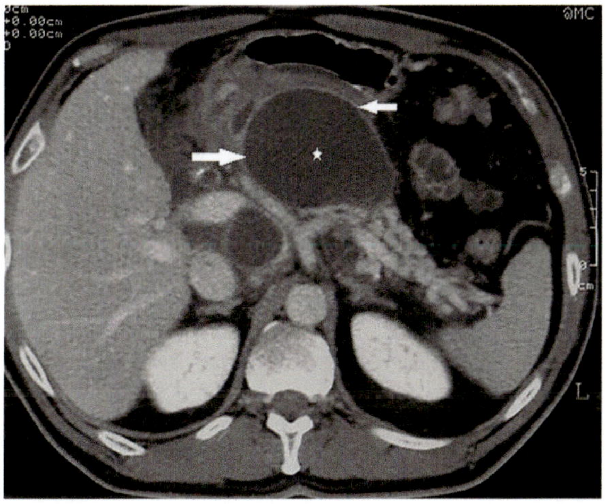

Figure 45.1 Axial CT image obtained 6 weeks after onset of gallstone pancreatitis, showing a large homogeneous fluid collection a thick enhancing wall (arrows).

systemic inflammatory response syndrome (SIRS) (**Table 45.2**).

Patients with persistent SIRS are at risk for failure of one or more organs (acute respiratory failure, shock and renal failure), which may be transient or persistent (>48 h). Involvement of multiple organs involved results in multi-organ failure, called multi-organ failure (MOF). The presence of SIRS and MOF significantly increases the risk of mortality.

Other Complications

Less frequent but frightening causes of severe acute pancreatitis are the formation of pseudoaneurysms near or within pancreatic necrotic collections, fistulae between the collections and the colon, colonic stenosis, abdominal abscesses, vascular thrombosis (portal vein, splenic artery).

CLINICAL AND THERAPEUTIC MANAGEMENT

Assessment of Disease Severity

At initial evaluation, the severity of acute pancreatitis should be assessed by clinical examination to assess for early fluid losses, organ failure (particularly cardiovascular, respiratory or renal compromise), and measurement of the systemic inflammatory response syndrome (SIRS) parameters (Table 45.2).

Assessment of Intensive Care Unit Monitoring Needs

In patients with severe acute pancreatitis, intensive care unit monitoring and support of pulmonary, renal, circulatory, and hepatobiliary function may minimize systemic sequelae.

Table 45.2 Features of systemic inflammatory response syndrome (SIRS).

Two or More of the Following Conditions	
Heart rate	>90 beats per minute
Temperature	>38.3 °C or <36.0 °C
Respiratory rate	>20 breaths per minute or $PaCO_2$ of <32 mmHg
White blood cell count	>12,000 cells per mL, <4000 cells per mL, or >10% immature

Initial Management

- Fasting.
- Fluid replacement: hydration at a rate of 5 to 10 mL/kg per hour of isotonic crystalloid solution (e.g., normal saline or lactated Ringer's solution) to all patients with acute pancreatitis, unless cardiovascular, renal or other related comorbid factors preclude aggressive fluid replacement. In the initial stages (within the first 12-24 hours) of the acute presentation, proper fluid therapy is associated with a reduction in morbidity and mortality.
- Pain control: abdominal pain is often the predominant symptom in patients with acute pancreatitis and should be treated with analgesics (also opioids). Uncontrolled pain can contribute to haemodynamic instability.
- Monitoring: patients with acute pancreatitis should be monitored (vital signs, urine output, electrolytes, serum glucose level, abdomen compartmental syndrome) closely in the first 24 to 48 hours. Patients with organ failure will need ongoing monitoring for other complications that might arise.
- Nutrition: patients with mild pancreatitis can often be managed with intravenous caloric support, as healing occurs quickly, allowing return to oral diet within a week. Nutritional support is often required, however, in patients with severe pancreatitis because it is unlikely that they will resume oral intake within 5-7 days. In this case, feeding with nasogastric or nasodigiunal tubes is preferable to total parenteral nutrition.
- Antibiotics: up to 20% of patients with acute pancreatitis develop an extrapancreatic infection (e.g., bloodstream infections, pneumonia, and urinary tract infections). These are associated with increased mortality. When an infection is suspected, antibiotics should be started while the source of the infection is being determined. However, if cultures are negative and no source of infection is identified, antibiotics should be discontinued. Prophylactic antibiotics are not recommended. Antibiotics should be used in patients with suspected infected pancreatic necrosis.

Management of Underlying Predisposing Conditions

In addition to treating pancreatic inflammation and its associated complications, it is important to address the underlying predisposing factors. For example, drugs associated with acute pancreatitis should be discontinued.

In patients with biliary pancreatitis, most of the stone go into the duodenum, but they can cause persistent obstruction (jaundice) and/or infection (cholangitis) of the biliary tract. In such cases, endoscopic treatment with endoscopic retrograde cholangiopancreatography (ERCP) should be performed within 24 hours to remove the stone (s) and/or treat the cholangitis. In the absence of obstruction of the common bile duct, the ERCP is not indicated. Cholecystectomy should be performed in all patients with a biliary cause after resolution of the acute clinical phas.

KEY CONCEPTS

- Acute pancreatitis can range from mild (80%) to severe forms (20%), associated with significant morbidity and mortality.
- The most frequent cause is biliary (up to 80% of cases) which must be carefully searched.
- To establish the cause of acute pancreatitis, all patients should undergo history, physical examination, laboratory evaluation (serum amylase or lipase, triglyceride, calcium, and liver biochemistries), and abdominal imaging (US or CT).
- At diagnosis, the severity of acute pancreatitis should be evaluated by clinical examination to assess for early fluid losses, organ failure, and SIRS score.
- Acute pancreatitis is treated with supportive care, including pain control, intravenous fluids especially during the first 24 hours, and correction of electrolyte abnormalities. Mild pancreatitis often requires no further therapy, and recovers within 3 to 7 days. Severe pancreatitis requires more intensive monitoring as transient (<48 hours) or persistent (>48 hours) organ failure and local or systemic complications may develop.

REFERENCES

- Banks PA, Bollen TL, Dervenis C, et al. Classification of acute pancreatitis – 2012: revision of the Atlanta classification and definitions by international consensus. Gut. 2013;62:102.
- Crockett SD, Wani S, Gardner TB, et al.; American Gastroenterological Association Institute Clinical Guidelines Committee. American Gastroenterological Association Institute guideline on initial management of acute pancreatitis. Gastroenterology. 2018;154:1096-101.
- Forsmark CE, Vege SS, Wilcox CM. Acute pancreatitis. New Engl J Med. 2016;17;375:1972-81.
- Greenberg JA, Hsu J, Bawazeer M, et al. Clinical practice guideline: management of acute pancreatitis. Can J Surg. 2016;59:128-40.
- Simons-Linares CR, Elkhouly MA, Salazar MJ. Drug-Induced Acute Pancreatitis in Adults: An Update. Pancreas. 2019 Nov/Dec;48(10):1263-73.

CHAPTER 46

CHRONIC PANCREATITIS

Armando Gabbrielli, Pietro Invernizzi

LEARNING OBJECTIVES

- To provide an anatomo-clinical definition of chronic pancreatitis and list its main types. To define its epidemiology, aetiology, and main risk factors.
- To define its pathogenesis.
- To describe its clinical picture and natural history.
- To describe the anatomo-clinical picture of autoimmune pancreatitis; define the complications of chronic pancreatitis.
- To define diagnostic procedures: bio-temporal and instrumental.
- To know the therapeutic goals in relation to aetiopathogenesis.

DEFINITION

Chronic pancreatitis (CP) is an irreversible disease, in which inflammation and fibrosis lead to a progressive reduction of the acinar and the endocrine component of the pancreas, with gradual deterioration of organ function. The pathogenesis of CP is not completely clarified, due to its multifactorial nature. However, acute pancreatitis (AP) is recognized as the initial event that initiates the processes that will lead to chronicity. At the onset and in the first years of illness, CP manifests itself clinically with episodes of abdominal pain, sometimes associated with isolated signs of AP, in a recurrent pattern. Progression of disease leads to a reduction in inflammation and a gradual increase in fibrosis, either segmental or widespread. Both phenomena are accompanied by painful symptoms and, frequent maldigestion/malabsorption (steatorrhea) and diabetes, due to the inevitable damage to the acinar and endocrine components.

Until recently, the majority of cases CP were thought to arise from chronic alcohol abuse. However, recent knowledge has reduced the aetiological weight of alcohol, which, however continues to represent, alongside cigarette smoking, an important factor in progression of the disease, the formation of pancreatic calcifications, and, more generally, the prognosis.

The evolution of diagnostics, through imaging methods (abdominal echotomography, endoscopy retrograde cholangiopancreatography [ERCP], computed tomography [CT], cholangiopancreatography-MR [CPMR], and echoendoscopy [EUS]), and bio-molecular have greatly expanded knowledge of CP. The disease, although uniform in the advanced stage, presents a completely different evolutionary dynamic in pathogenesis (**Table 46.1**) and clinical presentation, necessitating different therapeutic management.

EPIDEMIOLOGY, AETIOLOGY, RISKS FACTORS

The onset of the CP generally occurs between the fourth and fifth decade of age. It predominantly affects men, with a M/F ratio of 3:1. The incidence has been estimated around 10-15 new cases/100,000 inhabitants/year and is constantly increasing. The hereditary/familial form and, in general, the forms associated with genetic alterations are characterized by the young age of patients.

The risk factors are alcohol abuse (wine, beer, spirits) and cigarette smoking.

Dietary imbalances play a secondary role. The alcohol abuse is associated with the disease in 40% of patients with CP, is dose-dependent, and related to exposure, on average, 15-20 years. However, the risk factors are multiple and the TIGAR-O classification (**Table 46.2**) is the most commonly used to identify CP risk factors.

PATHOGENESIS

Although alcohol is the most common cause of CP, its pathogenesis is still not sufficiently defined because it is multifactorial. A sort of precipitation of aggregates (so-called plugs), caused by protein hypersecretion, not compensated by adequate intraductal production of bicarbonates, create the substrate for calcium to precipitate. This leads to multiple intraductal obstructions, from

Table 46.1 Different types of chronic pancreatitis.

Type of Disease	Pathophysiological Mechanism
Associated with papilla stenosis due to : • Biliary stones • Sphincter of Oddy dysfunction (SOD)	Pancreatic duct obstruction
Duct obstruction after episodes of acute severe pancreatitis (with gland necrosis)	Pancreatic duct obstruction
Paraduodenal	Inflammation of heterotopic pancreas in duodenal wall
Autoimmune	Antibodies against acinar/ductal pancreatic structures
Related to slow-growth tumours • Vater papilla • Neuroendocrine tumours • Intraductal papillary mucinous neoplasia (IPMN)	Pancreatic duct obstruction
Associated with • CFTR • PRSS1 (codons 122 and 29) • SPINK1 (codons 16,22,23)	Alteration of pancreatic juice composition ↓ autoinhibition trypsin activity Alteration of pancreatic secretory trypsin inhibitor (PSTI) with ↓ trypsin inhibition
Associated with pancreas *divisum*	Recurrent obstruction due to minor papilla dysfunction

Table 46.2 TIGAR-O Classification, Risk Factors for RAP.

Toxic-Metabolic (T) Alcohol consumption - Smoking Hypercalcemia/hyperparathyroidism – chronic renal failure Hypertrglyceridemia Organotin compounds (e.g., di-n-butyltin dichloride) Medications - phenacetin abuse – toxins	**Autoimmune (A)** Isolated autoimmune CP Associated with other autoimmune disorders • Sjogren's syndrome • Inflammatory bowel disease • Primary biliary cirrhosis
Idiopathic (I) Early onset Late onset Tropical	**Recurrent and Severe Acute Pancreatitis (R)** Post-necrotic (severe acute pancreatitis) Recurrent acute pancreatitis Ischaemic/vascular disease Post-irradiation
Genetic (G) Autosomal recessive/modifier genes CFTR mutations Spink 1 mutations Cationic trypsinogen (codon16, 22, 23 mutations) Anionic trypsinogen PRSS2, alfa1-antitrypsin deficency	**Obstructive (O)** Pancreas divisum Sphincter of Oddi disorders (controoversial) Duct obstruction (e.g., tumour, parasite) Preampullary duodenal wall cyst Post-traumatic pancreatic duct scars

which inflammation and fibrosis originate, leading to progressive atrophy not only of the exocrine acinar tissue but also, in the late phase, of endocrine tissue (Langerhans islets).

Among the various pathogenic hypotheses, Whitcomb recently (2013) proposed a two-phase pathogenetic model (hits): the first hit is an episode of acute pancreatitis that, through activation of the immune system, initiates pancreatic damage; the second hit results in alteration of the normal inflammatory response, as it involves prolonged activation of the stellate pancreatic cells, with irreversible outcome towards fibrosis.

Lithiasis in the main bile duct, through obstruction of the papilla of Vater, can lead to organic dysfunction of the sphincter of Oddi, such as a cicatricial stenosis, resulting in a chronic inflammatory process.

Paraduodenal pancreatitis is a rare form of disease involving the duodenal wall in the minor papilla associated with alcohol abuse and smoking. Inflammation of pancreatic islets within the duodenal wall creates an obstacle to normal pancreatic juice outflow with secondary obstructive chronic pancreatitis.

Autoimmune pancreatitis (AIP) affects less than 5% of CP patients; there are two different forms:

- Type 1, with intense infiltration of plasma cells and CD4+ T lymphocytes resulting in fibrosis and sclerosis; the plasma cells express on the surface IgG4 that increase in the serum, even if this does not imply their specific role in the predominantly cell-mediated pathogenesis;
- Type 2 only affects the pancreas, appears in the young, and is not associated with increased IgG4 expression.

In both forms, morphological impairment can be diffuse or segmental and associated with multiple stenoses of the intrapancreatic ducts.

CP can be associated with mutations in the cystic fibrosis gene (CFTR), the cationic trypsinogen-encoding gene (PRSS1), and the gene coding one for the pancreatic secretory trypsin inhibitor (SPINK1). Mutation of the CFTR gene, in heterozygosis or homozygosis, increases the viscosity of the pancreatic juice, impeding its flow into the duodenum. Mutation of the PRSS1 gene results in the intrapancreatic site in early activation of trypsin with repeated episodes of AP and CP. A similar mechanism is also hypothesized for mutations in the SPINK1 gene, responsible for alteration of the pancreatic secretory inhibitor of trypsin.

Pancreas divisum, still discussed as the aetiological factor of CP, is due to a defect in the fusion between the two embryonic ventral and dorsal buds, with the lack of fusion of the main ducts. The papilla minor, forced to drain the juice coming from a part of the head and from the tail, is structurally and functionally anomalous and therefore becomes an obstacle for the outflow of pancreatic juice.

CLINICAL ASPECTS

Pain at the epigastrum region is the main symptom in CP and is referred to continuously, with irradiation to both hypochondria also posteriorly ("belt").

It is exacerbated after a meal, especially if accompanied by alcoholic beverages, and can be associated with nausea and vomiting.

In the initial stages of the disease, pain is episodic, alternating with periods of apparent well being. In progression of the disease, it becomes continuous, though widely variabile among patients. This obviously poses problems for differential diagnosis with pancreatic cancer. The pain, more present in the early years, is reduced in intensity and frequency, associated with progressive glandular dysfunction both exocrine and endocrine. Therefore, in these more advanced phases, signs/symptoms of malabsorption secondary to maldigestion and diabetes occur. Weight loss, abdominal cramps, flatulence, abdominal swelling, alteration of the alvo, and steatorrhea (yellowish feces, unformed, greasy, abundant, foul-smelling) follow.

Steatorrhea, a manifestation of lipid malabsorption, involves vitamin deficiencies, in particular of fat-soluble vitamins (A, D, E, K). It is associated with azotorrhea due to protein malabsorption.

These signs appear when pancreatic enzyme secretion is less than 10% of its maximum capacity. In addition, more than 50% of patients with CP may develop diabetes due to partial or total destruction of the endocrine component of the organ.

Different from type 1 diabetes, is a secondary diabetes, therefore particular and defined as 3c DM (T3cDM).

The complications that can occur during exacerbations are presented in **Table 46.3**.

The cavitary lesions are pancreatic pseudocysts, the result of an episode of acute necrotizing pancreatitis, and retention cysts, secondary to obstruction of a secondary pancreatic duct caused by intraductal stones. In paraduodenal pancreatitis, the extent of inflammation in the duodenal lumen may lead to intestinal obstruction with post-prandial nausea and vomiting.

Jaundice appears due to obstruction of the intra-

Table 46.3 Chronic pancreatitis: complications.

Peripancreatic fluid collection	Fluid collection after acute pancreatitis, retention cysts
Duodenal obstruction	Obstruction of duodenal lumen due to inflammatory infiltration
Jaundice	Intrapancreatic bile duct stenosis due to inflammatory stricture
Digestive bleeding (oesophageal/gastric) varices	Secondary to thrombosis of splenic vein/portal vein
Pancreatic ascites	Secondary to rupture of main pancreatic duct lesion
Pancreatic adenocarcinoma	Secondary to chronic pancreatic inflammation

pancreatic tract of the common bile duct, which may be compressed by pseudocysts or by parenchymal inflammation of the pancreatic head associated with edematous/inflammatory changes in the peri-vaterian area.

Approximately half of the cases of AIP include other autoimmune/disimmune diseases: the digestive tract (ulcerative colitis and Crohn's disease), the biliary tract (primary sclerosing cholangitis and, less frequently, primitive biliary cholangitis) the salivary glands (syndrome of Sjögren) and extra-digestive (interstitial nephritis, systemic lupus erythematosus, vasculitis, interstitial pneumonitis).

Pancreatic adenocarcinoma is a late complication of CP, probably secondary to chronic inflammation.

DIAGNOSIS

Biochemical Parameters

The limited sensitivity and specificity of current bio-humoral examinations does not allow definitive diagnosis of CP. Amylase and lipase levels only allow diagnosis in case of exacerbation of the disease. However, the laboratory can be useful to test the exocrine and endocrine insufficiency of the pancreas.

Fat maldigestion can be measured with measurement of fecal fat in 24 h, but is of limited clinical use due to the complexity of the procedure. More specific and sensitive is measurement of fecal elastase-1: normal exocrine function values > 200 µg/g feces; slight exocrine insufficiency when between 100 and 200 µg/g feces; severe deficiency when < 100 µg/g feces. Endocrine function can be evaluated initially with post-prandial glycemic testing, while the glucose load curve with glucose determination, insulin level, and C-peptide allows to evaluate the insulin reserve and possible insulin resistance.

Radiological Parameters

The study of the pancreatic gland in the past was made difficult by its retroperitoneal position.

The introduction of non-invasive or relatively invasive modern imaging methods, such as US, CT, MRI with cholangiopancreatographic reconstructions (CPMR) and EUS, has relegated ERCP to a marginal diagnostic role of great therapeutic importance.

Diagnostic ERCP is burdened by important morbidity of which acute pancreatitis after ERCP is the most insidious, with an incidence of 5-15%. By reviewing the different methods we need to start with abdominal US that, with its low invasiveness and repeatability, represents the first evaluation exam. However, it is limited by being operator-dependent and by the not infrequent difficulty in visualizing the pancreatic gland in its entirety. It can visualize gland structure, calcifications of masses or collections and diameter of the Wirsung duct. In suspected lesions, ultrasound-guided biopsy can be performed.

CT and the MRI, with a possible secretin stimulus, are the radiological examinations of choice in this pathology.

The first choice exam is MRI because relatively invasive, while yielding information about typology (paraduodenal, autoimmune, ductal stenosis, sequelae of acute pancreatitis), stage of disease (early or advanced) and sphincter-pancreatic gland function via stimulation with secretin.

The hormone secretionic stimulus induces an increase in the liquid component of pancreatic secretion, allowing better visualization of the pancreatic duct (with visualization of secondary ducts, site of alterations in the early stages of the disease), facilitating the diagnosis of morphological alterations

such as pancreas divisum or functional alterations of the sphincter of Oddi (with impaired discharge of pancreatic juice in dynamic study) and indirect data about the function of the pancreatic gland given by the index of filling of the duodenal C-loop by the pancreatic juice. MRI is also able to diagnose cystic collections, complications of the disease, and their contents (liquid with or without necrotic or blood component) also for treatment. MRI is the method of choice in pediatric patients because it does not use ionizing radiation. However, MRI has a poor sensitivity in detecting intrapancreatic calcifications. CT with contrast is therefore a complementary examination of fundamental importance for highlighting with great accuracy the calcifications and their location and the possible presence of neoplastic transformations (rare but fearful complication of CP). It also visualizes edema or atrophy of the pancreatic gland.
EUS allows very accurate study, even in the earliest stages of the disease, of the duct and of the pancreatic parenchyma by means of an ultrasound transducer located at the tip of the endoscope. Its high resolution allows early diagnosis of small masses even less than one centimeter. Using an operator channel and thin needles inside it, it allows to perform ultrasound-guided cyto-histological sampling of solid lesions and lymph nodes or to characterize cystic lesions by aspirating and analyzing their contents. Since this is a transgastric and transduodenal approach, it is not burdened by the problem of intestinal gas, which often hinders abdominal US. The correct use of the methods allows a correct diagnosis in the majority of patients.

THERAPY

The goals of therapy are summarized in **Table 46.4**.

Table 46.4 Targets of medical therapy.

Management of acute phase
Pain treatment
Prevention of pain relapses
Treatment of complications
Treatment of maldigestion
Treatment of diabetes

Medical Therapy

Treatment of exacerbations is the same as acute pancreatitis. Abdominal pain is the predominant symptom of disease. Its genesis can be traced to three main mechanisms:

- hypertension from ductal stenosis resulting in parenchymal ischaemia;
- neuronal inflammation by infiltration of the nerve endings resulting in the release of algogenic cytokines;
- stenosis of the biliary pathway.

The first step in the treatment of pain is complete cessation of alcohol and smoking. Analgesics such as non-steroidal anti-inflammatory drugs (NSAIDs) or paracetamol are the second step, followed by combination with a minor opioid (e.g., tramadol). In case of failure, major opioids (morphine, buprenorphine) combined or not with drugs to raise the therapeutic threshold of pain (tricyclic drugs or serotonin reuptake inhibitors) may represent the final step.
Insufficient secretion of pancreatic enzymes causes hyperstimulation of pancreatic secretion and pain from ductal hypertension with a decrease in the degradation of cholecystokinin-releasing factor (CCK) and an increase in CCK. Hence, the use in selected patients of pancreatic enzymes with blocking the CCK action for a feedback mechanism. Few data with discordant results have been published on the use of antioxidant agents, such as selenium, vitamin C, beta-carotene, vitamin E, and methionine to decrease free radical concentrations.
Only in autoimmune pancreatitis, the therapy has an aetiologic rationale with the use of steroids that act with very positive results: methylprednisolone at a dose of 1 mg/kg/day for 2-3 weeks tapered by 5 mg per week is the standard therapy.
Pancreatic insufficiency with maldigestion involves the administration of pancreatic extracts at high doses (at least 30,000-40,000 U of lipase per main meal, 20,000U at breakfast and 10,000 at snacks) adapted according to clinical response. The recommended diet is a high-calorie type, limiting fats and administering vitamin complexes to supplement the malabsorption of fat-soluble vitamins.
The diabetes of the patient with CP is defined as type III, characterized by instability of glucose balance with frequent episodes of hypoglycemia linked to variable intestinal absorption and the concomitant hepatic disorder and absence of hormones against regulators (glucagon). The onset of diabetes is observed in advanced forms of disease and treatment with insulin rather than oral antidiabetics.

Endoscopic Therapy

The rationale for endoscopic therapy is its ability to resolve ductal hypertension, which is one of the basic mechanisms of pain in patients with CP. A dysfunction of the Oddian sphincter can be removed by performing sphincterotomy of the pancreatic side of the sphincter of Oddi associated or not with that of the biliary side. In lithiasis of the main pancreatic duct, stone fragmentation (often not extractable endoscopically because of their size) with extracorporeal shock wave lithotripsy (ESWL) should be combined with sphincterotomy. In distal stenosis (near the papilla) placement of a prosthesis can re-establish correct outflow of pancreatic juice into the duodenum, also resolving ductal hypertension. The advantage of endoscopic treatment is that it is repeatable and does not preclude surgical treatment. In intractable pain, neurolysis of the celiac ganglion can be performed by EUS, which has produced suboptimal results, especially in the long term. EUS can also be used to drain symptomatic pancreatic cysts by creating a fistula between the collection and the gastric or duodenal cavity (cystogastro-or cystoduodenostomia). Endoscopic therapy can be used in selected patients also to resolve with stent placement the inflammatory stenosis of the intrapancreatic distal tract of the bile duct.

Encouraging results were obtained by placement of metal stents, 8-10 mm in diameter, completely coated and easily removed after about one year.

Surgical Therapy

Surgical therapy is indicated for treating pain not responsive to medical therapy or endoscopy or arising from suspected or certain neoplasia complicating the chronic pancreatitis.

Other indications for surgical treatment are stenosis of the bile duct and duodenum due to fibrotic phenomena. Complications of cystic lesions (bile duct or compression of the intestinal lumen and the infection of lesion) are further indications for surgical treatment. Intralesional bleeding is usually treated with radiological embolization of the bleeding vessel. In pain, depending on its cause, surgical treatment includes:

- creation of anastomosis between the dilated main pancreatic duct and a jejunal (pancreatic-fasting) loop in ductal hypertension pain;
- resection of the diseased part of the pancreas (duodenocephaly or resection of the pancreatic tail) in inflammation.

In suspected neoplastic transformation, treatment can only be resective as in pancreatic neoplasia. Complications, such as stenosis of the biliary or duodenal ducts or non-aggressive endoscopic cystic lesions, involves combining specific derivative treatments with conventional techniques.

KEY CONCEPTS

- Chronic pancreatitis is a multifactorial and progressive disease that causes both exocrine (maldigestion) and endocrine (diabetes) insufficiency.
- It is important to define the type of disease: the therapeutic approach (medical, endoscopic and surgical) is different for the different forms of chronic pancreatitis.
- Clinically, the disease is characterized by recurrent episodes of abdominal pain in the epigastric area radiating to the hypochondria ("a bar") and also posteriorly ("belt").
- The diagnostic classification foresees identification of the causes of chronic pancreatitis (organic, metabolic, genetic) through evaluation of glandular function, both exocrine and endocrine, and determination by bio-humoral tests.
- Magnetic resonance imaging with secretin is the imaging method of choice in the evaluation of chronic pancreatitis, as it yields morphological and functional data.
- The main objective of medical therapy is to control of painful symptoms and correct pancreatic insufficiency.
- Endoscopic treatment restores emptying of pancreatic secretion in the duodenum and makes use of numerous techniques (sphincterotomy of the papilla of Vater, extraction of intraductal stones, placement of intraductal prostheses, extracorporeal lithotripsy).
- Pancreatic surgery is indicated in the treatment of pain not responsive to medical or endoscopic therapy for pain and dilatation of the Wirsung duct (> 6 mm). Radical pancreatic surgery is indicated for focal forms of disease with undiluted pancreatic duct.

REFERENCES

- Dumonceau JM, Delhaye M, Tringali A, et al. Endoscopic treatment of chronic pancreatitis: European Society of Gastrointestinal Endoscopy (ESGE) Clinical Guideline. Endoscopy. 2012;44:748-96.
- Frulloni L, Falconi M, Gabbrielli A, et al. Italian consensus guidelines for chronic pancreatitis. Dig Liver Dis. 2010;42 (Suppl 6):S381-406.
- Whitcomb DC. Genetic risk factors for pancreatic disorders. Gastroenterology. 2013;144:1292-302.

PANCREATIC NEOPLASMS AND PRECANCEROUS LESIONS

Pietro Fusaroli, Alessandro Repici

LEARNING OBJECTIVES

- To define the epidemiology of adenocarcinoma as the prevalent histotype of pancreatic cancer.
- To list the risk factors for adenocarcinoma of the pancreas and highlight possible genetic predisposition.
- To propose model of carcinogenesis and molecular classification of adenocarcinoma.
- To describe the screening of precancerous lesions in high-risk person.
- To describe the clinical presentation of pancreatic cancer and list the instruments for diagnosis, staging, and prognosis.
- To highlight the limits of therapies for pancreatic cancer and to describe methods of palliation.
- To describe the main anatomopathological and clinical connotations of cystic tumours of the pancreas and their prognosis.

ADENOCARCINOMA OF THE PANCREAS

Epidemiology

Pancreatic cancer as commonly understood corresponds to ductal adenocarcinoma, which represents more than 90% of malignant pancreatic neoplasms. Other malignant tumours of the pancreas, of more rare histotype and often with cystic appearance, are listed in **Table 47.1**. Pancreatic cancer is the fourth leading cause of cancer death in the United States. In Italy, approximately 13,700 new cases were estimated in 2017, given the continuous and parallel increase in both sexes of incidence and mortality (the curves, due to the poor prognosis, almost overlap) (**Figure 47.1**).

Table 47.1 Histological classification of epithelial tumours of the exocrine pancreas (modified by WHO 2010).

Benign	• Serous cystadenoma° • Mucinous cystadenoma° - Intraductal papillary mucinous adenoma° - Mature cystic teratoma°
Borderline (uncertain malignant potentianl)	• Mucinous cystic tumour with moderate dysplasia° • Mucinous intraductal tumour with moderate dysplasia° • Solid pseudopapillary tumour
Malignant	• Ductal adenocarcinoma • Mucinous non-cystic carcinoma ° • Signet ring cell carcinoma • Adenosquamous carcinoma • Undifferentiated carcinoma (anaplastic) • Undifferentiated giant osteoclastic cell carcinoma • Mixed ductal-endocrine carcinoma • Serous cystadenocarcinoma° • Mucinous cystadenocarcinoma° • Intraductal papillary mucinous carcinoma° • Acinar cell carcinoma - Acinar cell cystadenocarcinoma° - Mixed acinar-endocrine carcinoma • Pancreatoblastoma - solid - cystic° • Solid pseudopapillary carcinoma°

° cystic tumours

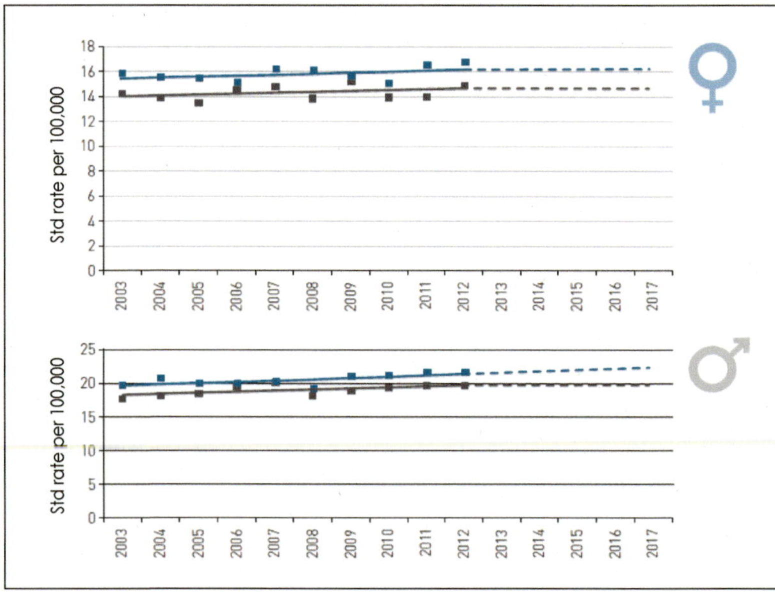

Figure 47.1 Time trend of incidence (blue) and mortality (black) from pancreatic cancer in Italy, in men and women (rates standardized for European population 2013).

The survival rate for patients is very low. In Italy, just over 20% of patients are alive 1 year from the diagnosis, while only 8.1% survive to 5 years. Of the patients surviving to 1 year, only 23% survive the next 5 years. These numbers include patients who can undergo surgery (15-20% of the total), for whom the 5-year survival rate is around 25%.

Risk Factors

Pancreatic cancer is more frequent in males and in advanced age (>80% of cases more than 60 years old). In addition to gender and age, risk factors for pancreatic cancer are smoking, family history, chronic pancreatitis, diabetes, obesity, and occupational exposure to solvents and nickel. A diet rich in fats and meat is also associated with increased risk, while a diet rich in fruits and vegetables has a protective effect.

The risk of disease for smokers is 2 to 4 times greater than for non-smokers and increases proportionately with the number of cigarettes smoked and the duration of habit. Approximately 20-30% of pancreatic cancers in men and 10% in women are attributable to cigarette smoking: this makes smoking the most important preventable factor for this disease.

Another risk factor that could be a target of prevention, by means of screening and surveillance of individuals at risk, is genetic predisposition to the disease, which accounts for about 10% of pancreatic cancers.

Family aggregation may be part of a hereditary syndrome genetically predisposing to cancer (**Table 47.2**), identifiable by looking for germline gene mutations, or can be framed in the so-called "family pancreas cancer" that simply defines the disease of an individual with at least two first-degree family members affected in the absence of known hereditary syndrome. First-degree family members of individuals belonging to families with familial pancreatic cancer have a risk of disease 9 times that of the general population. The gene mutations thus far associated with familial cancer are BRCA2 (5-17% of cases) and PALB2 (up to 3%). Based on these findings, it is now mandatory to acquire an accurate family history for each new patient diagnosed with pancreatic cancer.

Precancerous Lesions and Model of Carcinogenesis

Pancreatic cancer develops starting from precancerous lesions. The most typical one is pancreatic intraepithelial neoplasia (PanIN), which evolves into invasive cancer due to the progressive acquisition of invasive histopathological traits. Adenocarcinoma can also originate from mucinous neoplasms, such as the intraductal papillary mucinous neoplasm (IPMN) or mucinous cystic neoplasm (MCN). The progression from minimally dysplastic ductal epithelium (PanIN1A and 1B) to more severe dysplasia (PanIN 2 and 3) to invasive cancer parallels the accumulation of mutations or epigenetic alterations of the ductal cells (**Figure 47.2**). Activation of the K-RAS oncogene (90% of cases), together with shortening of telomeres, is the earliest genetic alteration and triggers aberrant activation of cell proliferation and survival signals. Inactivation of tumour suppressor genes such as

Table 47.2 Main familial syndromes, associated genetic mutations, and relative risk of developing pancreatic cancer.

Syndrome	Gene	Relative risk
Hereditary breast and ovarian cancer	BRCA 1 and 2	6-10 times
Peutz-Jeghers polyposis	STK11/LKB1	132 times
Lynch syndrome or hereditary non-polyposic colorectal cancer	(HNPCC)	MLH1, MSH2,
other DNA mismatch repair genes	8-9 times	
Hereditary pancreatitis	PRSS1, PRSS2, SPINK1, CTRC	26-60 times
Cystic fibrosis	CFTR	5-6 times
Atypical nevi melanomas (FAMM)	CDKN2A	13-22 times
Familial adenomatous polyposis (FAP)	APC	4-6 times

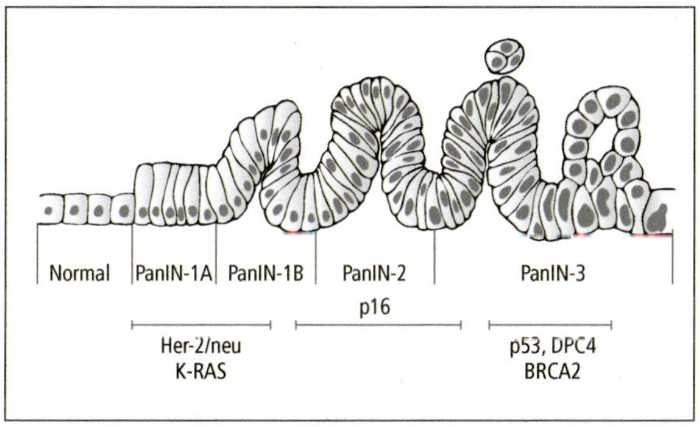

Figure 47.2 Model of genetic and histological progression of pancreatic intraepithelial neoplasm (PanIN).
(from: Hruban RH et al.; Am J Pathol 2000)

CDKN2A (90% of cases), with loss of the p16 protein, which regulates cell transition from phase G1 to phase S, contributes to the increased proliferative capacity of the cell, while the subsequent mutations of DPC4 (or SMAD, 85% of cases), p53, and BRCA2 correspond to the most advanced stages of dysplasia, resulting in inhibition of cell apoptosis and genomic instability.

Histopathology and Molecular Classification

Adenocarcinoma is localized primarily in the head of the pancreas (60-70% of cases), while localization in the body (10-15%) or the tail (5-10%) is more rare. Cephalopancreatic tumours are characterized by frequent obstruction and subsequent retrograde dilatation of the bile duct and pancreatic duct. They can also infiltrate the papilla of Vater or the duodenal wall. In non-cephalic tumours, the disease can extend to the spleen, stomach, and/or left adrenal gland.

At diagnosis, the majority of patients (80-90%) present locally advanced or metastatic disease. The locally advanced disease is defined by invasion of the portal vein or of the superior mesenteric vessels and/or invasion of the duodenal wall and/or other adjoining organs. The most frequent metastatic localizations are lymph nodes, liver, and peritoneum; less frequent localizations include the lungs, pleura, and bones.

Ductal adenocarcinoma can present good (G1), moderate (G2) or poor (G3) differentiation. A histological characteristic of the tumour is the presence of a dense stroma that can become the main tissue component. In any case, the interaction between fibroblasts and neoplastic epithelial cells is considered crucial for the initiation and progression of pancreatic cancer. Furthermore, the desmoplastic reaction could constitute a barrier to the penetration of chemotherapeutic drugs, contributing to their poor efficacy.

Another histological feature of pancreatic cancer is neuroinvasiveness, which determines the progression of the tumour along nerve endings and is believed to contribute to post-surgical metastases and recurrences. Based on its transcriptional profile, ductal adenocarcinoma of the pancreas is classified into 4 subtypes, which correlate the mutational pattern and histopathological traits:

- the first subtype, defined as squamous or quasi-mesenchymal, is characterized by the increased expression of TP63 and the mutation of TP53; it involves a significantly worse prognosis than that of the remaining subtypes;
- the second subtype, defined as classical or pancreatic progenitor, is characterized by the expression of transcription factors, in particular PDX1, crucial for the differentiation of pancreatic exocrine and endocrine cells. This subtype can express mucins typical of IPMNs, which

are therefore considered precancerous lesions specific to this subgroup;

- the third subtype, called immunogenic, shares many molecular characteristics with the previous one, from which it is distinguished by the infiltration of immune cells and the expression of transcription factors associated with B and T lymphocytes, cytotoxic or regulatory. The increased expression of tumour immunosuppression pathways mediated by CTLA4 and PD1 makes the immunogenic subtype a candidate for new immunotherapies;
- also the fourth subtype, called ADEX (aberrantly differentiated endocrine exocrine), is a variant of the classical subgroup, from which it differs by the concomitant expression of transcription factors typical of pancreatic endocrine or exocrine cells.

Screening for Diagnosis of Precancerous Lesions in High-Risk Asymptomatic Subjects

Screening of the general population for pancreatic cancer is not currently feasible due to the lack of an efficient biomarker and the limited window of time that elapses between diagnosable disease and advanced disease.

However, recent studies have proposed screening for precancerous lesions, in particular IPMN, in asymptomatic subjects defined as high-risk, being affected by a predisposing hereditary syndrome or as first-degree relatives of two or more patients suffering from pancreatic cancer. These pioneering screening programs have used imaging techniques such as magnetic resonance cholangio-pancreatography (MRCP) and endoscopic ultrasound, which have diagnosed cystic lesions referable to IPMN in a relevant fraction (30-50%) of the subjects enrolled, while solid lesions were found in less than 2% of individuals. While surveillance over time is recommended for cystic lesions, the finding of solid lesions may also indicate prophylactic surgery.

Clinical Presentation of Adenocarcinoma

Dyspepsia and asthenia are often initial non-specific symptoms. Jaundice, secondary to bile duct compression by a pancreatic head tumour, is present in 50-60% of patients at the time of diagnosis. Pain, present in about 3/4 of patients, is an expression of peripancreatic nerve structure infiltration by the neoplasm and has an epigastric localization with posterior irradiation. Weight loss, present in 90% of cases at diagnosis, is secondary to the onset of the cancer-related cytokine-related anorexia-cachexia syndrome. Diabetes, already mentioned as a risk factor and present in 50% of cases at diagnosis, can also be an early manifestation of cancer, preceding the appearance of symptoms. For this reason, patients with recent onset diabetes, especially in the absence of familiarity, should be evaluated for pancreatic cancer. Other conditions that might indicate pancreatic adenocarcinoma are acute pancreatitis of undefined aetiology and migratory thrombophlebitis (associated in about 10% of cases).

In advanced stage, the symptomatology is dominated by pain and symptoms related to local and metastatic progression (jaundice, ascites, vomiting from mechanical occlusion secondary to duodenal infiltration).

Diagnosis in Symptomatic Patients

Blood tests have a limited role in the diagnostic pathway of patients with suspected pancreatic cancer.

Routine laboratory tests can document elevation of bilirubin and movement of cholestasis indices in patients with pancreas head cancer. Occasionally, alterations of amylase and lipase can also be observed.

The CA19-9 tumour marker, still the most accurate biomarker of pancreatic adenocarcinoma (total sensitivity and specificity around 80%), is not synthesized by persons with double negative Lewis blood group (5-10% of the population), is not very sensitive for small malignancies (50% for tumours <3cm) and loses specificity in the presence of jaundice (high values also for cholecystitis and cholangitis) or pancreatitis. The combined dosage of the carcinoembryonic antigen (CEA) can improve the specificity of CA19-9. Due to these limitations, the diagnostic utility of CA19-9 in the initial diagnosis is confined to confirming the probable malignancy of pancreatic lesions identified with imaging techniques. Otherwise, in patients with a diagnosis, monitoring CA19-9 may be useful for evaluating the response to surgery and/or chemotherapy.

Transabdominal ultrasound, being an operator-dependent method and obstructed by obesity and meteorism, has variable sensitivity (75-89%) but good specificity (90-99%) in recognizing the hypoechoic pancreatic area typical of pancreatic cancer (**Figure 47.3A**). In any case, ultrasound can show indirect signs of neoplasia such as dilatation of the biliary tract and Wirsung (double-duct sign), distention of the gallbladder, liver metastases, and ascites. Because of its wide accessibility, ultrasound is the method that most often directs the diagnosis in patients with initial non-specific symptoms and those with jaundice.

Multilayered computed tomography (CT) with contrast medium is the current gold standard for the diagnosis of pancreatic cancer (overall sensitivity 89-97%), although its sensitivity in identifying small tumours remains unsatisfactory (77% for tumours <2 cm, 67% for those <1.5 cm). Image acquisitions take place in three phases (arterial, venous, and portal), allowing assessment of lesion ratios (typically hypodense in the late arterial or parenchymal phase) with peripancreatic vessels (as well as with adjacent organs) (**Figure 47.3B**).

Magnetic resonance imaging (MRI) has an overall diagnostic accuracy similar to CT. However, thanks to the better contrast enhancement of pancreatic tissue, MRI can identify about 80% of pancreatic neoplastic lesions that are not diagnostic at CT because of "low attenuation" compared to the surrounding parenchyma (**Figure 47.3C**).

Endoscopic ultrasound (EUS) is currently the most sensitive imaging technique for pancreatic cancer (>95%), enabling the identification of lesions of <2 cm in size. EUS is therefore recommended in all cases in which the suspicion of pancreatic cancer persists beyond the negativity of CT and MRI. EUS also makes it possible to obtain a cytological/histological diagnosis of lesions identified by means of fine needle aspiration (FNA. **Figure 47.3D**). Finally, EUS is at least equivalent and probably superior to CT in determining surgical resectability of pancreatic cancer.

Positron emission tomography with 18-fluoro-deoxyglucose (18FDG-PET) identifies pancreatic cancer by exploiting the increased glucose consumption of tumour tissue, with sensitivity and specificity comparable to those of CT and MRI. PET has a limited role in the first diagnosis of pancreatic cancer, whereas it may come into play to highlight relapses and/or metastases in patients who have undergone surgery.

Staging

The formal staging of pancreatic cancer makes use of the TNM classification based on: tumour size (T), lymph node localization (N), and presence of distant metastases (M).

The current classification (8th edition) of the American Joint Committee on Cancer (AJCC) includes 4 stages:

- Stage I - neoplasm confined to the pancreas without lymph node (N0) or distant (M0) metastasis, <2 cm (T1, stage IA) or between 2 and 4 cm (T2, stage IB);
- Stage II - neoplasm >4 cm no involvement of the celiac axis or the superior mesenteric artery (T3, "resectable") and free from lymph node metastasis (N0, stage IIA), or "resectable" neoplasm of any size (T1-T3) with ≤3 lymph node metastasis (N1, stage IIB), in any case without distant metastasis (M0);
- Stage III - non-resectable neoplasm (T4) or with ≥4 lymph node metastases (N2), without distant metastasis (M0);
- Stage IV - neoplasm with distant metastasis (M1).

In pancreatic cancer, the TNM classification, which is the typical tool of post-surgical prognosis, must be integrated with the "resectability" parameter, thus defined based on imaging:

- resectable disease: neoplasm not infiltrating the vascular structures and free of distant metastasis;
- borderline disease: neoplasm free of distant metastasis but in "limited" contact with vascular structures:
  - definition of "limited" in evolution with the progress of vascular reconstructive techniques;
  - current criteria: a) no contact with the ce-

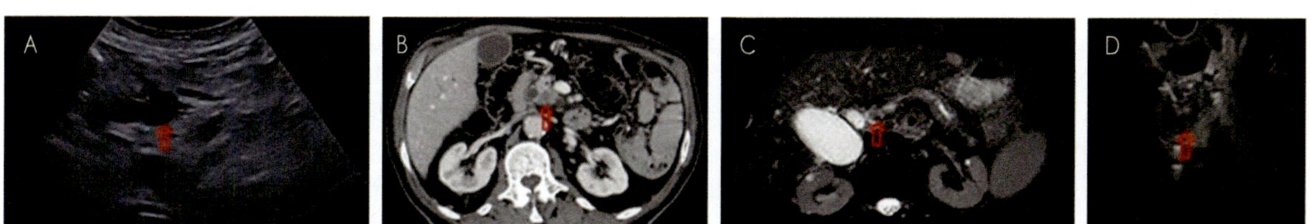

Figure 47.3 Images of pancreatic head cancer: A) ultrasound of the abdomen; B) CT abdomen with contrast medium; C) MRI with contrast medium; D) FNA during EUS.

liac tripod; b) segmentary contact with the common hepatic artery; c) <180° contact with the superior mesenteric artery; d) contact with the portal vein amenable of resection and reconstruction;
- resectability generally re-evaluated after neoadjuvant radiochemotherapy;
- non-resectable disease: neoplasm infiltrating adjacent "non-reconstructable" vessels or with distant metastasis.

Preoperative laparoscopy can be complementary to imaging as a staging tool for limiting the number of laparotomies that do not result in resection due to peritoneal disease or liver micrometastases not detected radiologically.

Therapy and Palliation

In patients with resectable tumours (~ 20% of new diagnoses), resective surgery (duodenal-cephalopancreasectomy for head tumours, distal resection for body and tail tumours, total pancreasectomy in patients at high risk of dehiscence of the pancreatic-jejunal anastomosis) is potentially curative and is therefore the first treatment option (operative mortality: 2-5% in high-volume centers).

Unfortunately, over 90% of resected patients relapse, so that a post-surgical treatment of adjuvant chemotherapy (gemcitabine and/or capecitabine) is currently part of the standard of care for these patients, with a median survival expectation of 26 months (30% alive at 5 years). We are awaiting the results of an adjuvant therapy trial with nab-paclixatel (nanoparticle albumin-bound paclitaxel) currently in progress. The possible therapeutic advantage resulting from the combined radiotherapy and chemotherapy in the adjuvant therapy setting is still controversial. Radiotherapy is now widely used in the United States, though it is not included in the European standard.

Despite the absence of evidence from randomized controlled trials, patients with borderline neoplasia have undergone preoperative/neoadjuvant therapy. The most common regimen is known as FOLFIRINOX (folic acid, 5FU, irinotecan, oxaliplatin), which enables the return of a high fraction of patients (~ 50%) to surgical resectability. The advantage of neoadjuvant therapy remains controversial and is currently being evaluated also for patients with resectable disease.

Nab-paclitaxel plus gemcitabine, or alternatively FOLFIRINOX, is the first-line treatment for patients with non-resectable disease (locally advanced or metastatic). Both these regimens provide an advantage of survival compared to the single therapy gemcitabine previously in use.

Therapies aimed at single molecular pathways of pancreatic cancer, in its various stages, have thus far not shown any clinical advantage. Therapies aimed at controlling the stroma and new generation immunotherapies, though promising, are not yet part of the therapeutic standard. Palliation of jaundice, duodenal obstruction, and pain is an integral part of the treatment of patients with inoperable cancer. Jaundice has three treatment options: endoscopy, radiology, and surgery. The first option, endoscopic retrograde cholangiopancreatography (ERCP) with placement of a plastic or metallic biliary prosthesis, is the one most frequently used to restore the outflow of bile into the duodenum. Currently this technique also allows duodenal stenosis to be treated by means of enteral prosthesis through which the biliary prosthesis is positioned. If the ERCP fails, it is possible to resort to biliary drainage guided by endoscopic ultrasound (EUS).

Thanks to advances in endoscopy, percutaneous drainage under radiological guidance and surgical derivation (biliary and intestinal) now have an increasingly smaller role in the palliation of these patients. Pain is generally controllable with medical therapy (non-steroidal anti-inflammatory drugs followed by or combined with parenteral, transdermal or epidural opioids). EUS-guided alcoholization of the celiac plexus may be considered in cases that cannot be managed pharmacologically.

PANCREATIC CYSTIC NEOPLASMS

Pancreatic cystic neoplasms (PCNs) comprise a heterogeneous group of lesions, present in 2-45% of the general population, with highly varied biological behavior, from benign to malignant. The wide use of sophisticated imaging techniques has led to increasingly frequent findings of this type of lesion in individuals who are asymptomatic for pancreatic disease and have undergone magnetic resonance imaging (MRI) or computed tomography (CT) for other clinical reasons. Correct clinical-instrumental classification of these patients is essential to prevent the progression of invasive forms of tumour and to limit the costs of excessive follow-up of lesions that never evolve into aggressive forms. PCNs are a large group of cystic lesions, including serous cystic neoplasm, mucinous cystic neoplasm (MCN), intraductal papillary mucinous neoplasm (IPMN) and solid pseudopapillary tumour.

Since PCNs often show overlapping morphological characteristics without typical clinical manifestations, the differential diagnosis between PCNs is not always easy.

As a result, in recent years various guidelines have been developed by experts, though only a few of these are evidence-based.

Among the guidelines most widely used and recognized for their validity, also internationally, are the Italian and European guidelines. The latter, updated in 2017, have the merit of being based on systematic reviews and on the GRADE methodology for the quality of the scientific evidence of the work and for the strength of the recommendations. To respond to relevant clinical questions, the guidelines address nine topics: biomarkers, radiology, endoscopy, IPMN, MCN, serous cystic neoplasms, rare cysts, (neo)adjuvant treatment, and pathology, and they provide indications for conservative treatment or surgery. A number of criticisms, however have been directed at the American guidelines for their inaccuracy in predicting the PCNs that will evolve into cancer, treating most PCNs in a similar way, with the result that patients with serous cystadenoma, which is benign, will be followed with MRI, at excessive cost for the healthcare system, while patients with malignancies or high-grade dysplasia risk not undergoing curative surgery.

Some of the studies that have compared the various guidelines propose an integrated approach that analyzes, in addition to the morphological aspect of PCNs, the cyst fluid content, in particular by means of molecular analysis, testing some hotspot mutations and deletions of HRAS, GNAS, VHL, PT53, PIK3CA, and PTEN.

Summarizing the approach of the European guidelines to PCNs:

- a conservative approach is recommended for asymptomatic patients with MCNs and IPMNs of secondary ducts <40 mm, without mural nodules;
- size >40 mm or a main pancreatic duct between 5 and 9.9 mm in diameter are relative indications for surgery;
- jaundice, mural nodules >5 mm, and the main pancreatic duct >10 mm in diameter are absolute indications for surgery.

In healthy patients with IPMN or MCN without signs of malignancy in which surgery is not ruled out a priori, radiological follow-up should never be interrupted, given the possible malignant evolution of these lesions.

Differential Diagnosis

Differential diagnosis of cystic lesions is based on morphological findings from instrumental investigations and analysis of cyst fluid. MRI is the exam of choice in identifying this type of lesion, especially in evaluating possible communication between the cystic lesion and the main pancreatic duct (in IPMN), whereas CT is less accurate but may play an important role in the presence of calcifications or malignant evolution, with solid mass infiltrating the parenchyma and vascular structures. Endoscopic ultrasound (EUS) is a valid method to integrate with MRI; however, as it is an operator-dependent technique based on ultrasound, it presents discordant values of accuracy in differentiating between benign and malignant PCNs, with significant differences in interobserver agreement.

The use of contrast medium in endoscopic ultrasound increases the diagnostic power of the method, especially in differentiating between mucoprotein plugs and mural nodules; moreover, the hyperenhancement of a mural nodule should raise the suspicion of malignant lesion evolution, for which needle aspiration may be indicated to confirm this nodule.

The main characteristics of PCNs are shown in **Table 47.3**.

Serous Cystadenomas

Serous cystadenomas are the most frequent type of benign cystic neoplasm.

They are generally asymptomatic but may cause abdominal pain and obstructive jaundice, especially if they become very large. They are more common in females in the sixth decade of life. The lesion consists of numerous small cysts separated by fibrous septa which give it a typical honeycomb appearance. A central star-shaped scar, sometimes calcified, it is typical of this cystic lesions, although it may be seen only in 10% of cases. Cyst fluid analysis highlights low CEA level (<5 ng/mL), high glucose values caused by glycogen-producing cells (PAS +) lining the septa, and

Table 47.3 Main characteristics of cystic lesions.

	Serous Cystadenoma	Mucinous Cystic Neoplasm (MCN)	IPMN	Cystic Tumour	Pseudopapillary Solid Tumour
Sex	75% F	F	F=M	F=M	90% F
Age	6th decade	5th-7th decade	7th decade	5th-7th decade	2nd decade
Distribution	Entire pancreas	Body-tail	Entire pancreas	Entire pancreas	Entire pancreas
Morphology	Microcystic/honeycomb	Unilocular, may have septa or calcified walls	Three variants: dilated main duct, dilated peripheral ducts (uni- or multifocal), mixed (involving the main and secondary ducts)	Solid, cystic or mixed	Solid or mixed (solid and cystic)
Cyst fluid	Low CEA, low amylase/lipase, high glucose	High CEA, variable amylase/lipase, low glucose	High CEA, high amylase/lipase, low glucose	Low CEA, low amylase/lipase	Low CEA, cytology often non-diagnostic
Behavior	Benign	Intermediate risk of malignancy	High risk of malignancy in IPMN of the main duct and in the mixed type; low risk in IPMN of the peripheral ducts	Low risk of malignancy; may be associated with multiple endocrine neoplasia type 1	Low risk of malignancy
Treatment	If asymptomatic, none	Surgical resection if >40 mm and/or mural nodules	Surgical resection in the main duct type; monitoring in the peripheral duct type (see ref guidelines)	Surgical resection in selected cases	Surgical resection

low viscosity. Cases of malignant degeneration are extremely rare. Surgical treatment is not indicated, except in cases that are symptomatic due to the size of the lesions.

Mucinous Cystic Neoplasms (MCN)

MCNs are cystic lesions that often affect women, with most frequently the body and tail of the pancreas.

An MCN is generally a single, unilocular lesion or with internal septations and ranging from a few millimeters to several centimeters in diameter. Biologically it is characterized by a potential for malignant evolution, with risk proportional to its volume and to the presence of solid nodules inside. The walls present an ovarian stroma, sometimes with calcific inclusions, and the cysts contain dense mucoid material. Unlike IPMNs, there is no communication between the cysts and the pancreatic ductal system. The cyst content is highly viscous with high glucose levels and CEA in general >192 ng/ml, though recent studies have demonstrated that this marker is not sufficiently accurate in diagnosing mucinous neoplasm or in differentiating between benign lesion and malignant evolution. Lesion size >4 cm, cystic wall thickening or intracystic septa, mural nodule, main pancreatic duct dilation and wall calcifications are characteristics associated to an increased risk of malignant transformation.

Intraductal Papillary Mucinous Neoplasms (IPMNs)

IPMNs are the most frequently diagnosed cystic neoplasms of the pancreas. They can involve the epithelial lining of the main pancreatic duct (main duct type), the secondary ducts (branch duct type), or both (mixed type), with hypersecretion of mucus that causes dilation of the ducts and consequent episodes of recurrent acute pancreatitis or evolution toward chronic obstructive pancreatitis.

In most cases, however, they are found incidentally during imaging performed for other clinical reasons. The most frequent form affects the peripheral ducts, which may be uni- or multifocal and has a low risk of progression into pancreatic cancer. The main duct type IPMN is less common but has a high rate of malignant transformation. The mixed type is quite rare and appears to have the same neoplastic risk as IPMN of the main duct. Cytological alterations are highly variable: from hyperplastic lesions to carcinomatous degeneration, through a sequence of mild, moderate, severe dysplasia and cancer.

From an anatomopathological point of view, IPMNs can be classified into 4 subtypes: intestinal, oncocytic, pancreatobiliary, and gastric, with different potential for evolution.

In the types involving the main pancreatic duct, radiological imaging shows uniform or segmental dilatation of the duct, whereas in the forms that mainly affect the secondary ducts, cystic dilatations communicating with the main pancreatic duct are observed. The presence of papilla of Vater open with mucus secretion is endoscopically pathognomonic. The treatment of choice for lesions of the main pancreatic duct is surgical resection for duct diameters >10 mm. For diameters between 5 and 9.9 mm, surgery is a relative indication and should be evaluated according to patient characteristics, age, comorbidity, and symptomatology. For the peripheral forms, an attentive surveillance plan by imaging can be implemented according to the guidelines.

Rare Cystic Tumours

Solid pseudopapillary tumours (SPTs) constitute approximately 1-2% of pancreatic neoplasms and 5% of PCNs. Despite a risk of malignancy of 8-20%, prognosis after surgical resection is excellent, with low risk of recurrence. They generally affect females and are more frequent around the third decade of life. At imaging SPT appear as an encapsulated lesion, with solid and cystic components and haemorrhagic areas. Lesions <3 cm are often without a capsule, with a higher solid component, and without signs of bleeding.

The cellular origin of SPTs is uncertain, as there is no clear benign counterpart in pancreatic cells. As they are much more common in women, like mucinous cystic neoplasms, a correlation has been suggested between these neoplasms and the embryogenetic development of the pancreas and the left ovary. On the other hand, the presence of proteins, such as A1AT and NSE together with vimentin, suggests an origin of totipotent pancreatic cells and neuronal precursors.

Cystic neuroendocrine tumours (NETs) account for less than 10% of all PCNs and are equally present in males and females between the fourth and the sixth decade of life. They are often found incidentally and are non-functioning tumours, i.e., they do not produce hormones.

At imaging, differential diagnosis with other PCNs is difficult, and only hyperenhancement of the wall at CT or at EUS with contrast can raise suspicion. They may be associated with genetic syndromes such as MEN1 and von Hippel-Lindau; however, in most cases they are sporadic and derive from cystic degeneration of a solid neuroendocrine tumour. The European guidelines suggest surgical treatment for cystic NETs >20mm, whereas those <20 mm, in the absence of malignancy characteristics, can be monitored with annual imaging.

KEY CONCEPTS

- Pancreatic adenocarcinoma is the fourth leading cause of cancer death, and its incidence is increasing.
- In most cases (> 80%), the disease is diagnosed at an advanced stage not amenable to surgery. The 5-year survival rate of operated patients is about 25%; the overall survival rate is 5-10%.
- The main risk factors for pancreatic adenocarcinoma are advanced age, smoking, familiarity, chronic pancreatitis, and diabetes.
- The cancer develops by means of the accumulation of gene mutations and precancerous lesions such as pancreatic intraepithelial neoplasms (PanIN), intraductal papillary mucinous neoplasms (IPMN) or cystic mucinous neoplasm (CMN). Precancerous screening could prevent cancer in high-risk individuals.
- The clinical presentation of pancreatic cancer includes jaundice (for tumours of the head), pain, weight loss, and new onset diabetes.
- Diagnosis and staging are based on imaging by ultrasound, computerized tomography, magnetic resonance, and endoscopic ultrasound. The latter also enables cyto-histological diagnosis by means of ultrasound-guided biopsies of the pancreas
- Surgical resection is the only potentially curative treatment. Adjuvant chemotherapy is indicated for improving post-surgical survival. Neoadjuvant chemotherapy can return to resectability a substantial fraction of neoplasms classified as borderline at imaging. Palliative chemotherapy can improve survival of patients with metastatic cancer.
- Endoscopy, via placement of a biliary prosthesis, has a prominent role in the palliation of jaundice secondary to pancreas head tumours.
- Pancreatic cystic tumours represent a large group of cystic lesions that may be benign and borderline (serous cystic neoplasm), or they may be malignant with metastatic potential (such as MCN, IPMN or solid pseupapillary tumour). Therefore, an accurate differential diagnosis is fundamental for a correct therapeutic approach.
- The analysis of cystic fluid and imaging exams (such as TC, RM and endoscopic ultrasound) are important for the differential diagnosis between pancreatic cystic lesions. Special attention should be given to the indentification of characteristics of malignant evolution such as enhancing mural nodule and main pancreatic duct dilation.
- Knowledge of pancreatic cystic tumours enables correct management, and the national and international guidelines are useful for starting patients on a course of radiological follow-up or surgical treatment.

REFERENCES

- Ducreux M, Cuhna AS, Caramella C, et al. Cancer of the pancreas: ESMO Clinical. Practice Guidelines for diagnosis, treatment and follow-up. Annals of Oncology. 2015;26 (Suppl5):v56-v68.
- Elta GH, Enestvedt BK, Sauer BG, et al. ACG Clinical Guideline: diagnosis and management of pancreatic cyst. Am J Gastroenterol. 2018 Apr;113(4):464-79.
- European Study Group on Cystic Tumours of the Pancreas. European evidence-based guidelines on pancreatic cystic neoplasms. Gut. 2018 May;67(5):789-804.
- Kamisawa T, Wood LD, Itoi T, Takaori K. Pancreatic cancer. Lancet. 2016 Jul 2;388(10039):73-85.
- Ryan DP, Hong TS, Bardeesy N. Pancreatic adenocarcinoma. N Engl J Med. 2014 Sep 11;371(11):1039-49.
- Tempero MA, Malafa MP, Al-Hawary M, et al. Pancreatic adenocarcinoma, Version 2.2017, NCCN Clinical Practice Guidelines in Oncology. J Natl Compr Canc Netw. 2017;15:1028-106.

GASTROINTESTINAL NEUROENDOCRINE TUMOURS

Edith Lahner, Massimo Claudio Fantini

LEARNING OBJECTIVES
- To gain knowledge about clinical and histological features of neuroendocrine tumours.
- To gain knowledge about diagnosis and treatment.

Neuroendocrine neoplasms (NEN) originate from the neuroendocrine system throughout the body; in two-thirds of cases the gastroenteropancreatic tract (GEP) is involved. These tumours are usually considered rare but their incidence has increased significantly in the last decades. To date, data on the actual epidemiology of NEN in Italy are scant. However, an estimate of the incidence and prevalence on NENs can be obtained from data obtained in other countries or from local (regional) registries in Italy. Collectively, these data indicate an incidence of about 0.3 cases per 100,000 inhabitants/year, and a prevalence 7-fold higher than the incidence (about 2 cases per 100,000 inhabitants). The lower incidence to prevalence ratio as compared to exocrine neoplasias is due to longer survival, making NEN a chronic oncologic disease. The main negative prognostic factors of NEN are the primary tumour site (pancreatic NEN generally have a worse prognosis than those localized in the intestine), TNM stage, WHO histopathological classification, which defines both the morphological appearance of the tumour and its proliferative activity in terms of number of mitosis or proliferation index (Ki67). The Ki67-based proliferation index tumour grading is considered the most solid prognostic factor for NEN. Indeed, it not only significantly correlates with overall survival, but also with progression of the disease in patients with advanced pancreatic NEN and tumour recurrence in patients undergoing curative surgery. Additional prognostic factors are expression of somatostatin receptors, SSRTs, which predicts a more favourable clinical behaviour than the absence of expression, tumour growth and patient's age at diagnosis. Clinically, GEP NENs are commonly divided into functional and non-functional, depending on the presence or not of a clinical syndrome related to the production and circulation of one or more hormonal substances. The therapy of these neoplasms will be described in the paragraphs on tumour location.

DIAGNOSIS

Histopathological Definition

The World Health Organization (WHO) classification considers all NENs as potentially malignant and distinguishes them based on location, differentiation, and proliferation index (**Table 48.1**). The GEP NENs are distinguished in "tumours" and "carcinomas". Neuroendocrine tumours (NETs) have a typical "organoid" structure (nests, trabeculae or solid) with very rare atypias. NETs are divided into two prognostic categories: G1 NET and G2 NET based on mitosis count and/or expression of proliferation marker Ki67 as evaluated by immunohistochemistry. Neuroendocrine carcinomas (NECs) exhibit wide spreading, solid growth with extensive necrosis and numerous cytological atypias. NECs can be subdivided in small and large cell subgroups. Based on recent scientific evidence, the 2016 European Guidelines on Neuroendocrine Tumours (ENETS) have proposed a new diagnostic cate- gory named NET G3, in which well differentiated neuroendocrine neoplasia (NEN) characterized by Ki-67 between 21% and 55% are included. The definitions of the WHO classification must necessarily be integrated and completed by the definition of the TNM staging system (extension of neoplastic invasion). Additional parameters are not mandatory for all GEP NEN histology records but may be useful in specific cases. They are: tumour size, multicentricity, presence of vascular and/or perineural invasion, surgical resection margins, distance of the tumour from the resection margins. For instance, in appendicular NET, macroscopic size of the tumour, description of the resection margins, and infiltration of the meso are all elements that must be recorded. In the sto-

Table 48.1 Morphological classification and grading (according to 2010 WHO classification).

Diagnosis	Grading	Mitotic Index	Ki67 Index	Differentiation
1. Neuroendocrine tumour (NET)	1	<2/10 hpf	≤ 2%	Well-differentiated
2. Neuroendocrine tumour (NET)	2	2-20/10 hpf	3-20%	Well/moderately differentiated
3. Neuroendocrine carcinoma (NEC)	3	>20/10 hpf	>20%	Poorly differentiated
4. Mixed adeno-neuroendocrine carcinoma (MANEC)	-	-	-	Poorly differentiated*
5. Hyperplastic and pre-neoplastic lesions	-	-	-	-

* in rare cases the neuroendocrine component may corrispond to NET G1 or G2.

mach, quantitative and qualitative evaluation of enterochromaffinlike cell (ECL) hyperplastic and/or dysplastic lesions in the context of chronic atrophic gastritis of the gastric body is recommended. Identification of the neuroendocrine phenotype requires immunohistochemical positivity for specific markers such as chromogranin A (CgA) and synaptophysin, whose expression is reduced in NEC. Based on Ki-67 (marker that quantifies tumour proliferation) or the number of mitoses on 10 high power fields (HPF, with a minimum magnification of 40x), three grade levels (G) have been identified: G1 (the least aggressive) to G3 (the most aggressive). In 2017 the revised WHO 2017 classification for pancreatic neuroendocrine tumours fixed the cut-off at 5% of Ki67-positive cells instead of 2%, to distinguish G1 from G2 (G1 <5%; G2 5-20%; G3> 20%).

BILIARY TRACT AND PANCREAS

TNM Staging System

The staging of NEN GEPs follows the TNM system proposed by the European Neuroendocrine Tumour Society (ENETS) that evaluates three parameters: T (local disease extension), N (lymph node involvement), and M (distant metastasis). The definitions of the stages (from I to IV) vary according to the location of the primary tumour. Stage IV (i.e., a metastatic tumour) is invariably associated with a worse prognosis than stages I to III, especially in extra-abdominal metastases (e.g., bony, pulmonary, cerebral metastasis).

Genetic Profile

Most NENs are sporadic. However, there are also rare genetic syndromes characterized by the association of various endocrine disorders. The multiple endocrine neoplasia syndrome (MEN1) is characterized by two or more neuroendocrine neoplasms in the pituitary, pancreatic or parathyroid glands (hyperplasia); possible additional sites are the thymus, lung, stomach, adrenal cortex, angiomas, and skin lipomas. In suspected MEN1 or established familiar aggregation of neuroendocrine tumours, a genetic test is performed on peripheral blood or on samples of tumour tissue for detecting mutation of the menin gene.

Laboratory Diagnostics

Plasma concentration of Chromogranin A (CgA) is used in both functional and non-functional NENs and its use should be restricted to follow-up, once diagnosis is made and not as a diagnostic or screening tool. Sensitivity of CgA testing varies between 70 and 90%, while specificity is affected by a high rate of false positives as in chronic atrophic gastritis (CAG), the concomitant use of proton pump inhibitors (PPI), and chronic renal failure. For functional forms, instead, there are specific markers. In the suspicion of "carcinoid syndrome" the 24-hour urinary concentration of 5-hydroxy-indolacetic acid (5-HIAA) is dosed. The accuracy of this test is high when the value is at least twice the maximum value of the reference range. Some recommendations are essential to reduce the false positive rate before collecting the sample (avoid pineapple, dried fruit, exotic fruit, alcohol, fermented cheeses, smoking). With these precautions sensitivity reaches 70% and specificity is close to 100%. During follow-up this test is used to monitor disease progression and response to therapy. In the Zollinger-Ellison syndrome (ZES), elevated basal blood levels of gastrin are found in 98% of patients, with values 10-fold higher than normal in 40% of cases. Possible false positives are due to the use of PPI and CAG. To increase its accuracy, the secretin test can be performed. During this test, gastrin blood levels are recorded at different time points after stimulation with secretin; an increase after stimulation of at least 120 pg/mL from baseline is indicative of ZES (sensitivity 94%, specificity 100%). If an insulinoma is suspected, the combination of high levels of insulin associated with elevated C-peptide values (>200 pmol/L) and hypoglycemia (<45 mg/dL) is diagnostic. The fasting test with measurement of the three aforementioned biochemical parameters in a 72-hour period, allows to achieve 100% diagnostic accuracy.

Endoscopic Diagnostics

Endoscopy with bioptic sampling has a fundamental role in the identification and characterization of primary GEP NEN. The stomach and the rectum are the most common sites in the gastrointestinal tract. In duodenal carcinoids, lesions are localized in the first or second duodenal sections in 70% of cases. Endoscopic ultrasound (EUS), using high ultrasonic frequencies, allows to accurately visualize the layers of the gastrointestinal wall, defining the depth of parietal invasion and lymph node involvement. Finally, ultrasound guided fine needle aspiration (EUS-FNA) of the suspected adenopathies, as well as of pancreatic NEN (PNEN), allows histological definition and calculation of Ki-67 positive cells.

Radiological Instrumental Diagnostics

Contrast enhanced CT scan is the most frequently used imaging technique to identify and stage GEP NENs. Magnetic resonance imaging (MRI), with hepatospecific contrast medium, allows study of the liver parenchyma and provides information on the nature of nodular lesions, although the diagnosis requires biopsy in most cases. Entero-CT and the entero-MRI allow to study the small intestine, after distension of the intestinal loops by oral negative and biphasic contrast, consisting of nonabsorbable iso-osmolar solutions (polyethylene glycol, PEG) and hyperosmolar solutions (mannitol, sorbitol), in CT and MRI, respectively.

Nuclear Diagnostics

The functional imaging techniques for NENs identify the expression of SSRTs (in particular subtype 2: SSRT-2). They include 111In-pentetreotide scintigraphy (or OctreoScan®) and positron emission tomography (PET) with somatostatin analogues labelled with 68Ga (68Ga-PET).
These techniques identify localization of the primary tumour, aid in staging especially for extra-abdominal lesions, and characterization of tumour lesions expression of SSTR, and in identifying patients eligible for somatostatinbased treatment. 68Ga-PET has higher diagnostic accuracy than OctreoScan®; it needs only one day instead of two and offers standardized quantification of positive areas based on the Standardized Uptake Value (SUV) parameter. Another functional test is 18F-FDG-PET, which identifies areas with high metabolic activity. Since high metabolic activity correlates with high proliferation and Ki67 expression, it is useful especially in the G3 NEC forms, with a negative prognostic value for positive cases.

CLASSIFICATION BY LOCATION

Neuroendocrine Tumours of the Stomach

Some 23% of all GEP NENs are gastric carcinoids, with an incidence of around 0.2 per 100,000 individuals.

Clinical Features

Gastric carcinoids can be divided in three subtypes: Type I carcinoids (**Figure 48.1**) accounts for 75-80% of all gastric NEN. Diagnosis is often incidental during oesophagogastroduodenoscopy (EGDS) performed for anaemia or dyspepsia.
Their pathogenesis is based on the presence of CAG with achlorhydria and hypergastrinemia. Since gastrin acts as a growth factor for enterochromaffin-like cells, gastrin induces in these cells an initial hypeproliferative phenotype followed by hyperplasia and dysplasia, generating a carcinoid neoplasia. Type I carcinoids are generally multiple, sub centimetric G1 NET, limited to the submucosa. Only 5% show invasive behaviour, they tend to recur (50% in 24 months) but with indolent behaviour.
Type II gastric carcinoids are found in 25- 35% of patients with MEN1 or ZES. They account for 6% of gastric carcinoids, they are generally G1 or G2 NETs,

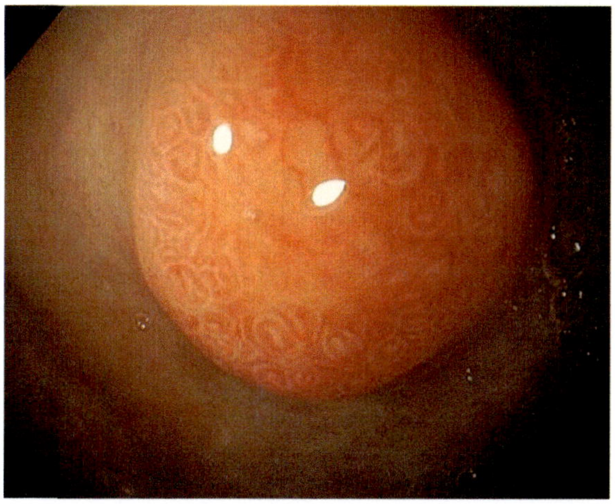

Figure 48.1 Endoscopic image of a type 1 gastric carcinoid of the body.

multiple and sub centimetric, indolent, and rarely malignant. Type III gastric carcinoids are not associated with any gastric disorder, are sporadic and characterized by adenocarcinoma-like malignant behaviour

Diagnosis
The gold standard for the diagnosis of gastric carcinoids is oesophagogastroduodenoscopy (EGDS) with biopsy of the lesions and the surrounding mucosa of the gastric body and fundus to determine the presence of CAG. Loco-regional staging of polyps >1 cm is performed by EUS; based on findings, endoscopic resection is then chosen (for type I and II NETs). For type III, staging is based on contrast enhanced CT.

Therapy
For type I carcinoids, management with endoscopic follow-up and resection of all visible lesions with polypectomy, mucosectomy or endoscopic submucosal dissection is recommended. Generally, EGDS is recommended every 6-12 (in recurrent multiple lesions) or 24 months, with complete biopsy mapping given the possible coexistence of CAG. Monitoring of iron and vitamin B12 blood levels every 6 months and supplantation if needed might be useful in these patients. Surgery is indicated only in the rare cases of locoregional invasion or distant metastasis. For type II carcinoids, endoscopic/surgical management is indicated. Therapy with PPI for ZES and possibly with somatostatin analogues (SSA) in advanced disease is also recommended. Type III gastric carcinoids are managed by surgery and chemotherapy.

Neuroendocrine Tumours of the Pancreas
NPCs have an incidence of 1/100,000/year and account for 10% of all pancreatic tumours.

Clinical Features
About 70% of NPC are non-functional and often diagnosed at advanced stage. In other cases the clinical picture is related to non-specific symptoms (e.g., loss of appetite, weight loss, diabetes) or due to growth of the mass (obstructive jaundice if the lesion is in the head of the pancreas, pain if in the tail). These NEN have a poorer prognosis than intestinal ones; in G3 NEC, the behaviour is similar to pancreatic adenocarcinoma. The remaining 30% of PNEN are functional and the clinical presentation differs according to the secreted hormone.
The gastrinoma can be found at the duodenal or pancreatic level and accounts for 12-15% of all functional NENs. It is responsible for the ZES in which acid hypersecretion resulting from hypergastrinemia results in a clinical picture of peptic ulcers nonresponsive at standard doses of PPIs and diarrhoea; the latter caused by increased volume of gastrointestinal secretion, inactivation of digestive enzymes, damage of the intestinal mucosa by the acid, and direct action on the enterocytes by gastrin.
Insulinoma originates in the beta cells of the pancreatic islets and accounts for about 15-18% of all functional NEN. It is found predominantly in adults and if diagnosed in young patients MEN1 should be suspected. The diagnosis of insulinoma is based on:

- the presence of hypoglycaemia that meets Whipple's criteria;
- signs and symptoms of hypoglycaemia Concomitant low blood glucose levels (<45 mg/dL);
- regression of symptoms after administration of sugars;
- inappropriately high insulin and peptide C levels for glycaemic values.

Hypoglycaemia occurs clinically with nausea, sweating, mental confusion, and loss of consciousness. Furthermore, the fasting test in a 72-hour period has 100% diagnostic accuracy: when symptoms appear or when glycaemic values are <40 mg/dL, peptide C and insulin levels are also measured. Not suppressed insulin levels (insulin/glycemia ratio >0.3 in hypoglycaemia) document an inappropriate insulin secretion, supporting the diagnosis of insulinoma.

Diagnosis
The gold standard for the diagnosis is histological evaluation of samples obtained by EUS (from the primary tumour) or echo- or CT-guided biopsy of metastasis. Staging is performed by contrast enhanced total body CT scan. To study the pancreaticobiliary system, MRI combined with a cholangiopancreato-MR sequence is indicated. In addition, evaluation of SSRTs expression by scintigraphy and tumour metabolic activity (PET-Gallium DOTANOC and/or PET-FDG) is recommended.

Therapy
In PNEN without locoregional invasion, surgical resection with lymphadenectomy is the gold standard therapy and has a curative intent. If the lesion is > 2 cm, simple surgical enucleation or radiological follow-up may be considered due to its slow evolution/progression. In young persons and

especially in functional lesions, surgical debulking, even in advanced/metastatic stage, can improve clinical manifestations (and quality of life) and disease prognosis. If OctreoScan® or 68Ga-DOTA-PET returns positive results, SSAs (octreotide or lanreotide) are the first line of therapy, with high efficacy in stabilizing the disease and good tolerability for the patient. In case of failure, peptide receptor radionuclide therapy (PRRT), an endovascular radiotherapy based on the combination of somatostatin labelled with radioisotope (177-Lutetio), is indicated. Recently approved in Italy for the treatment of gastroenteropancreatic neuroendocrine tumours, this therapy provides long term control of the disease by acting via a cytotoxic mechanism. Another type of treatment is based on new generation of oral administered drugs: the "targeted therapies". Everolimus acts on the mTOR pathway by controlling tumour proliferation. Sunitinib has an antiangiogenic action. Both are approved for the treatment of advanced pancreatic neuroendocrine tumours and tumour progression. Chemotherapy (usually combinations with streptozolocin or temozolomide/capecitabine) remains a valuable option for poorly differentiated and/or high Ki-67-expressing tumours. Clinical studies demonstrated the efficacy of these therapies in reducing tumour mass, although no significant improvement of on overall survival was observed.

Intestinal Neuroendocrine Tumours

Intestinal carcinoids account for 8-10% of all GEP NENs and predominantly arise in the leum. Their incidence is 0.30/100,000, with an average age at diagnosis of 65.4 years. These neoplasms have a better prognosis than PNEN of comparable stage. Moreover, tumours of the colon are generally more aggressive than those of the small intestine.

Clinical Features

Non-functional tumours are characterized by non-specific symptoms related to the tumour mass (bleeding, anaemia, recurrent sub occlusive episodes); often diagnosis is made during emergency surgery performed for intestinal obstruction. Functional tumours, on the other hand, can cause carcinoid syndrome due to the massive blood release of serotonin and its derivatives. It is characterized by skin flushing (63-94%: red-violet complexion the face and neck, associated with hot flashes, often triggered by stress or alcohol intake), diarrhoea (68-84%), abdominal pain (10-55%), telangiectasia (25%), and bronchospasm (3-19%). Moreover, in 15-20% of cases it can be accompanied by "carcinoid heart disease" caused by fibrotic damage to the endocardium lining the tricuspid and pulmonary valves. This syndrome, which may also be present in pulmonary NETs, usually occurs in metastatic disease and is associated with a urinary increase in 5-HIAA.

Diagnosis

Histological evaluation of samples obtained during rectosigmoidocolonscopy (RSCS) or more sophisticated techniques such as double or single balloon enteroscopy, is the gold standard for diagnosis. In the presence of metastatic disease, tissue samples can be obtained by US- or CT-guided biopsy. The study of the primitive site can be aided by entero-CT or entero-MRI. Staging is based on a total body CT scan with contrast, which reveals a starry image produced by the "stretching" of the mesentery caused by the abundant desmoid reaction that characterizes ileal carcinoids. Functional imaging to identify the expression of SSTRs complete the diagnostic workup.

Therapy

Due to the high risk of intestinal obstruction, surgical resection of the primary tumour is indicated even in metastatic disease. Surgery entails segmental resection combined with enlarged lymphadenectomy that can be extended to include superior mesenteric artery lymph nodes in some cases. If SSRTs are expressed, the SSAs are used for their antiproliferative action and for controlling carcinoid syndrome with good clinical and biochemical response. In the most advanced SSRT-positive forms that lose response to SSA, PRRT can be undertaken. As for targeted therapies, everolimus is approved for this form of carcinoids. Chemotherapy remains the mainstay therapy for G3 NEC.

Neuroendocrine Tumours of the Rectum

Clinical Features

Rectal carcinoids only rarely manifest with rectorrhagia or subocclusive symptoms (if large) but are generally asymptomatic and occasionally diagnosed during RSCS. Recent data report a detection rate of one rectal carcinoid every 2,500 screening colonoscopies. They are usually subcentimetric, arise in the submucosa and protrude in the lumen like small polypoid nodules. Follow-up is often negative after endoscopic resection. However, cases of infiltration beyond the submucosa, lymph node involvement, and distant metastasis characterise up to 14% of these neoplasms. Risk factors for malignant behaviour are diameter >2 cm, blood vessel invasion, high Ki-67 expression, poor differentiation, and metastasis.

Diagnosis

The gold standard diagnostic procedure is RSCS with bioptic sampling of the identified lesions, accompanied, in case of polyps >1 cm, by EUS for locoregional staging to define appropriate endoscopic resection technique. Pelvic floor MRI can complete staging of advanced forms; contrast enhanced total body CT scan and functional imaging. Follow-up should be programmed based on findings from RSCS, especially in lesions or after surgical treatment.

Therapy

Endoscopic resection followed by endoscopic follow-up is an effective management for small G1 NETs.

For polyps between 1 and 2 cm, surgery with anterior resection of the rectum should be considered. In general, surgery is indicated in tumour involvement beyond the submucosa and/or locoregional lymph nodes and more extensive resections (similar to those for adenocarcinoma) in the forms with high Ki-67 expression and in the poorly differentiated forms. In metastatic tumours, removal of the primary lesion should be limited to cases at high risk of occlusion. In the metastatic forms expressing SSRT, SSA can be prescribed, as well as PRRT, even if published evidence in this regard is scarce. Chemotherapy is used for the G3 NEC forms.

KEY CONCEPTS

- Neuroendocrine neoplasms (NEN) affect the gastroenteropancreatic tract (GEP) in two thirds of cases.
- These tumours are rare but their incidence is increasing.
- The main negative prognostic factors of NEN are: site of the primary tumour; TNM stage; WHO histopathological class (morphological appearance of the tumour and proliferation index (Ki67).
- Clinically, NEN GEPs are commonly divided into functional and non-functional, depending on the presence or absence of a clinical syndrome related to the production of one or more hormones.
- The 2010 World Health Organization (WHO) classification considers all NENs as potentially malignant and they are classified based on location, differentiation, and proliferation index.
- NEN GEPs are distinguished in "tumours" (NET) and "carcinomas" (NEC).

REFERENCES

- Delle Fave GF, O'Toole D, Sundin A, et al.; Vienna Consensus Conference participants. ENETS Consensus guidelines update for gastroduodenal neuroendocrine neoplasms. Neuroendocrinology. 2016;103(2):119-24.
- Falconi M, Eriksson B, Kaltsas G, et al.; Vienna Consensus Conference participants. Consensus guidelines update for the management of functional p-NETs (F-p-NETs) and non-functional p-NETs (NF-p-NETs). Neuroendocrinology. 2016; 103(2): 153-71.
- Garcia-Carbonero R, Sorbye H, Baudin E, et al.; Vienna Consensus Conference participants. Consensus guidelines for high grade gastro-entero-pancreatic (GEP) neuroendocrine tumours and neuroendocrine carcinomas (NEC). Neuroendocrinology. 2016;103(2):186-94.
- Linee Guida AIOM. Edizione 2016. http://www.aiom.it/professionisti/documenti-scientifici/linee-guida.
- Niederle B, Pape UF, Costa F, et al. Vienna Consensus Conference participants. ENETS Consensus guidelines update for neuroendocrine neoplasm of the jejunum and ileum. Neuroendocrinology. 2016;103(2):125-38.
- O'Toole D, Kianmanesh R, Caplin M. ENETS 2016 Consensus guidelines for the management of patients with digestive neuroendocrine tumours: an update. Neuroendocrinology. 2016;103(2):117-8.
- Pavel M, O'Toole D, Costa F, et al. Vienna Consensus Conference participants. Consensus guidelines update for the management of distant metastatic disease of intestinal, pancreatic, bronchial neuroendocrine neoplasms (NEN) and NEN of unknown primary site. Neuroendocrinology. 2012;95(2):157-76.
- Ramage J, De Herder WW, Delle Fave GF, et al. Vienna Consensus Conference participants. Consensus guidelines update for colorectal neuroendocrine neoplasms (NEN). Neuroendocrinology. 2016;103(2):139-43.

GASTROINTESTINAL BLEEDING

Paolo Giorgio Arcidiacono, Alessandra Dell'Era

LEARNING OBJECTIVES

- To describe the main causes of acute and chronic gastrointestinal bleeding.
- To identify the principal methods for investigating bleeding location and source.
- To be aware of the principles of therapy for the main causes of bleeding.

DEFINITION

The term "gastrointestinal bleeding" (GIB) describes any episode of bleeding that originates from the digestive tract. Two typologies of GIB are distinguished: upper GIB (UGIB), which originates above the ligament of Treitz, and lower GIB (LGIB), originating below it. In about 5% of cases, however, it is difficult to identify the site of bleeding by conventional endoscopic examinations (upper endoscopy and ileocolonoscopy); in such cases the bleeding is defined obscure.

EPIDEMIOLOGY

According to data from the Italian Ministry of Health, in 2005 the incidence of hospitalizations was 60/100,000 for UGIB and 30-40/100,000 for LGIB. The mortality related to an episode of upper GIB is about 8-10%, which has remained stable for the last 40 years and is strongly dependent on the bleeding cause and the presence of comorbidities.
LGIB has a better prognosis with a mortality rate of less than 5%. Obscure bleeding generally has a chronic/intermittent nature and a lower mortality rate.

CLINICAL PRESENTATION

Clinical presentation depends on the bleeding site, the volume, and the rate of blood loss. The following presentations are distinguished:
Haematemesis: emission of blood with vomit; bright red or brown-black (coffee ground vomit) when the blood has been altered by hydrochloric acid.
Melena: emission of black (as haemoglobin is degraded into haematin in the intestinal tract) liquid or semiliquid stool, typically malodorous.
Haematochezia and proctorrhagia: emission of bright red blood, respectively of minimal or abundant entity, alone or mixed with faeces.
Occult bleeding: blood traces detectable only by fecal occult blood test.
Clinical signs secondary to blood loss in the absence of evident bleeding (for example, in the massive acute haemorrhage, when blood has not yet been emitted by natural orifices): Orthostatic hypotension, angina, dyspnea, shock.
In general, melena is a manifestation of an upper digestive bleeding, whereas haematochezia or proctorrhagia a manifestation of lower digestive bleeding. In massive bleeding from the upper digestive tract, the blood, which has a cathartic effect, flows rapidly through the intestinal tract, with emission of reddish blood from the anus (red melena).
Conversely, in slowed intestinal transit, bleeding from the ileum or the right colon can occur with the appearance of melena.

CLASSIFICATION OF A PATIENT WITH GASTROINTESTINAL BLEEDING

In GIB patient, it is essential to focus on haemodynamic stabilisation first and then on diagnosis and therapy of the source of bleeding. Orthostatic hypotension is evaluated by measuring systolic blood pressure and heart rate in standing and supine position. It may be useful to calculate the shock-index (heart rate in beats per minute/systolic blood pressure in mmHg); values between 0.5-0.7 are normal; values between 0.7 and 1 denote a need for close monitoring and values >1 are indicative of haemodynamic instability. Other parameters to monitor are oxygenation and hourly diuresis. In haematemesis, possible obstruction of the airways must be excluded.

Blood loss must be estimated (evaluating alterations in blood pressure and heart rate and appearance of signs and symptoms), so that it can be suitably reintegrated.
It is necessary to cannulate at least two peripheral veins; optionally, in massive bleeding, place a central venous catheter, and take blood samples for haematocrit, clotting test (PT, PTT), platelets, blood typing, and compatibility testing. The initial value of haematocrit is a poor indicator of acute blood loss, as bleeding causes the cellular and liquid part of the blood to be lost in equal proportions.
In about 24-72 hours, the recall of liquids from the extravascular compartment tries to restore the blood volume, while the haematocrit value declines. Contrarily, in chronic blood loss, the haematocrit is a good indicator of blood loss.
The decision to transfuse the patient is based on pulse and pressure instability, signs of persistent bleeding (haematemesis, red blood from the nasogastric tube, haematochezia), advanced age, comorbidities making an ongoing anemia dangerous (ischaemic heart disease, cerebrovascular insufficiency). Packed red blood cells are preferred for maintaining haematocrit values above 30% in elderly patients and 20% in young patients. The transfusion of plasma and/or platelets should be reserved for transfusion of large quantities of blood or coagulation disorders. Alterations of acid-base balance must also be monitored, as cellular hypoxia may lead to the production of lactate resulting in the onset of metabolic acidosis. In severe hypotension, sympathomimetic amines should be administered (dopamine, adrenaline or noradrenaline).

CLINICAL EVALUATION AND LOCATION OF THE SITE OF BLEEDING

When the patient is stabilized, it is necessary to perform medical history and accurate physical examination. Assessment includes:
Patient age, as the most frequent causes of bleeding differ depending on age (for example, the most frequent causes of lower GIB in elderly patients are diverticula, angiodysplasia, and polyps of the colon, while in children and adolescents it is Meckel's diverticulum); previous episodes of bleeding and their location; concomitant symptoms (e.g., abdominal pain, dyspepsia, vomiting...); comorbidities (e.g., cirrhosis, neoplasia, etc.); previous surgery; consumption (and type) of drugs or alcohol.
Physical examination will look for signs of cirrhosis (e.g., spider nevi, hepatosplenomegaly, ascites) and abdominal masses or areas of abdominal pain. Increased bowel sounds is usually indicative of upper gastrointestinal bleeding.
The use of a nasogastric tube (NGT), positioned after initial evaluation, provides indications about the bleeding site, allows the gastric cavity to be irrigated, facilitates endoscopy, and allows the stomach to be emptied, thus preventing massive vomiting that could cause pneumonia ab ingestis. In haematemesis, the tube will allow to evaluate cessation/resumption of bleeding. In melena, the color of the aspirated liquid can help in differential diagnosis of superior or inferior bleeding. A bright red or coffee blood aspirate is indicative of upper bleeding; if the aspirate is clear, upper bleeding can not be excluded, as it could be bleeding of duodenal origin with a competent pylorus that prevents the backflow of material from the duodenum to the stomach. Finally, if bile is present in the aspirate, bleeding of proximal origin to the Treitz can be considered unlikely. SNG also has a prognostic value: mortality in patients with "coffee-ground" tubes and melena is <9%, while for patients with aspirates with bright red blood and haematochezia, mortality can reach 30%.
Rectal exploration allows to verify the presence and characteristics of rectal blood and to verify the coexistence of haemorrhoidal varices and possible rectal masses. A finding of bright red blood on the finger indicates that the bleeding probably originates in the lower GI, whereas melena probably indicates upper GI bleeding. However, 50-100 mL of blood in the stomach are enough to produce black stools and blood losses >1000 mL cause acceleration of intestinal transit, with the emission of bright red or dark red stools, even if the bleeding originates in the upper GI tract.
Finally, if the blood tests result in a disproportionate increase in blood nitrogen compared to creatinine, the site of bleeding is likely to be the upper GI tract.

ACUTE UPPER GASTROINTESTINAL BLEEDING

Endoscopic Examination

Digestive endoscopy is the gold standard to check for upper gastrointestinal bleeding (UGIB), identify the site and nature of the lesion, perform treatment, if necessary, and define the required level of support and need for hospitalization. Scoring systems such as the Glasgow-Blatchford or the

Rockall scores are among the most widely used to predict the risk of repeated bleeding and mortality after UGIB. The former is based on clinical parameters (presence of shock, comorbidities), the latter on endoscopic findings (diagnosis of bleeding source and signs of recent bleeding), on demographics (age) and clinical parameters (presence of shock, comorbidities).
For the exploration of the upper digestive tract, upper endoscopy is the gold standard endoscopic examinationy.
Upper endoscopy must be performed urgently, after restoration of haemodynamic stability. In patients with clinical signs suggestive of higher risk (persistence of haemodynamic instability despite reanimation maneuvers, relapsing haematemesis or contraindications to anticoagulation withdrawal) upper endoscopy must be performed even earlier.
It is possible to observe patients with mild bleeding, especially if young, and delay the upper endoscopy. It performed by intubation under direct endoscopic vision with the patient in left lateral position, so as to explore the pharyngo-laryngeal district. The complete upper digestive tract should be explored without stopping at the first lesion, since there may be more than one lesion and the first encountered lesion may not be the bleeding source. The type of blood present in the lumen can provide useful information: fresh, bright red and liquid blood is strongly indicative of active bleeding; dark red blood with clots is indicative of a very recent bleeding.

Aetiology, Evolution, and Prognosis

Various causes may explain upper GIB (Table 49.1). In 80% of cases the bleeding is self-limiting; in the remaining 20% of cases, however, bleeding may continue or recur.
The mortality rate is about 8-10%, strongly dependent on prognostic factors: advanced age, source of bleeding, severity of bleeding and/or the need for urgent surgery, presence of other serious concurrent illnesses, occurrence or recurrence of in-hospital bleeding, endoscopic signs of recent bleeding and emission of red or dark red blood from the rectum.

Table 49.1 Causes of upper gastrointestinal bleeding

Diagnosis	% of total
Peptic Ulcer	47.1
Gastritis	18.1
Oesophagitis	15.2
Angiodysplasia	6.2
Mallory-Weiss lesion	6.9
Neoplasia	3.7
Oesophageal varices	1.8
Dielafoy's lesion	1.5

Source: Wuerth, B.A. & Rockey, D.C. Dig Dis Sci 2018; 63:1286-1293

Causes of Upper Digestive Bleeding

Peptic Ulcer

A peptic ulcer is the cause of approximately 50% of UGIB (see Table 49.1).
The use of NSAIDS is probably the single most important risk factor. The frequency of hospital admissions for a bleeding ulcer has decreased over the years for younger patients; it has, conversely, increased in person aged over 65 years, probably due to the use of NSAIDS. The majority of ulcers stops bleeding spontaneously and does not require specific therapy.
Table 49.2 presents the most widely used endo-

Table 49.2 Forrest classification of bleeding ulcers in relation to rebleeding risk and need for surgery.

Forrest Class	Endoscopic Aspect	Rebleeding Risk %	Need for Surgery %
Ia	Active Spurting bleeding	50-70	35
Ib	Active Oozing bleeding	50-70	35
IIa	Ulcer with non-bleeding visible vessel	50-70	35
IIb	Ulcer with adherent clot	33-36	10
IIc	Haematin (black) flat spot on ulcer base	18-25	5
III	Clean base ulcer	1-3	0

scopic classification of bleeding ulcers (Forrest classification) with the corresponding incidence of recurrent bleeding and the need for surgical intervention. It is now believed that patients with Forrest III classification can be dismissed early after therapy for the ulcer has been initiated.
Patients with Forrest classification Ia to IIc should be admitted for at least 3 days because the majority of recurrences occurs within this period; patients with Forrest classification IIb and IIc may be observed in general wards, while those with Forrest Ia, Ib, and IIa treated with endoscopic haemostasis and observed in the intensive care unit for about 24 hours.

Medical Therapy
Medical therapy with proton pump inhibitors (PPI) before endoscopy (e.g., omeprazole 40 mg/12 hours for 5 days or 80 mg bolus followed by infusion of 8 mg/h for 72 h) has significantly reduced the number of patients with active bleeding or recent bleeding during endoscopic evaluation.

Endoscopic Therapy
Different endoscopic methods (diathermocoagulation, injection of vasoconstrictive substances such as 1:10,000 adrenaline, injection of hypertonic solution, injection of sclerosing substances such as, polydocanol, thrombin injection, clip placement) have been used effectively and with equivalent results for the control of haemorrhage from peptic ulcer disease.

Prevention of Long-Term Bleeding Recurrences
Therapy with oral PPI (full dose initially and minimal effective dose thereafter) and *Helicobacter pylori* eradication, particularly in patients taking NSAIDS, significantly reduces both short- and long-term bleeding recurrence. There is no convincing evidence of the efficacy of long-term therapy with H2 blockers.

Gastric Erosions
Gastric erosions are the second cause of UGIB (see Table 49.1).
Erosive gastropathy is typically associated with three main aetiological factors: consumption of NSAIDS, alcohol abuse, and stress. Erosive gastropathy caused by NSAIDS and alcohol generally causes self-limiting bleeding. The therapy is based on the removal of the noxa and on PPI therapy.
Stress gastropathy occurs only under extremely serious conditions: multiple traumas, vast surgical intervention, extensive burns, severe intracranial lesions, sepsis, and coagulopathies.
The mortality rate is high due to the severity of the underlying conditions, but in recent years its incidence has greatly reduced, probably due to routine adoption of prophylactic PPI, H2 blockers, and/or sucralfate.

Gastrointestinal Bleeding from Portal Hypertension
In patients with portal hypertension, GIB may be caused by oesophageal varices, gastric varices and, rarely, ectopic varices (duodenal, colic) or a portal hypertensive gastropathy.
Oesophageal varices sooner or later develop in all cirrhotic patients, but only about 30% will bleed. Oesophageal varices are a cause of bleeding in 10 to 30% of patients (Table 45.1), with a mortality rate <20% (more than 50% in the past). Mortality depends on the degree of hepatic insufficiency. It is essential to provide prophylaxis of haemorrhagic relapses because the one-year risk of repeated bleeding is 60% in the absence of prophylactic maneuvers (the risk is higher in the first 6 weeks after initial bleeding).
Bleeding from gastric varices is less frequent (about 10% of all UGIB in patients with portal hypertension) but is usually more severe than that caused by oesophageal varices.
Portal hypertensive gastropathy, which is present in 90% of patients with portal hypertension, may cause bleeding, which is clinically insignificant but often relapsing. **Figure 49.1** presents the algorithm for diagnosis and treatment of variceal bleeding in cirrhotic patients.

Prevention of First Variceal Bleeding and Bleeding Recurrences
Patients with oesophageal varices and high bleeding risk, according to the classification of varices (dimensions and presence of red signs) and the severity of hepatic insufficiency based on the Child-Pugh index, should begin preventive therapy using non-selective beta-blockers (propranolol, nadolol, carvedilol, started at a low dose then progressively increased to obtain a heart rate of approximately 50-55 beats/minute or until the occurrence of side effects), which lower the portal pressure through the reduction of cardiac flow and splanchnic vasoconstriction, or endoscopic variceal band ligation (elastic compression and consequent ischemia of the varicose veins through the application of rubber elastic bands).
In patients with contraindications or intolerance to beta-blockers, endoscopic variceal ligation is

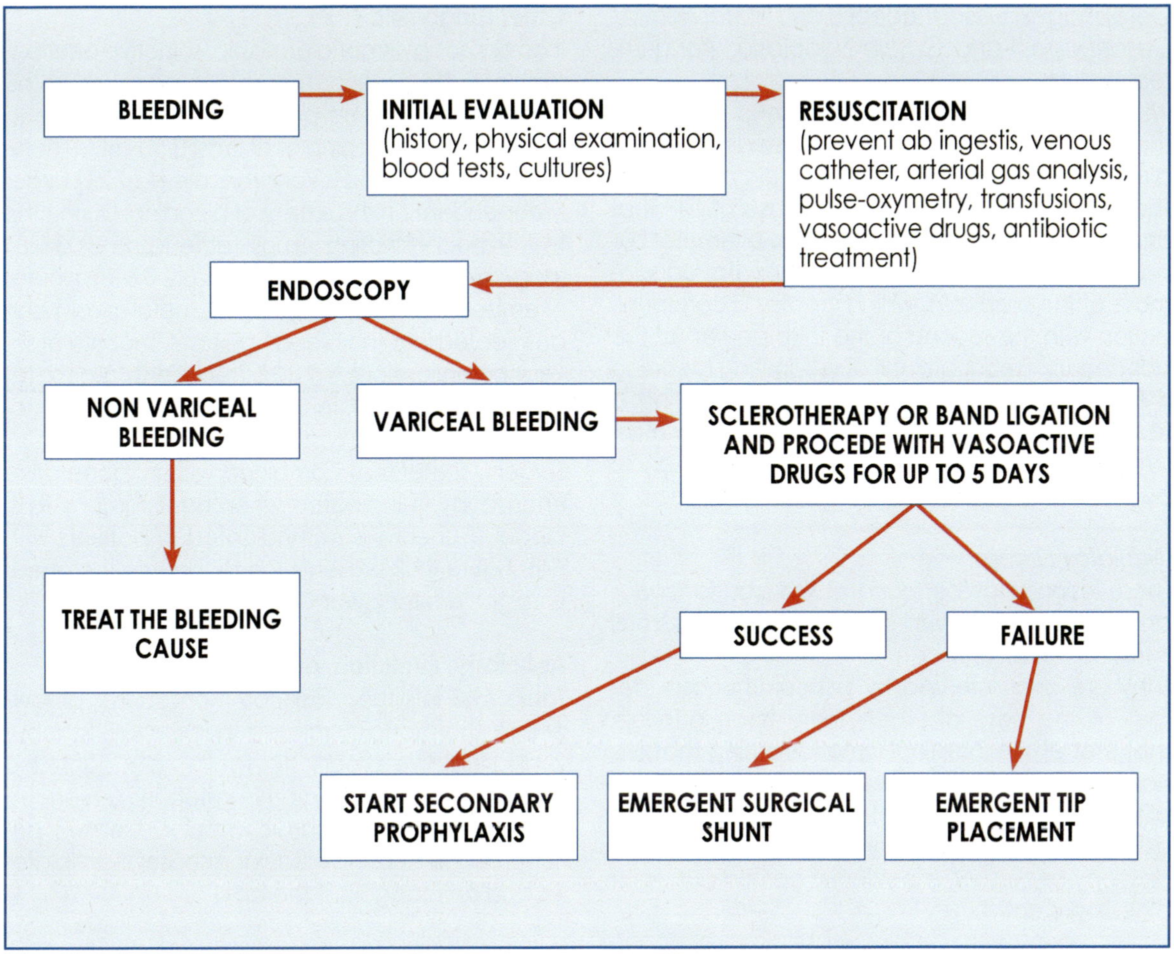

Figure 49.1 Algorithm for the diagnosis and treatment of acute variceal in cirrhotic patients.

performed.
Finally, in secondary (but not primary) prophylaxis, it is possible to combine a non-selective beta-blocker with isosorbide mononitrate (20 mg bid).

Treatment of Acute Haemorrhage
First-line therapy of acute variceal bleeding consists in the combined use of vasoactive drugs (splanchnic vasoconstricting drugs): terlipressin (slow bolus of 2 mg every 4-6 hours for 2-5 days; after the first 24 hours the use of 1 mg every 6 hours is possible); somatostatin (slow bolus of 250 mcg iv repeatable up to 2 times; infusion: 250 mcg/hour for 5 days); octreotide (slow bolus of 50 mcg iv repeatable up to 2 times; infusion: 25-50 mcg/hour for 5 days); endoscopic therapy (sclerotherapy or, preferably, endoscopic ligation) and antibiotic prophylaxis. Bleeding is stopped in 70-85% of cases with the administration of vasoconstrictor drugs that reduce portal pressure secondary to splanchnic vasoconstriction.
Success rates of 90-95% are obtained with endoscopic ligation or sclerotherapy (injection of irritant substances in varices and their surroundings, causing thrombosis and inflammation of varices) when ligation is impossible. In the rare eventuality in which pharmacological and endoscopic therapy fails or has a higher risk of failure, a radiologically placed transjugular intrahepatic portosystemic shunt (TIPS) may be performed to decompress the portal system by creating an intrahepatic shunt between a suprahepatic vein and the portal vein, through the insertion of a metal stent.

Mallory-Weiss Lesion
Mallory-Weiss lesion is a longitudinal tear of 5-15 mm in the gastro-oeasophageal junction mucosa, which often occurs on the gastric side and causes about 5-10% of upper GIB (see Table 49.1), more frequently in alcoholics. Typically, the patient reports haematemesis after empty retching. Generally, the bleeding stops spontaneously and requires only support therapy; in ongoing bleeding the treatments are local injection of adrenaline (1:10,000), cauterization or clip positioning.

Oesophagitis, Oesophageal Ulcer, Hiatal Hernia, Oesophageal and Gastric Neoplasia, Aorto-Enteric Fistula

With the exception of aorto-enteric fistula, all these lesions rarely cause acute bleeding but are a relatively common cause of chronic bleeding.

The aorto-enteric fistula is a rare case of GIB that usually occurs in patients with aorto-bifemoral bypass, due to dehiscence of the proximal anastomosis of the prosthesis, which creates a communication with the second or the third portion of the duodenum. Frequently, initial self-limiting bleeding is followed by a bleeding-free interval lasting a few hours to a few weeks, followed by a new massive bleeding. Diagnosis is made by endoscopy or by abdominal CT and the treatment is surgical.

Dieulafoy Lesions

These lesions may be found at the gastric fundus and duodenum, as well as in the colon and small intestine.

They are characterized by a small mucosal defect at the base of which there is an arteriole that erodes the intestinal lumen, causing massive haemorrhage. The bleeding site is generally very difficult to find because of the minute size of the defect, making angiography or videocapsule endoscopy necessary, especially if carried out whilst bleeding is active.

ACUTE LOWER GASTROINTESTINAL BLEEDING

Lower GIB is often intermittent and self-limiting. In the adult population, episodes of mild or moderate haematochezia happen in 8-10% of cases, frequently due to benign lesions such as anorectal disease (60-70%) and diverticula (35-60%), even if they can be caused by more serious lesions such as adenomatous polyps and/or malignancy.

Endoscopic Examination

The gold standard examination is colonoscopy, possibly extended to exploration of the terminal ileum, which is performed as soon as the patient is stabilized and after appropriate bowel cleansing using cathartic solutions (PEG electrolytic solutions). Only by doing so the procedure will be carried safely and may simultaneously be diagnostic and therapeutic.

The diagnostic rate of colonoscopy is between 70 and 90%, with a low incidence of complications (about 1%).

Other Diagnostic Tests

If colonoscopy is not diagnostic, selective arteriography of the superior mesenteric artery or of the celiac tripod can be performed, which is able to detect active bleeding of at least 0.5-1 mL/minute. The diagnostic yield is very variable (12-72%) largely dependent on the extent of bleeding. During the test, vasoconstricting drugs (adrenaline 0.03-0.04 mcg/kg/minute, vasopressin at 0.2-0.6 U/minute) or embolizing material (gelfoam, metal spirals) can be injected into the bleeding vessel. The rate of severe complications is 9-10% (reactions to contrast media, renal failure, femoral artery thrombosis, laceration of intestinal vessels).

Surgery, sometimes combined with intraoperative endoscopy, is indicated when arteriography fails. Opaque enema is not indicated in patients with GIB. **Figure 49.2** presents the diagnostic-therapeutic algorithm for lower GIB.

Aetiology, Evolution, and Prognosis

Table 49.3 lists the most common causes of lower GIB. The mortality related to lower GIB is about 2-4%. Negative prognostic factors are: signs and symptoms of haemodynamic instability, advanced age, comorbidities (cardiovascular diseases, peripheral and cerebrovascular diseases), antiplatelet and anticoagulant therapy.

Cause

Colonic Diverticula

Only about 3% of patients with colonic diverticula bleed; however, given the very high prevalence of diverticula in the population, these represent the cause of bleeding in approximately 30% of LGIB (see Table 49.3).

Bleeding is generally sudden, painless, and abundant; it often, but not always, originates from the right colon. It is believed that the cause of bleeding is a lesion of the wall of an arteriole penetrating in the surroundings of a diverticulum. In addition, in 80% of cases the bleeding ceases spontaneously, while the remaining 20% require urgent therapy. The bleeding site can be identified with colonoscopy, angio-CT, angiography or labelled red blood cell scintigraphy.

Endoscopic treatment entails injective, mechanical or thermal haemostasis for identifying the bleeding diverticulum; alternatively, arteriographic treatment can be performed, which is usually effective, or a surgical resection if bleeding does not stop.

Anal Diseases

Internal haemorrhoids, affecting at least 50% of the population, are the most frequent cause of haematochezia, which is typically intermittent, often mild, and is noticed by the patient during defecation. Bright red blood colors the feces or the toilet paper or drops directly into the toilet. Only occasionally do patients report massive bleeding.

Anal fissures, tears of the squamous epithelium of the anal canal, are common causes of mild rectal bleeding and anal pain in young persons.

Ischaemic Colitis

Ischaemic colitis can manifest with haematic diarrhoea, abdominal pain and vomiting. Colonoscopy shows segmental involvement of the colon

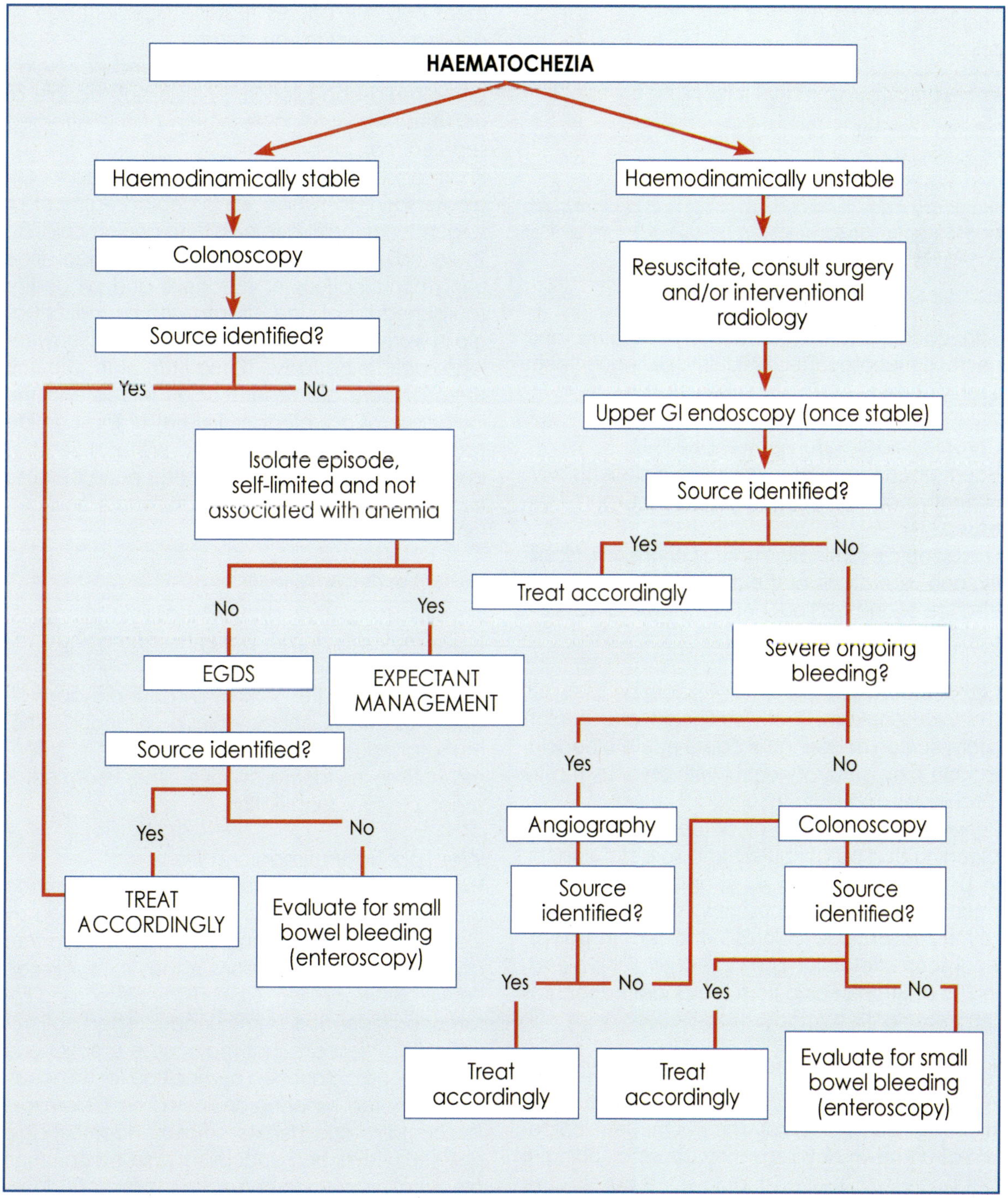

Figure 49.2 Diagnosis and treatment of lower gastrointestinal tract bleeding.

Table 49.3 Causes of lower gastrointestinal bleeding.

Diagnosis	% of total
Diverticula	26.4
Benign anorectal diseases	16.1
Colitis (infective, ischaemic, IBD, undetermined)	13.6
Neoplasia	6.1
Polyps	2.5
Angiodysplasia	1
Following endoscopy	3
Following surgery	1.7
Miscellaneous	3.4
Unknown	22.8

Modified from: Oakland K, Guy R, Uberoi R, et al. Gut 2018;67:654–662.

with edematous, erythematous, ulcerated and necrotic mucosa, often difficult to distinguish from Crohn's colitis.

Chronic Inflammatory Bowel Diseases

Haematochezia is more frequent in patients with ulcerative colitis than in patients with Crohn's disease.

Endoscopic examination reveals erythema, friability, and ulcerations of the mucosa. However, the chance of an infectious aetiology must always be considered.

Colorectal Tumours

Colonic neoplasms, both malignant and benign (polyps), can occasionally cause acute bleeding, though they generally occur with chronic, mostly occult bleeding.

Between 2% and 18% of acute lower GI tract bleeding can be attributed to colorectal cancer. In patients older than 40 years presenting with haematochezia, colonoscopy should be performed to exclude colonic neoplasia. In polyps, endoscopic resection allows to control the bleeding. In acute bleeding from malignant neoplasms the treatment is surgical.

Solitary Rectal and Other Ulcers

A solitary rectal ulcer can sometimes cause acute bleeding. Cecal ulcers or ulcers of the terminal ileum of unknown aetiology may cause bleeding. It has been hypothesized that in some cases these ulcers are due to the toxic effect of NSAIDS.

Angiodysplasia

Angiodysplasia comprises vascular abnormalities presenting as cherry-red flat spots, usually multiple, <5 mm in diameter, more frequent in the right colon and elderly patients. The aetiology of angiodysplasia is unknown. It is responsible for approximately 20% of LGIB (see Table 49.3) and can bleed chronically. Acute bleeding is usually self-limiting, but often recurrent. Angiodysplasia requires treatment only if it causes massive haemorrhage or anemia resistant to iron therapy.

The treatment of isolated lesions is endoscopic argon-plasma coagulation. If this is not feasible or not effective, surgical resection of the affected segment can be performed.

Pharmacological therapy is usually reserved for angiodysplasia, for which endoscopic treatment or surgery is not feasible (e.g., diffuse angiodysplasia). There have been reports of therapeutical trials using combinations of estrogens and progestins (burdened by of side effects such as metrorrhagia in women and gynecomastia in men), slow-release octreotide (dose 10 mg im/month; with this therapy there are reports of an increase in the incidence of gall bladder lithiasis) or thalidomide (dose 100 mg/day; to be used with caution because of its teratogenicity), but for none of these treatments is there evidence of certain and prolonged efficacy.

Radiation Colitis/Proctitis

Similar to angiodysplasia, post-actinic telangiectasias may develop in patients undergoing radiation therapy for pelvic tumours, in particular for rectum or prostate cancer. Endoscopic appearance resembles angiodysplasia, although other mucosal lesions may be associated, such as edema, diffuse erythema, friability. The treatment is argon plasma coagulation.

Infectious Haemorrhagic Colitis

The most common causes of acute diarrhoea are haemorrhagic intestinal infections caused by *Campylobacter jejuni* and *Salmonella*. More rare causes are *Shigella* infections, some strains of *E. coli*, *Yersinia enterocolitica*, *Clostridium difficile* and *Entamoeba histolytica*. In immunodepressed patients with AIDS, infections that may cause proctitis and haemorrhagic diarrhoea also include rectal gonorrhea, venereal lymphogranuloma from *Chlamydia trachomatis*, and *Herpes simplex*. Haemorrhagic colitis with fever and abdominal pain is a common presentation of cytomegalovirus infections. In infectious colitis with haemorrhagic diarrhoea, colonoscopy findings are often similar and sometimes indistinguishable from those of ulcerative colitis and Crohn's disease. For differential diagnosis it is useful to consider potential risk factors, associated symptoms, and stool cultures. It is useful to recall that infectious colitis, unlike inflammatory bowel diseases, are self-limiting by nature and endoscopic appearance tends to normalize within few weeks.

Vasculitis

Vascular inflammation and necrosis may cause ischemia and severe acute bleeding. Polyarteritis nodosa, Schönlein-Henoch purpura, systemic lupus erythematosus, rheumatoid vasculitis, Behçet's disease can all cause haematochezia.

Colinic Varices and Hypertensive Portal Colopathy

Ileal, colic or rectal varices, which sometimes tend to form around anastomotic orifices, can sometimes cause massive bleeding. Diagnosis is made by endoscopy or angiography. If the cause is portal hypertension, advised therapy is surgical decompression or TIPS.

Meckel's Diverticulum

Meckel's diverticulum is the most frequent congenital abnormality of the digestive tract, with an incidence of 0.3-3.0%. In 50% of cases, it is covered with normal ileal mucosa, while in the remaining 50% of cases it may contain gastric mucosa. The gastric mucosa secretes hydrochloric acid and can cause ulcers in the ileal mucosa, with possible bleeding. Bleeding, which occurs more often at a young age, is usually painless and can be melanic or bright red. Diagnosis is made by scintigraphy with technetium-99m-labeled red blood cells, which are picked up by the gastric mucosa present in the diverticulum. The treatment is surgical resection.

NSAID$_s$ Enteropathy

NSAIDs may cause ulcerative or stenosing, often bleeding, lesions even in the small intestine. The therapy is based on the discontinuation of NSAIDs, argon plasma coagulation of bleeding lesions during enteroscopy or surgical resection of stenosing lesions.

CHRONIC LOWER GASTROINTESTINAL BLEEDING

The term chronic LGIB describes bleeding lasting for days or weeks and usually implies intermittent or slow blood loss. It can occur with modest haematochezia or occult bleeding (see next paragraph). In most cases, the cause of haematochezia is an anal lesion (hemorrhoids, anal fissures), while most of the more proximal lesions are rectal or sigmoid erosions. Diagnostic evaluation is based on examination of anal region, digital rectal examination, and flexible sigmoidoscopy. If these investigations do not disclose a likely cause for the bleeding, colonoscopy is performed to exclude more proximal lesions.

OBSCURE GASTROINTESTINAL BLEEDING

If the location and the source of bleeding are not identifiable with common examinations (upper endoscopy or colonoscopy), bleeding is defined as being of obscure origin. Obscure gastrointestinal bleeding with visible bleeding is defined obscure-overt GIB; vice versa, if the bleeding is detected with the fecal occult blood test or is assumed due to chronic iron deficiency anemia, it is defined as obscure-occult GIB.

The patient's history and physical examination may provide useful clues. The patient should be asked about the consumption of drugs that may damage the mucosa or worsen the bleeding; a family history of GIB should prompt considering genetic forms (for example, hereditary haemorrhagic telangiectasia). Physical examination can disclose cutaneous lesions, Plummer-Vinson syndrome, pseudoxanthoma elasticum, some polyposis syndromes (Peutz-Jeghers, Gardner, Cronkhite-Canada).

Evaluation of Occult GIB

Fecal Occult Blood Detection

Since only about 10% of polyps and 50-60% of carcinomas bleed, a positive predictive value of fecal occult blood detection is approximately 20% for colonic carcinoma and about 25% for polyps.

Results of the test are strongly influenced by the type of test used (guaiac-based versus immunochemical method), by the method of collection of fecal samples, and by the adoption of dietary restrictions in the days immediately preceding the collection of feces. In fact, it has been demonstrated that in minor bleeding from the upper digestive tract the guaiac-based test may return a positive result, while the immunochemical test, more indicated in colorectal cancer screening, is not very sensitive.

Endoscopy

Upper endoscopy and ileocolonoscopy are the principal diagnostic and potentially therapeutic investigations in patients with positive fecal occult blood test or iron deficiency anemia.

The bleeding source is more often found in the upper digestive tract (29-56%) than in the colon (20-30%), but traditional endoscopy fails to detect the bleeding cause in approximately half of cases. In this case, it is likely that the lesion is in the small intestine.

The current diagnostic algorithm includes repetition of both upper endoscopy and colonoscopy to identify lesions missed at the first round (from 28 to 75%). In case of repeated negativity it may be useful to perform the procedures described below.

Videocapsule Endoscopy

Videocapsule endoscopy (VCE) is the first diagnostic examination to perform in the event of negative traditional endoscopy.

VCE consists of an orally administered capsule (27x11 mm) that contains six light-emitting diodes, a lens, a chip for acquisition of images, two small batteries, and an antenna for transmission. Acquired images (2 per second) are transmitted to a recorder attached to the hip of the patient and are transferred to a computer equipped with software that converts them into a video for analysis by a specialist. On average, after 8 hours the capsule is inactive and is expelled with the feces (in over 95% of cases). The diagnostic yield is very variable (around 75-80% in most studies, range 38-93%).

Double Balloon Enteroscopy

Double-balloon enteroscopy (DBE) is performed when there is a need for endoscopic evaluation of the small intestine, together with biopsies and/or therapeutic maneuvers (e.g., endoscopic haemostasis, polypectomy, dilations). The endoscope, approximately 2.2 metres long, slides inside an overtube.

At the apex are two latex balloons that are alternately inflated and deflated with a pump maneuvered by the operator during the examination. The endoscope is advanced the small intestine and the intestinal portion is folded on the overtube like an accordion. Each step allows the examination of approximately 40 cm. The exam takes approximately 2 hours and the patient is under deep sedation.

The method is well tolerated and safe (the complication rate is substantially equivalent to traditional endoscopy). A possible complication specific to DBE, of unknown cause, is an isolated increase in amylase and lipase or the occurrence of pancreatitis. With the oral approach it is usually possible to examine about 2-3 metres of small intestine, while with the anal approach about 1-2 metres of intestine are typically examined; therefore, the complete exploration of the small intestine is achieved in about 40-50% of cases (in Europe) using a combination of the two approaches. The diagnostic yield varies from 38 to 75%.

"Push" Enteroscopy

"Push" enteroscopy (now almost completely replaced by DBE) involves the oral insertion of an endoscope for observation of maximum 160 cm of small intestine.

Intraoperative Enteroscopy

Intraoperative enteroscopy is carried out in case of failure of the previous methods; during the operation an enteroscope is inserted into the small intestine by the surgeon.

Contrastographic Radiological Techniques

There are two methods for small intestine radiological investigation, both use contrast medium: small bowel follow through (SBFT) and small bowel enema which uses double contrast (i.e., duodenal infusion of barium and subsequent air insufflation) for evaluating filling and distension of small intestinal loops and, if possible, to reveal the aspect of the folds. These methods poorly show flat or small lesions.

Scintigraphy

Scintigraphy with technetium-99m-labelled red blood cells may aid in locating the site of GIB when the rate of bleeding is equal to or greater than 0.1-0.4 ml/minute. The diagnostic yield in obscure gastrointestinal bleeding is of 37-65%.

Angiography

A angiography, which must always be performed after angio-CT, is able to identify whether a bleeding is active at the time of examination if the blood flow is equal to or higher than 0.5 mL/min. In obscure gastrointestinal bleeding, the diagnostic value of the examination varies from 27 to 77% (mean 47%).

Exploratory Laparotomy

Nowadays, exploratory laparotomy is performed almost always in combination with intraoperative enteroscopy (see above).

Computed Tomographic (CT) Enterography

CT-enterography provides digital reconstruction of sectional images of analyzed region. With the latest software, it is also possible to spatially reconstruct images by different planes, obtaining three-dimensional images. CT-enterography is performed by preparing the patient with a macrogol solution (orally or by nasoduodenal tube) to obtain optimal filling and distension of bowel loops and then abdominal CT. The diagnostic yield is about 47% and must be weighted against exposure to high doses of radiation.

Magnetic Resonance (MR) Enterography

The advantages of magnetic resonance over CT is the absence of ionizing radiation and the flexibility of the technique in image and spatial resolution in multiple planes, as well as the excellent contrast resolution of soft tissues with the possibility to better distinguish normal from pathological tissues.

Causes of Gastrointestinal Occult and Obscure Bleeding

The most common causes of obscure gastrointestinal bleeding are angiodysplasia (70-80% of cases) and tumours (5-10% of cases). Other causes (10-25%) are small intestine iatrogenic bleeding by NSAIDS, infections (TB), small intestine Crohn's disease, celiac disease, Meckel's diverticulum, vasculitis, Zollinger-Ellison syndrome, actinic enteritis, jejunal diverticula, chronic mesenteric ischemia. The predominant causes are vascular lesions in patients older than 50 years, and small intestinal tumours in younger persons.

KEY CONCEPTS

- Overt GIB is a frequent and clinically relevant event.
- In the management of the haemorrhagic patient, precedence must be given to reanimation to achieve stabilization.
- Diagnosis of the location and the source of GIB has a fundamental therapeutic and prognostic importance.
- The investigations for diagnosis of GIB are endoscopy, CT-angiography, angiography, and scintigraphy with labelled albumin or red blood cells. The decision of which technique to used first is clinical and does not preclude alternative techniques later.
- GIB is self-limiting in most cases. Otherwise, endoscopic therapies are able to control bleeding in a high percentage of cases.
- Obscure GIB occurs when the cause of bleeding is not identified with traditional bidirectional endoscopy and is divided in obscure/occult and obscure/overt.
- Videocapsule endoscopy for studying the small intestine is the examination of choice in obscure/occult or obscure/overt intestinal bleeding.

REFERENCES

- de Franchis R, Bosch J, Garcia-Tsao G, Reiberger T, Ripoll C. Baveno VII Faculty. Baveno VII - Renewing consensus in portal hypertension. J Hepatol. 2022; 76(4):959-74.
- Gralnek IM, Stanley AJ, Morris AJ, et al. Endoscopic diagnosis and management of nonvariceal upper gastrointestinal hemorrhage (NVUGIH): European Society of Gastrointestinal Endoscopy (ESGE) Guideline - Update 2021. Endoscopy. 2021;53(3):300-32.
- Laine L, Barkun AN, Saltzman JR et al. ACG Clinical Guideline: Upper Gastrointestinal and Ulcer Bleeding. Am J Gastroenterol. 2021; 116(5):899-917.
- Pennazio M, Spada C, Eliakim R, et al. Small-bowel capsule endoscopy and device-assisted enteroscopy for diagnosis and treatment of small-bowel disorders: European Society of Gastrointestinal Endoscopy (ESGE) Clinical Guideline. Endoscopy. 2015; 47(4):352-86.
- Triantafyllou K, Gkolfakis P, Gralnek IM et al. Diagnosis and management of acute lower gastrointestinal bleeding: European Society of Gastrointestinal Endoscopy (ESGE) Guideline. Endoscopy 2021;53(8):850-68.

CHAPTER 50

ACUTE LIVER FAILURE

Francesco Azzaroli, Olivia Morelli

LEARNING OBJECTIVES

- To know the definition of acute liver failure (ALF) and acute on chronic liver failure (Acute on Chronic Liver Failure, ACLF).
- To know prevalent causes, pathogenesis, and clinical picture of ALF.
- To know how to recognize the diagnostic elements and to evaluate the prognosis of ALF.
- To know the fundamental elements of ALF therapy.

DEFINITION

Acute liver failure (Acute Liver Failure, or ALF) is a dramatic, rare clinical syndrome, characterized by a sudden onset of functional liver failure in a patient without a previous history of liver disease. The clinical picture is common, irrespective of the aetiology of ALF, and is characterized by the development of jaundice, coagulopathy (INR >1.5) and liver encephalopathy. The development of infectious complications often determines the onset of a multi-organ failure (MOF), a clinical picture that results in the death of the patient in most cases. For this reason, urgent liver transplantation today represents the optimal therapy in the majority of cases of ALF, having dramatically improved the prognosis. The growing understanding of the causes and pathogenic mechanisms of ALF, its earlier recognition and improvement of intensive care, have recently allowed to obtain an improvement of prognosis even in the absence of transplantation. Based on the interval elapsing between the onset of jaundice and hepatic encephalopathy ALF is divided into hyperacute (<7 days), acute (8-28 days) and subacute forms (5-12 weeks) that present different clinical manifestations and chances of spontaneous recovery (**Table 50.1**). The absence of encephalopathy with presence of coagulopathy and jaundice defines the condition of Acute liver injury (ALI) that may lead to ALF.

EPIDEMIOLOGY

The incidence of ALF is very low and is reported as less than 10 cases per million people per year in developed countries. The main causes of ALF in adult patients differ between the US and the countries of northern Europe on one hand, and the countries of the Mediterranean area, Africa, and Asia on the other. In the first, especially in Britain, the most prevalent cause of ALF is drug induced liver injury including the voluntary ingestion, for suicidal purpose, of paracetamol, which alone is involved in over 50% of cases. Within the countries of the Mediterranean area, including Italy, the most frequent cause is still represented by fulminant HBV hepatitis, though this infection is generally in reduction, thanks to the diffusion of vaccination. Other less common causes of ALF are autoimmune hepatitis, acute hepatitis from

Table 50.1 Main causes of ALF in adults.

	Hyperacute ≤1 week	**Acute** 1-4 weeks	**Subacute** 4-12 weeks
Severity of coagulopathy	+++	++	+
Severity of jaundice	+	++	+++
Degree of intracranial hypertension	++	++	+/-
Possibility of spontaneous recovery	Good	Moderate	Poor

HAV, HEV, EBV or HSV, Wilson's disease, ischaemic liver injury and poisoning by Amanita phalloides. It remains however a significant proportion of ALF from unknown causes.

AETIOLOGY

The possible causes of ALF are numerous ranging from virus to drugs and toxics or rarer causes.
A list of the main causes of ALF in adults is reported in **Table 50.2**.

BASICS OF PHYSIOPATHOLOGY

The pathogenesis of ALF varies depending on the specific cause. In general, ALF develops when the hepatocyte necrosis exceeds the liver capacity of regeneration determining organ damage and failure. The ALF can develop even without necrosis, as in acute liver fat of pregnancy or Reye's syndrome. In general, oxidative stress and ATP depletion determine massive necrosis, while the ATP is preserved in apoptosis. The discrimination between a prevailing necrosis vs apoptosis in ALF could be useful in the future to evaluate prognosis and therefore the need of transplantation.
One of the most frequent causes of acute damage from drugs is paracetamol. In this case the severity is dose dependent. Paracetamol is metabolized by glucuronidation and sulphonation and, to a lesser extent, through the cytochrome P450. The way of the cytochrome P450 leads to the production of a toxic metabolite (NAPQ; N-acetyl-benzoquinone imine) which is conjugated with glutathione. In case of intoxication the cellular glutathione is depleted resulting in hepatocyte toxicity given by NAPQ. The induction of the P450 (alcohol, barbiturates) favours a greater production of toxic metabolite and thus of hepatotoxicity from paracetamol, especially in malnourished patients.

CLINICAL PICTURE

The diagnosis of ALF is based on detection of INR >1.5 and encephalopathy in a patient without a pre-existing history of liver cirrhosis. The trend is rapidly progressive with a predominance of the aspects related to cytolysis and coagulopathy in hyperacute/acute forms while jaundice prevails in the subacute ones. These events are accompanied by the presence of a systemic inflammatory response (**Table 50.3**) with peripheral vasodilatation which can progress to multiorgan failure. The unfavourable evolution of the patient with ALF is mainly due to the consequences of cerebral oedema, respiratory dysfunction requiring mechanical ventilation, renal failure, and to bacterial and fungal infections which lead to multi-organ failure. The main clinical and laboratory manifestations are shown in **Table 50.4**.
One type of acute liver failure not to be confused with the ALF is represented by the "acute-on-chronic liver failure", a term which refers to a rapid deterioration of liver function in a patient with a pre-existing compensated chronic liver disease. Such event is much more frequent than ALF and typically is observed in a cirrhotic patient whose clinical picture precipitates for a intervening cause such as: severe infection, gastrointestinal bleeding, portal vein thrombosis, superimposed acute hepatitis, acute damage from alcohol or drugs.

Table 50.2 Main causes of ALF in adults.

Viral	A, B, C, D, E viruses, herpes simplex, cytomegalovirus, Epstein-Barr, herpes zoster, haemorrhagic fevers, seronegative
Medications/Drugs	Paracetamol, anti-tuberculosis, antibiotics, NSAIDs, aspirin (Reye's syndrome in children), antiepileptic drugs, chemotherapy, cocaine, ecstasy
Toxic Substances	Alcohol, *Amanita phalloides*, herbs (eg., Kava), carbon tetrachloride
Vascular	Budd-Chiari and veno-occlusive disease, ischaemia, right heart failure, hyperthermia
Pregnancy	Acute fatty liver, HELLP (haemolysis, elevated liver enzyme levels, and low platelet levels) syndrome
Miscellaneous	Sepsis, autoimmune hepatitis, Wilson disease, neoplastic infiltration, primary non-function of transplanted liver

Table 50.3 Criteria for the definition of Systemic Inflammatory Response Syndrome (SIRS).

Two or More of the Following Criteria
Body temperature >38 °C or <36 °C
Heart rate >90/min
Respiratory rate >20/min or PaCO2 <4.3 kPa or 32 torr
White blood cell count >12,000/mm^3, <4000/mm^3 or >10% immature neutrophils

Table 50.4 Major clinical and laboratory manifestations oin ALF.

Clinical	Laboratory
Asthenia Nausea/Vomiting Pain in the right upper quadrant Hepatomegaly Encephalopathy Jaundice Ascites Digestive haemorrhage (haematemesis or melena) Hypotension and tachycardia Cerebral Oedema: papilledema, hypertension, bradycardia	INR >1.5 Hypertransaminasemia (often very high) Hyperbilirubinaemia Thrombocytopenia (<150x103/mm^3) Anemia LDH increased Increased serum creatinine and BUN Hyperamylasemia and hyperlipasemia Hypoglycaemia Hyperammonemia Electrolyte disturbances (hypophosphatemia, hypomagnesemia, hypokalemia) pH alterations (acidosis or alkalosis)

The prognosis is generally better in some acute forms, such as in acetaminophen poisoning (spontaneous survival 65%), acute fulminant hepatitis with HAV or shock (50-60%) compared to subacute ones including idiosyncratic reactions to drugs (29%) or from unknown causes (25%). In developed countries, acute hepatitis B infection is drastically reduced as a result of vaccination and spontaneous survival has improved with the advent of antivirals that have favourably changed the prognosis which remains, however, influenced by possible superinfection with HDV.

Early identification of patients that will require liver transplantation is essential to ensure early intervention and to improve survival. In particular, rapidly worsening patients that are potential candidates to liver transplantation must be referred to transplantation centres before the development of encephalopathy in order to facilitate patient management. There are several prognostic scores among which the most commonly used in clinical practice are the King's College criteria (**Table 50.5**) and the MELD (based on INR, bilirubin and creatinine that can be calculated online). A MELD greater than 30 identifies patients at higher risk. These criteria were developed to select patients at higher risk of death from ALF, however, since these criteria have limitations, the American Society for Study of the Liver recommended to not rely only on these prognostic scores to evaluate patient eligibility for liver transplantation.

Therefore, prognosis is critically influenced by the speed with which the case is identified and transferred into an intensive care unit which should be connected with a transplant centre in order to ensure both optimal intensive care and a timely or urgent organ transplant as needed. When the transplant is performed within 24 hours of the onset of coma survival is usually of 70-80%.

Table 50.5 King's College Criteria.

Paracetamol	Not Paracetamol
Arterial pH <7,3 or Arterial Lactates >3.0 mmol/L after adequate fluid infusion	Prothrombin time >100 s (INR >6.5)
or all 3 of the following criteria	*or 3 of the following criteria*
Hepatic encephalopathy grade 3 or 4	age <10 or >40 years
Prothrombin time >100 s (INR >6.5)	unfavorable aetiology: hepatitis seronegative (non-A non-B), idiosyncratic drug reactions, Wilson disease
Serum creatinine >3.4 mg/dL (300 micromol/L)	duration of jaundice before encephalopathy >7 days INR >3.5 (PT >50 s) bilirubin >300 micromol/L (>17.6 mg/dL)

ACUTE ON CHRONIC LIVER FAILURE

Much more common in clinical practice is the finding of a rapid deterioration of liver function in a compensated cirrhotic patient, a form of ALF which represents a complication of chronic liver disease (ACLF). Generally, it arises as a result of an acute decompensation event such as infection, haemorrhage, portal vein thrombosis, acute damage from drugs or a superimposed acute hepatitis. The European Association for the Study of the Liver–Chronic Liver Failure (EASL-CLIF) has proposed criteria to define the various degrees of ACLF associated with different probabilities of death (**Tables 50.6**, **50.7**). Calculation of the score can be done online at the address https://www.efclif.com/scientific-activity/score-calculators/clif-c-aclf where entering the data gives back the degree of ACLF and the probability of death.

THERAPY

The patient with ALF should be hospitalized in a hepatological intensive care unit or a general intensive care unit and requires close monitoring of vital signs and of laboratory parameters.
The therapy is based both on general measures, common to the various forms of ALF, and on specific therapies that vary according to aetiology (**Table 50.8**), whose identification is therefore vitally important for therapeutic and prognostic purposes. For example, N-acetyl-cysteine (NAC) infused intravenously at high doses (10 g/day) acts as a specific antidote in the control of liver

Table 50.6 EASL-CLIF criteria to define the various degrees of ACLF.

	Score 1	Score 2	Score 3
Bilirubin	<6 mg/dL	**6.0-11.9 mg/dL**	**≥12 mg/dL**
Creatinine	<1.5 mg/dL 1.5-1.9 mg/dL	**2.0-3.4 mg/dL**	**≥3.5 mg/dL or renal replacement therapy**
Encephalopathy (West Haven Criteria)	Grade 0	**Grade 1-2**	**Grade 3-4**
INR	<2.0	**2.0-2.4**	**≥2.5**
Mean blood pressure	≥70 mmHg	**<70 mmHg**	**Vasoactive drugs**
PaO_2/FIO_2 SpO_2/FIO_2	>300 >357	**201-300** **215-357**	**≤200** **≤214**

Blue: criteria that define organ dysfunction
Red: criteria that define organ failure

Table 50.7 ACLFM mortality by grade.

Definition	28-Day Mortality
No ACLF • Absence of organ failures • Single organ failure (liver, coagulation, circulatory, respiratory) + Creatinine <1.5 mg/dL and absence of encephalopathy • Encephalopathy and Creatinine <1.5 mg/dL	4.4-6.3%
ACLF grade 1 • Single renal failure • Single organ failure (liver, coagulation, circulatory, respiratory) + Creatinine 1.5-1.9 mg/dL and/or Grade 1-2 encephalopathy • Grade 3-4 encephalopathy + Creatinine 1.5-1.9 mg/dL	18.6-27.8%
ACLF grade 2 Two organ failures	32%
ACLF grade 3 Three or more organ failures	68-88.9%

Table 50.8 Principles of therapy for ALF.

General Measures
Haemodynamics - Maintaining adequate pressure values (fluid infusion; vasopressors)
Respiratory function - Possible intubation and ventilation
Hydroelectrolytic alterations - Monitoring and correction
Renal function - Haemodialysis if necessary
Coagulopathy - Give at least one dose of Vitamin K Use fresh frozen plasma, platelet preparations or recombinant clotting factors if invasive procedures are necessary
Infection - Careful monitoring and treatment of infections
Metabolic problems - Monitoring blood sugar Enteral or parenteral nutrition if possible
Stress ulcer prophylaxis - Proton pump inhibitors / anti-H2
Encephalopathy/Cerebral oedema - Avoid stimulation/sedation if possible Monitor intracranial pressure (possible use of mannitol) Immediate treatment of possible convulsions Transfer to an intensive care unit and inclusion on the liver transplant waiting list

Specific Measures	
Amanita phalloides	Penicillin G/silibinin
Autoimmune hepatitis	Immunosuppression (eg. Methylprednisolone)
Hepatitis B	Nucleos(t)ide analogs
Herpes viruses	Acyclovir
Neoplasms	Chemotherapy
Paracetamol	N-acetylcysteine
Budd-Chiari syndrome	Anticoagulants/TIPS

damage from acetaminophen being a source, for the hepatocyte, of glutathione whose sulfhydryl groups restrict the formation of a highly reactive intermediate compound of paracetamol that binds to the cellular proteins, leading to the formation of cysteine adducts. However, its effectiveness decreases if not used within 24-48 hours from intentional or accidental overdose of paracetamol. The use of NAC is continued up to 72 hours.

In the past, extracorporeal liver support systems have been developed to replace liver function deficiency; however, they have not changed patients' survival. Recently, a randomized prospective study showed a better survival of patients with ALF who are not candidates for transplantation with high volume plasma exchange. The procedure consists in the removal of the patient's plasma (15% of the patient's ideal body weight) at a rate of 1-2 litres per hour with fresh frozen plasma infusion in an equivalent volume. In the study it corresponded to about 8-12 litres of fresh frozen plasma for each procedure that was repeated for 3 consecutive days.

Liver transplantation is the definitive treatment of ALF with excellent long-term survival. Another strategy to reduce the mortality of patients is represented by auxiliary liver transplantation in which a partial liver transplant (left lobe of the liver or right liver) is performed as a temporary support to the functional recovery of the native liver. This type of transplant is however burdened by a high rate of post-operative mortality, and in more than 15% of the cases re-transplantation is needed.

KEY CONCEPTS

- Acute liver failure is a rare clinical syndrome characterized by the rapid appearance of a functional failure of the liver in a patient without a previous history of liver disease.
- The pathogenesis of ALF varies depending on the aetiology, it generally arises when hepatocytes death prevails over liver regeneration.
- The main aetiology of ALF in the US and in the northern European countries is the accidental or deliberate poisoning by acetaminophen and the drug induced liver injury (DILI), while in the Mediterranean countries, Africa and Asia is represented by acute viral hepatitis (HBV, HAV, HDV, HEV). Less frequent causes are autoimmune hepatitis, Wilson's disease, acute liver ischemia and mushroom poisoning.
- The clinical picture is dramatic with jaundice, severe coagulation deficit and hepatic encephalopathy leading to coma. The occurrence of brain oedema and infections usually leads to the development of MOF which is associated with a high mortality rate (>90%).
- NAC i.v. infusion is effective if started within 24-48 hours of acetaminophen poisoning and reduces the need for transplantation.
- Urgent liver transplantation represents the definitive treatment of ALF with good survival rates (>70%) after transplantation
- Acute decompensation in advanced liver cirrhosis constitutes a much more common type of ALF, known as Acute-on-chronic liver failure (ACLF). Generally, in the cirrhotic patient, it follows the onset of infection, bleeding, portal vein thrombosis, superimposed acute hepatitis, acute damage from alcohol or drugs (DILI).

REFERENCES

- Arroyo V, Moreau R, Jalan R. Acute-on-Chronic Liver Failure. Longo DL, editor. N Engl J Med. 2020;382(22):2137-45.
- EASL Clinical Practical Guidelines on the management of acute (fulminant) liver failure. J Hepatol. 2017; 66(5):1047-81.
- Hernaez R, Solà E, Moreau R, Ginès P. Acute-on-chronic liver failure: An update. Gut. 2017;66(3):541-53.
- Gambino C, Piano S, Angeli P. Acute-on-Chronic Liver Failure in Cirrhosis. J Clin Med. 2021;10(19):4406.
- Germani G, Theocharidou E, Adam R, Karam V, Wendon J, O'Grady J, Burra P, Senzolo M, Mirza D, Castaing D, Klempnauer J, Pollard S, Paul A, Belghiti J, Tsochatzis E, Burroughs AK. Liver transplantation for acute liver failure in Europe: outcomes over 20 years from the ELTR database. J Hepatol. 2012;57(2):288-96.
- Stravitz RT, Lee WM. Acute liver failure. Lancet. 2019;394 (10201):869-81.

ACUTE ABDOMEN

Monia Baldoni, Giovanni Sarnelli

LEARNING OBJECTIVES
- To understand the clinical assessment of patients with acute abdomen.
- To know the main laboratory and instrumental tests for a fast diagnosis.
- To be aware of differential diagnosis between main causes.

Acute abdomen is a medical and/or surgical syndrome responsible for around 7% Emergency Department visits.
Acute abdomen refers to severe abdominal pain with sudden onset. A wide range of intra- or extra-abdominal disorders of variable severity may cause it: from a mild and self-limiting degree to real urgency/emergency, which can rapidly become life-threatening events. The management of patients with acute abdomen relies on correct assessment, rapid diagnosis, and prompt medical and/or surgical treatment. It often involves the collaboration and coordination of health professionals to prevent complications and improve patient outcomes. Making the right diagnosis is challenging for physicians, since the patient's history, clinical presentation, and laboratory and radiological data do not always lead to an unequivocal conclusion.

PATHOPHYSIOLOGY OF ABDOMINAL PAIN

Pain is the key symptom in acute abdomen; it is a subjective reaction to tissue and/or visceral organs damage, which makes the patient aware of an active pathological state. Understanding its features and estimating objectiveness is fundamental to achieve a correct diagnosis. From a pathophysiological point of view, it can be classified into visceral, somatic, and referred pain.
Visceral pain originates from internal organs and it can be caused by different stimuli, such as distension, stretching, contraction and ischemia; it is transmitted to the central nervous system via unmyelinated C fibers and Aβ fibers. It arises as a diffuse and poorly defined sensation in the midline of the body. Pain from foregut organs (stomach, pancreas, liver, biliary tract, and proximal duodenum) is typically localized to the epigastrium. The remaining small bowel and proximal third of the colon, including the appendix, is perceived to the periumbilical region. Pain of hindgut organs (distant two-thirds of the colon, bladder, pelvic and genitourinary organs) is usually localized to the hypogastrium. Moreover, visceral pain is often associated with marked autonomic phenomena, including pallor, profuse sweating, nausea, vomiting, and changes in vital signs.
Somatic-parietal pain is caused by irritation of the parietal peritoneum due to inflammatory or chemical stimuli (blood, infected fluids, and gastric content) and it is transmitted via spinal nerves. Unlike visceral pain, somatic pain is well defined, localized, and abrupt with typical signs of peritoneal involvement (see below).
Referred pain, or visceral-parietal pain, originates from the viscera but is perceived in somatic areas different from the onset site, also distant from it. This occurs because of a common embryologic origin between the internal organ and the symptomatic dermatome.
An example of this is Kehr's sign, which is right shoulder tip pain associated with pain in the right hypochondrium in a patient with cholecystitis, or violent left shoulder tip pain occurring after abdominal trauma, which often indicates a damaged or a ruptured spleen.

EPIDEMIOLOGY

The major causes of acute abdomen are listed in **Table 51.1**. Their incidence varies in relation to age, sex, and predisposing conditions. The most common causes in adults are acute appendicitis,

*The Authors wish to thank Dr. Carlo Romano Settanni for his assistance.

Table 51.1 Causes of acute abdomen.

Abdominal	Extra-Abdominal and Systemic
Intestinal Appendicitis, Diverticulitis, Perforated Peptic Ulcer, Severe Acute Gastritis, Bowel Obstruction and Perforation (intestinal tumours, hernia or volvulus), Colitis and Enteritis (ischaemic, infective), Complications of IBD	**Cardiovascular** Myocardial Ischemia and Infarction, Myocarditis, Endocarditis, Pericarditis, Congestive Heart Failure, Aortic Dissection, Aortic Aneurysm Rupture
Liver and Biliary tract Biliary Duct Obstruction, Cholecystitis, Cholangitis, Liver Abscess, Hepatitis	**Endocrine and Metabolic** Uremia, Diabetic Ketoacidosis, Porphyria, Acute Adrenal Failure (Addisonian Crisis), Hyperlipidemia, Hyperparathyroidism
Spleen Splenic Rupture, Splenic Abscess, Splenic Torsion	**Thoracic** Pulmonary Embolism and Infarction, Pneumonia, Pleuritis and Pleural Empyema, Pneumothorax, Oesophagitis, Oesophageal Motor Disorders, Oesophageal Rupture (Boerhaave Syndrome) Haematological, Immunological, Allergic and Connective
Pancreas Pancreatitis, Pancreatic Tumours	**Tissues** Sickle Cell Anemia, Haemolytic Anemia, Henoch -Schönlein Purpura, Acute Leukemia, Lymphomas, Systemic Lupus Erythematosus, Dermatomyositis, Nodous Polyarteritis, Vasculitis, Allergies (drugs, food, hymenoptera and arachnid stings and bites), Eosinophilic Enteritis, Hereditary Angioedema
Urinary tract Nephrolithiasis, Pyelonephritis, Ureteral Calculosis, Renal Infarction, Infections	**Toxins** Hypersensitivity Reactions, Insect Bites, Reptile Poison, Plumb Poisoning
Vascular Abdominal Aortic Dissection or Rupture, Superior Mesenteric Artery Obstruction or Dissection, Splenic Infarction and Aneurysm, Adrenal Infarction, Abdominal or Retro-Peritoneal Bleeding (spontaneous or iatrogenic)	**Infections** Herpes zoster, Typhoid Fever, Tuberculosis, Brucellosis
Obstetrical, Gynecological and Urologic Extra-Uterine Pregnancy, Endometriosis, Ovarian Cyst Rupture, Ovarian Torsion, Ovarian Abscess, Complicated Ovarian Tumours, Pelvic Peritonitis, Adnexitis, Prostatitis, Epididymitis, Testicular Torsion	**Musculoskeletal and Neurological** Radiculopathies, Medullary or Peripheral Nerve Tumours, Discitis, Arthritis of the Spine, Costochondritis, Osteomyelitis, Tabes Dorsalis, Iliopsoas Abscess
Various Abdominal Organ Rupture	**Various** Narcotic Abstinence Syndrome, Mediterranean Familial Fever, Psychiatric Disorders, Heat Stroke, Foreign Body

IBD inflammatory bowel diseases

diverticulitis, cholecystitis, pancreatitis, and adnexitis. The prevalent surgical cause in children is acute appendicitis, whereas the most common non-surgical cause is gastroenteritis. The most frequent abdominal causes in the elderly are bowel obstruction (from colon or stomach cancer), diverticulitis and cholelitiasis with its complications. In any case, the prevalence of cardiovascular, pulmonary, and neurological diseases is high in such patients, making diagnosis is more challenging and the outcome is worse. Mortality rates are high in acute abdomen due to cardiovascular diseases (myocardial infarction, mesenteric ischemia, and abdominal aortic aneurysm rupture). More generally, higher mortality and morbidity have been associated with vital signs abnormalities, old age, use of corticosteroids, organ failure, and recent surgery.

CLINICAL ASSESSMENT

Patient Evaluation

The patient's general conditions, vital parameters, and pain characteristics are evaluated to establish the severity of the clinical case and the need for prompt action.

Vital Signs and General Conditions

Evaluation begins by measuring the patient's vital signs: blood pressure, cardiac frequency, respiratory rate, oxygen saturation, body temperature and state of consciousness. The mnemonic ABC (Airway, Breathing, and Circulation) is useful to memorize initial steps to identify unstable patients who need immediate action. Tachypnea is associated with chest diseases, cardiorespiratory failure, intestinal ischemia, sepsis, and diabetic ketoacidosis. Orthopnea is associated with cardiopathies and ascites. Fever may indicate bacteraemia but it may be absent in anergic, immunocompromised or elderly patients. In the global assessment of the patient, it is also important to consider posture: for example, patients with peritonitis usually assume a forced position, often in lateral decubitus with legs flexed to the abdomen (typically in patients with acute pancreatitis), and generally refuse to change posture because movement (coughing, breathing) exacerbates the pain originating from peritonitis. In contrast, patients with bilious or renal colic are restless and continuously change body position.

Remote History

An accurate investigation of the patient's history is always necessary: previous intra- or extra-abdominal diseases (some are recurrent, such as nephrolithiasis, cholelitiasis, and peptic disease) and surgery (patients may suffer from bowel obstruction due to adherence syndrome). The physician should investigate if the patient has an allergic diathesis. Moreover, it is helpful to enquire into diet, recent travels, and possible pregnancy and menstrual period in women of reproductive age. Accurate history taking is not always possible in patients with severe pain and instability of vital signs: in such cases, a brief history is sufficient to record key information.

Pharmacological History

Physicians should always ask about patient's current medications and use of addictive drugs. In fact, peptic ulcer and its complications (bleeding and perforation) are frequently associated with the use of non-steroidal anti-inflammatory drugs (NSAIDs), whereas recent antibiotic therapy may give rise to a toxic megacolon, which is a complication of pseudomembranous colitis due to *Clostridium difficile*. The use of cocaine is associated with intestinal and cardiac ischemia. Alcohol abuse is linked with many gastrointestinal disorder (gastritis, pancreatitis, hepatopathies).

Medical History of the Present Illness

Knowing the features of abdominal pain, its mode of onset (spontaneous, post-traumatic, related to food intake, etc.) and associated symptoms is essential for establishing a correct diagnosis.

- Site. The site and the possible radiation or migration of pain are very relevant data, as shown in **Figure 51.1**.
- Intensity. Generally, the intensity of pain is linked to the severity of the disease. Pain threshold is subjective and varies depending on attitude, pain experience, age, and cognitive state.
- Features. The modes of pain onset (abrupt, acute and/or stabbing, dull, deep and oppressive), the duration and course (worsening, continuous or intermittent) are important information. For example, continuous pain, persistent or worsening, is mostly associated with inflammatory disease (as in acute pancreatitis). In bowel perforation the pain is acute and abrupt, and quickly reaches its extreme (referred as "stabbing pain"), just as the pain from aortic aneurysm rupture or aortic dissection. Even pain caused by acute biliary tract obstruction (cholelitiasis) has a rapid onset and gradually fades. This pain is typically severe and continuous, but, even if it is commonly named "biliary colic", it isn't intermittent pain; it is usually evoked by high-fat meals. A colicky pain, cramplike, with paroxysms of variable duration followed by remission periods, is typical of gastroenteritis and intestinal obstruction at early stage (becomes continuous as abdominal distension progresses and somatic with perforation).
- Associated signs and symptoms. Patients with acute abdomen often have relevant associated symptoms. For example, vomiting is frequent and it is indicative of many conditions: it may be associated with bowel obstruction (mechanical ileus) or with peristalsis blockage, in excessive stimulation of peritoneal and mesenteric nerves (paralytic ileus) or with psychiatric and metabolic diseases and even more. Vomiting may be diagnostically useful to

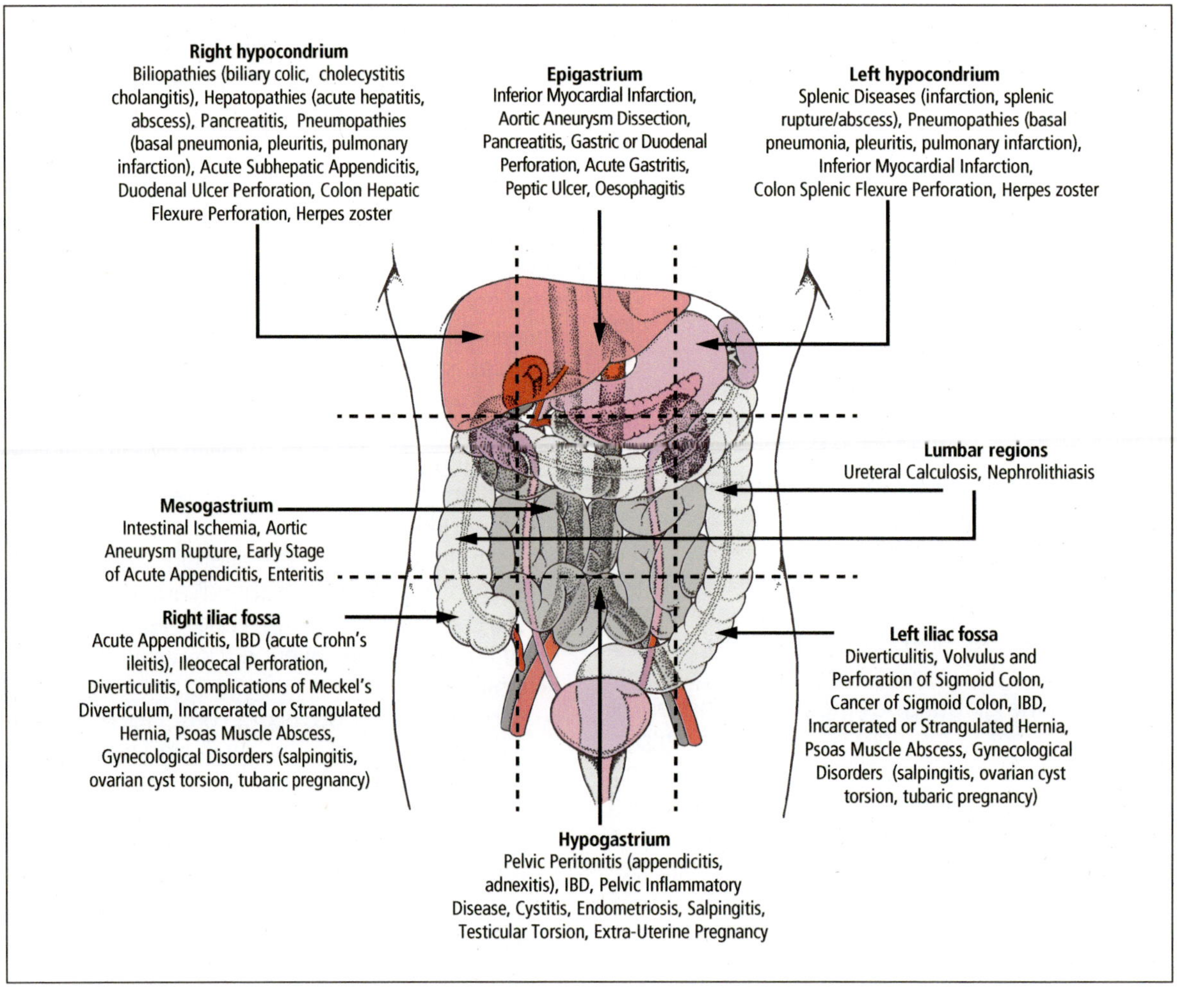

Figure 51.1 Main causes of acute abdomen and relative location IBD Inflammatory Bowel Diseases.

understand the possible aetiology: fecal vomiting is frequently present in small or large bowel obstruction; early, postprandial or non bilious vomiting may indicate gastric obstruction; blood or coffee ground emeses may be present in patients with peptic disease, stomach or oesophageal tumours, but also liver cirrhosis (variceal bleeding); a massive haematemesis in a patient with prior abdominal aortic aneurysm surgery may be indicative of aortoenteric fistula. Infectous gastroenteritis should be suspected in patients with vomiting and diarrhoea. Melena is usually found in patients with upper gastrointestinal bleeding, but in patients with slow peristalsis it may be due to small bowel and/or right colon bleeding lesions. Rectal bleeding and haematochezia, associated or not with abdominal pain, are found in bowel ischemia or diverticular bleeding. Acholic stools and hyperchromic urine in patients with jaundice are associated with cholestatic disorders. Halted bowel movements and gas pass are associated with mechanical or paralytic ileus.

Physical Examination

Physical examination includes the abdomen, chest, urogenital apparatus, and rectum.

Abdominal examination may disclose: distension because of ileus, mechanical or paralytic or ascites (umbilical hernia may be present in cirrhotic patients), typical dermatomal herpes zoster rash, periumbilical or flank ecchymosis (Cullen's and Grey Turner's signs in acute haemorrhagic necrotic pancreatitis), surgical scars, hernias and/or masses, etc. Sub-icterus or icterus may be indicative of cholestasis or massive haemolysis. Auscultation can reveal a bowel obstruction in case of hyperperistalsis with high-pitched tinkles and splashes or a paralytic ileus in the absence of bowel sounds. Superficial palpation appreciates tenson of the abdominal wall muscles,

which is indicative of peritonitis (abdominal guarding) and which can be limited to a single region in localized peritonitis.
Even a positive Blumberg sign (pain elicited upon sudden removal of pressure during palpation) and tenderness to percussion are indicative of peritonitis. Deep palpation may reveal visceromegaly or abdominal masses. A central abdominal pulsating mass is highly indicative of abdominal aortic aneurysm (AAA).
Percussion may reveal tympanic sounds due to meteorism in mechanical or paralytic ileus, or disappearance of liver dullness in pneumoperitoneum.
Murphy's sign (breath held during deep palpation of right hypochondrium) may be associated with acute cholecystitis. Suspicion of acute appendicitis may be supported by tenderness to pressure at McBurney's point (one-third of the distance from the right anterior superior iliac spine to the umbilicus) and by Rovsing's sign (pain elicited in the right iliac fossa on deep pressure at the left iliac fossa).
Rectal examination is helpful to reveal stool consistency (to exclude fecalomas), signs of bleeding (melena or rectal bleeding), anal and peri-anal disorders (haemorrhoids, fistulas, anal hyper- or hypotonia), abnormal masses (rectal or prostate cancer) or of prostatitis. Male genital examination may disclose testicular diseases (e.g., infection or torsion); gynecological examination is useful in females with low abdominal pain.

Diagnostic Tests

Laboratory and instrumental tests are essential to support diagnosis.

Laboratory Tests

The most widely used tests are listed in **Table 51.2**.

Instrumental Tests

A diagnostic hypothesis (**Figure 51.2**) should be supported by findings from specific instrumental tests:

- Electrocardiography (ECG). ECG is a primary fundamental diagnostic test if cardiovascular disease is suspected, especially in pain in upper regions in patients with no abdominal guarding. ECG abnormalities can be observed also in patients with abdominal disorders.
- Radiography (Rx). Plain abdominal Rx is helpful as preliminary test in many situations, for example in case of suspicion of bowel obstruction or ileus (air-fluid levels of small or large bowel), gastrointestinal perforation (sub-diaphragmatic free gas), urinary tract calculosis, emphysematous lesions or detectable foreign bodies. Chest x-ray is useful if a thoracic disease is suspected.
- Ultrasonography. Abdominal ultrasonography is often recommended as a screening test for acute abdomen, since it yields copious information, is fast, can be performed at the bedside, and can be freely used in young people

Table 51.2 Laboratory tests.

Common Blood Tests	CBC	WBC, RBC, Hb, Ht, MCV, MCH, MCHC, Platelets
	Electrolytes	Na, K, Cl, Ca, Mg, Phosphorus
	Kidney	Creatinine, BUN, Clearance
	Inflammation	CRP, ESR
	Various	Blood Sugar Level, LDH, CK, SGOT, and SGPT
Blood Tests for Specific Diseases	Liver	Transaminases (SGOT and SGPT), Alkaline Phosphatase, γ-GT, Total Bilirubin, Direct and Indirect Bilirubin
	Pancreas	Lipase, Amylase
	ACS	Cardiac Troponin T, CK, CPK-MB, Myoglobin
	Heart Failure	BNP
	Coagulation	PT, aPTT, INR, Fibrinogen, D-dimer
	Blood Gas Analysis	pH, PaO2, PaCO2, HCO3-, BE, Lactate
	Pregnancy	hCG
	Urine Test	pH, Leukocytes, Haemoglobin, Bacteria, Nitrites, Glucose, Ketone Bodies, Sediment Study

CBC complete blood count, WBC white blood cells, RBC red blood cells, Hb haemoglobin, Ht haematocrit, MCV mean corpuscular volume, MCH mean corpuscular haemoglobin, MCHC mean corpuscular haemoglobin concentration, Na sodium, K potassium, Cl chloride, Ca calcium, Mg magnesium, BUN blood urea nitrogen, CRP C reactive protein, ESR erythrocyte sedimentation rate, LDH lactate dehydrogenase, CK creatine kinase, SGOT serum glutamic-oxaloacetic transaminase, SGPT serum glutamic-pyruvic transaminase, γ-GT γ-glutamyl transpeptidase, ACS acute coronary syndrome, CPK-MB creatine phosphokinase muscle-brain, BNP brain natriuretic peptide, PT prothrombin time, aPTT activated partial thromboplastin time, INR international normalized ratio, Pa partial pressure, O2 oxygen, CO2 carbon dioxide, HCO3- bicarbonate ion, BE base excess, hCG human chorionic gonadotropin.

and pregnant women, as it does not involve radioactive exposure. It plays a key role in diagnosis of AAA rupture, acute appendicitis, diverticulitis, pancreatitis, cholecystitis, biliary tract pathologies (calculosis), uropathies (ureterohydronephrosis or renal calculosis), obstetric and gynecological diseases, abdominal abscesses and ascites. FAST- ultrasonography (focused assessment with sonografy for trauma) is a rapid and reliable test to detect fluids (blood) in the abdominal cavity.

- Computed Tomography (CT). Abdominal CT, with or without contrast, is a second step imaging test with high sensitivity and specificity; it has high diagnosability for organ ischemia, vascular lesions, gastrointestinal perforation, acute appendicitis, pancreatitis, diverticulitis, biliary tract calculosis, intestinal volvulus or aortic dissection with thrombosis.
Side effects associated this test are related to radioactive exposure (increased risk of cancer) and contrast administration (allergies, nephropathies, lactic acidosis in diabetic patients on therapy with biguanides).
- Magnetic Resonance (MR). MR is recommended when acute abdomen from hepatobiliary diseases and gynecological disorders are suspected if screening tests are inconclusive

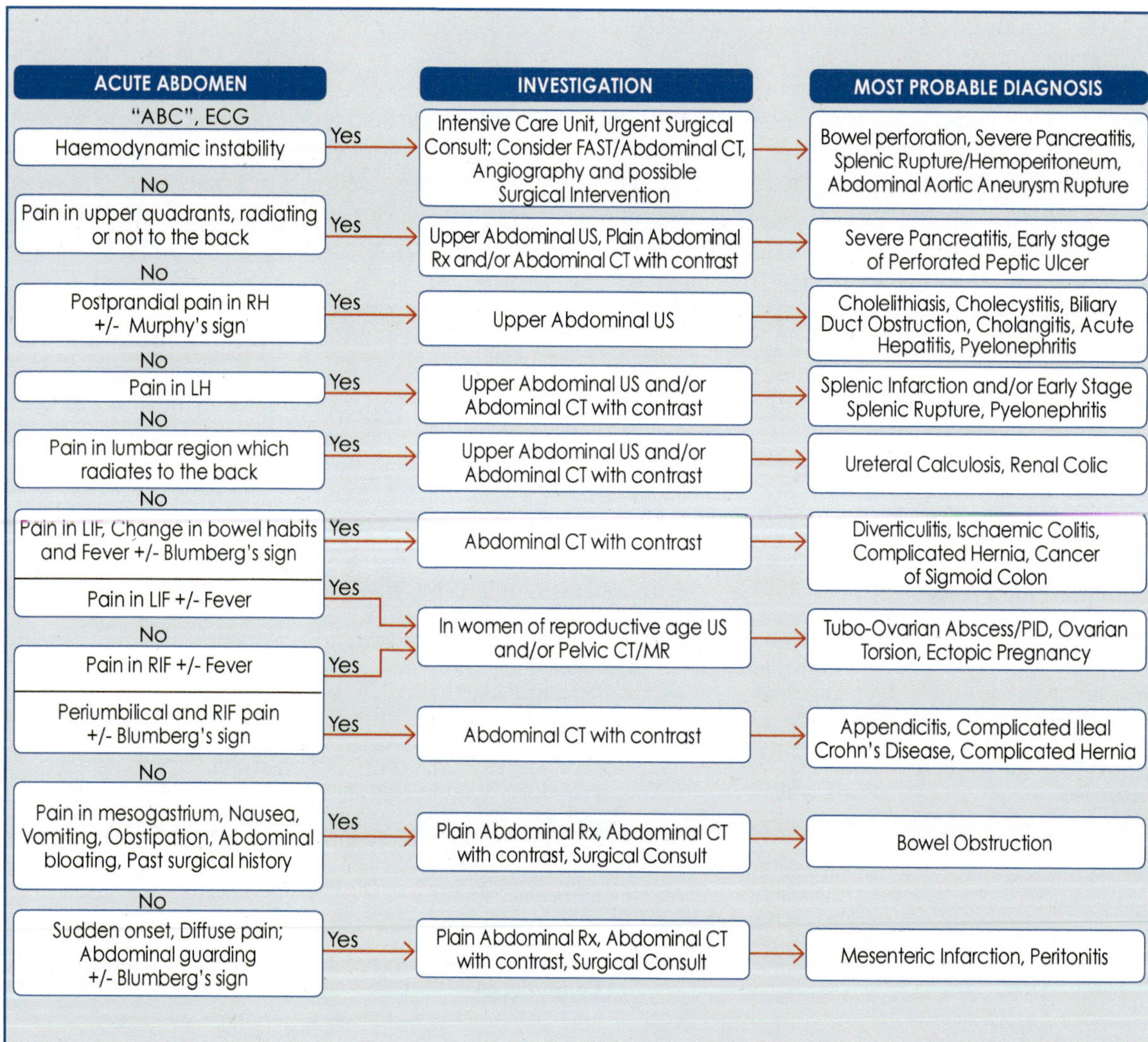

Figure 51.2 Urgent approach to acute abdominal pain. Symptoms and objective findings lead to the most probable diagnostic hypotheses that must be confirmed with appropriate instrumental investigations. ABC airways, breathing and circulation, ECG electrocardiography, FAST focused assessment with sonography for trauma, RIF right iliac fossa, LIF left iliac fossa, RH right hypochondrium, LH left hypochondrium, PID pelvic inflammatory disease, MR magnetic resonance, Rx radiography, CT computed tomography, US ultrasonography.

(pelvic inflammation, ovarian torsion, ovarian haemorrhage) and in pregnant women. Even here, contrast, usually gadolinium-based, must be used with caution in patients with allergic diathesis and nephropathies.

- Surgery. Besides its therapeutic role in many diseases causing acute abdomen, surgical intervention (laparoscopic or laparotomic if necessary) may be recommended if the diagnostic procedures mentioned above are inconclusive or if the patient's condition is critical and rapidly worsening, requiring immediate attention. In such cases a delay in action while waiting for test results may increase the risk of morbidity and mortality.

KEY CONCEPTS

A rapid clinical assessment is fundamental when dealing with a patient with acute abdomen because the patient's condition can suddenly deteriorate, making it necessary to proceed with urgent surgical intervention. It is essential:

- first, to measure vital signs and assess the state of consciousness, with prompt intervention if the patient's conditions are critical;
- to know the main causes of acute abdomen related to the pattern of symptom onset;
- to obtain accurate history;
- to perform complete assessment;
- to order appropriate diagnostic laboratory and instrumental tests;
- to integrate information for prompt diagnostis, with the help of other medical specialists.

REFERENCES

- Macaluso CR, McNamara RM. Evaluation and management of acute abdominal pain in the emergency department. International Journal of General Medicine. 2012;5:789-97.
- Mayumi T, Yoshida M, Tazuma S, Furukawa A, et al. Practice Guidelines for Primary Care of Acute Abdomen 2015. Jpn J Radiol. 2016:34:80-115.
- Sikandar S, Dickenson AH. Visceral Pain – the Ins and Outs, the Ups and Downs. Curr Opin Support Palliat Care. 2012 March;6(1):17-26.
- Feldman, Friedman, Brandt. Sleisenger and Fordtran's Gastrointestinal and Liver Disease. Pathophysiology, Diagnosis, Management. 10th edition. Elsevier, 2016 pp. 161-174

INDEX

B

C

D

I

J

K

L

M

N

O

P

R

S

T

U

V

W

Y

Z